Diagnosis and Treatment of Pineal Region Tumors

Diagnosis and Treatment of Pineal Region Tumors

Edited by

Edward A. Neuwelt, M.D.

Associate Professor of Neurosurgery
Assistant Professor of Biochemistry
Division of Neurosurgery
Oregon Health Sciences University
Portland, Oregon

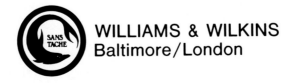

WILLIAMS & WILKINS
Baltimore/London

Editor: Carol-Lynn Brown
Copy Editor: Shirley Riley Smoot
Design: Bert Smith
Illustration Planning: Lorraine Wrzosek
Production: Ann G. Seitz
Cover: Joel Ito

Copyright ©, 1984
Williams & Wilkins
428 East Preston Street
Baltimore, MD 21202, U.S.A.

Accurate indications, adverse reactions, and dosage schedules for drugs are provided in this book, but it is possible that they may change. The reader is urged to review the package information data of the manufacturers of the medications mentioned.

Made in the United States of America

Library of Congress Cataloging in Publication Data

Diagnosis and treatment of pineal region tumors.

  Bibliography: p.
  Includes index.
  1. Pineal body—Tumors—Surgery. 2. Pineal body—Tumors. I. Neuwelt, Edward A. [DNLM: 1. Pineal body. 2. Brain neoplasms—Therapy. 3. Brain neoplasms—Diagnosis. WK 350 D536]
RD594.D53 1984   617'.44   84-3625
ISBN 0-683-06438-X

Composed and printed at the
Waverly Press, Inc.

*To P.C.—a terrific wife
and mother*

Foreword

Doctor Edward Neuwelt and his contributors, with this book, have made an outstanding contribution to the neurosurgical literature. As he points out the management of pineal region tumors is most controversial, especially in the United States. A major reason for that controversy is the lack of a definitive reference for the physician who is confronted with a patient harboring one of these unusual lesions. The book does not dictate a course of action; indeed, it should not. Instead it very successfully accomplishes the goal of the authors which is "to review the diagnosis and treatment of these tumors so that the practitioner can make an intelligent decision as to the proper course of treatment in an individual patient."

It successfully outlines, in depth, current understanding of both the basic science and clinical science of these disorders. I would not do the authors justice by trying to comment on their individual contributions. Suffice it to say the book is extremely well written and illustrated. Unlike most multi-authored texts it is well balanced with no anemic chapters. This is a tribute to the genius of the editor, Dr. Neuwelt, and the qualifications and expertise of his contributors. As a surgeon I was most impressed by the anatomical description of the pineal region and the technical detail of the surgical procedures. I believe all neurosurgeons who peruse this book will second my opinion. The basic scientists and nonsurgeons who wish a comprehensive survey of the subject will likewise be satisfied. It will serve as the standard reference on this topic for years to come, both for the student and the practitioner.

Clark Watts, M.D.
Columbia, Missouri

Preface

Although tumors of the pineal gland are not the most common tumors of the central nervous system, they are certainly one of the most controversial. The controversy in part relates to the fact that current neurodiagnostic techniques are sensitive in picking up even small lesions, but are not specific as to the underlying type of pathology. As a result, the standard mode of therapy for lesions of the pineal in the past, empiric radiation without a tissue diagnosis, is called into question. This is particularly true in the United States where a very significant proportion of tumors in the pineal region are either benign lesions or lesions in which a gross total excision can be achieved. Indeed our current series of malignant pineal region tumors shows 9 of 13 successful gross total excisions. Only 3 of these 13 patients had pure germinomas. Seven of the nine with a gross total removal remain tumor free in a 3 month–6 yr follow-up. An initial surgical approach is probably less applicable in Japan where the highly radiosensitive germinoma remains by far the most common tumor. Thus, a major area of the controversy in the United States relates to whether the 20 or so pathological types of tumor that can be found in the pineal region should first be diagnosed with tissue histology or alternatively, be treated with an initial trial of empiric radiotherapy.

Because of the magnitude of this controversy, as evidenced by the plethora of recent publications on the topic, the purpose of this monograph is to review the diagnosis and treatment of these tumors so that the practitioner can make an intelligent decision as to the proper course of treatment in an individual patient.

The monograph begins with a review of the pathology and epidemiology of tumors of the pineal region and then proceeds to the diagnosis of these lesions. Diagnosis, neuro-ophthalmology and neuroradiology are particularly important and are therefore emphasized. The question of therapy is then discussed in the following chapters commencing with an historical overview. Because the anatomy of veins in this region is so key to surgery, a separate chapter on the microsurgical anatomy of this region is given, followed by chapters relating to surgical approaches to the pineal gland. In separate chapters written by both neurosurgeons and radiotherapists, an alternative form of initial therapy, empiric radiation, is presented. Finally, some more recent advances with regard to tumor markers and chemotherapy as well as postoperative radiotherapy in the treatment of lesions in the pineal region are discussed. It is our feeling that making this information available to the practicing physician in a complete and coordinated fashion will have a significant impact on improving the diagnosis and treatment of tumors in the pineal region.

To facilitate the use of this text as a reference, the bibliographies of all the chapters are combined at the end of the book and each paper is listed alphabetically by the last name of the senior author.

The editor gratefully acknowledges the assistance of Virginia Kirby in manuscript preparation.

EDWARD A. NEUWELT

Contributors

Eustacio O. Abay III, M.D.
Neurosurgeon
Bel-Air Village
Makati, Metro Manila
Philippines

Robert E. Anderson, M.D.
Professor and Director
Neuroradiology Section
Department of Radiology
University of Utah School of Medicine
Salt Lake City, Utah

Erik-Olof Backlund, M.D., Ph.D.
Professor and Chairman
Department of Neurosurgery
Universitetet I Bergen
Haukeland Hospital
Bergen, Norway

H. Hunt Batjer, M.D.
Assistant Professor
Neurological Surgery Service
University of Texas Southwestern
   Medical School
Dallas, Texas

James E. Bruckman, M.D.
Clinical Assistant Professor
Department of Radiation Therapy
Bishop Clarkson Memorial Hospital
Omaha, Nebraska

Barbara Danoff, M.D.
Associate Professor
Department of Radiation Therapy
University of Pennsylvania School of Medicine
Philadelphia, Pennsylvania

Lawrence H. Einhorn, M.D.
Professor
Department of Medicine
Indiana University School of Medicine
University Hospital
Indianapolis, Indiana

Glenn S. Forbes, M.D.
Associate Professor of Radiology
Department of Diagnostic Radiology
Mayo Clinic
Mayo Medical School
Rochester, Minnesota

Eugene P. Frenkel, M.D.
Professor
Department of Internal Medicine
University of Texas Health Science Center
Dallas, Texas

Rebecca Gelman, Ph.D.
Assistant Professor
Department of Biostatistics
Dana-Farber Cancer Institute
Harvard School of Public Health
Boston, Massachusetts

Gordon L. Grado, M.D.
Clinical Assistant Professor
Department of Radiation Therapy
Bishop Clarkson Memorial Hospital
Omaha, Nebraska

Mary Kay Gumerlock, M.D.
Assistant Professor
Division of Neurosurgery
Oregon Health Sciences University
Portland, Oregon

Maie Kaarsoo Herrick, M.D.
Neuropathologist
Santa Clara Valley Medical Center
San Jose, California
Clinical Assistant Professor
Pathology (Neuropathology) and Neurology
Stanford University Medical Center
Stanford, California

Fred Hochberg, M.D.
Assistant Professor
Neurology Service
Massachusetts General Hospital
Boston, Massachusetts

Harold J. Hoffman, M.D., F.R.C.S.(C)
Professor of Surgery
Division of Neurosurgery
Hospital for Sick Children, Toronto
University of Toronto
Toronto, Ontario
Canada

Mark T. Jennings, M.D.
Memorial Sloan-Kettering Cancer Center
New York, New York

Claude Lapras, M.D.
Professor
Neuro-Chirurgien des Hopitaux de Lyon
Lyon, Cedex
France

Edward R. Laws, Jr, M.D.
Professor
Department of Neurological Surgery
Mayo Clinic
Mayo Medical School
Rochester, Minnesota

Richard P. Moser, M.D.
Assistant Professor of Surgery
Department of Head and Neck Surgery
University of Texas Cancer Center
M. D. Anderson Hospital and Tumor Institute
Houston, Texas

Edward A. Neuwelt, M.D.
Associate Professor of Neurosurgery
Assistant Professor of Biochemistry
Division of Neurosurgery
Oregon Health Sciences University
Portland, Oregon

Gerhard Pendl, M.D.
Associate Professor of Neurosurgery
Allgemeines Krankenhaus der Stadt Wien
Neurochirurgische Univ. Klinik
Vienna, Austria

Russel J. Reiter, Ph.D.
Professor
Department of Anatomy
The University of Texas Health Science Center-
San Antonio
San Antonio, Texas

Mark Scott, Ph.D.
Stuart Pharmaceuticals
Wilmington, Delaware

Glenn E. Sheline, M.D.
Professor
Department of Radiation Oncology
University of California Medical School
San Francisco, California

William T. Shults, M.D.
Physician and Surgeon
Chief, Neuro-Ophthalmology
Good Samaritan Hospital and Medical Center
Assistant Professor
Department of Ophthalmology
Clinical Associate Professor
Department of Neurology
Oregon Health Sciences University
Portland, Oregon

Bennett M. Stein, M.D.
Byron Stookey Professor and Chairman
Department of Neurological Surgery
The Neurological Institute
Columbia University College of Physicians and
  Surgeons
Director of Neurosurgery
Presbyterian Hospital
New York, New York

Kintomo Takakura, M.D.
Professor and Chairman
Department of Neurosurgery
University of Tokyo Hospital
Hongo, Bunkyo-ku, Tokyo
Japan

Clark Watts, M.D.
Professor and Chief
Division of Neurosurgery
University of Missouri
Health Sciences Center
Columbia, Missouri

Benton M. Wheeler, M.D.
Fellow
Department of Hematology/Oncology
Indiana University School of Medicine
University Hospital
Indianapolis, Indiana

Stephen D. Williams, M.D.
Associate Professor
Department of Medicine
Indiana University School of Medicine
University Hospital
Indianapolis, Indiana

Contents

CHAPTER 1

The Challenge of Pineal Region Tumors

EDWARD A. NEUWELT, M.D. and MARY KAY GUMERLOCK, M.D.

INTRODUCTION

Pineal region tumors offer the neurosurgeon a challenge of no small magnitude. The patients may present at any age usually with symptoms and signs of obstructive/noncommunicating hydrocephalus. This initial pattern is complicated by the wide range of tumors arising in this region, each with its own course, prognosis, and optimal treatment. Neuroradiologic evaluation is sensitive but nonspecific regarding etiology. When surgery is a part of the management, further technical challenge is encountered. Because the pineal gland has been relatively unapproachable until recently, little is understood about the malfunctioning human pineal, its clinical presentation, and implications thereof. Much is yet to be learned about its role in circadian rhythms and reproduction. How specific tumor pathology relates to these remains to be studied as well. Thus, besides being a microneurosurgical challenge, pineal region tumors provide new avenues of basic clinical investigation. The following cases emphasize each of these various aspects in treating pineal region tumors.

CASE 1

"Jet Lag" as the Presenting Symptom in a Pineoblastoma

A 51-yr-old neurosurgeon presented with inability to regain his day/night diurnal variation after two transatlantic trips in 6 months. In addition to increased fatiguability, the patient began having episodes of intractable nausea with some vomiting. A CT scan was obtained which showed a 2 cm calcium-containing contrast-enhancing tumor in the pineal region (Fig. 1.1). Angiography showed minimal tumor blush. A ventriculoperitoneal shunt was placed and the patient symptomatically improved. Serum and CSF levels of beta human chorionic gonadotropin (β-HCG) and alpha fetoprotein (AFP) were normal. Ten days later, he was taken to the operating room where gross total excision of a semiencapsulated pineal tumor was carried out. Final pathologic diagnosis returned pineoblastoma. The patient tolerated surgery well but was left with a definite Parinaud's syndrome and a dense hemianopsia both of which resolved over a year. One month following resection, the patient returned to the hospital with evidence of increased intracranial pressure and a CT scan showed an epidural hygroma. This was drained at which time his ventriculoperitoneal shunt was also ligated. The shunt was later removed. Three months postoperatively the patient received radiation therapy (4000-rad whole head, 1500-rad boost to pineal region, and 4000 to 4500-rad spinal). Currently 2 yr after surgery, the patient is quite functional and is swimming every day. His CT scan continues to show a small amount of pineal region calcification, but no evidence of tumor (Fig. 1.2). For obvious reasons he has opted not to return to his profession as a neurosurgeon at this point.

Studies in basic pineal gland function suggest a role in diurnal variation (44). However, it is rare to see a patient with a pineal region tumor complain of insomnia or difficulty with day/night cycles. Perhaps this is in part secondary to the lack of data on human pineal function. While Moore-Ede et al (28) mention melatonin in their review of circadian rhythms in health and disease, there is no mention of pineal region tumors. Nonetheless early work in "diurnal treatment" of such disorders is being reported (20).

It is also unusual for a patient of this age to have such a primitive neuroectodermal tumor. Prognosis is guarded but currently this patient is without evidence of disease clinically or radiographically. Regarding his preoperative "jet lag" symptoms, the patient has not been on any long airplane trips postoperatively to test his diurnal variability. Diurnal melatonin and hormone se-

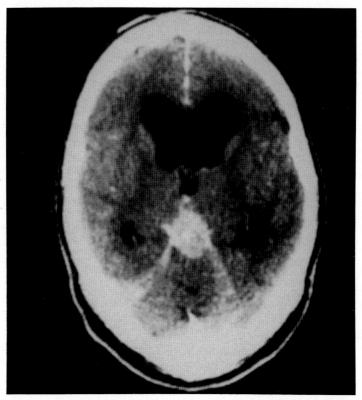

Figure 1.1.   Uniformly enhancing pineal region tumor which at the time of surgery was found to be a pineoblastoma.

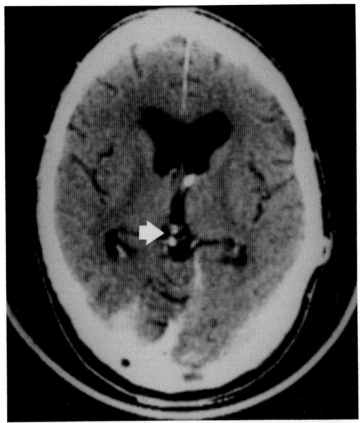

Figure 1.2. Postoperative CT scan 9 months following surgery and radiotherapy, no longer demonstrating an enhancing pineal region tumor. There is a small amount of calcification that remains in the pineal region (*arrow*).

cretion might be interesting to check and follow in a patient such as this.

CASE 2

Disappearance of Plasma Melatonin after Removal of a Neoplastic Pineal Gland

This 17-yr-old white male presented in August of 1981 with progressively severe nocturnal headaches, but no abnormal findings on either general physical or neurologic exam were observed. A CT scan revealed a calcified enhancing partially cystic tumor in the region of the pineal gland. In addition, the CT ventriculogram showed clear evidence of obstructive hydrocephalus (Fig. 1.3). CSF cytology was negative. CSF and serum levels of AFP, and β-HCG were undetectable. Anterior pituitary function was within the normal range. A ventriculoperitoneal shunt was placed and 4 weeks later gross total excision of a well encapsulated pineal tumor was carried out. Microscopic examination revealed a predominantly low grade astrocytoma with Rosenthal fibers (Fig. 1.4A). It also contained some less differentiated cells thought to be rests of pineoblastoma (Fig. 1.4B). Postoperatively, the patient had a transient left homonymous hemianopsia and Parinaud's syndrome. He subsequently received a localized port of mega-voltage radiation for a total of 5040 rad. Two years postoperatively, aside from some diplopia on far lateral gaze, the patient is doing well and CT scan shows no evidence of tumor.

If complete pinealectomy of a diseased pineal gland is attempted microsurgically, it would be very worthwhile to document complete excision with a marker. In many germ cell tumors of the pineal, for example, the beta subunit of human chorionic gonadotropin and alpha fetoprotein can be useful both diagnostically and in following therapeutic efficacy (31,32,34). In this case, a young man presenting with a typical pineal region tumor was evaluated both pre- and postoperatively for 24-hr variations of plasma me-

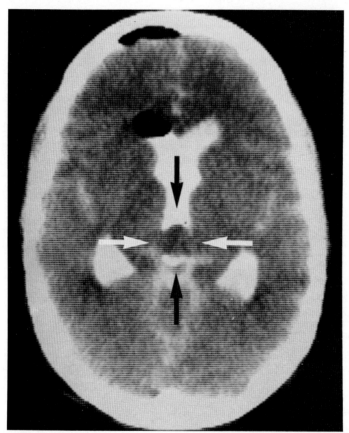

Figure 1.3. Preoperative transaxial CT metrizamide ventriculogram at the level of the lateral ventricles demonstrating a spherical pineal region mass (*arrows*). The low density in the left anterior lateral ventricle is air. (From Neuwelt EA, Levy A: *New England Journal of Medicine*. 308:1132–1135, 1983 (33).)

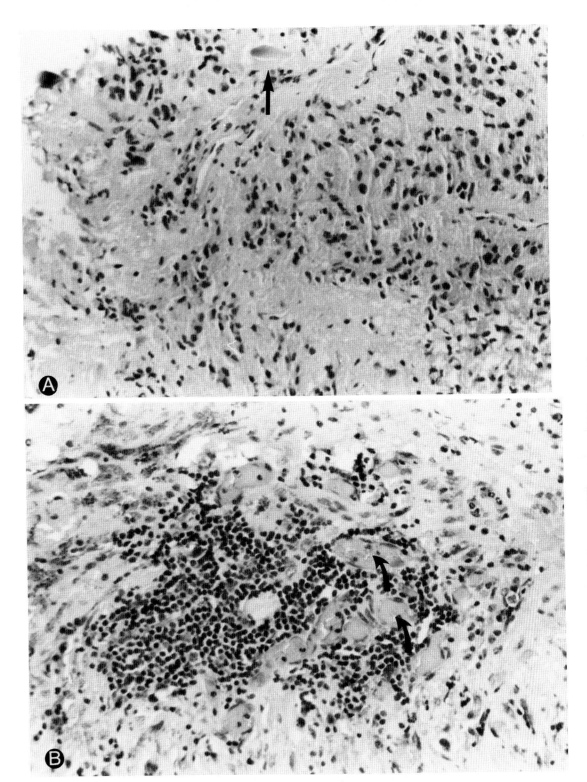

Figure 1.4. *A*, photomicrograph (H & E × 100) of that portion of the well encapsulated pineal tumor thought to be a low grade astrocytoma with Rosenthal fibers (*arrows*). *B*, photomicrograph of that portion of the tumor thought to be pineoblastoma (small dark-staining cells). It also shows capillary proliferation (*arrow*). (From Neuwelt EA, Levy A: *New England Journal of Medicine*. 308: 1132–1135, 1983, (33).)

latonin levels using the gas chromatography-negative chemical ionization mass spectrometric (GC-MS) assay of Lewy and Markey (24). This assay has received increasing recognition for its high degree of accuracy (specificity), sensitivity, and precision (2,17,26,46). Preoperative melatonin plasma levels drawn every 2 hr showed a normal circadian secretory rhythm with levels increasing during the night to 70 pg/ml and decreasing during the day to between 1.5 and 10 pg/ml (Fig. 1.5). Six weeks postoperatively plasma levels were again evaluated every 2 hr over a 24-hr period: at no time could melatonin be detected in the plasma (Fig. 1.5). The patient was on the same drug regimen (phenytoin) during both study periods and was not irradiated until after the second study.

The results of these studies demonstrate that, despite the presence of a pineal tumor, the preoperative circadian variation of plasma mela-

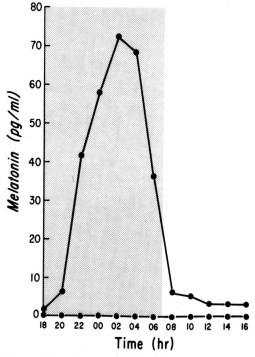

Figure 1.5. Human plasma melatonin levels before and after removal of a tumor-infiltrated pineal gland. Plasma was obtained at 2-hr intervals before (*solid line*) and after (*dashed line*) resection of the pineal tumor. Levels determined by mass spectral assay. The *shaded area* depicts nighttime. The minimal detectable plasma melatonin level by the mass spectral assay is < 1 pg/ml. (From Neuwelt EA, Levy A: *New England Journal of Medicine.* 308: 1132–1135, 1983, (33).)

tonin levels was normal. Following gross total tumor resection, plasma melatonin levels disappeared, suggesting that a complete pinealectomy had been performed. More recently another patient (Case 7) was found to have undetectable urinary 6-hydroxymelatonin (a metabolite of melatonin) levels both pre- and postoperatively. The results of his plasma melatonin levels are pending, but it appears that this latter patient's tumor *did* affect pineal function in contrast to the present case.

Plasma melatonin levels may be useful as a marker for neoplasms and other lesions of the pineal gland (3,4,18,56). In previous work using this assay, Lewy and associates (21) and Markey and co-workers (27) were not able to detect any melatonin in the plasma of pinealectomized rats. While such studies have been done in a variety of mammals (1,23,37,38,55,57) they have been difficult to do in man, because pinealectomy is not a common operation. Although the precise utility of melatonin as a tumor marker remains unclear, the fact that the pineal gland appears to be the sole source of plasma melatonin in man indicates that measurement of this hormone may be a reliable means of assessing the completeness of pinealectomy. Moreover, our findings help to validate the measurement of plasma melatonin as a marker for the adrenergic innervation of the pineal gland (54), the phase and period of its endogenous circadian pacemaker (56), and the effects of light in man (22,25).

By age, sex, and neuroradiologic criteria, our patient had a preoperative presumptive diagnosis of germinoma (48,49). At surgery, a well encapsulated pineal tumor with elements of both low grade astrocytoma and pineoblastoma was found and completely removed with little permanent sequelae. Indeed, this patient highlights three crucial issues in the diagnosis and therapy of pineal tumors. First is the danger of presuming that a young male with a pineal tumor has a germinoma or even a radiosensitive tumor. A very similar young patient was recently reported by DeGirolami and Armbrustmacher (5) who was treated with a VP shunt and empiric radiotherapy for a presumed germinoma. The patient expired 7 months after a shunt and radiotherapy, and at autopsy was also found to have a "sharply demarcated, encapsulated" low grade astrocytoma. Clearly, radiotherapy and a shunting procedure alone in our patient would have been a less than adequate therapy. Second, as has been reported previously (32,52), pineal tumors can be of mixed histology. Thus, a stereotactic needle biopsy of a pineal tumor can be not only dangerous due to its proximity to the deep venous system which surrounds the pineal gland (i.e. the vein of Galen, the internal cerebral veins, and the basilar vein of Rosenthal), but also may not provide an adequate tissue sample. Finally, with the advent of microsurgery which can minimize damage to the deep venous drainage system, benign and even malignant pineal tumors can often be completely excised with minimal morbidity and mortality.

On the basis of a 30 month follow-up in one patient, no untoward clinical sequelae have been associated with what appears to be a complete pinealectomy. With regard to the usefulness of melatonin as a tumor marker, further studies are underway.

CASE 3

Presence of Lymphocyte Membrane Surface Markers on "Small Cells" in a Pineal Germinoma

A 16-yr-old boy was first seen with an 18-month history of progressive blurred vision, bifrontal headaches, ataxia, and difficulty with higher cortical functions. About 2 weeks prior to admission he developed projectile vomiting. Physical examination revealed that the left pupil was slightly larger than the right. Both pupils reacted sluggishly to light. There was paralysis of upward gaze; attempts at upward gaze were accompanied by retraction nystagmus. The patient had a decreased ability to converge, although on conjugate lateral gaze to either side he was able to adduct his eyes normally. Motor examination revealed mild right-sided weakness. The remainder of the neurological examination was normal. The patient's CT scan (Fig. 1.6) revealed a massive pineal lesion that enhanced markedly with contrast. Angiography showed the tumor to be essentially avascular. Occipital transtentorial exploration of the lesion and subtotal decompression were carried out. Histological examination showed a germinoma; sections revealed diffuse proliferation of large cells amidst a background of small mononuclear cells (Fig. 1.7). Beta human chorionic gonadotropin and alpha fetoprotein were undetectable by radioimmunoassay in serum and cerebrospinal fluid samples obtained at surgery.

In some series, germinomas account for as many as 50% of tumors in the pineal region (6). Histologically (14) and ultrastructurally (53),

the tumor is identical to seminoma of the testes (34). It is characterized by the presence of two types of cells: large cells with abundant clear cytoplasm and sharp cytoplasmic borders; and small mononuclear cells with only scanty cytoplasm. Both histologically (14) and ultrastructurally (53) the "small cells" appear to be lymphoid, although at least at the level of the light microscope they are somewhat similar to pinealoblasts and medulloblasts. To characterize this small cell population further, we assayed for surface markers of lymphocytes in a single-cell suspension prepared from this patient's pineal germinoma.

In this single-cell suspension (32), 81% of the small cells formed rosettes with sheep erythrocytes. The rosetted cells were centrifuged onto slides and stained with Leishman's-Giemsa stains (15). The rosette-forming population (T lymphocytes) was composed exclusively of small mononuclear cells (Fig. 1.8).

The presence of surface immunoglobulins, a B lymphocyte marker (41), was determined using a fluorescence-activated cell sorter. As determined with the cell sorter, 15% of the single-cell suspension bore surface κ-light chains and 18% bore surface λ-light chains. The cells possessing the surface immunoglobulins were of approximately the same diameter as peripheral blood lymphocytes as determined by the laser beam scatter distribution provided by the cell sorter.

Thus, the majority of the small cells have a T cell surface marker. A smaller number of the cells possess surface immunoglobulins characteristic of B cells. Also of interest, a number of plasma cells were seen on the Leishman's-Giemsa stained slides prepared with the cytocentrifuge. Similar studies on a pineocytoma and on a pineoblastoma were negative for B and T cell markers.

The results obtained in this study were confirmed on frozen sections of this patient's germinoma. The hanging drop technique was used to show that the tumor contained many erythrocyte rosette-forming cells and few complement receptor-bearing cells. Thus, these frozen section studies also indicate that the majority of the small cells are T lymphocytes and that a few are B lymphocytes. In addition surface marker studies in a suprasellar germinoma ("ectopic pinealoma") have also confirmed that the small cells are T lymphocytes (34).

Lymphocyte infiltration is characteristic of a number of malignant tumors (40), particularly

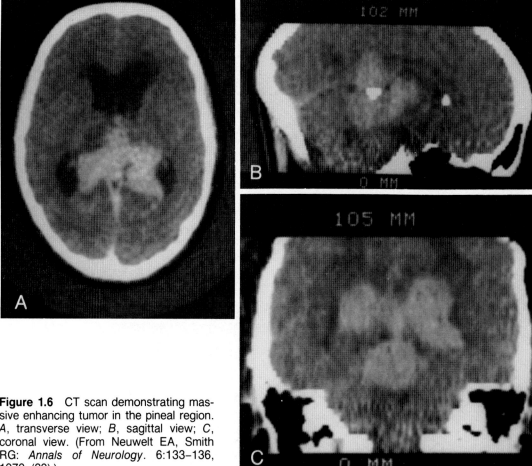

Figure 1.6 CT scan demonstrating massive enhancing tumor in the pineal region. *A*, transverse view; *B*, sagittal view; *C*, coronal view. (From Neuwelt EA, Smith RG: *Annals of Neurology*. 6:133–136, 1979, (29).)

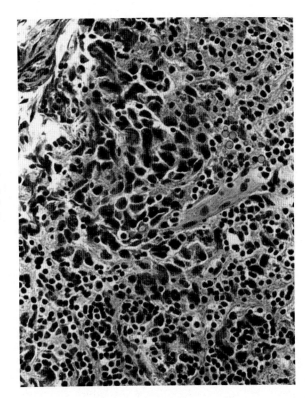

Figure 1.7. Photomicrograph demonstrating characteristic two-cell pattern of a pineal germinoma (H & E, × 420 before 10% reduction). (From Neuwelt EA, Smith RG: *Annals of Neurology.* 6:133–136, 1979, (29).)

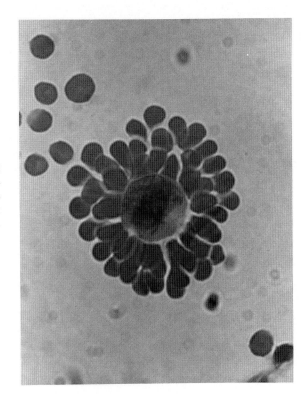

Figure 1.8. Typical sheep red blood cell rosette around "small cell" of pineal dysgerminoma (H & E, × 1050 before 10% reduction). (From Neuwelt EA, Smith RG: *Annals of Neurology.* 6:133–136, 1979, (29).

carcinoma of the breast (12) and malignant melanoma (9). Evaluation of cell membrane markers on these lymphoid cells in primary melanoma indicates that they are predominantly T cells, although in metastatic melanoma B cells are more common (9). Stavrou et al (51) have reported detecting T lymphocytes in gliomas. The current studies indicate that the small cells so characteristic of the pineal germinoma are predominantly T lymphocytes. The possibility that the small cells in pineal germinomas have lymphocyte surface markers but are not lymphocytes appears highly unlikely on the basis of the light (14) and electron microscopic (53) appearance of these cells. The biological significance of such lymphocytic infiltrates in germinomas and other neural (29) and extraneural (9,12) tumors remains unclear.

CASE 4

Pineal Tumor in an Infant

A 6-month-old female was the term product of a normal pregnancy and delivery. Her birth weight was 3900 g and her head circumference 35 cm. She was tachycardic at birth and an electrocardiogram showed paroxysmal atrial tachycardia for which she subsequently received digoxin. Her growth and development were normal until age 5½ months when she became irritable, her development seemed to stagnate, and she began vomiting. The patient was then noted to have sunset eyes, a tense fontanelle, and a head circumference in the 90th percentile. Aside from sunset eyes and the inability to look up, the patient had no other focal neurologic deficit. CT scan showed a ring-enhancing lesion in the region of the pineal (Fig. 1.9). A ventriculoperitoneal shunt was then inserted which decreased her irritability, spasticity and inability to look up. However, within 24 hours the symptoms recurred and the shunt was revised. This resulted in transient improvement, but again 3 days later, the patient's anterior fontanelle was tense, she was unable to look up and she was irritable and vomiting. A repeat CT scan at that time showed a dramatic increase in both the ventricular size and the size of the ring-enhancing pineal tumor (Fig. 1.10). Serum and CSF levels of AFP and β-HCG were within normal limits. CSF cytology was unremarkable. The patient was taken to the operating room and the tumor was removed via an occipital transtentorial approach. The tumor was surprisingly well encapsulated and with the aid of the cavitron (an ultrasonic aspirator), a gross total tumor resection was accomplished (Fig. 1.11). Pathologic evaluation revealed the tumor to be primarily pineoblastoma, but some areas were more consistent with low grade astrocytoma (Fig. 1.12). Nine days following the craniotomy, the ventriculoperitoneal shunt was ligated and aside from some transient irritability at 24 hr, the patient showed no evidence of recurrent hydrocephalus. The shunt was later removed and an asymptomatic chronic subdural hematoma drained. A myelogram was normal as was the lumbar CSF cytology. A cranial CT scan, done after the metrizamide myelogram, showed normal subarachnoid spaces with contrast agent entering the entire ventricular system, and a rather large surgical cavity (Fig. 1.13). Because of the patient's young age and what appeared to be a gross total tumor resection, no further therapy such as radiation and/or chemotherapy was planned. She is now 14-months-old, and is beginning to show CT scan evidence of tumor recurrence but is developing normally. She will receive chemotherapy.

The controversy as to therapy of pineal region tumors in very young children is particularly difficult. While CT scan is the mainstay of diagnosis and follow-up in patients such as this, angiography is important in infants to rule out vein of Galen aneurysms which by CT scan can erroneously be diagnosed as tumors (see Fig. 1.17). Indeed, Lazar and Clark (19) explored a patient who was found at surgery to have a thrombosed vein of Galen aneurysm.

In this present case, the tumor grew dramatically over a period of several days. Although it was felt that this lesion was most likely neoplastic in origin, the possibility of an abscess in the area could not be ruled out. In addition, as recently reviewed by Demakas et al (7), in very young patients, approximately 50% of pineal region tumors are benign and amenable to surgical resection. They reported three infants with pineal region tumors: a hemangioma, a ganglioglioma, and a pineoblastoma. Resection was accomplished in all but the last patient.

The sequelae of radiation therapy in the very young has been clearly documented (8,10,13,19,36,42,43), and complications of radiotherapy appear to be marked in children less than 1 yr of age. Intellectual and psychological sequelae, hypothalamic dysfunction, and/or anterior pituitary dysfunction are common. As shown by Shalet et al (50) poor growth in young children who undergo cranial irradiation occurs

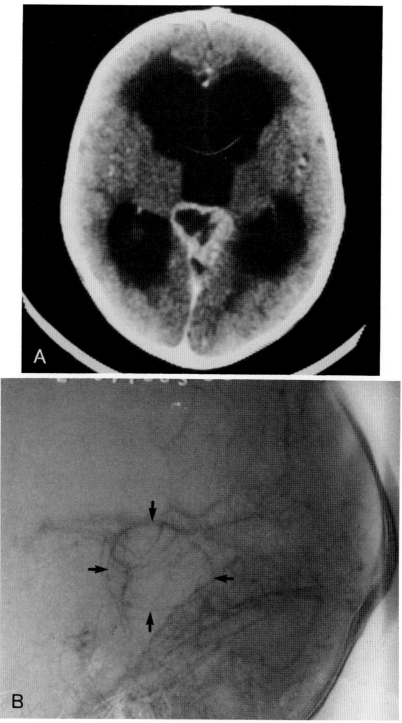

Figure 1.9. *A*, enhanced transverse section CT scan at the time of presentation of this 6-month-old child demonstrating a ring-enhancing lesion in the pineal region and enlarged ventricles. *B*, late arterial vertebral angiogram at the time of presentation showing avascular mass in the pineal region (*arrows*).

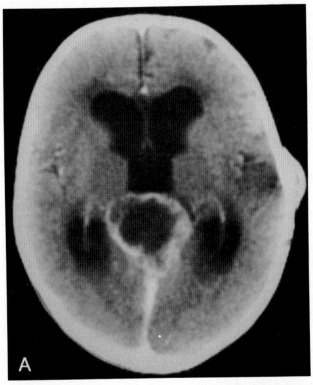

Figure 1.10. Enhanced CT scan after an insertion of a ventriculoperitoneal shunt with dramatic increase in the size of the ring-enhancing pineal region mass. *A*, transverse section.

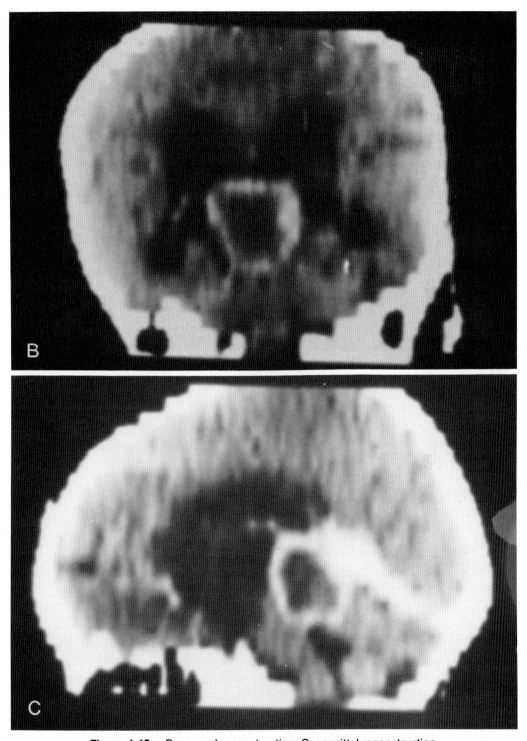

Figure 1.10. *B*, coronal reconstruction; *C*, saggittal reconstruction.

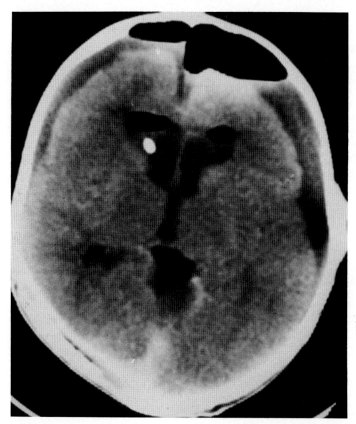

Figure 1.11. Enhanced CT scan following a gross total resection of the pineal region tumor with no evidence of residual enhancing tumor.

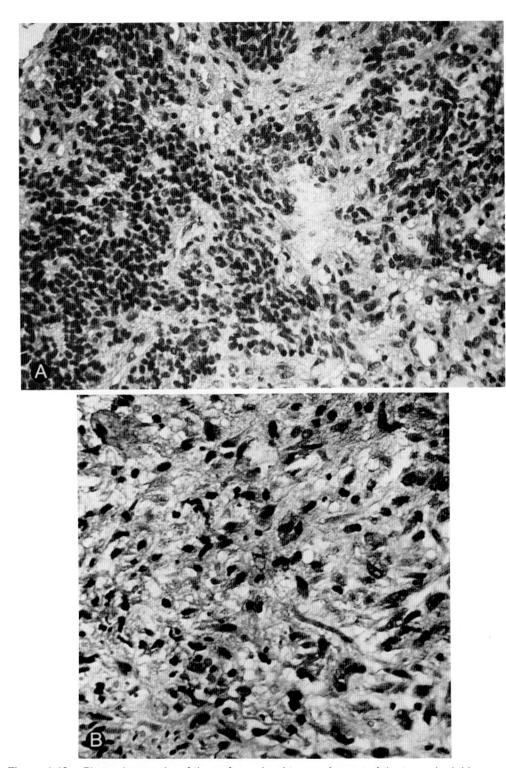

Figure 1.12. Photomicrographs of tissue from pineal tumor. *A*, most of the tumor had this appearance of a pineoblastoma (H & E, × 300). *B*, some of the tumor had this appearance of a low grade astrocytoma (H & E, × 405).

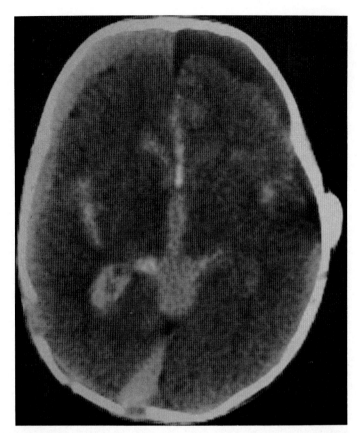

Figure 1.13. Metrizamide CT cisternogram 2 weeks postoperatively, and 1 week after the ligation of the patient's ventriculoperitoneal shunt. This CT scan was done following the patient's metrizamide myelogram which was within normal limits. Note that the metrizamide refluxes into both lateral ventricles and fills the tumor cavity in the pineal region.

irrespective of whether radiation-induced growth hormone deficiency develops.

Hoffman et al (13) in their series of 42 pineal region tumor patients treated with radiation, had 2 deaths associated with radiation damage, 4 patients had diffuse cerebral atrophy on CT scan, and 11 patients had significant mental impairment. At least six patients required hormone replacement therapy, many of these showed panhypopituitarism.

On the other hand, Deutsch (8) has recently reviewed radiotherapy in 91 children with primary brain tumors. He reports that tumor doses of at least 4000 rad seem to be necessary for any likelihood of tumor control. Of the patients treated at least 5 yr prior to his evaluation, 43% were still alive and the majority of the survivors were leading normal lives, although many had what he referred to as "mild impairment." The utilization of chemotherapy in the treatment of pineal region tumors is at such an early stage of evaluation that this modality should also be

avoided in the rapidly developing brain. In summary, in very young children with pineal region tumors, the moribidity of radiation and/or chemotherapy is increased because of the rapidly developing brain and these risks must be weighed against the risks of a surgical exploration.

CASE 5

Lipomas of the Pineal Region

A 35-yr-old licensed vocational nurse presented with a 7-yr history of headaches, a tendency to fall backwards when her eyes were closed, and mild problems with concentration. Physical and neurologic examinations were remarkable only for a positive Rhomberg test. A CT scan without contrast showed a fat density lesion in the region of the pineal which did not enhance following the administration of intravenous contrast (Fig. 1.14), and there was no evidence of hydrocephalus. The patient is doing

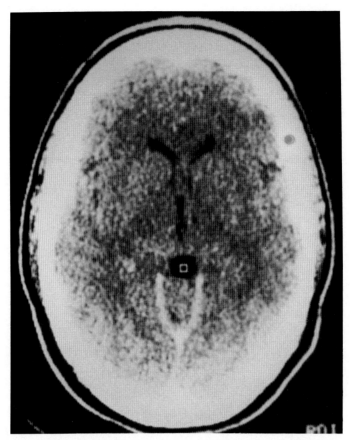

Figure 1.14. Enhanced CT scan in a patient with a presumed pineal region lipoma. The small *white square* at the center of the pineal region lipoma was used for determination of CT number by region of interest analysis. By this technique the CT number was determined to be −70.

well under conservative management for her headache.

Although there is certainly controversy as to the correct CT diagnosis in many pineal region tumors (11), there are a few pineal lesions in which the presumptive diagnosis is fairly clear-cut. One of these is the pineal region lipoma. While fat density on CT scan certainly can be seen in various teratomas and dermoids, when the entire lesion appears to be fat density the diagnosis is most likely lipoma. The diagnosis and treatment of intracranial lipomas has recently been reviewed by Kazner et al (16). As stated in that communication there is usually no problem in differentiating lipomas from teratomas and dermoid tumors. The authors also conclude that in the case of intracranial lipoma a direct surgical approach is seldom necessary although these lesions sometimes result in aqueductal occlusion and hydrocephalus. In that circumstance they recommend merely a ventriculoperitoneal shunt.

CASE 6

Pineal Region Meningioma

A 56-yr-old Caucasian female was referred in January 1981 with the insidious onset over several months of mentation difficulty and problems with balance. More recently she had developed headaches, decreased visual acuity, and progressive nausea and vomiting. On examination the patient was alert with a rather flat affect. She had bilateral papilledema but no abnormalities of extraocular movement, and in particular, there was no deficit of upward gaze. Her pupils were midsized and reacted sluggishly. Her motor examination showed a rather marked right palmar drift. She had bilateral extensor plantar responses. CT scan showed an increased-density lesion containing calcium. After administration of intravenous contrast the lesion markedly and uniformly enhanced (Fig. 1.15). Four-vessel arteriography revealed no ab-

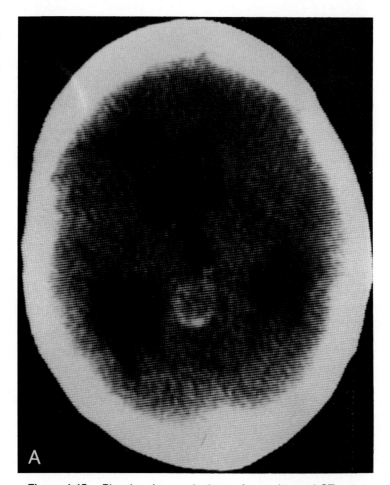

Figure 1.15.   Pineal region meningioma. *A*, unenhanced CT scan.

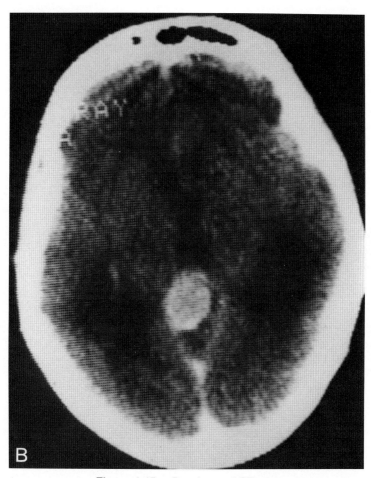

Figure 1.15. *B*, enhanced CT scan.

normal vascularity or tumor blush (Fig. 1.16). The patient underwent a ventriculoatrial shunt with prompt resolution of her mental problems and improvement in her balance. Subsequently, an occipital transtentorial craniotomy was performed with exposure of the pineal region and a gross total excision of a well encapsulated meningotheliomotous meningioma. The patient had a transient homonymous hemianopsia which cleared in 6 weeks.

Generally the diagnosis of meningioma is fairly straightforward. The patients usually have a slowly progressive course of neurologic deficit referable to the location of the lesion. Neuroradiologic evaluation is quite specific. The density of these tumors is generally somewhat higher than that of the surrounding brain and there is often calcification. Enhancement with intravenous contrast is usually marked and uniform. Angiographically there is usually a characteristic tumor blush during the capillary phase and the tumor is often fed by hypertrophied branches of the external carotid artery.

Unfortunately, when meningiomas arise in the pineal region, the diagnosis may not be straightforward. The patient can rather abruptly develop increased intracranial pressure due to obstruction of the cerebral aquaduct. The CT scan appearance can be virtually identical to that of numerous other pineal region tumors. In addition, meningiomas in the pineal are not necessarily attached to the dura and may arise from the arachnoidal cells of the velum interpositum. Hence, they may not necessarily demonstrate a capillary blush and/or hypertrophied dural arterial feeders. Even if they are attached to the dura they may be avascular. For instance, we recently operated on an enhancing tumor in the pineal region which like the present case did not produce a capillary blush, but at surgery was found to be a falcotentorial meningioma. It was also an atypical pineal region mass in that it arose above the internal cerebral veins and anterior to the vein of Galen. The vast majority of pineal tumors arise below the vein of Galen and internal cerebral veins.

As pointed out by Stein (Chapter 13), patients with pineal region meningiomas often present with altered higher cortical function (i.e. dementia, depression, psychiatric symptoms), which may or not be associated with hydrocephalus. Unlike other tumor types, patients with pineal region meningiomas have a decreased frequency of Parinaud's syndrome. For instance, Roda et al (45) reviewed pineal region meningiomas and was able to find only 3 of 11 patients who had

Parinaud's syndrome. In the recent report by Rozario and associates (47) of two patients with meningioma without dural attachment, one of the patients at angiography demonstrated an avascular mass and the other patient had a 2 cm vascular blush which was fed predominantly by the medial and lateral posterior choroidal arteries. One of the most recent reports of meningiomas of the pineal region is that by Piatt and Campbell (39). This report is of interest since one of the two tumors they report had a dural attachment and thereby could be referred to as a tentorial or falx meningioma rather than a true pineal region meningioma. In the discussion of this paper Stein states that, "The free-lying meningioma attached to the tela should receive its blood supply from the posterior choroidal arteries and occasionally the anterior choroidal artery if the tumor is large. However, the tentorial origin of meningioma gives rise to a blood supply that is extracerebral and related to the tentorium or falx arteries" (39).

In summary, meningiomas of the pineal region are tumors without clear dural attachment and probably arise from arachnoidal cells from the velum interpositum. Unlike most meningiomas, evaluation by computerized tomography does not clearly differentiate them from a number of other types of pineal region tumors since they are often well defined in size, have calcium, and uniformly enhance. Patients with these tumors who undergo angiography may or may not have a vascular blush and/or dural feeders as is typical of most other meningiomas. The CT appearance of vein of Galen aneurysms can mimic the appearance of pineal region meningioma (Fig. 1.17).

Pineal region meningiomas are an excellent example of a benign tumor which cannot be differentiated from other types of malignant pineal region tumors, and for which the only reasonable therapeutic intervention is surgery. Unfortunately, these tumors are sometimes empirically irradiated which increases the scarring of the already-dense arachnoid around the tumors, thus increasing the chances of damaging the deep venous structures in this region when they are subsequently approached surgically.

CASE 7

A Pineal Tumor Containing Elements of Germinoma and Astrocytoma

A 17-yr-old white male presented with weight loss, fatigue, and a 2-week history of progres-

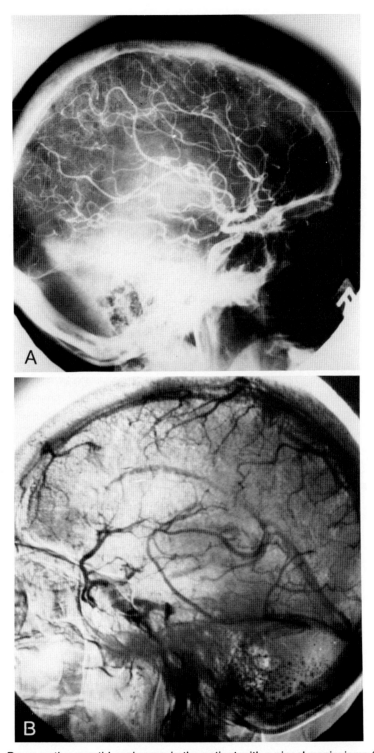

Figure 1.16. Preoperative carotid angiogram in the patient with a pineal meningioma (see Fig. 1.15) with filling of the anterior, middle, and posterior cerebral arteries. A vertebral artery angiogram (not shown) was also unremarkable. *A*, arterial phase showing no abnormal tumor vascularity. *B*, Venous phase showing no tumor blush or significant displacement of venous structure.

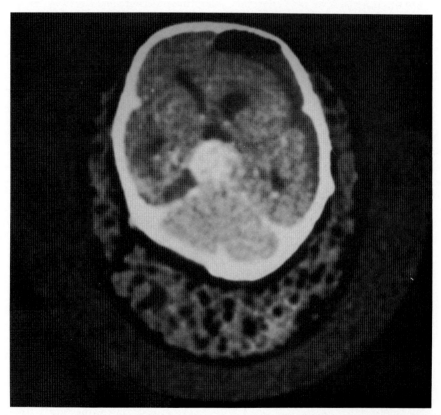

Figure 1.17.   Enhanced CT scan following ligation of a vein of Galen aneurysm showing the similarity of the enhanced CT scan of the vein of Galen aneurysm to the pineal region meningioma illustrated in Figure 1.15.

sively severe intermittent headaches. Upon examination he was noted to have papilledema and an emergency CT scan demonstrated a large pineal region tumor with nonuniform enhancement (Fig. 1.18*A*). The patient underwent a ventriculoperitoneal shunt which alleviated his symptoms. Studies of his cerebrospinal fluid obtained at the time of shunt insertion were negative for neoplastic cells, AFP and β-HCG. An angiogram showed an essentially avascular tumor. Surgery was delayed 2 weeks to allow the hydrocephalus to resolve. At surgery, the tumor was well encapsulated and a gross total resection was obtained via an occipital transtentorial exposure (Fig. 1.18, *B* and *C*). The tumor was of mixed histology. Postoperatively the patient had a significant hemianopsia and an increase in his Parinaud's syndrome. However, these findings were much less apparent 6 weeks postoperatively when the patient was readmitted for a myelogram (which was normal) and removal of his ventriculoperitoneal shunt.

Histopathologic evaluation of the tumor (Fig. 1.19) revealed, (1) areas with large epithelial cells and small lymphoid-appearing cells consistent with germinoma, (2) other areas that were clearly astrocytic as confirmed by immunoperoxidase staining using antibody to glial fibrillary acidic protein (GFAP), and (3) other areas of tumor cells with large vesicular nuclei and scant cytoplasm which taken in isolation could be neoplastic cells of pineal parenchymal cell origin (pineocytoma). These were GFAP negative. Because of the presence of malignant elements in the tumor, the patient is receiving postoperative whole head irradiation with a boost to the tumor bed. Because of the normal myelogram, normal cytology, and the prospect that chemotherapy may be necessary in the future, it was decided not to employ full craniospinal irradiation.

Pineal tumors containing elements of both neoplastic pineal parenchymal cells (i.e. pineocytoma or pineoblastoma) and astrocytoma have been reported as have germ cell tumors of mixed histology. On the other hand, mixed tumors of germ cell origin, and astrocytic origin have not been previously reported. In addition the frequency of such mixed lesions is probably not well appreciated. Hoffman et al (13) in reviewing the Toronto experience of 61 pineal region tumors mention a 3% mixed histology rate. In our own series of 15 primary malignant pineal tumors this is the fourth tumor with a mixture of neoplastic elements. The three previous cases were a combination of pineoblastoma and astrocytoma (see Chapter 14).

The existence of such a lesion in this patient and the fact that it was sufficiently encapsulated to permit total excision is important in regard to the controversy over appropriate initial therapy for pineal region tumors. This controversy revolves around whether to treat the hydrocephalus symptomatically, which may require a shunting procedure and then to administer empiric radiotherapy without a tissue diagnosis; to do a stereotactic needle biopsy; or to do an open surgical procedure with the intent of not only obtaining sufficient pathologic tissue but also of excising the lesion even if it is malignant.

Therefore, the key question with regard to this lesion is *what its history would have been* had this patient either undergone a shunting procedure and empiric radiation or a stereotactic biopsy prior to shunting and radiation. Since neoplastic cells of pineal parenchymal cell origin as well as germinoma elements are radiosensitive, it is likely that the tumor would have significantly decreased in size with radiotherapy. However, as was clearly pointed out by DeGirolami and Armbrustmacher (5) patients with encapsulated low grade glial tumors in the pineal gland can expire in a distressingly short period of time despite aggressive radiotherapy. On the other hand, as has been demonstrated by Lapras (see Chapter 15), the pineal glial tumors are often very well encapsulated and patients can survive for long periods if the tumor is excised even without postoperative radiotherapy. Our experience with glial tumors arising within the pineal gland is similar to that of Lapras.

An alternative initial diagnostic step in this young man would have been stereotactic biopsy. As illustrated in the chapter by Moser and Backlund (Chapter 12), stereotactic biopsies of pineal lesions in experienced hands can be done with minimal morbidity and mortality despite the fact that these tumors are surrounded by large thin-walled deep draining veins. The problem with stereotactic biopsy as illustrated by this case is the adequacy of the tissue sample and the importance of tumor debulking. Had the stereotactic biopsy been done and a pathologic diagnosis of either pineocytoma and/or low grade astrocytoma been made, then a consideration of an aggressive surgical attack may have been considered, whereas, if the pathologic di-

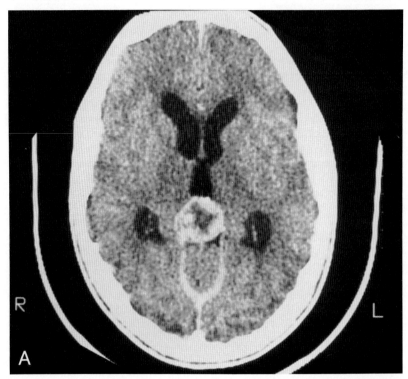

Figure 1.18.   Transverse cut CT scan of a pineal tumor which consisted of germinoma, pineocytoma and astrocytoma. *A*, preoperative enhanced CT scan.

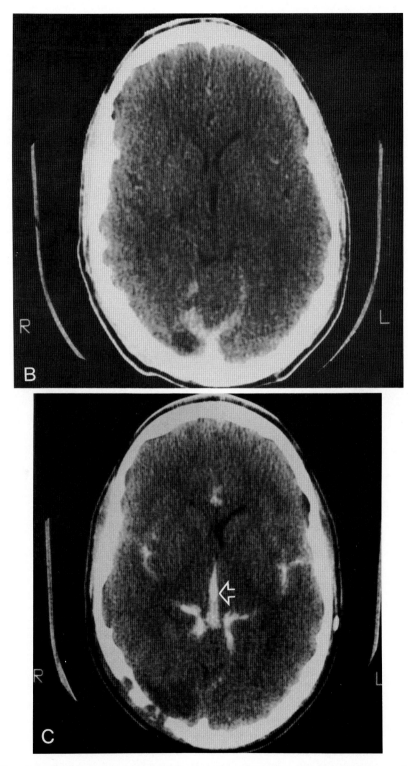

Figure 1.18. *B*, postoperative enhanced CT scan. *C*, postmetrizamide myelogram cranial CT scan showing contrast entering the third ventricle via the operative site.

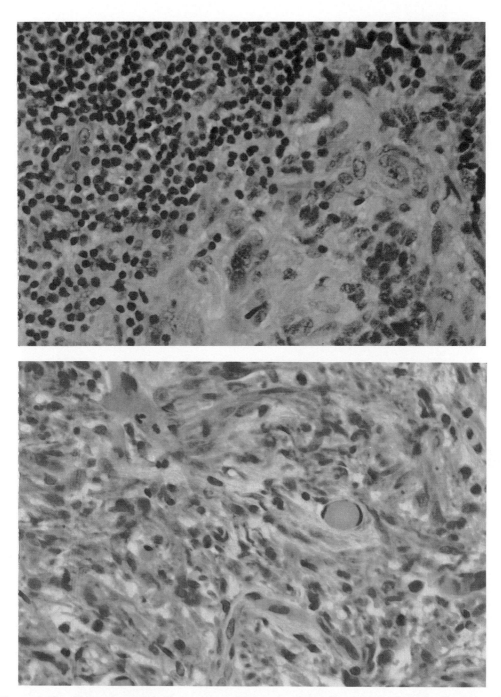

Figure 1.19. Photomicrograph of pineal tumor tissue. *A*, areas with a large and small cell component consistent with germinoma (H & E, × 100). *B*, and *C*, areas staining brown with the antiglial fibrillary acidic protein (GFAP) immunoperoxidase-hematoxylin technique are consistent with astrocytoma (× 100). **D**, islands of cells which are consistent with pineocytoma and are GFAP negative (× 40).

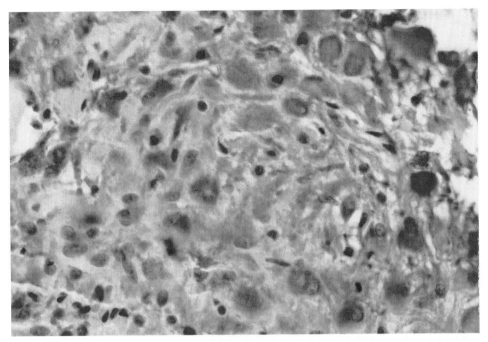

Figure 1.19. C

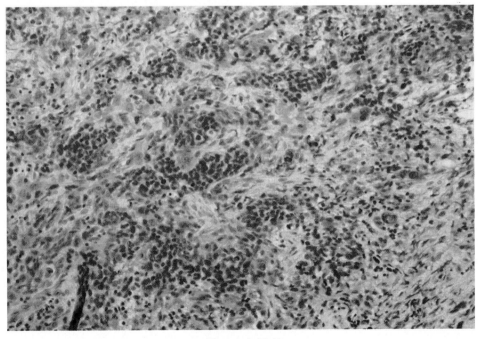

Figure 1.19. D

agnosis was that of germinoma almost certainly the patient would have received radiotherapy without additional surgical intervention. In the latter case this would certainly have shrunk the tumor but in all likelihood the long-term prognosis would have been limited.

Finally, with regard to the importance of debulking tumors of the pineal, minimizing the tumor burden considerably improves the prognosis of pineal region tumors. This is certainly consistent with the current approach to medulloblastoma in which children with this highly malignant tumor seem to do considerably better if an aggressive initial surgical approach is used prior to the initiation of radiotherapy (35).

CONCLUSION

These preceding case studies serve to emphasize various facets of pineal region tumors. The first case highlights the possible effect of such tumors on pineal physiology. Dr. Reiter in Chapter 4 notes a clear relationship between pineal function and diurnal rhythms. While the pineal gland has been studied extensively in various mammals, basic investigation *in man* is somewhat lacking. However, with the development of an accurate, sensitive, and specific melatonin assay, more can be learned in the clinical setting. Application of this basic work is seen in the second case.

Another aspect of clinical investigation focuses on the immunopathology of pineal tumors. The small cells of a pineal germinoma in the third case seem to be primarily T lymphocytes. Does this particular new insight suggest possibilities for future therapy?

Clinical management of infants with pineal region tumors is addressed in Case 4. The questions range from surgical approach as discussed by Dr. Hoffman in Chapter 11 to the role of stereotaxic biopsy (see Chapter 12) and radiation therapy (see Chapter 16).

Tumors of the pineal region can be "benign" and/or radio-insensitive. Some require surgical treatment, others do not. Lipomas as in Case 5 may well be diagnosed radiographically (see Chapter 3) and do not necessarily require surgical intervention, while meningiomas (see Case 6) can often be surgically cured. Dr. Stein discusses the surgical therapy of benign pineal tumors in Chapter 13.

Throughout the case presentations several themes recur. Mixed histology is not uncommon (see Chapters 2 and 14) even to the point of three tumor types in a single lesion as seen in Case 7. Rational therapy would ideally be tailored to tumor type; hence it is essential to accurately and fully diagnose the lesion. Primitive tumors can be seen in adults (Case 1) and germ cell tumors are not limited to the teenage male.

Indeed germ cell tumors alone raise several questions. What constitutes optimal management considering nationality or geographic location (i.e. the Japanese experience, Chapter 17), tumor location (Chapter 20) and the natural history of these lesions (Chapter 6)? The role of chemotherapy in this tumor is becoming more definite (Chapters 19 and 21).

Regardless of pathology, tumors in the pineal region present rather stereotypically with symptoms of hydrocephalus and neuro-opthalmologic signs (see Chapter 5). Management of pineal region tumors follows a basic scheme of hydrocephalus treatment followed by surgical approach for diagnosis, and further therapy individually tailored to the pathology. Technical advances such as microscope, ultrasonic aspirators (Cavitron Ultrasonic Surgical Aspirator Coopervision Medical, Stamford, CT), and laser are utilized, thus allowing surgical approach to an historically prohibitive area.

Acknowledgments. Case 2 has been published previously (33) and is reprinted with permission.

Case 3 has been published previously and is reprinted with permission (29).

Case 5 was kindly contributed by Dr. Rick Pratt.

Case 6 was kindly referred by Dr. Charles W. Sternberg.

References

1. Arendt J, Forbes JM, Browm WB, Marston A: Effect of pinealectomy on immunoassayable melatonin in the sheep. *J Endocrinol* 85:1P–2P, 1980.
2. Arendt J: Current status of assay methods of melatonin. In Birau N, Schloot W (eds): *Melatonin–Current Status and Perspectives* (Advances in the Biosciences). New York, Pergamon Press, 1981, vol 29, pp 3–7.
3. Barber SG, Smith JA, Hughes RC: Melatonin as a tumour marker in a patient with pineal tumour. *Br Med J* 2:328, 1978
4. Barber SG, Smith JA, Cove DH, Smith SCH, London DR: Marker for pineal tumours? *Lancet* 2:372–373, 1978.
5. DeGirolami U, Armbrustmacher VW: Juvenile pilocytic astrocytoma of the pineal region: Report of a case. *Cancer* 50:1185–1188, 1982.
6. DeGirolami U, Schmidek H: Clinicopathological study of 53 tumors of the pineal region. *J Neuro-*

surg 39:455–462, 1973.

7. Demakas JJ, Sonntag VKH, Kaplan AM, Kelley JJ, Waggener JD: Surgical management of pineal area tumors in early childhood. *Surg Neurol* 17:435–440, 1981.

8. Deutsch M: Radiotherapy of primary brain tumors in very young children. *Cancer* 50:2785–2789, 1982.

9. Edelson RL, Hearing VJ, Dellon AJ, et al: Differentiation between B cells, T cells, and histiocytes in melanocytic lesions: Primary and metastatic melanoma and halo and giant pigmented nevi. *Clin Immunol Immunopathol* 4:557–568, 1975.

10. Eiser C: Psychological sequelae of brain tumors in childhood: A retrospective study. *Br J Clin Psycholog* 20:35–38, 1981.

11. Futrell NN, Osborn AG, Cheson BD: Pineal region tumors: Computed tomographic-pathologic spectrum. *AJR* 137:951–956, 1981.

12. Hamlin IME: Possible host resistance in carcinoma of the breast, a histological study. *Br J Cancer* 22:383–401, 1968.

13. Hoffman HJ, Yoshida M, Becker LE, Hendrick EB, Humphreys PR: Pineal region tumors in childhood. *Concepts Pediatr Neurosurg* 4:360–386, 1983.

14. Jellinger K: Primary intracranial germ cell tumours. *Acta Neuropathol* 25:291–306, 1973.

15. Kaplan ME, Clark C: An improved rosetting assay for detection of human T lymphocytes. *J Immunol Methods* 5:131–135, 1974.

16. Kazner E, Stochdorph O, Wende S, Grumme T: Intracranial lipoma: Diagnostic and therapeutic considerations. *J Neurosurg* 52:234–245, 1980.

17. Kenneway DJ, Frith RG, Phillipou G, Matthews CD, Seamark RF: A specific radioimmunoassay for melatonin in biological tissue and fluid and its validation by gas chromatography-mass spectrometry. *Endocrinology* 101:119–127, 1977.

18. Kennaway DJ, McCulloch G, Matthews CD, Seamark RF: Plasma melatonin, luteinizing hormone, follicle-stimulating hormone, prolactin, and corticoids in two patients with pinealoma. *J Clin Endocrinol Metab* 49:144–145, 1979.

19. Lazar ML, Clark K: Direct surgical management of masses in the region of the vein of Galen. *Surg Neurol* 2:17–22, 1974.

20. Lewy AJ, Kern HA, Rosenthal NE, Wehr TA: Bright artificial light treatment of a manic-depressive patient with a seasonal mood cycle. *Am J Psychiatry* 139:1496–1498, 1982.

21. Lewy AJ, Tetsu M, Markey SP, Goodwin FK, Kopin IJ: Pinealectomy abolishes plasma melatonin in the rat. *J Clin Endocrinol Metab* 50:204–205, 1980.

22. Lewy AJ, Newsome DA: Different types of melatonin circadian secretory rhythms in some blind subjects. *J Clin Endocrinol Metab*, 56:1103–1107, 1983.

23. Lewy AJ: Biochemistry and regulation of mammalian melatonin production. In Relkin R (ed): *The Pineal Gland.* New York, Elsevier, 1983, pp 77–128.

24. Lewy AJ, Markey SP: Analysis of melatonin in human plasma by gas chromatography negative

25. Lewy AJ, Wehr TA, Goodwin FK, Newsome DA, Markey SP: Light suppresses melatonin secretion in humans. *Science* 210:1267–1269, 1980.

26. Lynch H, Assay methodology. In Relkin R (ed): *The Pineal Gland.* New York, Elsevier, 1983, pp 129–150.

27. Markey SP, Buell PE: Pinealectomy abolishes 6-hydroxymelatonin excretion by male rats. *Endocrinology* 111:425–426, 1982.

28. Moore-Ede MC, Czeisler CA, Richardson GS: Circadian timekeeping in health and disease: Part I. Basic properties of circadian pacemakers. *N Engl J Med* 309:469–476, 1983; Part II. Clinical implications of circadian rhythmicity. *N Engl J Med* 309:530–536, 1983.

29. Neuwelt EA, Smith RG: Presence of lymphocyte membrane surface markers on "small cells" in a pineal germinoma. *Ann Neurol* 6:133–136, 1979.

30. Neuwelt EA, Clark K: *Clinical Aspects of Neuroimmunology.* Baltimore, Williams & Wilkins, 1978, pp 93–94.

31. Neuwelt EA, Batjar H: Surgical management of pineal region tumors. *Contemp Neurosurg* 4:1–5, 1982.

32. Neuwelt EA, Glasberg M, Frenkel E, Clark WK: Malignant pineal region tumors. *J Neurosurg* 51:597–607, 1979.

33. Neuwelt EA, Lewy A: Disappearance of plasma melatonin after removal of a neoplastic pineal gland. *N Engl J Med* 308:1132–1135, 1983.

34. Neuwelt EA, Frenkel EP, Smith RG: Suprasellar germinoma (ectopic pinealoma): Aspects of immunologic characterization and successful chemotherapeutic responses in recurrent disease. *Neurosurgery* 7:352–358, 1980.

35. Norris DG, Bruce DA, Byrd RL, Schut L, Littman P, Bilaniuk LT, Zimmerman RA, Capp R: Improved relapse-free survival in medulloblastoma utilizing modern technique. *Neurosurgery* 9:661–662, 1981.

36. Onoyama Y, Abe M, Takahashi M, Yabumoto E, Sakamoto T: Radiation therapy of brain tumors in children. *Radiology* 115:687–693, 1975.

37. Ozaki Y, Lynch HJ: Presence of melatonin in plasma and urine of pinealectomized rats. *Endocrinology* 99:641–644, 1976.

38. Pelham RW, Ralph CL, Campbell IM: Mass spectral identification of melatonin in blood. *Biochem Biophys Res Commun* 46:1236–1241, 1972.

39. Piatt Jr, JH, Campbell GA: Pineal region meningioma: Report of two cases and literature review. *Neurosurgery* 12:369–376, 1983.

40. Preud'homme JL, Seligman M: Surface-bound immunoglobulins as a cell marker in human lymphoproliferative diseases. *Blood* 40:777–794, 1972.

41. Raff MC, Steinberg M, Taylor RB: Immunoglobulin determinants on the surface of mouse lymphoid cells. *Nature* 225:553–554, 1970.

42. Raimondi AJ, Tomita T: Pineal tumors in childhood. *Childs Brain* 9:239–255, 1982.

43. Rappaport R, Brauner R, Czernichow P, Thibaud E, Renier D, Zucker JM, Lemerle J: Effect of hypothalamic and pituitary irradiation on puber-

tal development in children with cranial tumors. *J Clin Endocrinol Metab* 54:1164–1168, 1982.

44. Relkin R: Pineal-hormonal interactions. In Relkin R (ed): *The Pineal Gland.* New York, Elsevier, 1983, pp 225–246.

45. Roda JM, Perez-Higueras A, Oliver B, Alvarez MP, Blazquez MG: Pineal region meningiomas without dural attachment. *Surg Neurol* 17:147–151, 1982.

46. Rollag MD: Methods for measuring pineal hormones. In Reiter R (ed): *The Pineal Gland: Anatomy and Biochemistry.* Boca Raton, CRC Press, 1981, vol 1, pp 273–302.

47. Rozario R, Adelman L, Prager RJ, Stein BM: Meningiomas of the pineal region and third ventricle. *Neurosurgery* 5:489–495, 1979.

48. Sano K, Matsutani M: Pinealoma (germinoma) treated by direct surgery and postoperative irradiation. *Childs Brain* 8:81–97, 1981.

49. Schmidek HH (ed): *Pineal Tumors.* New York, Masson Publishing USA, Inc, 1977, pp 1–138.

50. Shalet SM, Beardwell CG, Aarons BM, Pearson D, Jones PHM: Growth impairment in children treated for brain tumors. *Arch Dis Childhood* 53:491–494, 1978.

51. Stavrou D, Anzil AP, Wiedenback W, et al: Immunofluorescence study of lymphocytic infiltration in gliomas. Identification of T-lymphocytes. *J Neurol Sci* 33:275–282, 1977.

52. Stein BM: The infratentorial supracerebellar approach to pineal lesions. *J Neurosurg* 35:197–202, 1971.

53. Tabuchi K, Yamada O, Nishimoto A: The ultrastructure of pinealomas. *Acta Neuropathol* 24:117–127, 1973.

54. Tapp E, Skinner RG, Phillips V: Radioimmunoassay for melatonin. *J Neural Transm* 48:137–141, 1980.

55. Tetsuo M, Perlow MJ, Mishkin N, Markey SP: Light exposure reduces and pinealectomy virtually stops urinary excretion of 6-hydroxymelatonin by rhesus monkeys. *Endocrinology* 110:997–1003, 1982.

56. Wurtman RJ, Kammer H: Melatonin synthesis by an ectopic pinealoma. *N Engl J Med* 274:1233–1237, 1966.

57. Yu HS, Pang SF, Tang PL, Brown GM: Persistence of circadian rhythms of melatonin and N-acetylserotonin in the serum of rats after pinealectomy. *Neuroendocrinology* 32:262–265, 1981.

CHAPTER 2

Pathology of Pineal Tumors

MAIE KAARSOO HERRICK, M.D.

HISTOLOGY OF THE NORMAL PINEAL GLAND

The lobular pattern of the pineal gland (Fig. 2.1) becomes defined during the second half of the first decade of life, when connective tissue septae containing blood vessels penetrate the parenchyma and separate it into anastomosing cords. The pineal parenchymal cells, or pineocytes, are a special type of neuroepithelial cells, closely related to neurons, but lacking axons. They have large, round to oval, or kidney-shaped pale nuclei with conspicuous nucleoli and fine chromatin. When stained with hematoxylin and eosin (H & E), the cytoplasm is fibrillary and poorly defined. The silver carbonate impregnation technique for pineal parenchymal cells (31), however, will demonstrate a characteristic black cytoplasm and a pale nucleus. The cells in the central part of the lobules are irregularly stellate with a few prolongations extended to the edge of the lobule. The peripheral cells tend to send all their processes to the edges of the lobules (Fig. 2.2). These processes end in club-shaped enlargements forming a radiating marginal zone in close relationship to the interlobular vessels. In aging individuals, occasional monstrous cells, presumably hypertrophic pineocytes, may be found. Melanin has been demonstrated to be present in fetal pineal cells (34, 77), and in scattered cells in the stroma of adult human pineal glands (95).

A small astrocytic component is normally found in the pineal gland. These glial cells have darker nuclei than the pineocytes, and processes which take up glial stains and contain glial fibrillary acidic protein (GFA) (69). Most of these astrocytes are fibrous, but apparently transitional forms between protoplasmic and fibrous cells also are seen. These cells are dispersed throughout the pineal gland, but focal aggregates may form glial islands. The astrocytes can vary greatly in numbers at any time of life, but tend to increase with age.

Only rarely can true ganglion cells be found in the human pineal postnatally. Small groups of undifferentiated neuroblast-like cells, however, have been identified in the human fetal pineal gland (77), and the older literature contains unverified descriptions of small collections of ganglion cells in the pineal of the neonates, but not the adult (70), and in the tissue at the tip of the pineal in children and adults (91).

Other components of the pineal gland are fibroblasts, usually situated next to the vascular adventitia, a few lymphocytes, plasma cells, mast cells, and lipid containing macrophages. The presence, within lobules or interlobular trabeculae, of concretions called acervuli, corpora arenaceae, or calcospherites, is well recognized. The mechanisms of formation and pathophysiological significance of these structureless, laminated or mulberry-shaped mineralized bodies, is not known. They contain iron and calcium, and have a hydroxyapatite or carbonate apatite structure. Although they may be sometimes found in infants, they are constantly present by the age of 16 and increase in numbers throughout life.

Studies of the ultrastructure of the human pineal gland have been performed on fetal material (65, 77–79) and on postmortem tissue from a 3-yr-old girl (65), but descriptions are lacking in adults. Besides the usual cytoplasmic organelles, prominent 50–80 Å filaments, few microtubules, bulbous cell processes, and cilia with a 9 + 0 microtubular pattern were described in the fetal pineocytes (77). In the poorly preserved material from the young child (65), intracellular structures suggestive of synaptic ribbons were reported. These findings are in agreement with the voluminous information available on histology of the pineal glands of a great variety of animal species. An extensive review of the accumulated data, along with a reprint of del Rio-Hortega's classic description of the pineal gland has been recently published by Haymaker et al (46).

31

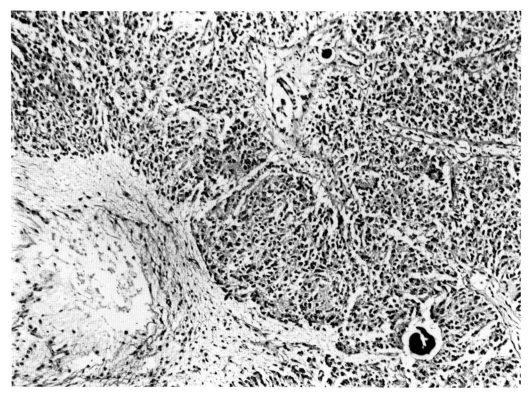

Figure 2.1.   Normal pineal gland, 44-yr-old man. Lobulated pattern with small cyst in glial island, *lower left*; calcospherite, *lower right*. (H & E, × 115.)

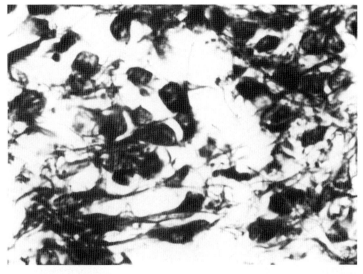

Figure 2.2.   Normal pineal gland, 44-yr-old man. Pineocytes with pale nuclei and argyrophilic, expanded cell processes extended toward blood vessel, *lower left*. (Silver carbonate impregnation for pineal parenchyma (31), × 730.)

TUMORS OF THE PINEAL REGION

The study of pineal tumors has been greatly hampered by their rarity. The incidence of neoplasms arising at the pineal site has been reported in large series to range from 0.4–1.0% of all intracranial neoplasms (146). Since many of the growths, however, are found in the younger age groups, their incidence in children is higher. For reasons not understood, pineal tumors are more frequent in Japan, where they have been reported to comprise 4.5 (6), 6.23 [as quoted by Koide and associates (63)], and even 8.4% (61) of all intracranial tumors [9.3%, if the suprasellar growths are included (61)].

The development of a rational classification of pineal region tumors has been slow and tortuous, and fraught with conceptual errors. As the histogenesis of these neoplasms has become better understood, the nomenclature applied to the various tumor types has changed. The true nature of many of the pineal tumors described in the older literature by a variety of names can only be discerned when descriptions and illustrations are sufficiently adequate. The historical details (15) and evolution of the current pineal nomenclature (29) have been thoroughly documented, and will not be repeated. A few brief comments, however, need to be made about the past and present terminology.

The name pinealoma, introduced by Krabbe (64), was for a long time used to designate the most common pineal tumor which we now know, does not rise from the pineal parenchymal cell, but is really a germinoma. The term ectopic pinealoma referred to tumors of similar histologic type when found at other, mainly midline locations, in the cranial cavity. Even now, some authors still incorrectly use these names in the above sense, while others have applied the term pinealoma as a generic designation for any neoplasm which arises in the pineal region. If it were to be used at all, the name pinealoma would be appropriate for tumors of pineal cell origin. However, in order not to perpetuate the past confusion, the deletion of this name altogether is to be recommended.

The basis for the modern classification of pineal tumors was provided by Russell (107) when she pointed out that the pinealoma was histologically similar to a common testicular neoplasm. She used the name atypical teratoma for these tumors, because of the frequent finding in them of teratomatous elements such as smooth muscle, cysts lined by low cuboidal, co-

lumnar mucus-secreting, and squamous epithelium, cartilage, and even choriocarcinoma. Subsequent studies (36) verified the similarity between the histological appearance and biological behavior of the so-called pinealoma and atypical teratoma, and the extragonadal germinoma, testicular seminoma, and ovarian dysgerminoma. The classification of neoplasms arising in the pineal region follows that of Russell and Rubinstein (108) (Table 2.1).

TUMORS OF GERM CELL ORIGIN

Hypotheses regarding the origin of this group of tumors are varied, but in the forefront are the theories suggesting that they arise from germ cells, or from even less differentiated embryonal cells, or from either (42). The germ cells are believed to originate in the yolk sac endoderm and migrate widely through the embryo. Although they localize in the gonadal ridges, sometimes they can find their way into other, usually midline sites, of the embryo, including the brain. In the case of tumors at extragonadal locations, these cells are believed to have been misplaced during early development. Such a concept helps to explain why neoplasms, which present a histological spectrum similar to those found in the pineal region, can also occur elsewhere in the cranial cavity, and at other diverse locations, including the mediastinum, retroperitoneum, and gonads. This hypothesis is also consistent with the fact that tumors of germ cell origin may arise not only in, but next to, the pineal gland.

The histological types of germ cell tumors, and their biological behavior, outlined in Table 2.2, is modified from Teilum's concept of differentiation of germ cell neoplasms in the testis and their relationship to each other (127). The

Table 2.1
Classification of Pineal Tumors[a]

1. Tumors of germ cell origin
    Germinomas (atypical teratoma) and other closely related tumors
    Teratomas
2. Tumors of pineal parenchymal cells
    Pineoblastomas
    Pineocytomas
3. Tumors of glial and other cell origin
4. Non-neoplastic cysts and masses

[a] From Russell DS, Rubinstein LJ (eds): *Pathology of Tumors of the Nervous System*, 4th ed. Williams & Wilkins, Baltimore, 1977, (108).

Table 2.2
Histological Types of Tumors of Germ Cell Origin and Their Biological Behavior[a]

Malignant	I. Germinoma (atypical teratoma, dysgerminoma, seminoma)
Malignant	II. Embryonal carcinoma
	A. Extraembryonic structures
Malignant	1. Endodermal sinus tumor (yolk sac tumor)
Malignant	2. Chriocarcinoma
	B. Embryonic endo-, meso-, ectoderm
Malignant or benign	1. Teratoma—immature
Benign	2. Teratoma—mature

[a] Adapted from Teilum: *Acta Pathol Microbiol Scand* 64:407–429, 1965, (127).

same scheme is applicable to this class of neoplasms when found intracranially. It is a characteristic of this group of neoplasms that frequently combinations of more than one histologic type may exist in a single tumor. For this reason, accurate figures documenting the incidence of some of the rarer subtypes of germ cell neoplasms are not available. The tumors which have been reported under the various names, often have other components as well. When an assessment of a small surgical biopsy is made, the possibility has to be kept in mind, that the specimen may not always reflect the total nature of the entire growth. It is also vital to remember, that when a diagnosis of an intracranial tumor of germ cell origin is made, a primary gonadal neoplasm must be ruled out.

Germinoma

The most common neoplasm of germ cell origin, as well as the most frequently occurring tumor in the pineal region, is the germinoma. It accounts for more than 50% of all neoplasms arising at the pineal site (103). A somewhat smaller figure of 46% was found among 100 pineal tumors by Davis (27), while in other smaller series, 10 (33%) of 31 (30) and 10 (29%) of 34 (28) histologically verified pineal growths were germinomas. In Japan, where the incidence of pineal tumors has been reported to be as high as 8.4% (61), the proportion of neoplasms of germ cell origin among them is also believed to be greater (63) than found elsewhere.

The germinoma is a tumor of the first three decades of life, with a peak incidence in the middle of the second decade. There is a marked predominance of affected males (103, 108). Among a series of 87 pineal germinomas, 77 occurred in male, and 10 in female patients (28). While still present, the difference is not as marked among patients with suprasellar germinomas (28, 100).

An association between germinoma and teratoma is well recognized (28, 103, 107, 108), but has been estimated to occur in less than one-fifth of all reported cases (28). Instances have also been described of multifocal tumors of the germ cell series. A germinoma of the floor of the third ventricle was associated with a small pineal dermoid cyst in Russell's Case 1 (107). A separate pineal region teratoma and foci of germinoma infiltrating the infundibulum and optic tract have also been documented (56). Case 4 of Kageyama and Belsky (60) was a patient with a pituitary teratoma, who also had germinoma in the pituitary stalk and tuber cinereum, along with microscopic foci of germinoma in the pineal gland. Association of a hypothalamic germinoma and mediastinal malignant teratoma (28), and a pineal teratoma, dermoid cyst of testis, and choriocarcinoma of the mediastinum in a 16-yr-old boy have also been recorded (103).

The germinoma is similar to the testicular seminoma in its biological behavior. Untreated, it is rapidly fatal. The germinoma is highly radiosensitive, and with irradiation, instances of survival are documented. Among 33 patients with biopsy-proven pineal and suprasellar germinomas in the Children's Cancer Study Group, 72% survived follow-up periods ranging from 2–15 yr (137).

Elevated levels of β-subunit of human chorionic gonadotropin (HCG) have been demonstrated in the serum or CSF of some patients with pineal or suprasellar germinoma (82, 83). Generally considered a marker for choriocarcinoma, the finding of HCG may indicate the prsence of foci of that tumor. An increased HCG level has also been reported in 9–10% of patients with pure testicular seminoma (57), and by analogy, such a finding may be true for the intracranial counterparts of this tumor.

A search in germinomas for substances indigenous to the pineal parenchymal cells, such as melatonin and one of its synthesizing enzymes, hydroxyindole-*O*-methyltransferase (HIOMT), or serotonin, has yielded conflicting, surprising results. As expected, no serotonin or catecholamine was detected by fluorescent histochemical reaction for monoamines in one germinoma (63). On the other hand, HIOMT was found in the dural extension of a suprasellar germinoma of an 18-yr-old girl (143), and HIOMT, melatonin, and serotonin were present in the subcutaneous metastases of a 14-yr-old boy with a pineal germinoma (141). The latter patient appears to be the same one who was subsequently reported by Borden and associates (14) after an 11-yr survival with widespread systemic metastases. Further investigations in this field are needed, including assays of extracranial germinomas and other tumors of germ cell origin.

PATHOLOGICAL FEATURES

The germinoma is a gray or pink granular, somewhat opalescent, solid tumor (28). Hemorrhage and necrosis are not common, but may occur. Calcification, although infrequent, has been described (28, 29). Cysts are usually not present. The tumor forms a poorly circumscribed mass at the pineal site, either obliterating the pineal gland or sparing it. Posteriorly, the tumor will compress the quadrigeminal plate and sometimes invade it. Hydrocephalus due to aqueductal compression is a common early complication. Anteriorly, the tumor mass may bulge into the posterior part of the third ventricle. In more than half of the cases (28) the tumor has spread into the anterior part of the third ventricle and may invade the infundibulum, optic nerves, and sella. The spread of tumor is either by direct extension or by metastasis. The entire ventricular system may become lined by neoplasm. At times, it is not possible to be certain whether the tumor arose in the pineal or suprasellar region, and multifocal origin can also not always be excluded. It is uncommon, however, for a patient with a pineal tumor to first present with symptoms referable to the suprasellar region (29).

Dissemination of tumor cells throughout the cerebrospinal pathways may result in distal leptomeningeal metastases and may be detected by cytological examination of the CSF (38). Direct extension into lumbar epidural fat and sacral bone (28), and direct invasion of the adventitia of the internal carotid arteries and gasserian ganglia have also been reported by Lewis and co-workers, Case 1 (68).

Surgical procedures have been followed by distal metastases in several instances. A mixed teratocarcinoma and germinoma was surgically removed from a 34-yr-old man, but local recurrence, invasion of the vein of Galen and hematogenous pulmonary metastases of the germinomatous component of the neoplasm occurred (128). In another patient, a 21-yr-old man, pulmonary metastases developed after partial removal of a pineal germinoma.

A unique case was recorded by Borden et al (14). The patient was a currently tumor-free man, who at the age of 9½ yr was treated by radiotherapy and ventriculocisternostomy for a pineal region mass. Over the subsequent 11 yr, he developed histologically verified metastatic deposits of germinoma deep to his gluteus maximus, in the spinous processes of cervical vertebrae, bone, lymph nodes, and pleura. Another case is that of a 17-yr-old boy with a ventriculoatrial shunt for an unbiopsied pineal mass, who died after developing metastases of germinoma to the lumbar muscles and supraclavicular lymph nodes (101). At least three instances of histologically verified peritoneal metastases of germinoma have also been reported in patients treated with ventriculoperitoneal shunts for unbiopsied pineal tumors [Wood et al, Cases 1 and 2 (140); Neuwelt et al, Case 2 (82, 83)]. Lethal hemorrhage into a germinoma within the subarachnoid space has been reported by Lewis and associates, Case 3 (68).

Upon microscopic examination, the tumor has a distinctive pattern consisting of sheets of large polygonal cells separated into lobules by blood vessels and connective trabeculae which are extensively infiltrated by small lymphocytes (Fig. 2.3). The large cells have big, round nuclei with scanty, vesicular chromatin and prominent eosinophilic nucleoli. The cell membranes are distinct, and the cytoplasm may be clear, or pink with the hematoxylin and eosin stain. The cytoplasm of the cells is rich in glycogen granules which can be demonstrated with the periodic acid-Schiff (PAS) reaction, and which disappear when treated with diastase. The histochemical reaction for alkaline phosphatase is positive (63). Mitotic figures are usually numerous.

The inflammatory response is intriguing, and in rare instances may be so severe as to obscure the true neoplastic nature of the process. In one patient with a pineal, and another with suprasellar germinoma, the lymphocytes have been shown to be predominantly T cells (82, 84). The lymphocytes may even form nodules with germinal centers. Frequently, scattered plasma cells, polymorphonuclear neutrophils, and macrophages may be found. There may be a granulomatous process, complete with epithelioid cells and multinucleated foreign-body and Langhans'-type giant cells. Inclusions in giant cells, comparable to asteroids and Schaumann bodies found in sarcoidosis have been documented (28).

The ultrastructure of the intracranial germinoma has been described by a number of investigators (26, 49, 71, 122, 125). There is general agreement that the cytoplasmic features resemble the dysgerminoma and seminoma. The primary tumor cells have a large ovoid, lightly osmiophilic granular nucleus with one or more prominent nucleoli. The cytoplasm contains a sparse granular endoplasmic reticulum, large numbers of ribosomes, sparse to well developed Golgi profiles, and many glycogen particles. A variable number of mitochondria, with scanty, often vesicular cristae, occasional centrioles, and few microtubules are found. Annulated lamellae, a variant of rough endoplasmic reticulum have been observed (45, 49, 63). The latter structures

are present in a variety of tumors, but are a common component of oocytes and ovarian dysgerminomas (49). Tight and gap junctions and desmosomes can be found between tumor cells.

The lymphocytic nature of the small cells in the germinoma is verified by the ultrastructural studies. Variable numbers of plasma cells, polymorphonuclear cells, and macrophages also have been identified. In at least one study of a third ventricular germinoma, macrophage activity was prominent and included phagocytosis of tumor cells (45). Whether or not the various types of inflammatory cell activity represent an immune response to the tumor remains at this time a matter of speculation.

Embryonal Carcinoma

In analogy to germ cell tumors elsewhere, embryonal carcinoma can be expected to arise also at the pineal site. Indeed, small foci of embryonal carcinoma have not infrequently been identified within various pineal tumors of germ cell origin. Neoplasms, whose major com-

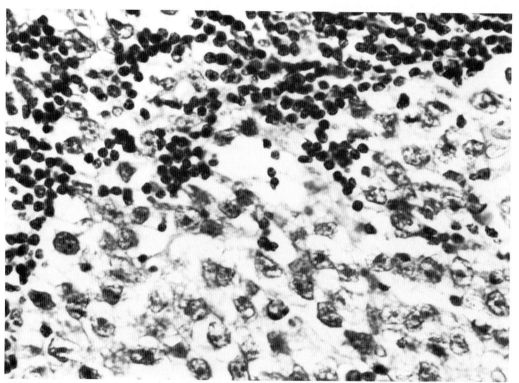

Figure 2.3. Germinoma, 11-yr-old girl. Cells with large nuclei and prominent nucleoli, *below*; lymphocytic infiltrate, *above*. (H & E, × 730.)

ponent is embryonal carcinoma are, however, exceedingly rare. Accurate analysis of the older literature poses difficulties since in the past, the endodermal sinus tumors were often classified as embryonal carcinoma.

Three pineal region embryonal carcinomas reported by Jellinger (58) contained additional areas of endodermal sinus tumor, germinoma, and choriocarcinoma. Endodermal sinus tumor was present in Borit and co-worker's case (16), and teratomatous elements were found in the tumor reported by Arita et al (7). All of the above patients were male, and ranged from 8–19 yrs in age.

Gonadal embryonal carcinomas possess the capacity to secrete human chorionic gonadotropin as well as α-fetoprotein. A search for these tumor markers would be useful in the pineal counterpart of this neoplasm.

PATHOLOGICAL FEATURES

Embryonal carcinoma may present as a large hemorrhagic, necrotic tumor mass in the pineal region (7). Extensive metastases throughout the CSF pathways in Borit and associates' case (16) consisted largely of endodermal sinus tumor (personally reviewed). Sakata et al (109) reported an 8-yr-old patient, with a pineal tumor consisting of benign teratoma, malignant ependymoma, and embryonal carcinoma. A ventriculoperitoneal shunt was followed by extensive subarachnoid as well as hematogenous extraneural metastases of the embryonal carcinoma component to lung, urinary bladder and pancreas. Unfortunately, the illustration of the embryonal carcinoma component of the tumor is not diagnostic, and the verbal description could fit either that neoplasm or an endodermal sinus tumor.

Microscopically, the tumor is composed of large embryonal, malignant-appearing epithelial cells. The size, shape, and arrangement of cells may be variable. The nuclei of the cells have a coarse, irregular nuclear membrane, varying degrees of nuclear vacuolization, and one or more prominent nucleoli. The cytoplasm may lack distinct cell borders and is amphophilic or vacuolated. Mitoses are frequent. The tumor cells grow in solid sheets or form large acinar, tubular, or papillary structures lined by cuboidal or columnar cells. The stroma is scanty, loose and edematous, or fibrous and hyalinized. Hemorrhage and necrosis are frequent. Detailed pho-

tomicrographs of embryonal carcinoma are depicted by Burger and Vogel (21).

Endodermal Sinus Tumor

This neoplasm of the germ cell series is believed to represent extraembryonic differentiation of the totipotential cells, and is characterized by growth of extraembryonic mesoblast and yolk sac endoderm. Found more frequently than the embryonal carcinoma, about two dozen instances of endodermal sinus tumors arising at the pineal site have been identified and extensively reviewed (51, 80, 117, 126). More than half of the tumors have contained elements of other germ cell neoplasms.

With the exception of a 24-yr-old man illustrated by Burger and Vogel (21) and a 20-month-old girl (80), all the patients have been in their second decade, and two-thirds have been males. The prognosis is almost uniformly dismal, and most patients have died within 2 yr. Only one patient with an endodermal sinus tumor at the pineal site was alive and tumor free 3½ yr after surgery (80). Another patient, a 13-yr-old girl (12) with a suprasellar endodermal sinus tumor, is reported by Albrechtsen and associates (2) to have survived 5½ yr.

The presence of AFP has been demonstrated in the CSF and serum of patients with endodermal sinus tumor (8, 117, 144) and in the serum, but not CSF of a 17-yr-old boy. His tumor contained both endodermal sinus tumor and choriocarcinoma, and also secreted HCG (43).

PATHOLOGICAL FEATURES

At autopsy, the endodermal sinus tumor is described as a firm, gray, hemorrhagic, and necrotic mass. This tumor invades extensively locally and disseminates widely throughout the subarachnoid space. Extension into the subdural lumbar space after surgery (114) and peritoneal implants from shunt procedure have been recorded (123, 139). Massive hemorrhage into the tumor may take place [Burger and Vogel, Fig. 4.221 (21)].

The microscopic appearance is distinctive (Fig. 2.4), and characterized by a loose, reticular pattern with many small cystic cavities, communicating channels lined by flat cells or columnar, mucin-secreting epithelium, and a myxoid to fibrous cellular primitive stroma. Schiller-

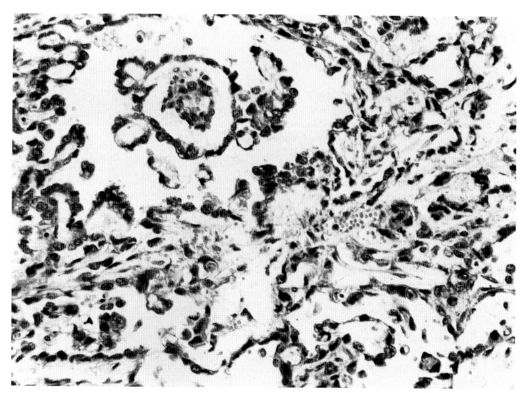

Figure 2.4. Endodermal sinus tumor, 5-yr-old boy. Delicate blood vessels and anastomosing channels lined by cuboidal cells. (H & E, × 290.)

Duval bodies may be seen, and consist of glomerular-like structures composed of delicate blood vessels covered by a single layer of cuboidal cells, projecting into a cavity lined by flattened epithelial cells. Lipid droplets may be present in the cellular cytoplasm. Eosinophilic, PAS-positive, and diastase-resistant hyaline globules can be found both within the cells and in the extracellular spaces. These globules have been demonstrated to contain AFP by the immunofluorescent (114) and by the peroxidase-antiperoxidase (PAP) immune complex method (43, 80, 117). Mucin stains may verify mucin production by some of the cells, and within the stroma (19). Admixtures of other types of germ cell tumor may be present. Teratomatous structures, such as foci of ducts lined by columnar epithelium, or dermoid or epidermoid cysts have also been identified.

In one instance, the ultrastructure of a pineal endodermal sinus tumor has been reported (117). The tumor nuclei were large, oval, or indented, with prominent nucleoli and delicate chromatin. The cells were cuboidal or irregularly shaped, with numerous microvilli, and rested on a basement membrane. Prominent rough endoplasmic reticulum, numerous mitochondria, and inconspicuous Golgi complexes and lysosomes were noted. Large amounts of electron-dense material were seen both within the dilated rough endoplasmic reticulum and in extracellular locations. Tight junctions and interlocking cytoplasmic protrusions were also present.

Choriocarcinoma

Choriocarcinoma, like the endodermal sinus tumor, is believed to represent extraembryonic differentiation of the primitive totipotential cells. As with all tumors of germ cell origin, choriocarcinoma is most likely to be found in combination with elements of other tumors in this group. Cases also exist where this neoplasm seems to have been present in apparently pure form [Fujii et al (37); Hutchinson et al (54); Nishiyama et al, Cases 4 and 13 (86); and Stowell et al (120)].

The number of reported cases of choriocarcinoma is somewhere in the region of the endodermal sinus tumor. The majority of affected patients are boys in the first or second decade. This is a highly malignant neoplasm, with a very poor prognosis. Sexual precocity has been reported in a number of instances (20, 54) in which a choriocarcinomatous component was present in the neoplasm.

In patients with histologically proven choriocarcinoma of the pineal region, elevated levels of gonadotropin have been reported in CSF, metastatic tumor tissue and urine (120); and urine and tumor at the primary site (20). Increased levels of HCG have also been documented in the CSF [Allen et al, Cases 3 and 4 (3)], serum [Allen et al, Case 3 (3), Fujii et al (37)], and in the CSF and serum of a patient whose neoplasm also contained components of endodermal sinus tumor and secreted AFP (43).

PATHOLOGICAL FEATURES

Characteristically, choriocarcinoma is described as granular, mottled reddish brown, and nearly always hemorrhagic and necrotic (37, 54, 120). It may appear circumscribed, but may invade the adjacent brain and has been known to infiltrate the tentorium, falx, and superior sagittal sinus (120). Hematogenous metastases have been documented to lungs [Goldzieher (41), Stowell et al (120), and Nishiyama et al, Case 13 (86)] and to liver (41), hilar nodes (86), both without (41) and after (86, 120) surgical procedures.

The microscopic features of a choriocarcinoma are those of a tumor composed of two cell types. The cytotrophoblastic cells are medium sized, uniform, with distinct cell borders and clear cytoplasm, and a vesicular nucleus. The syncytiotrophoblastic cells are large and multinucleated. The nuclei are irregular and hyperchromatic, and the cytoplasm is usually eosinophilic and contains vacuoles. A villous-like formation is suggested by the capping of cytotrophoblastic cells by the syncytiotrophoblast. The peroxidase immunoperoxidase (PAP) technique has been used to demonstrate AFP in the tumor cells (43) and was present in the syncytio- , but not cytotrophoblastic cells in one instance (37).

Teratomas—Typical and Teratoid

The capacity of the tumors of germ cell derivation to form tissues of great variety and combination, ranging from extraembryonal to immature and mature embryonal structures, has caused them to be designated in a broad sense as teratomas (42, 103, 108). In a sense, a tumor of germ cell origin, when composed of tissue of one histological type might be regarded as a teratoma exhibiting either undetermined or unilateral differentiation. In the following discussion, the term teratoma will be used to describe tumors in which elements derived of all three, or two germ layers, respectively, can be identified.

Among the pineal region tumors of germ cell origin, the teratomas are second to germinoma in frequency. These tumors occur almost exclusively in males, usually in the first two decades, with a peak incidence in the second decade. The pineal region is the most common intracranial site for teratomas. In a review of 93 intracranial teratomas reported up to 1940, 39 were found at the pineal, 15 at the pituitary, and 10 in the posterior fossa (121) region. The remainder were situated in a variety of locations. This is in marked contrast to intracranial teratomatous neoplasms of the newborn and infants, which have a female preponderance and generally do not originate from the pineal site (42, 124). Other reviews of the older literature concerning intracranial and pineal teratomas are contained in the papers by Hosoi (52) and Bochner and Scarff (13), and an extensive current discussion of this topic is presented by Gonzales-Cruzzi (42). Pineal teratomas in two brothers have been described (135), and separate pineal and fourth ventricular teratomas were reported in a 2-yr-old boy (4).

PATHOLOGICAL FEATURES

The tumor may involve the pineal gland or may be parapineal. Teratomas are usually circumscribed, may be round or lobulated, and will compress the surrounding structures (Fig. 2.5). The cut surface is characteristically a mixture of solid and cystic areas. The solid portions may range in color and consistency. The cysts of various sizes may contain watery, mucoid, or sebaceous material. Bone, cartilage, or hair may be identified, and presence of teeth has been reported (13, 73). In some instances, the majority of the mass may consist of a dermoid or epidermoid cyst. A rare complication is the apparent rupture of a pineal region tumor containing tooth-like structures, as diagnosed on the basis of clinical and radiological findings (73). The microscopic features are usually even more varied than the macroscopic appearance. Any combination of elements of all three, or two

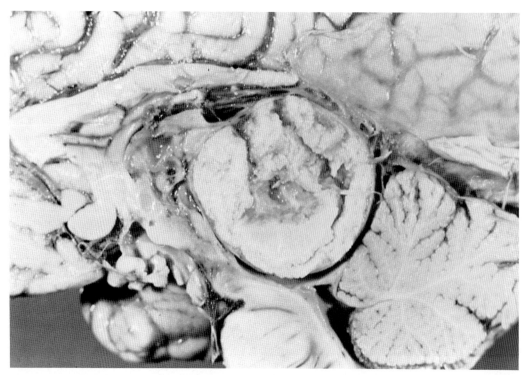

Figure 2.5. Mature teratoma, 13-yr-old boy. Much of the tumor is a circumscribed, encapsulated mass with a friable center. Additional neoplasm extends anteriorly into the third ventricle. There is pronounced compression of the midbrain. Used with permission from Wilkins RH, Rangachary SS (eds): *Neurosurgery.* (In press). New York, McGraw-Hill Book Company.

germ cell layers may be present, and may range from immature to mature in development (Figs. 2.6 and 2.7). Endodermal elements may consist of gastrointestinal and respiratory tissue and a variety of mucous-secreting glands. Mesodermal components, such as bone, cartilage, and muscle may be seen, along with undifferentiated mesenchyme and unidentifiable immature elements. Ectoderm is frequently represented by squamous epithelium and by neural tissues.

Tissues of neuroectodermal derivation are among the most common components of teratomas (42) and have also been described in the intracranial examples. The morphology of the neural tissues may range from the immature to well differentiated. Sheets of neuroblastic cells, neurons in various stages of maturation, primitive neuroepithelium-forming tubules (Fig. 2.6), islands of glial tissue, and choroid plexus may be recognized.

The presence of immature somatic tissue components in a teratoma does not in itself denote malignancy (42). It is presumed, that incom-

pletely differentiated tissues have the capacity to mature, yet that they are also potentially malignant. Willis (138) points out that the immature neuroepithelial tissues sometimes have the capacity to metastasize. Guidelines for predicting the future behavior of teratomas have been outlined by Gonzales-Cruzzi (42).

Malignant potential is imparted to pineal teratomas by the occasinal presence of foci of germ cell tumors such as choriocarcinoma (40) or germinoma (33, 135). Rhabdomyosarcoma has also been reported (40, 92) and in the older literature, reference has been made to pineal teratomas containing areas of "spindle cell sarcoma" (121). The diagnosis of Wilms tumor in a partially resected pineal neoplasm of an 8-yr-old boy (134) may well represent a component of a teratoma, as this tumor has been sometimes found in sacrococcygeal teratomas (42).

Intracranial dissemination of pineal teratomas has not been reported. Distal intracranial subarachnoid metastases, similar histologically to the primary tumor, were observed in a 10-yr-

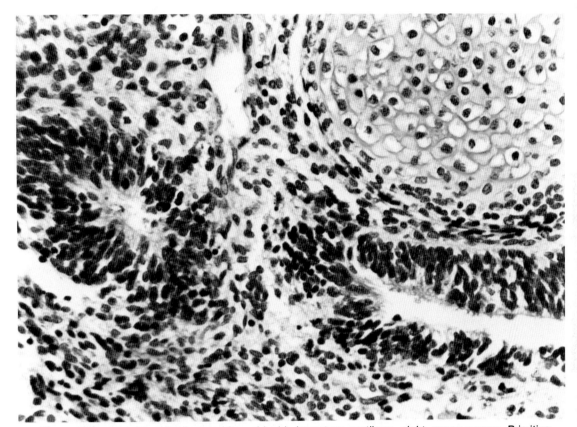

Figure 2.6. Immature teratoma, 11-yr-old girl. Immature cartilage, *right upper corner*. Primitive neuroepithelial tubules, *below and left*. (H & E, × 460.) Courtesy of Dr. R. W. R. Archibald, San Jose, CA.

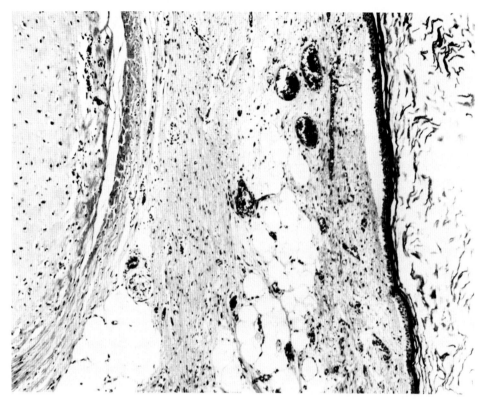

Figure 2.7.   Mature teratoma, 13-yr-old boy (same patient as Fig. 2.5). From left to right; cartilage, collagenous connective tissue and fat, keratinized squamous epithelium. (H & E, × 115.)

old girl with an immature teratoma of the optic chiasm (53). The coexistence of spinal subarachnoid cysts lined by keratinized epithelium and cuboidal cells, and massive congenital intracranial teratoma (50), poses a question of metastasis or multicentric origin.

TUMORS OF PINEAL PARENCHYMAL CELLS

Neoplasms arising from the pineal parenchyma are not as rare as has been thought in the past. McGovern estimated their incidence to be 20% of 236 pineal tumors reported in the literature prior to 1946 (75). In a review of histologically verified pineal region neoplasms, 8 (25.8%) of the 31 were derived from the pineal parenchyma (30), while in another series, 10 (29.4%) of 34 were of pineal cell origin (33).

The apparent ability of the neoplastic pineal parenchymal cell to produce tumors of great histological variety is explained by its intimate phylogenetic relationship to both photoreceptor cells and neurons. Several lines of evidence support the belief, that during evolution the neu-

rosensory photoreceptor function of fish and amphibians is gradually lost in reptiles and birds, and that the mammalian pineal gland has an exclusively neurosecretory function.

Rudimentary photoreceptor differentiation in the form of bulbous cell processes containing vesicles and cilia with a 9 + 0 microtubular configuration have been demonstrated in the pineal glands of fetal, but not adult, rat and hamster (24), and in the neonatal rat (145). Similar structures have been found in the pineals of lower vertebrates (25, 88). Bulbous cell processes, with 9 + 0 cilia have been observed in the fetal human pineocytes (77). Although present in cells of various embryonal origin as reviewed by Clabough (24), similar cilia are also a component of many neurons (93), thus forming a morphological link between photoreceptor cells, pineocytes, and neurons.

The adult mammalian (142) and lower vertebrate pineocytes (25, 88) are also related to the retina (35) through the common possession of synaptic ribbons (vesicle-coated lamellae), structures of unknown significance found in some cells of sensory type. Synaptic ribbons were not found in fetal human pineal glands (66, 77), but were believed to be present in the pineocytes of a 3-yr-old girl (65).

Increasing evidence is accumulating to support the suggestion made by Rubinstein (102) that the neoplastic pineal parenchymal cells are capable of divergent differentiation into tumors with astrocytic or ganglionic components. Rubinstein further remarked on the relationship of the pineal gland to the neurosecretory system, which is emphasized by the report of a unique pineal neoplasm with the histological features of a chemodectoma (133). The spectrum of differentiating capacity was broadened even more by subsequent recognition of pineal parenchymal tumors with retinoblastomatous elements. The latter finding is in agreement with the presumed phylogenetic derivation of the pineocytes from photoreceptor cells (47, 104, 105). Collaborative data about the multipotential nature of the neoplastic pineal cells has been gained from the study of human, as well as experimental pineal tumors. The finding in many of the human pineal parenchymal neoplasms, of cells of several histological types, and in at least two instances [Herrick and Rubinstein, Case 11 (47), Sobel et al, Case 2 (114)], the entire spectrum of pineoblast-like cells, ganglion cells, abortive photoreceptor elements, and astrocytes, strongly supports the concept of multidirectional differentiation. In agreement is also the demonstration by immunocytochemical methods of cells containing either the 68K neurofilamentous subunit or glial fibrillary acidic protein in a pineoblastoma (99). The former is considered to be a neuronal and the latter an astrocytic component. Photoreceptor-like differentiation has also been observed in one such hamster pineocytoma (133), while the pineal functional capacity has been verified in seven similar neoplasms by the demonstration of hy-droxyindole-O-methyltransferase (96). Not enough data are available yet regarding the possible usefulness of HIOMT assays in patients with pineal parenchymal neoplasms.

The following description of the pathology and biological behavior of pineal parenchymal tumors is based on a total of 40 pathologically verified cases [28 examined personally and 12 collected from the literature (47)]. The findings are similar to another series of cases reported by Borit (18), and consistent with additional case reports which have subsequently appeared in the literature (39, 63, 72, 81, 82, 114, 129).

The histological types of pineal parenchymal tumors and their biological behavior is outlined in Table 2.3. An accurate assessment of the morphology of these neoplasms is of more than academic interest. The clinical behavior which ranges from highly malignant to benign, and the expected response to various modalities of therapy may be predicted from the morphological appearance.

An effective method for demonstrating the neoplastic pineal parenchymal cell is the De-Girolami and Zvaigzne (31) modification of the Achúcarro-Hortega silver carbonate impregnation for pineal parenchymal cells applicable to paraffin-embedded tissue. This technique is highly reliable, but in a small control series, gave a positive reaction in three cerebral neuroblastomas while three medulloblastomas were negative.

Pineoblastoma

The pineoblastoma is the least differentiated of the pineal parenchymal neoplasms, and constituted 17 (43%) cases of the pineal parenchymal tumors.

The majority of pineoblastomas occur during the first two decades of life, with the highest incidence in the first 10 yr. There is no appreciable predilection to either sex. These neo-

Table 2.3
Histological Types of Pineal Parenchymal Tumors and Their Biological Behavior[a]

Malignant	Pineoblastoma
Malignant	Pineoblastoma with pineocytic differentiation
Malignant	Pineoblastoma with retinoblastomatous differentiation
Malignant	Pineocytoma
Malignant or benign	Pineocytoma with astrocytic differentiation
Benign	Pineocytoma with neuronal differentiation
Benign	Pineocytoma with neuronal and astrocytic differentiation

[a] From Herrick MK, Rubinstein LJ: *Brain.* 102:289–320, 1979, (47).

plasms are highly malignant, and no survivals beyond 2 yr were documented among the cases reviewed.

PATHOLOGICAL FEATURES

Usually the pineal gland is replaced by the tumor mass, although rarely the pineal may be only minimally enlarged or even of normal size, although always microscopically involved. When cut, the tumors are pink, white, or gray, smooth or granular, and occasionally contain cysts filled with gelatinous material. Foci of hemorrhage and necrosis are frequent. Although the growth might appear rather circumscribed, seeding throughout the cerebrospinal fluid pathways may take place very early, and was present in every instance. Hematogenous metastases to cranial bones, lungs and lymph nodes have been documented (10) in a 3-yr-old girl who had not received any treatment.

The pineoblastoma is a highly cellular neoplasm consisting of sheets of small, primitive cells, very similar in appearance to the medullo-blastoma (Fig. 2.8). The tumor cells have round to oval nuclei which contain coarse chromatin. The cytoplasm is scant and ill defined but at times, may be drawn into a single process oriented toward thin walled blood vessels. Homer Wright rosettes, consisting of a circular arrangement of tumor cells around a pink fibrillary center, are sometimes seen (Fig. 2.9). The number of mitotic figures is variable. Focal necrosis, hemorrhage, and punctate calcifications are not uncommon. With the silver impregnation for pineal parenchymal cells, a thin rim of black cytoplasm with a short, usually single process, can be demonstrated around a pale staining nucleus (Fig. 2.10). Not infrequently, better differentiated areas, indistinguishable from pineocytoma, may be present.

Ultrastructural studies of pineoblastomas are rare [Glasberg et al (39); Kline et al (62); Markesbery et al (72); Neuwelt et al, Cases 4 and 5 (83); Sobel et al, Case 1 (114)]. The predominant cells of pineoblastomas are poorly differentiated, with prominent nuclei and thin cytoplasmic rims containing few organelles. Rare dense core

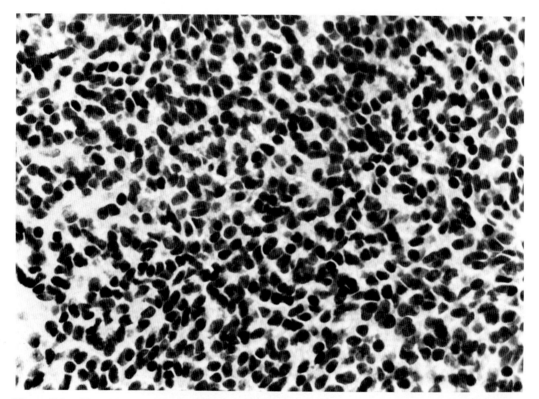

Figure 2.8. Pineoblastoma, 51-yr-old man. Highly cellular tumor composed of small, darkly staining uniform nuclei and poorly defined cytoplasm. (H & E, × 730.) Courtesy of Dr. M. R. Glasberg, Abbington, PA.

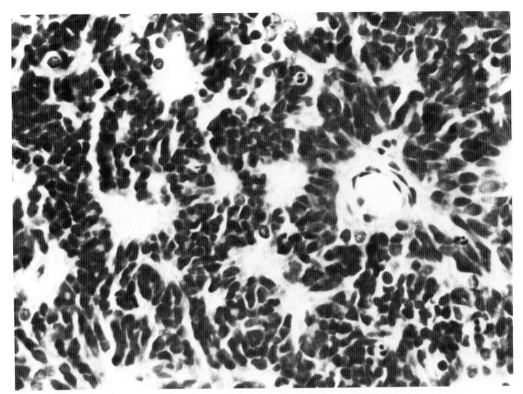

Figure 2.9. Pineoblastoma, 21-yr-old man. Highly cellular tumor with Homer Wright rosettes. Perivascular orientation of tumor cells, *right*. (H & E, × 730.) Courtesy of Dr. M. R. Glasberg, Abbington, PA.

and clear vesicles have been described in some cell processes (39, 72, 83), and cilia (83) with 9 + 0 microtubular configuration have also been seen (62, 72).

The remarkable similarity, both by light microscopy and ultrastructurally, between the cells of fetal cerebellum and cerebrum, the pineoblastoma, medulloblastoma, primitive cerebral neuroectodermal tumor, and cerebral neuroblastoma, has been reviewed by Markesbery and associates (72). These findings suggest a common primitive neuroectodermal origin. The report of a pineoblastoma in one, and a medulloblastoma in another member of a pair of infant monozygotic twins (136) further serves to emphasize this relationship.

Pineoblastoma with Retinoblastoma Differentiation

Retinoblastomatous differentiation in a pineoblastoma has been observed on at least six occasions. Five of the children were boys, aged 1¾ [Sobel et al, Case 2 (114)]; 2½ (118); 2¾

(Herrick and Rubinstein, Case 11 (47)]; 3 (63); and 1½ (personally examined) yr. The sixth was a 3-yr-old girl (63). In two (10, 63), the retinoblastomatous features were not recognized as such. In all instances, the tumor had disseminated widely throughout the subarachnoid pathways. Only in one were retinoblastomatous structures seen in the metastatic components of the tumor (118). Retinoblastomatous differentiation has also been documented in a 57-yr-old man who survived 6 months with an unusual pineocytoma which had a papillary pattern and had remained localized at the pineal site (129).

Of additional interest are reports of children with bilateral retinoblastomas in early infancy, who concomitantly, or later, develop primary pineal neoplasms (9, 55, 59), so-called trilateral retinoblastomas (9). In an analysis of 11 such patients (9), a positive family history was often elicited. The retinoblastomas presented at a mean age of 6 months, and the pineal neoplasm at 4 yr of age. In five instances, the tumor was examined histologically. In three instances, the pattern was that of a small-celled, undifferen-

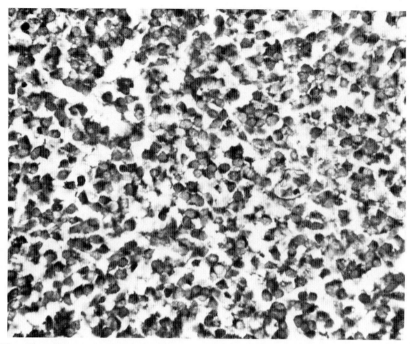

Figure 2.10.   Pineoblastoma, 4-yr- and 7-month-old boy [Case 7 of Herrick and Rubinstein (47)]. Tumor cells with pale nuclei and a thin, black rim of cytoplasm, sometimes extended into a single process. (Silver carbonate impregnation for pineal parenchyma (31), × 500.) Photograph courtesy of Dr. L. J. Rubinstein, University of Virginia School of Medicine, Charlottesville, VA.

tiated neoplasm, similar to pineoblastoma. One tumor resembled retinoblastoma, and one was said to show a tendency to formation of rosettes. In addition, reports also exist of three trilateral retinoblastomas with the intracranial tumor located in the supra- or parasellar region (9, 55).

PATHOLOGICAL FEATURES

The gross appearance of the tumors is similar to pineoblastomas. Microscopic examination discloses features characteristic of neuroepithelial variants of retinoblastoma, consisting of fleurettes and Flexner-Wintersteiner rosettes. The fleurettes consist of a semicircular arrangement of columnar cells with basal nuclei and horizontal apical membranes through which project club-shaped processes (Figs. 2.11 and 2.12). The Flexner-Wintersteiner rosettes are tubular arrangements of columnar cells with apical limiting membranes (Fig. 2.12). The fleurettes are believed to represent attempts by neoplastic cells to form photoreceptors (130–132). The Flexner-Wintersteiner rosettes are thought to indicate a less advanced stage of retinal differentiation than the fleurettes. The existence of this rare subgroup of pineoblastomas serves

to emphasize the evolutional relationship between the photoreceptor function of the pineal of fishes and amphibians and the neurosecretory activity of the mammalian pineal gland.

Ultrastructural studies of pineoblastomas with fleurettes and Flexner-Wintersteiner rosettes are lacking. In the pineoblastoma studied by Kline and associates (62), however, rosette-forming cells with bulb-shaped cytoplasmic protrusions and cilia with 9 + 0 microtubular structure were felt to suggest an attempt at photoreceptor differentiation. Ultrastructural evidence of rudimentary photoreceptor-like differentiation was also found in an experimental hamster pineocytoma induced by human papovavirus (JC virus) (133).

Neuronal and astrocytic differentiation has also been found in two of the pineoblastomas with retinoblastomatous differentiation [Herrick and Rubinstein, Case 11 (47); Sobel et al, Case 2 (114)].

OTHER VARIANTS OF PINEOBLASTOMA

Two other very rare variants of pineoblastoma have been described. In one, a lobular arrangement of larger, more mature cells is surrounded

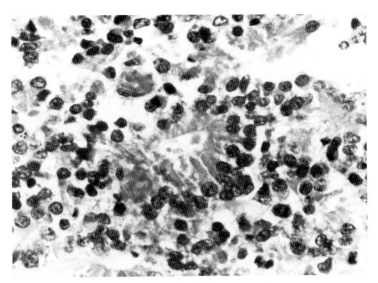

Figure 2.11. Pineoblastoma with retinoblastomatous differentiation, 2-yr- and 9-month-old boy [Case 11 of Herrick and Rubinstein (47)]. Fleurette, *center*. (H & E, × 400.) Photo courtesy of Dr. L. J. Rubinstein, University of Virginia School of Medicine, Charlottesville, VA.

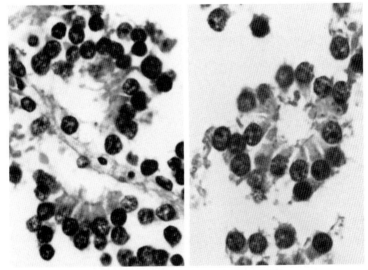

Figure 2.12. Pineoblastoma with retinoblastomatous differentiation, same case as Figure 2.11. Fleurettes, *left*; Flexner-Wintersteiner rosette, *right*. (H & E, × 730.)

by smaller, less mature cells, resembling the mosaic pattern of the fetal pineal gland [Herrick and Rubinstein, Case 4 (47); Russell, Case 5 (107)]. Although a superficial similarity exists, these tumors are distinct from germinoma.

In two instances, cells containing melanin pigment have been noted in pineoblastomas [Best (11); Herrick and Rubinstein, Case 5 (47)]. Melanin granules have been described in cells of human fetal pineal glands (34, 77) and

in a variety of neuroepithelial tumors (108). Melanin-containing cells also have been identified in the stroma of the adult human pineal glands (95).

Pineocytoma

A considerable amount of overlap of both clinical and pathological features exists between the pineoblastoma and the pineocytoma. Among the tumors in our combined series, 10 (25%) were classified as pineocytomas. The peak incidence of pineocytomas was later than that of pineoblastomas and occurred in the third decade, and the age of affected individuals was more varied, ranging from 5–69 yr. Again, both sexes were about equally affected. The only patient who survived beyond 2 yr after the onset of symptoms had a neoplasm in which astrocytic differentiation had taken place.

PATHOLOGICAL FEATURES

The gross appearance of the pineocytoma is similar to the pineoblastoma, except there may be a tendency for the tumor to appear more circumscribed (Fig. 2.13). In four of the nine patients available for follow-up, the tumor disseminated widely along the cerebrospinal fluid pathways. Recurrent subarachnoid hemorrhage in one patient with pineocytoma and another with a pineal tumor with less well defined histology has been described (119).

Microscopically, very frequently, areas of pi-neoblastomatous charges are present in pineocytomas and transitional features between the two histological types are common. The lobulated appearance of the normal pineal gland is mimicked by the tendency of the tumor cells in a pineocytoma to be divided into islands by delicate connective tissue septae and thin-walled blood vessels (Fig. 2.14). The pineocytoma is less cellular than the pineoblastoma, and the cell nuclei are slightly larger. The cytoplasm of the cells, while still wispy and delicate, is more abundant. Arrangement of cells around blood vessels with cell processes directed toward vessel walls may be seen, along with occasional Homer Wright rosettes. As in the pineoblastoma, the number of mitotic figures may be variable, and necrosis, and hemorrhage are common. With the silver impregnation technique for pineal parenchyma, the cells of the pineocytomas have a pale nucleus and argyrophilic cytoplasm, often elongated into a prominent single process (Fig. 2.15).

One pineocytoma with papillary features has been described (129). This locally invasive tumor occurred in a 57-yr-old man who died 6

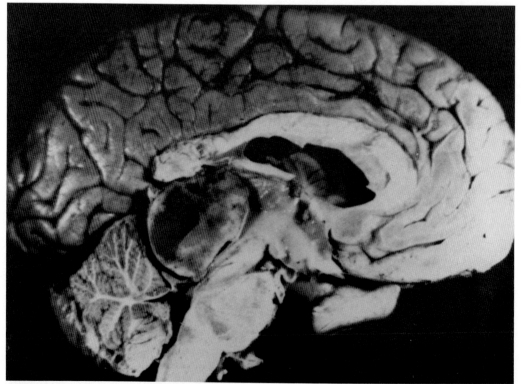

Figure 2.13.   Pineocytoma, 69-yr-old woman [Case 18 of Herrick and Rubinstein (47)]. Circumscribed tumor with cystic, gelatinous degeneration, compressing midbrain and bulging into third ventricle. Used with permission of *Brain* 102:289–320, 1979; and Oxford University Press, Oxford.

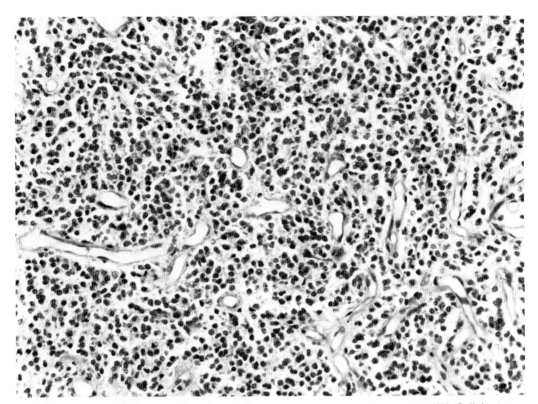

Figure 2.14. Pineocytoma, 62-yr-old man [Case 20 of Herrick and Rubinstein (47)]. Cellular tumor with tendency to lobular arrangement. In other areas, this neoplasm had an astrocytic component. (H & E, × 290.)

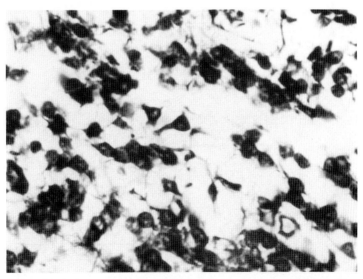

Figure 2.15. Pineocytoma, same patient as Figure 2.13. Tumor cells with argyrophilic, scant cytoplasm, extended sometimes into a single process (*center*). (Silver carbonate impregnation for pineal parenchyma (31), × 730.)

months after onset of symptoms, in spite of radiation therapy. In addition to the papillary component of the neoplasm, fleurettes and Flexner-Wintersteiner rosettes, indicative of differentiation towards the neuroepitheliomatous variant of retinoblastoma, also were present.

Ultrastructural studies of pineocytoma are confined to one tumor with transitional features between pineoblastoma and pineocytoma (72). In addition to the poorly differentiated cells seen in the pineoblastoma, larger, more pleomorphic cells were present. The cytoplasm of these larger cells had a well developed Golgi apparatus, many dense core vesicles, and cilia with a 9 + 0 microtubular pattern. Cell processes containing microtubules and clear and dense core vesicles were also seen. The findings were believed to suggest a potential for ganglion cell differentiation. In this tumor, both light and ultrastructural evidence of astrocytic differentiation also was present.

Pineocytoma with Astrocytic Differentiation

Two of the 10 pineocytomas contained an astrocytic component. Both patients were male, one was 62, the other 48 yr of age. The astrocytic part of the neoplasm was benign in the first man who survived 8 yr. The glial cells in the tumor of the second patient were malignant, and participated in the widespread dissemination along the neuraxis, resulting in death 1½ yr after the onset of symptoms. Astrocytic differentiation has also been described in a pineocytoma with neuronal differentiation (15), and was noted both by light and electron microscopy in the patient with pineoblastoma with transitional pineocytomatous features studied by Markesbery and associates [Case 2 (72)]. A focus of pilocytic astrocytoma in a pineoblastoma of a 38-yr-old woman also was described by Neuwelt et al [Case 5 (83)]. It appears then, that astrocytic differentiation is not limited to the pineocytoma but can be found even in the less differentiated pineoblastoma. Since astrocytes are part of the normal structure of the pineal gland, their presence in pineal parenchymal neoplasms can be interpreted either as entrapment or simultaneous neoplasia of a second cell line. More likely, the astrocytic tumor component reflects the ability of the neoplastic cells to differentiate in several directions. In support of the latter hypothesis, is the recent demonstration by immunocytochemical methods, of cells containing either neurofilamentous 68K subunits or glial fibrillary acidic protein (99) in a pineoblastoma.

By light microscopy, the astrocytes are identifiable by their larger, paler nuclei and either fibrillary or plump, eosinophilic cytoplasm. Rosenthal fiber formation may take place. Conventional techniques, such as a phosphotungstic acid hemotoxylin stain (PTAH), or an immunoperoxidase stain for glial fibrillary acidic protein (GFA) (Fig. 2.16) will verify the astrocytic

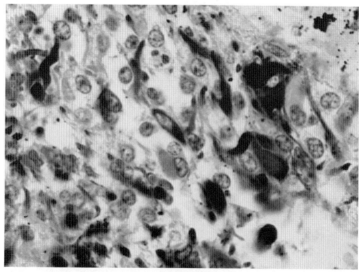

Figure 2.16. Pineocytoma with astrocytic differentiation, same case as Figure 2.14. Astrocytes with darkly stained cytoplasm. (Immunoperoxidase stain for GFA, counterstained with hematoxylin, × 730.)

nature of the cells, which are usually scattered among the neoplastic pineal parenchymal cells. In only one instance, have the astrocytes exhibited the malignant features of nuclear hyperchromasia, pleomorphism, and mitotic activity [Herrick and Rubinstein, Case 19 (47)].

Pineocytoma with Neuronal or Neuronal and Astrocytic Differentiation

Thirteen (32%) of the patients had pineocytoma composed entirely of mature neuronal elements, with or without an astrocytic component. These tumors tend to occur in adults of any age. Because they are slowly growing and do not disseminate, long survivals, up to 8 yr [McGovern, Case 3 (75)] have been documented among this group of patients. Since these tumors are composed of mature cells, they are not expected to be radiosensitive.

PATHOLOGICAL FEATURES

Although direct invasion of surrounding structures may take place, these tumors do not undergo distant dissemination. At least one in-

stance of massive hemorrhage into the neoplasm has been reported (22) (Fig. 2.17).

Microscopically, two distinct morphological patterns may be seen, and at times may be intimately intermingled in the same neoplasm. Tumor cells with small, dark, rather monotonously uniform nuclei may form bands and trabeculae, and become arranged into giant rosettes around pink fibrillary acellular centers (Fig. 2.18). These rosettes are much larger than the usual neuroblastic Homer Wright rosettes, and are believed to represent a manifestation of mature, small neuronal elements. Such an interpretation is supported by the demonstration of argyrophilic, often club-shaped fibrillary processes within the central portions of the rosettes. In further support of this belief is the not infrequent finding of large, often atypical ganglion cells among the small, uniform ones (Fig. 2.19). The mixture of apparently transitional cell forms, and a change from a rather monotonous to a rather pleomorphic pattern of ganglion cells intermingled with astrocytes results in a typical appearance of ganglioglioma (106).

Another view was taken by Borit et al (16) who suggested the name pineocytoma for the

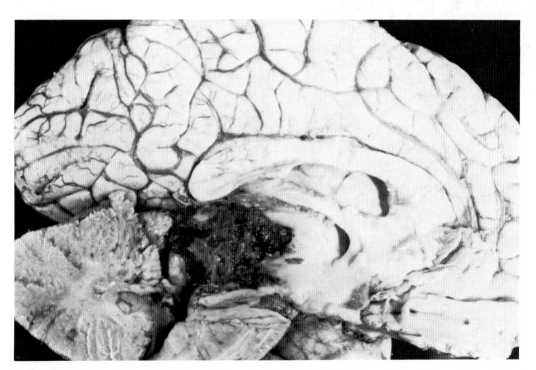

Figure 2.17.   Pineocytoma with neuronal and astrocytic differentiation, 55-yr-old man [Case 20 of Herrick and Rubinstein (47), Burres and Hamilton (22)]. Pineal apoplexy. Courtesy of Dr. Lysia S. Forno, Stanford University Medical Center, Stanford, CA.

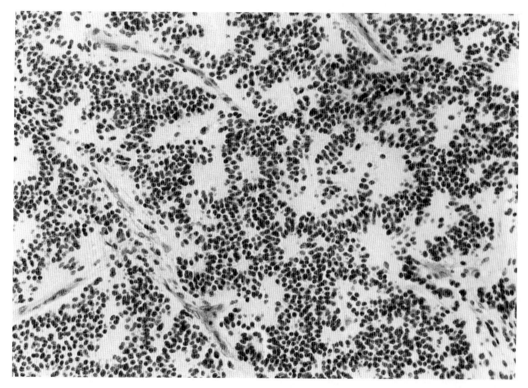

Figure 2.18.   Pineocytoma with neuronal differentiation, 58-yr-old man. Cells with darkly staining, small nuclei, arranged around fibrillary acellular areas, sometimes forming giant rosettes. (H & E, × 290.) Courtesy of Dr. M. R. Glasberg, Abbington, PA.

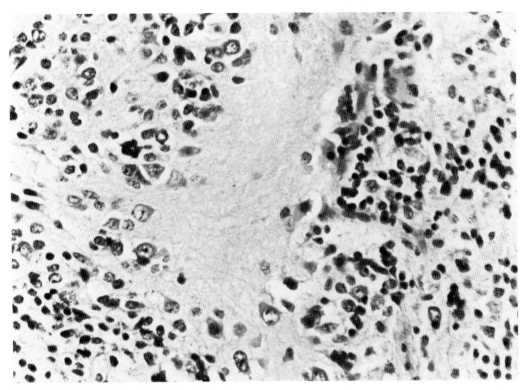

Figure 2.19. Pineocytoma with neuronal differentiation, 1-yr- and 7-month-old girl. Large, mature ganglion cells among cells with small dark nuclei and acellular fibrillary areas. (H & E, × 730.) Courtesy of Dr. M. R. Glasberg, Abbington, PA.

tumors with giant rosettes and relatively benign behavior. In their material, the distinction was not apparent between the malignant tumors of pineal parenchyma growing in sheets and a lobular pattern, leading Borit et al (16) to include as pineoblastoma, both the malignant pineal tumors designated as pineoblastoma and pineocytoma in the present classification.

The ultrastructural features of pineocytomas with neuronal and astrocytic differentiation have been studied in four instances. Synaptic complexes, clear and dense core vesicles, and numerous closely packed neuritic processes filled with microtubules confirmed the ganglionic nature of many of the tumor cells [Herrick and Rubinstein, Case 27 (47)] (Fig. 2.20). In another tumor (85), processes containing microtubules, filaments, and rare dense core vesicles, as well as cell processes similar to fibrous astrocytes suggested differentiation along the lines of pineocytes or neurons and astrocytes. Neuronal like appearance of tumor cells with densely packed processes rich in microtubules were also noted in a brief description of a pineocytoma

with giant rosettes [Neuwelt et al, Case 7 (83)], also reported in abstract form by Glasberg et al (39). Neuronal and astrocytic features were also present in the case of Nakazato et al (81).

TUMORS OF GLIAL AND OTHER CELL ORIGIN

Occasional pineal neoplasms of assorted histological type have been documented. Most of these belong to the spectrum of glial tumors, such as astrocytoma, astroblastoma, glioblastoma, oligodendroglioma, ependymoma, and even choroid plexus papilloma. These tumors presumably arise from structures in the vicinity of the pineal gland, although some of the astrocytic neoplasms may actually have their origin from the astrocytes normally present in the pineal itself.

Among the 31 histologically verified pineal region tumors reported by DeGirolami and Schmidek (29), 4 were astrocytomas, 3 glioblastomas, 2 ependymomas, and 1 an oligodendroglioma, while in another series of approximately similar size (33), no gliomas were found. Among

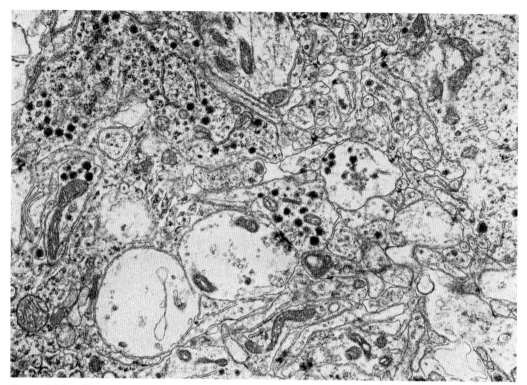

Figure 2.20.   Pineocytoma with neuronal differentiation, 51-yr-old woman [Case 27 of Herrick and Rubinstein (47)]. Tumor cell processes demonstrating numerous dense core vesicles and one synapse, *center*; × 14,500). Courtesy of Dr. Mary Herman, University of Virginia School of Medicine, Charlottesville, VA.

the 65 pineal neoplasms documented by Ringertz et al (97), 6 were astrocytomas and polar spongioblastomas, 1 was a glioblastoma, and 6 were ependymomas and choroid plexus papillomas. A small asymptomatic pineal astrocytoma (90) and a glioblastoma with leptomeningeal metastases (87) have been reported recently. A picture of a pineal glioblastoma is depicted by Burger and Vogel (21).

Meningiomas of the pineal region may arise from the falx and tentorium near their junction. Tumors unattached to dura are thought to originate from the velum interpositum located at the roof of the third ventricle, or from the connective tissue of the pineal gland. In addition to one case of their own, Roda et al (98) were able to collect 10 previously documented cases of pineal region meningiomas without dural attachment. The series included three children aged 3, 8, and 14 yr, and the average age of the patients was 28, which is lower than that re-

ported for meningiomas on the whole. All histological subtypes of meningioma have been described, including fibroblastic, psammomatous, transitional, endotheliomatous, and angioblastic (hemangiopericytomatous) patterns (100).

Other rare tumors reported in the pineal area include a chemodectoma (113) and craniopharyngioma (115).

Infrequent reports of metastases to the pineal gland from systemic malignancies exist in the literature. In many instances, more than one intracranial tumor deposit was present. In a series of 130 autopsied patients (89) with disseminated neoplastic disease, the pineal gland was involved in five. The growth was solitary in three of these patients, while additional cerebral foci were present in two. Three patients were men with bronchogenic carcinoma, and two were women with breast cancer (89). Among 99 patients with malignant systemic neoplasms, only one pineal contained a metastasis from bronchogenic carcinoma (68). A pineal metastasis from small cell bronchogenic carcinoma is illustrated in Figure 2.21.

NON-NEOPLASTIC CYSTS AND MASSES

Small, single, or multiple cysts filled with watery or proteinaceous material are not infrequently seen in the pineal gland at autopsy. Some of the mechanisms proposed to explain the pathogenesis of these cysts are that they result from degenerative changes in a glial plaque (Fig. 2.1), or in the pineal parenchyma, or are formed by sequestration of the pineal diverticulum from the pineal recess. In the latter case, the cyst may be lined at least partially by ependyma. Usually, the pineal is not enlarged by the cysts, but occasionally slight enlargement may result (Fig. 2.22).

A symptomatic pineal cyst is extremely rare, and in the reported cases, often a relationship between its presence and the patient's clinical course is not clear. A historical review of this topic and six patients were reported by Carr (23), and Ringertz and associates (97) mentioned two bean-sized cysts in their series of pineal tumors. A large pineal cyst, which acted as a mass lesion, was removed from a 21-yr-old woman, who died after surgery (112). Megyeri (76), who searched for cysts in pineal glands, estimated that 34 previously reported cases existed in the literature previous to 1960. Among 41 of 104 individuals he examined, in only four patients was there actually some enlargement of the gland, and only one of these was considered to be responsible for slight hydrocephalus from aqueductal compression. An asymptomatic pineal cyst, demonstrated by computed tomographic scan in a woman with polycystic kidney disease, represents probably a fortuitous coincidence (1). The nature of this lesion was never determined histologically. Multicystic change, but only slight pineal gland enlargement, was reported in 31 of a series of 275 patients with cancer (44). These were mostly children and adolescents, and the majority had acute granulocytic or lymphocytic leukemia. Hemorrhage into a well-verified (5), and probable (48) pineal cyst, has been documented.

As an independent finding, dermoid or epidermoid cysts in the pineal region are extremely rare (108), and more often represent components of a teratoma. This possibility must be

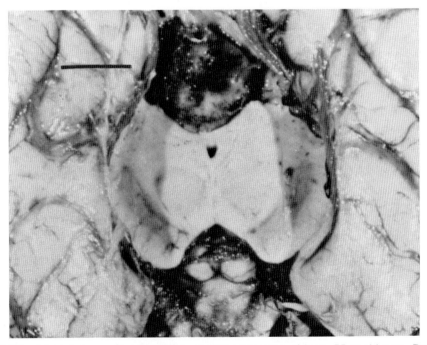

Figure 2.21. Metastatic small cell undifferentiated carcinoma of lung, 55-yr-old man. Patient had other cerebral metastases. *Bar* equals 1 cm.

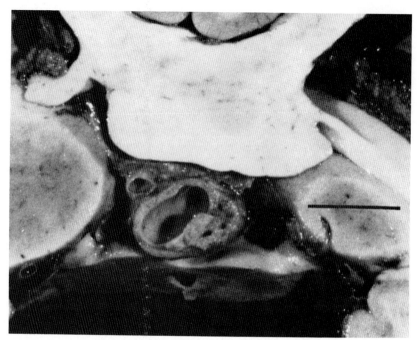

Figure 2.22. Cystic pineal, 35-yr-old man, incidental finding. For orientation, the corpus calloseum is above the pineal and the cerebral aqueduct can be seen below it. *Bar* equals 1 cm.

kept in mind when a diagnosis is made on the basis of surgical removal of only portions of the cyst wall (74, 110).

Among additional rare pineal region space occupying lesions mentioned in the literature are arachnoid cyst (92) and cysticercus of the quadrigeminal cistern (83). The glial-vascular mass in a 4-week-old infant, called a hemangioma, had the histological appearance of a malformation of small blood vessels of capillary and cavernous type [Demakas et al, Case 1 (32), Sonntag et al (116)]. A unique case of a 14-yr-old boy who was well 2 yr after the removal of a solitary "plum-sized" sarcoid granuloma (111) has also been described.

HEMORRHAGE AS A COMPLICATION OF PINEAL REGION NEOPLASM

Intracranial hemorrhage is a rare, but well documented complication of tumors of the pineal region. The bleeding may manifest itself as pineal apoplexy, subarachnoid hemorrhage, or a combination of both, and has occurred into neoplasms of a variety of histological types as well as into non-neoplastic masses.

Massive hemorrhage into choriocarcinomas (37, 120) and endodermal sinus tumor [Burger

and Vogel, Fig. 4.221, (21)] has been described. Tumors of pineal parenchyma are usually vascular, and may also invite apoplexy. Catastrophic bleeding occurred into a pineocytoma with neuronal and astrocytic differentiation (22) and into a pineocytoma with an astrocytic component [Herrick and Rubinstein, Case 20 (47)]. Pineal cysts are also not exempt (5, 48). One of these patients had been on anticoagulant therapy (5).

Insidious, sometimes repeated subarachnoid hemorrhage, was associated with a germinoma [Lewis and associates, Case 3 (68)] and two cases of pineocytoma (119). One of these was a tumor with neuronal differentiation while the other one was histologically not well defined. More acute symptoms from subarachnoid hemorrhage were experienced by a patient with an angioblastic meningioma (100).

References

1. Abreo K, Steele TH: Pineal cyst associated with polycystic kidney disease: case report. *Am J Kidney Dis* 1:106–109, 1981.
2. Albrechtsen E, Klee JG, Møller JE: Primary intracranial germ cell tumours, including five cases of endodermal sinus tumour. *Acta Pathol Microbiol Scand*, 233[Suppl 80]:3238, 1972.
3. Allen JC, Nisselbaum J, Epstein F, Rosen G, Schwartz MK: Alpha-fetoprotein and human

chorionic gonadotropin determination in cerebrospinal fluid. *J Neurosurg* 51:368–374, 1979.

4. Aoyama I, Makita Y, Nabeshima S, Motomichi M: Intracranial double teratomas. *Surg Neurol* 17:383–387, 1982.

5. Apuzzo MLJ, Davey LM, Manuelidis EE: Pineal apoplexy associated with anticoagulant therapy. *J Neurosurg* 45:223–226, 1976.

6. Araki C, Matsumoto S: Statistical reevaluation of pinealoma and related tumors in Japan. *J Neurosurg* 30:146–149, 1969.

7. Arita N, Bitoh S, Ushio Y, Hayakawa T, Hasegawa H, Fujiwara M, Ozaki K, Par-khen L, Mori T: Primary pineal endodermal sinus tumor with elevated serum and CSF alphafetoprotein levels. *J Neurosurg* 53:244–248, 1980.

8. Arita N, Ushio Y, Abekura M, Koshino K, Hayakawa T: Embryonal carcinoma with teratomatous elements in the region of the pineal gland. *Surg Neurol* 9:198–203, 1978.

9. Bader JL, Meadows AT, Zimmerman LE, Rorke LB, Voute PA, Champion LAA, Miller RW: Bilateral retinoblastoma with ectopic intracranial retinoblastoma: trilateral retinoblastoma. *Cancer Genet Gytogenet* 5:302–313, 1982.

10. Banerjee AK, Kak VJ: Pineoblastoma with spontaneous intra and extra-cranial metastasis. *J Pathol* 114:9–12, 1973.

11. Best PV: A medulloblastoma-like tumour with melanin formation. *J Pathol* 110:109–111, 1973.

12. Bestle J: Extragonadal endodermal sinus tumor originating in the region of the pineal gland. *Acta Pathol Microbiol Scand* 74:214–222, 1968.

13. Bochner SJ, Scarff JE: Teratoma of the pineal body. Classification of embryonal tumors of the pineal body: Report of a case of teratoma of the pineal body presenting formed teeth. *Arch Surg* 36:303–309, 1979.

14. Borden IV S, Weber AL, Toch R, Wang CC: Pineal germinoma. *Am J Dis Child* 126:214–216, 1973.

15. Borit A: History of tumors of the pineal region. *Am J Surg Pathol* 5:613–619, 1981.

16. Borit A, Blackwood W, Mair WGP: The separation of pineocytoma from pineoblastoma. *Cancer* 45:1408–1418, 1980.

17. Borit A, Blackwood W: Pineocytoma with astrocytomatous differentiation. *J Neuropathol Exp Neurol* 38:253–248, 1979.

18. Borit A: Embryonal carcinoma of the pineal region. *J Pathol* 97:165–168, 1969.

19. Brown NJ: Yolk-sac tumor ('orchioblastoma') and other testicular tumors of childhood. In Hugh RCB (ed): *Pathology of the Testis*. Oxford, Blackwell Scientific Publications, 1976, pp 364–365.

20. Bruton OC, Martz DC, Gerard ES: Precocious puberty due to secreting chorionepithelioma (teratoma) of the brain. *J Pediatr* 59:719–725, 1961.

21. Burger PC, Vogel SF: Neoplasms in the pineal region. In *Surgical Pathology of the Nervous System and its Coverings*, ed 1. New York, John Wiley, 1976, pp 398–407.

22. Burres KP, Hamilton RD: Pineal Apoplexy. *Neurosurg* 4:264–268, 1979.

23. Carr JL: Cystic hydrops of the pineal gland. *J Nerv Dis* 99:552–572, 1944.

24. Clabough JW: Cytological aspects of pineal development in rats and hamsters. *Am J Anat* 137:215–230, 1973.

25. Collin JP: Differentiation and regression of the cells of the sensory line in the epiphysis cerebri. In Wolstenholme GEW, Knight J (eds): *The Pineal Gland*. Edinburgh-London, Churchill Livingstone, 1971, pp 127–146.

26. Cravioto H, Dart D: The ultrastructure of "pinealoma". *J Neuropathol Exp Neurol* 32:552–565, 1973.

27. Davis RL: Personal communication in Smith RA III, Eastridge MN. Pineal tumors. In Vinken PJ, Bruyn GW (eds): *Handbook of Clinical Neurology*, Amsterdam, North-Holland Publishing Co., 1974, vol 17, pp 648–665.

28. Dayan AD, Marshall AHE, Miller AA, Pick FJ, Rankin NE: Atypical teratomas of the pineal and hypothalamus. *J Pathol Bacteriol* 92:1–28, 1966.

29. DeGirolami U, Schmidek H: Clinicopathological study of 53 tumors of the pineal region. *J Neurosurg* 39:455–462, 1973.

30. DeGirolami U: Pathology of tumors of the pineal region. In Schmidek HH (ed): *Pineal Tumors*. New York, Masson Publishing USA, 1977, pp 1–19.

31. DeGirolami U, Zvaigzne O: Modification of the Achúcarro-Hortega pineal stain for paraffin-embedded formalin-fixed tissue. *Stain Technol* 48:48–50, 1973.

32. Demakis JJ, Sonntag VKH, Kaplan AM, Kelley JJ, Waggener JD: Surgical management of pineal area tumors in early childhood. *Surg Neurol* 17:435–440, 1981.

33. Donat JF, Okazaki H, Gomez MR, Reagan TJ, Baker HL, Laws ER: Pineal tumors. *Arch Neurol* 35:736–740, 1978.

34. Dooling EC, Chi Je G, Gilles FH: Melanotic neuroectodermal tumor of infancy. Its histological similarities to fetal pineal gland. *Cancer* 39:1535–1541.

35. Fine BS, Yanoff M: Ocular Histology. *A Text and Atlas*, ed 2. Hagerstown, Harper & Row, 1979, p 74.

36. Friedman NB: Cerminoma of the pineal. Its identity with germinoma ("seminoma") of the testis. *Cancer Res* 7:363–368, 1947.

37. Fujii T, Itakura T, Hayashi S, Komai N, Nakamine H, Saito K: Primary pineal choriocarcinoma with hemorrhage monitored by computerized tomography. Case report. *J Neurosurg* 55:484–487, 1981.

38. Gindhart TD, Tsukahara YC: Cytologic diagnosis of cerebrospinal fluid and sputum. *Acta Cytol* 23:341–346, 1979.

39. Glasberg MR, Kirkpatrick JB, Neuwelt EA: Pineal parenchymal cell tumors. A light microscopic and ultrastructural study. *J Neuropathol Exp Neurol* 38:314, 1979.

40. Glass RL, Culbertson CG: Teratoma of the pineal gland with choriocarcinoma and rhabdomyosarcoma. *Arch Pathol* 41:552–555, 1946.

41. Goldzieher M: Über eine Zirbeldrüsengeschwulst. *Virchows Arch [Pathol Anat]* 213:353–365, 1913.

42. Gonzales-Cruzzi F: Extragonadal Teratomas. *Atlas of Tumor Pathology*, 2nd series, Fascicle 18. Washington DC, Armed Forces Institute of Pathology, 1982.

43. Haase J, Neilsen K: Value of tumor markers in the treatment of endodermal sinus tumors and choriocarcinomas in the pineal region. *Neurosurgery* 5:485–488, 1979.

44. Hajdu SI, Porro RS, Lieberman PH, Foote FW, Jr: Degeneration of the pineal gland of patients with cancer. *Cancer* 29:706–709, 1972.

45. Hassoun J, Gambarelli D, Choux M, Toga M: Macrophagic activity in intracerebral germinoma: Ultrastructural study of a case. *Hum Pathol* 2:207–210, 1980.

46. Haymaker W, Liss L, Vogel FS, Johnson Jr JE, Adams RD, Scharenberg K: The pineal gland. In Haymaker W, Adams RD (eds): *Histology and Histopathology of the Nervous System*. Springfield, Charles C Thomas, 1982, vol II, pp 1801–2023.

47. Herrick MK, Rubinstein LJ: The cytological differentiating potential of pineal parenchymal neoplasms (true pinealomas). *Brain* 102:289–320, 1979.

48. Higashi K, Katayama S, Orita T: Pineal apoplexy. *J Neurol Neurosurg Psychiatry* 42:1050–1053, 1979.

49. Hirano A, Llena JF, Chung HD: Some new observations on intracranial germinoma. *Acta Neuropathol* 32:103–113, 1975.

50. Hirsch LF, Rorke LB, Schmidek HH: Unusual cause of relapsing hydrocephalus. Congenital intracranial teratoma. *Arch Neurol* 34:505–507, 1977.

51. Ho K-L, Rassekh ZS: Endodermal sinus tumor of the pineal region. Case report and review of the literature. *Cancer* 44:1081–1086, 1979.

52. Hosoi K: Teratoma and teratoid tumors of the brain. *Arch Pathol* 9:1207–1219, 1930.

53. Hübner G: Intracerebral metastatic malignant teratoma in the region of the optic chiasm. *Beitr Pathol* 157:189–199, 1976.

54. Hutchinson JSM, Brooks RV, Barratt TM, Newman CGH, Prunty FTG: Sexual precocity due to an intracranial tumour causing unusual testicular secretion of testosterone. *Arch Dis Child* 44:732–737, 1969.

55. Jakobiec FA, Tso MO, Zimmerman LE, Danis P: Retinoblastoma and intracranial malignancy. *Cancer* 39:2048–2058, 1977.

56. James W, Dudley HR: Teratoma in the region of the pineal body. Report of a case. *J Neurosurg* 14:235–241, 1957.

57. Javadpour N: The role of multiple tumor markers in the diagnosis and management of seminoma. In Anderson CK, Jones WG, Ward AM (eds): *Germ Cell Tumors*. New York, Alan R Liss Inc., 1981, pp 297–311.

58. Jellinger K: Primary intracranial germ cell tumours. *Acta Neuropathol* 25:291–306, 1973.

59. Judisch GF, Shivanand RP: Concurrent heritable retinoblastoma, pinealoma, and trisomy X. *Arch Ophthalmol* 99:1767–1769, 1981.

60. Kageyama N, Belsky R: Ectopic pinealoma in the chiasmal region. *Neurology* 11:318–327, 1961.

61. Katsura S, Suzuki J, Wada I: A statistical study of brain tumors in the neurosurgical clinics in Japan. *J Neurosurg* 16:570–580, 1959.

62. Kline KT, Damjanov I, Katz SM, Schmidek H: Pineoblastoma: An electron microscopic study. *Cancer* 44:1692–1699, 1979.

63. Koide O, Watanabe Y, Sato K: A pathological survey of intracranial germinoma and pinealoma in Japan. *Cancer* 45:2119–2130, 1980.

64. Krabbe KH: The pineal gland, especially in relation to the problem of its supposed significance in sexual development. *Endocrinology* 7:379–414, 1923.

65. Kurumado K, Mori W: Synaptic ribbon in the human pinealocyte. *Acta Pathol Jpn* 26:381–384, 1976.

66. Kurumado K, Mori W: A morphological study on the pineal gland of human embryo. *Acta Pathol Jpn* 27:527–531, 1977.

67. Legait H, Legait E: Contribution a l'etude de la glande pineale humaine; etude faite a l'aide de 747 glandes. *Bull Assoc Anat* 61:107–121, 1977.

68. Lewis I, Baxter DW, Stratford JG: Atypical teratomas of the pineal. *Can Med Assoc J* 89:103–110, 1963.

69. Lowenthal A, Flament-Durand J, Karcher D, Noppe M, Brion JP: Glial cells identified by anti-α-albumin (anti-GFA) in human pineal gland. *J Neurochem* 38:863–865, 1982.

70. Marburg O: Zur Kenntnis der normalen und pathologischen Histologie der Zirbeldrüse. Die Adipositas cerebralis. *Arb Neurol Inst Wien Univ* 17:217–279, 1909.

71. Markesbery WR, Brooks WH, Milsow L, Mortara RH: Ultrastructural study of the pineal germinoma *in vivo* and *in vitro*. *Cancer* 37:327–337, 1976.

72. Markesbery WR, Haugh RM, Young AB: Ultrastructure of pineal parenchymal neoplasms. *Acta Neuropathol* 55:143–149, 1981.

73. McCormack T, Plassche WM, Lin Shu-Ren: Ruptured teratoid tumor in the pineal region. *J Comput Assist Tomogr* 2:499–501, 1978.

74. McDonnell DE: Pineal epidermoid cyst: Its surgical therapy. *Surg Neurol* 7:387–391, 1977.

75. McGovern VJ: Tumors of the epiphysis cerebri. *J Pathol Bact* 61:1–9, 1949.

76. Megyeri L: Cystische Veränderungen des Corpus pineale. *Frankfurt Z Pathol* 70:699–704, 1960.

77. Møller M: Presence of a pineal nerve (nervus pinealis) in the human fetus; a light and electron microscopical study of the innervation of the pineal gland. *Brain Res* 154:1–12, 1978.

78. Møller M: The ultrastructure of the human fetal pineal gland. I. Cell types and blood vessels. *Cell Tissue Res* 152:13–30, 1974.

79. Møller M: The ultrastructure of the human fetal pineal gland. II. Innervation and cell junctions. *Cell Tissue Res* 169:7–21, 1976.

80. Murovic J, Ongley JP, Parker JC, Page LK: Manifestations and therapeutic considerations in pineal yolk-sac tumors. Case report. *J Neurosurg* 55:303–307, 1981.

81. Nakazato Y, Ishida Y, Kawabuchi J: Ganglioneuroblastic differentiation in a pineocytoma. *J Neuropathol Exp Neurol* 37:665, 1978.

82. Neuwelt EA, Smith RG: Presence of lymphocyte membrane surface markers on "small cells" in a pineal germinoma. *Ann Neurol* 6:133–136, 1979.

83. Neuwelt EA, Glasberg M, Frenkel E, Clark WK: Malignant pineal region tumors. *J Neurosurg* 51:597–607, 1979.

84. Neuwelt EA, Frenkel EP, Smith RG: Suprasellar germinomas (ectopic pinealomas): Aspects of immunological characterization and successful chemotherapeutic responses in recurrent disease. *Neurosurgery* 7:352–358, 1980.

85. Nielsen SL, Wilson CB: Ultrastructure of a "pineocytoma." *J Neuropathol Exp Neurol* 34:148–158, 1975.

86. Nishiyama RH, Batsakis JG, Weaver DK, Simrall JH: Germinal neoplasms of the central nervous system. *Arch Surg* 93:342–347, 1966.

87. Norbut AM, Mendelow H: Primary glioblastoma multiforme of the pineal region with leptomeningeal metastases: A case report. *Cancer* 47:592–596, 1981.

88. Oksche A: Sensory and glandular elements of the pineal organ. In Wolstenholme GEW, Knight J (eds): *The Pineal Gland*, Edinburgh-London, Churchill Livingstone, 1971, pp 127–146.

89. Ortega P, Malamud N, Shimkin MB: Metastasis to the pineal body. *Arch Pathol* 52:518–528, 1951.

90. Papasozomenos S, Shapiro S: Pineal astrocytoma: Report of a case, confined to the epiphysis, with immunocytochemical and electron microscopic studies. *Cancer* 47:99–103, 1981.

91. Pastori G: Ein bis jetzt hoch nicht beschriebenes sympathetisches Ganglion zum nervus conari sowie zur Vena magna Galeni. *Z Gesamte Neurol Psychiat* 123:81–90, 1930.

92. Pecker J, Scarabin JM, Vallee B, Brucher JM: Treatment of tumours of the pineal region: Value of stereotaxic biopsy. *Surg Neurol* 12:341–348, 1979.

93. Peters A, Palay SL, Webster HDF: The fine structure of the nervous system. *The Neurons and Supporting Cells*. Philadelphia, Saunders, 1976.

94. Preissig SH, Smith MT, Huntington HW: Rhabdomyosarcoma arising in a pineal teratoma. *Cancer* 44:281–284, 1979.

95. Quast P: Beiträge zur Histologie und Cytologie der normalen Zirbeldrüse des Menschen. II. Zellen und Pigment des interstitiellen Gewebes der Zirbeldrüse. *Z Mikrosk Anat Forsch* 24:38–100, 1931.

96. Quay WB, Ma Y-H, Varakis JN, ZuRhein GM, Padgett BL, Walker DL: Modification of hydroxyindole-O-methyltransferase activity in experimental pineocytomas induced in hamsters by a human papaovavirus (JC). *J Natl Cancer Inst* 58:123–126, 1977.

97. Ringertz N, Nordenstam H, Flyger G: Tumors of the pineal region. *J Neuropathol Exp Neurol* 13:540–561, 1954.

98. Roda JM, Perez-Higueras A, Oliver B, Alvarez MP, Blazquez MG: Pineal region meningiomas without dural attachment. *Surg Neurol* 17:147–151, 1982.

99. Roessmann U, Velasco ME, Gambetti P, Autilio-Gambetti L: Neuronal and astrocytic differentia-

tion in human neuroepithelial neoplasms. An immunohistochemical study. *J Neuropathol Exp Neurol* 42:113–121, 1983.

100. Rozario R, Adelman L, Prager RJ, Stein BM: Meningiomas of the pineal region and third ventricle. *Neurosurgery* 5:489–495, 1979.

101. Rubery ED, Wheeler TK: Metastases outside the central nervous system from a presumed pineal germinoma. *J Neurosurg* 53:562–565, 1980.

102. Rubinstein LJ: Tumors of the central nervous system. *Atlas of Tumor Pathology*, 2nd series, Fascicle 6. Washington DC, Armed Forces Institute of Pathology, 1972.

103. Rubinstein LJ: Tumors of the central nervous system. *Atlas of Tumor Pathology*, 2nd series, Fascicle 6, (Suppl). Washington DC, Armed Forces Institute of Pathology, 1982.

104. Rubinstein LJ: Cytogenesis and differentiation of pineal neoplasms. *Hum Pathol* 12:441–448, 1981.

105. Rubinstein LJ: Cytogenesis and differentiation of primitive central neuroepithelial tumors. *J Neuropathol Exp Neurol* 31:7–26, 1972.

106. Rubinstein LJ, Okazaki H: Gangliogliomatous differentiation in a pineocytoma. *J Pathol* 102:27–32, 1970.

107. Russell DS: The pinealoma: Its relationship to teratoma. *J Pathol Bact* 56:145–150, 1944.

108. Russell DS, Rubinstein LJ: *Pathology of Tumors of the Nervous System*, ed 4. Baltimore, Williams & Wilkins, 1977, pp 287–290.

109. Sakata K, Yamada H, Sakai N, Hosono Y, Kawasako T, Sasaoka I: Extraneural metastasis of pineal tumor. *Surg Neurol* 3:49–54, 1975.

110. Sambasivan M, Nayar A: Epidermoid cyst of the pineal region. *J Neurol Neurosurg Psychiatry* 37:1333–1335, 1974.

111. Schaefer M, Lapras C, Thomalske G, Grau H, Schober R: Sarcoidosis of the pineal gland. *J Neurosurg* 47:630–632, 1977.

112. Sevitt S, Schorstein J: A case of pineal cyst. *Br Med J* 11:490–492, 1947.

113. Smith WT, Hughes B, Ermocilla R: Chemodectoma of the pineal region, with observations on the pineal body and chemoreceptor tissue. *J Pathol Bact* 92:69–76, 1966.

114. Sobel RA, Trice JE, Neilsen SL, Ellis WG: Pineoblastoma with ganglionic and glial differentiation. *Acta Neuropathol* 55:243–246, 1981.

115. Solarski A, Panke ES, Panke TW: Craniopharyngioma in the pineal gland. *Arch Pathol Lab Med* 102:490–491, 1978.

116. Sonntag VKH, Waggener JO, Kaplan AM: Surgical removal of a hemangioma of the pineal region in a 4-week-old infant. *Neurosurgery* 8:586–588, 1981.

117. Stachura I, Mendelow H: Endodermal sinus tumor originating in the region of the pineal gland. *Cancer* 45:2131–2137, 1980.

118. Stefanko SZ, Manschot WA: Pinealoblastoma with retinoblastomatous differentiation. *Brain* 102:321–332, 1979.

119. Steinbok P, Dolman C, Kaan K: Pineocytomas presenting as subarachnoid hemorrhage. Report of two cases. *J Neurosurg* 47:776–780, 1977.

120. Stowell RE, Sachs E, Russell WO: Primary in-

tracranial chorionepithelioma with metastases to the lung. *Am J Pathol* 21:787–801, 1945.

121. Sweet WH: A review of dermoid, teratoid and teratomatous intracranial tumors. *Dis Nerv Syst* 1:228–238, 1940.

122. Tabuchi K, Yamada O, Nishimoto A: The ultrastructure of pinealomas. *Acta Neuropathol* 24:117–127, 1973.

123. Takei Y, Mirra SS, Miles ML: Primary intracranial yolk sac tumor: report of three cases and an ultrastructural study. *J Neuropathol Exp Neurol* (Abstr) 36:633, 1977.

124. Tamura H, Kury G, Suzuki K: Intracranial teratomas in fetal life and infancy. *Obstet Gynecol* 27:134–141, 1966.

125. Tani E, Ikeda K, Kudo S, Yamagata S, Nishiura M, Higashi N: Specialized intercellular junctions in human intracranial germinomas. *Acta Neuropathol* 27:139–151, 1974.

126. Tavcar D, Robboy SJ, Chapman P: Endodermal sinus tumor of the pineal region. *Cancer* 45:2646–2651, 1980.

127. Teilum G: Classification of endodermal sinus tumor (mesoblastoma vitellinum) and so-called "embryonal carcinoma" of the ovary. *Acta Pathol Microbiol Scand* 64:407–429, 1965.

128. Tompkins VN, Haymaker W, Campbell EH: Metastatic pineal tumors. A clinico-pathologic report of two cases. *J Neurosurg* 7:159–169, 1950.

129. Trojanowski JQ, Tascos NA, Rorke LB: Malignant pineocytoma with prominent papillary features. *Cancer* 50:1789–1793, 1982.

130. Tso MOM, Fine BS, Zimmerman LE: The nature of retinoblastoma. I. Photoreceptor differentiation: A clinical and histopathologic study. *Am J Ophthalmol* 69:339–349, 1970.

131. Tso MOM, Fine BS, Zimmerman LE: The nature of retinoblastoma. II. Photoreceptor differentiation: An electron microscopic study. *Am J Ophthalmol* 69:350–359, 1970.

132. Tso MOM, Fine BS, Zimmerman LE, Vogel MH: Photoreceptor elements in retinoblastoma. *Arch Ophthalmol* 82:57–59, 1969.

133. Varakis JN, ZuRhein GM: Experimental pineocytoma of the Syrian hamster induced by a human papovavirus (JC). A light and electron microscopic study. *Acta Neuropathol* 35:243–264, 1976.

134. Vuia O: Embryonic carcinosarcoma (mixed tumour) of the pineal gland. *Neurochirurgia* 23:47–54, 1980.

135. Wakai S, Segawa H, Kitahara S, Asano T, Sano K, Ogihara R, Tomita S: Teratoma in the pineal region in two brothers. Case reports. *J Neurosurg* 53:239–243, 1980.

136. Waldbaur H, Gottschaldt M, Schmidt H, Neuhäuser G: Medulloblastom des Kleinhirns und Pineoblastom bei eineiigen Zwillingen. *Klin Padiatr* 188:366–371, 1976.

137. Wara WM, Jenkin RDT, Evans A, Ertel I, Hittle R, Ortega J, Wilson CB, Hammond D: Tumors of the pineal and suprasellar region: Childrens cancer study group treatment results 1960–1975. *Cancer* 43:698–701, 1979.

138. Willis RA: Nervous tissue in teratomas. In Minckler J (ed): *Pathology of the Nervous System*. New York, McGraw-Hill, 1979, vol 2, pp 1937–1943.

139. Wilson ER, Takei Y, Bikoff WT, O'Brien M, Tindall GT: Abdominal metastases of primary intracranial yolk sac tumors through ventriculoperitoneal shunts: Report of three cases. *Neurosurgery* 5:356–364, 1979.

140. Wood BP, Haller JO, Berdon WE, Lin SR: Shunt metastases of pineal tumors presenting as pelvic mass. *Pediatr Radiol* 8:108–109, 1979.

141. Wurtman RJ, Axelrod J, Kelly DE: *The Pineal.* New York, Academic Press, 1968, p 31.

142. Wurtman RJ, Kammer H: Melatonin synthesis by an ectopic pinealoma. *N Engl J Med* 274:1233–1237, 1966.

143. Wurtman RJ, Axelrod J: Demonstration of hydroxyindole-O-methyltransferase, melatonin, and serotonin in a metastatic parenchymatous pinealoma. *Nature* 204:1323–1324, 1964.

144. Yoshiki T, Itoh T, Shirai T, Noro T, Tomino Y, Hamajima I, Takeda T: Primary intracranial yolk sac tumor. Immunofluorescent demonstration of alpha-fetoprotein synthesis. *Cancer* 37:2343–2348, 1976.

145. Zimmerman BL, Tso MOM: Morphologic evidence of photoreceptor differentiation of pinealocytes in the neonatal rat. *J Cell Biol* 66:60–75, 1975.

146. Zülch KJ: Biologie und Pathologie der Hirngeschwülste. In Oliverona H, Tönnis J (eds): *Handbuch der Neurochirurgie.* Berlin, Springer Verlag, 1965, p 348.

CHAPTER 3

Diagnostic Radiology of Pineal Tumors

ROBERT E. ANDERSON, M.D.

INTRODUCTION

A number of radiological imaging methods have been employed over the years to examine the pineal region. Plain skull films were occasionally useful in a screening role, if abnormal calcification in the pineal region was present (visible under the age of 6 or covering more than 1 cm in diameter), if spread sutures were present, or if erosion of the sellar floor secondary to chronic increased intracranial pressure was seen.

Prior to the availability of computed tomographic (CT) scanning, further radiological workup for a suspected pineal region mass might have included an isotope brain scan, air or positive contrast ventriculography, and cerebral angiography (Figs. 3.1, 3.14–3.25). Several of these studies were generally required to determine the extent of the lesion. Since CT head scanning has become widely available, this imaging method has become the screening method of choice, as well as the most versatile imaging tool for the investigation and characterization of pineal region masses (Figs. 3.2–3.13).

CT SCAN

CT scans through the pineal region, before and after intravenous contrast enhancement, have replaced all other radiological imaging methods for the detection of pineal region tumors. The high degree of sensitivity of the CT scan in detecting calcium has resulted in redefinition of abnormal calcification in the pineal area. Older data from plain skull film examinations indicate that only 5% of normal children younger than 10 yr of age will show any sign of pineal calcification. More recent CT scan data indicate that the percentage is approximately twice that found with plain films—approximately 10% of normal children age 10 yr or under may show physiologic calcification. However, the youngest patient with normal pineal calcification found in a review of 725 patients was 6½-yr-old. All of those cases with calcification below age 6 had neoplasms (14).

A normal pineal gland, with or without physiologic calcification, can be seen routinely on CT scans through the area. The posterior third ventricle and the quadrigeminal plate portion of the circum-mesencephalic cistern provide low-density markers for the localization of the normal gland. Intravenous contrast enhancement produces clear definition of the larger vascular structures in the area, especially the internal cerebral veins/vein of Galen complex (Figs. 3.2, 3.3, and 3.5).

Tumors of the pineal gland may grow anteriorly into the third ventricle, posteriorly into the quadrigeminal plate cistern and midline cerebellar structures, or laterally into the thalamus. Upward growth is restricted by the splenium of the corpus callosum. The close proximity of the pineal gland to the cerebral aqueduct results in obstructive hydrocephalus with relatively small pineal region tumors. Pineal region masses may be detected on plain CT scans if they distort the posterior third ventricle or quadrigeminal plate cistern, or if they exhibit abnormal calcification. Many of the histologic types of pineal region neoplasms show strong contrast enhancement, a fact that makes intravenous contrast infusion mandatory in these cases (Figs. 3.3–3.13).

In view of the hazards of approaching the pineal region for biopsy using traditional methods, some investigators have attempted to arrive at a specific tumor diagnosis from radiologic evidence alone, so that therapy might be instituted without a histologic diagnosis. Chang et al (1) emphasized the differential diagnostic value of calcification within a pineal region mass. They found 100% calcification in cases of pineal germinoma, a variable rate in cases of pineal teratoma, and a small percentage of calcification

(text continues on p. 66)

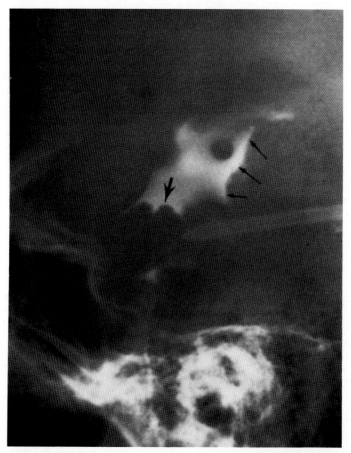

Figure 3.1.   Positive contrast ventriculogram. Contrast outlines the margins of the third ventricle. A mass indents the posterior third ventricle (*arrows*). Note also the distortion of the anterior third ventricle (*large arrow*), which indicates the presence of a sizeable suprasellar "ectopic pinealoma" in this patient. The suprasellar lesion was not apparent on an early generation enhanced CT scan. This examination is rarely used at the present time, due to the versatility of present-day CT equipment (see Figs. 3.2–3.13).

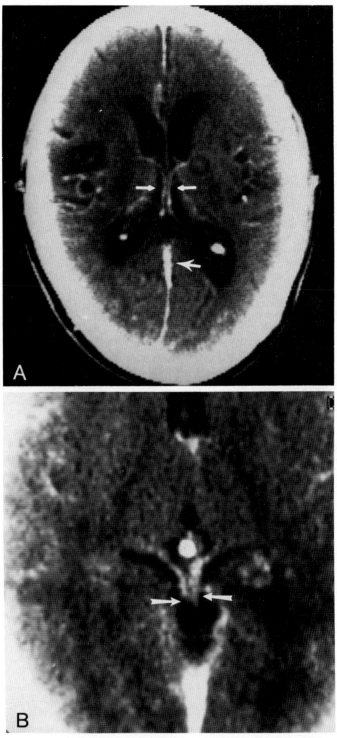

Figure 3.2.   Normal vessels about the pineal region: *A*, internal cerebral veins (*small arrows*) and straight sinus (*large arrow*) are generally well demonstrated on contrast enhanced CT scan of the pineal region. *B*, internal cerebral veins converge to join the vein of Galen immediately posterior to the pineal gland (*arrow*). Note the small amount of eccentrically placed calcification in this normal pineal gland.

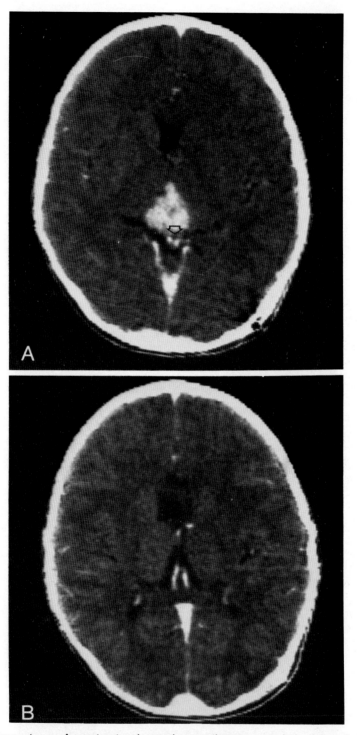

Figure 3.3. Pineocytoma: *A*, contrast enhanced scan shows a regularly enhancing mass at the pineal region with paired internal cerebral veins visible along its posterior margin (*arrow*). *B*, CT section slightly higher shows that the internal cerebral veins lie parallel to each other and pass directly over the tumor mass.

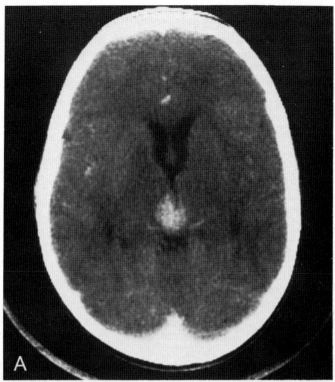

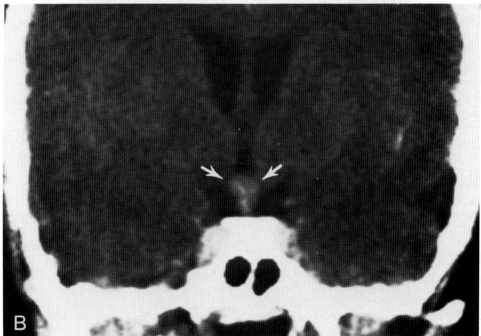

Figure 3.4. Pineal and suprasellar mass germinoma. *A*, enhancing pineal region tumor. *B*, a careful search for a suprasellar lesion should be made in any patient showing a pineal region mass. A Small suprasellar germinoma (*arrows*) is best visualized on coronal CT scan.

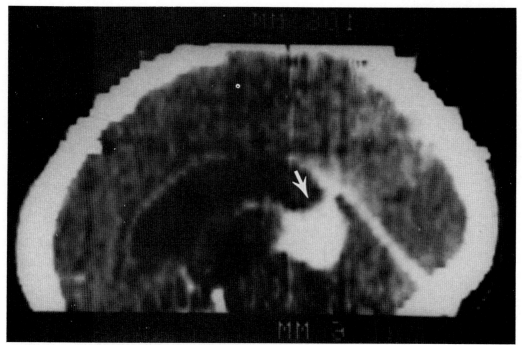

Figure 3.5. Sagittal reconstruction. Pineocytoma causing ventricular obstruction. Note that the mass effect caused by dilatation of the lateral ventricles pushes the distal internal cerebral vein and vein of Galen downward more than the tendency of the tumor to push it upward (*arrow*). The tumor has grown posteriorly and inferiorly to broadly indent the midline posterior fossa structures. Compare the shape and position of the posterior margin of the mass with the position of the precentral cerebellar vein in this same case (see Fig. 3.24).

in cases of teratoma mixed with germinoma or embryonal carcinoma (1). Zimmerman et al (14) found that CT characteristics, along with considerations of the patient's age and sex, led to a correct histologic prediction in most cases. Teratomas might contain fat, calcium, or bone. Pineal tumors were slightly hyperdense on plain scan and generally enhanced strongly following intravenous contrast infusion. Glial element tumors, on the other hand, were hypo-dense or iso-dense on the plain scans (13). Both Takeuchi (11) and DuPont et al (2) felt that the CT finding of tumor infiltration along the margins of the ventricular system might be diagnostic of germinoma. Inoue et al (4) consider that typical CT findings, plus a rapid decrease in tumor size with low doses of radiation, are "virtually diagnostic of germinoma."

Others feel that the CT findings in an individual case are not reliable in predicting tumor histology, and feel that surgery is indicated (5, 6, 8–10, 12). Local experience supports this view-

point. A series reported by Futrell (3) included two germinomas, two teratocarcinomas, and one pineal hamartoma, benign teratoma, astrocytoma, and neurilemmoma. One case was considered to be a pineal lipoma from the characteristic low density on CT scan. The divergent histologic patterns found in this group were reflected in a wide variety of CT scan appearances. The authors concluded that a presumptive histologic diagnosis on the basis of the CT scan was not possible, nor were characteristics of contrast enhancement, calcification, tumor size, position, etc., helpful in distinguishing benign from malignant neoplasms.

CT scan findings in a number of diverse lesions are presented in Figures 3.6–3.13, to emphasize the difficulty in predicting histology from scan appearance.

ANGIOGRAPHY

Cerebral angiography remains an essential feature of the radiologic evaluation of patients

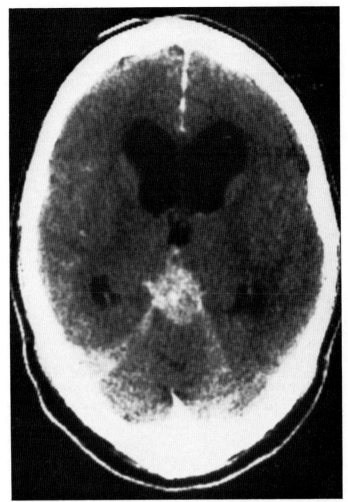

Figure 3.6. Pineoblastoma. Contrast enhanced scan showing irregular tumor mass at the pineal level with coarse calcification.

with a mass in the pineal region. As illustrated by the case in Figure 3.13, the lesion seen on CT scan may not even be a neoplasm, but rather a collection of abnormal blood vessels. Angiography is also useful in determining the position of cortical veins in the vicinity of the planned surgical approach, of displaced normal vessels in relation to the mass, and the degree of tumor vascularity (7). A tumor stain seen on the angiogram may influence the surgical plan, and may also have some diagnostic significance. Chang et al (1) feel that the visualization of tumor vessels on angiography is suggestive of either a teratoma or an embryonal cell carcinoma.

Since the angiogram is intended as an aid in planning the surgical approach, it is necessary for the clinician to be familiar with normal and abnormal angiographic anatomy in this area. Cases showing mass effects are compared to normal examples so that the reader can more readily appreciate the vascular patterns frequently seen in lesions of the pineal region.

The arterial phase of the vertebral angiogram is frequently very helpful in determining the position of a mass in relation to normal vascular structures. The posterior medial choroidal artery, a branch of the posterior cerebral artery, courses anteriormedially past the pineal gland (Figs. 3.14–3.17). It may be displaced posteriorly or anteriorly by a pineal tumor, depending on

(text continues on p. 80)

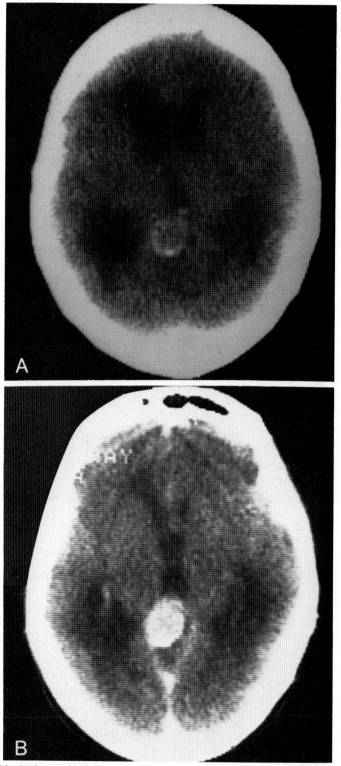

Figure 3.7.   Meningioma: *A*, plain scan of a mass at the pineal region shows partial calcification of the margins of the lesions. *B*, following contrast infusion, dense uniform enhancement occurs. Neither carotid nor vertebral arteriograms showed a tumor stain to suggest the diagnosis of meningioma. Case courtesy of Dr. C. Sternberg, Chattanooga, TN.

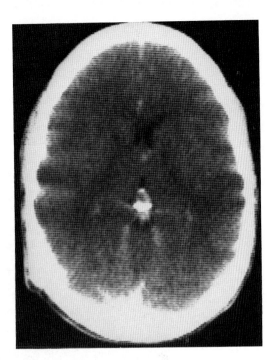

Figure 3.8. Pineal gland tumor. The tumor contained both astrocytoma and pineoblastoma elements.

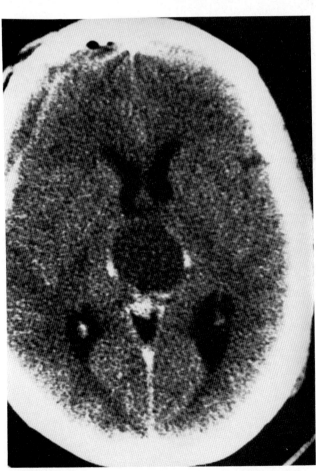

Figure 3.9. Craniopharyngioma. The most conspicuous abnormality in this case was this cystic mass at the pineal level. Case courtesy of Dr. R. Sherry, Syracuse, NY.

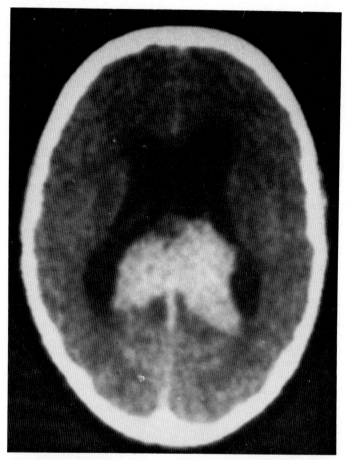

Figure 3.10.   Germinoma. Large mass mimics corpus callosum glioma.

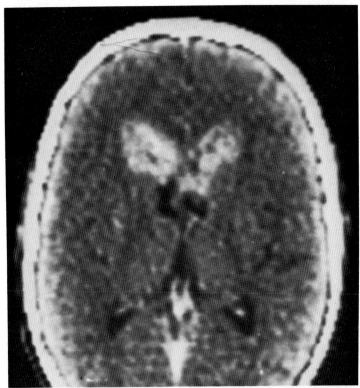

Figure 3.11. Metastases from medulloblastoma. Enhancing tumor deposits along frontal horns in a pattern considered by some to be pathognomonic of germinoma.

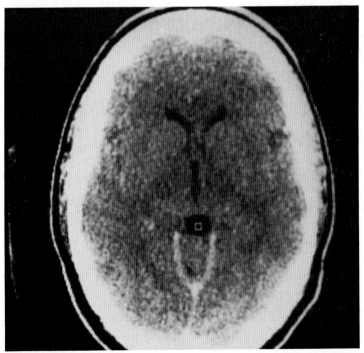

Figure 3.12. Lipoma. Hounsfield numbers in square have a mean of −71. Case courtesy of Dr. Richard Pratt, Abilene, TX.

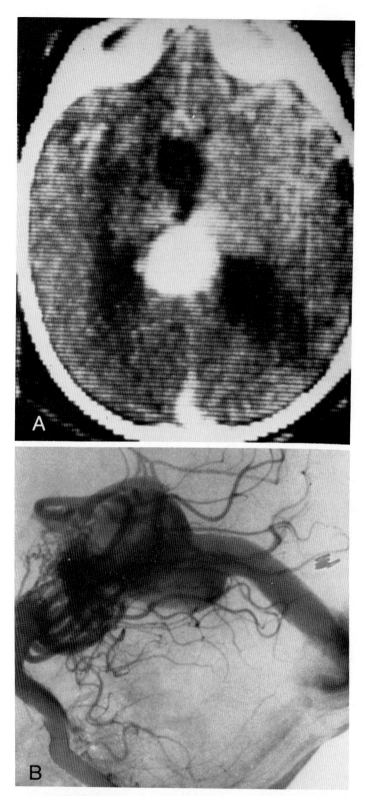

Figure 3.13. Arteriovenous malformation (AVM) at the vein of Galen; *A*, contrast enhanced CT scan shows an enhancing mass at the pineal region with hydrocephalus. *B*, vertebral arteriogram shows hypertrophied branches of the basilar artery filling a large vein of Galen aneurysm.

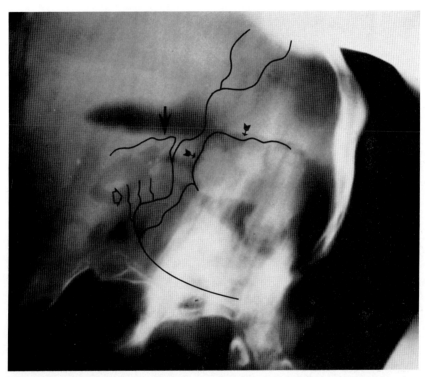

Figure 3.14. Schematic diagram. Arterial phase, vertebral angiogram: arteries which may be displaced by a pineal region tumor include the posterior medial choroidal artery (*large arrow*), the posterior thalamo-perforating arteries (*open arrow*), and the superior vermian branches of the superior cerebellar arteries (*small arrows*). Compare with normal arteriogram, Figure 3.15, and abnormal studies, Figures 3.16, 3.17 and 3.25.

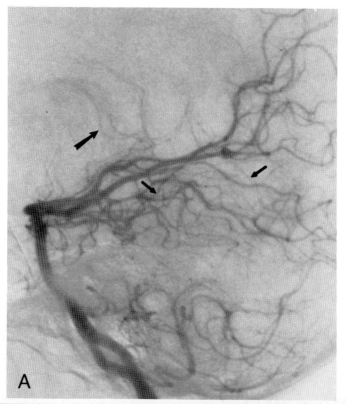

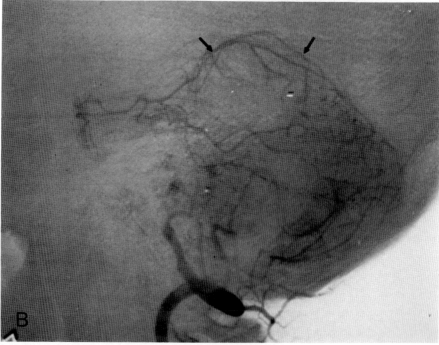

Figure 3.15.   Normal lateral vertebral angiogram, arterial phase: *A*, note the configuration of the posterior medial choroidal arteries (*larger arrow*), and the superior vermian arteries outlining the margins of a normal vermis (*small arrows*). *B*, nonfilling of posterior cerebral branches in this normal example shows superior vermian branches clearly (*arrows*). Compare with Figures 3.16, 3.17 and 3.25.

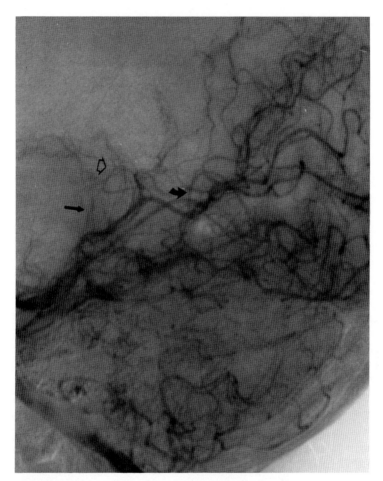

Figure 3.16. Vertebral study, lateral view. Thalamoperforator branches are stretched (*arrow*). Posterior medial choroidal artery is tilted backward (*open arrow*). The initial segment of the posterior cerebral artery on either side has lost its normal undulations. Compare with normal example, Figure 3.15. Note also backward shift of the superior vermian arteries (*curved arrow*).

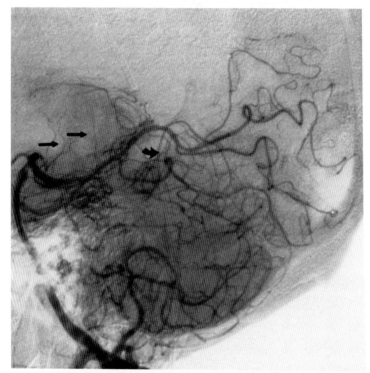

Figure 3.17. Example of hypertrophied, irregular, stretched posterior thalamoperforating arteries supplying a tumor in the pineal region (*arrows*). Superior vermian arteries are displaced by this large mass (*curved arrows*). Compare with Figure 3.5.

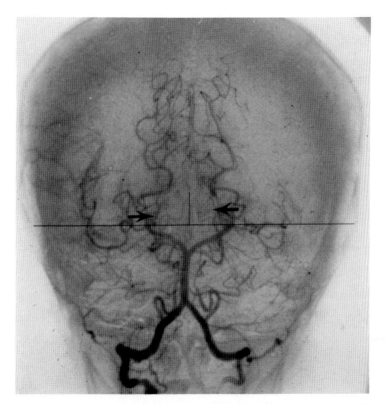

Figure 3.18.   Vertebral study AP view. Arterial branches are used to assess the midline, as marked by the superior and inferior vermian arteries. Since pineal masses are usually at the midline, these structures are not usually displaced across the midline. Instead, a mass near the midline effaces the normal undulations of the superior cerebellar and posterior cerebral artery branches proximally as they encompass the midbrain structures and pass near the pineal region (*arrows*). Compare with Figures 3.19 and 3.25.

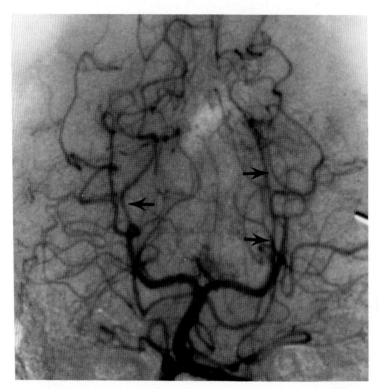

Figure 3.19. Anteroposterior vertebral study, arterial phase. Large mass at the pineal level shows typical effacement and stretching of superior cerebellar and posterior cerebral artery branches as they course along the margin of the mass (*arrows*).

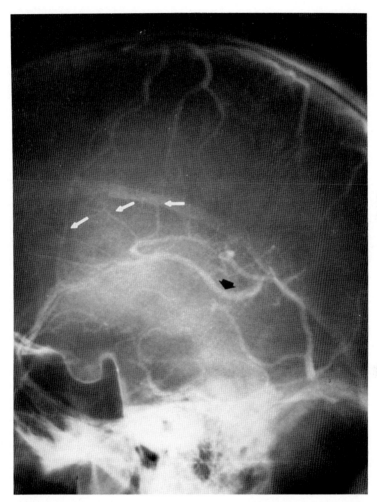

Figure 3.20. Carotid arteriogram, normal venous phase. In addition to the normal, smoothly s-shaped curvature of the internal cerebral vein running along the roof of the third ventricle (*large arrow*) immediately superior to the pineal gland, subependymal veins are frequently visible (*small arrows*) which provide a good estimate of lateral ventricular size on the lateral projection.

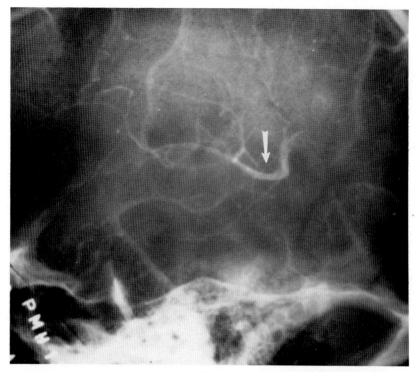

Figure 3.21. Abnormal carotid venous phase. Compare with normal example, Figure 3.20. The smooth curve of the internal cerebral vein has been lost. Instead of being elevated by the tumor mass, it appears to be shifted downward (*arrow*). This apparent paradoxical shift is due to the fact that obstruction and dilatation of the lateral ventricles has produced a mass effect which predominates over the local effects of the pineal mass. Compare with Figure 3.5.

whether the mass grows forward or extends primarily downward into the quadrigeminal plate region. Posterior thalamoperforate branches of the posterior cerebral artery may become stretched by a pineal region mass, and may also become hypertrophied if the tumor spreads into the thalamic region on either side (Figs. 3.14–3.17). Larger masses may affect the main trunks of the posterior cerebral arteries and superior cerebellar arteries as they course around the mass (Figs. 3.19 and 3.25). Posterior extension of a large pineal region tumor results in posterior displacement of the superior vermian arteries as the mass indents the vermis (Figs. 3.16 and 3.17).

The venous plate of both carotid and vertebral studies show venous displacements by a pineal region tumor. Dense opacification of the internal cerebral veins after carotid injection reveals displacements of internal cerebral veins and vein of Galen, either by the pineal tumor itself (tending to elevate the posterior portion of the internal cerebral complex) or by secondary hydrocephalus (which tends to depress this venous complex) (Figs. 3.5, 3.21, and 3.24). The precentral cerebellar vein passes close to the pineal region on its way to the vein of Galen, and therefore exhibits a characteristic posterior bowing with larger pineal tumors in a manner similar to the displacement of the superior vermian arteries (Figs. 3.5 and 3.24). Angiographic tumor staining is unusual in many of the neoplasms in this region; but when present, helps to outline the mass in relation to adjacent vascular structures (Fig. 3.25).

MYELOGRAPHY

Tumors of the pineal region are among those metastasizing via the CSF pathways to both the intracranial and spinal subarachnoid spaces. In one review of 61 cases, 10% of tumors of the pineal gland itself showed spread via CSF pathways, as did 37% of suprasellar germinomas. Radiotherapy to the spinal axis is therefore recommended by some authors for large pineal tumors, simultaneous pineal and hypophyseal lesions, and all biopsy proven germinomas (10). Others are reluctant to subject these young pa-

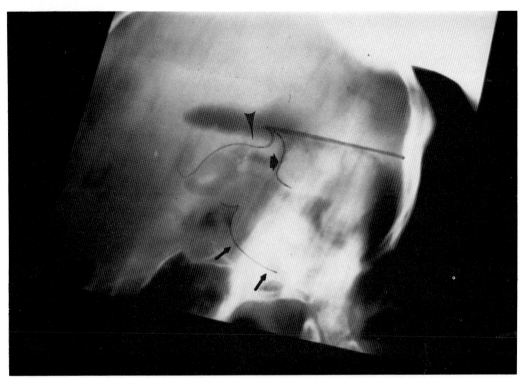

Figure 3.22. Schematic diagram, vertebral angiogram, venous phase. Internal cerebral veins course over the pineal region (*large arrow*). A large pineal mass may displace the precentral cerebellar vein posteriorly (*wide arrow*). Ponto-mesencephalic vein marks the surface of the pons (*small arrows*). Compare with normal study, Figure 3.23, and abnormal example, Figure 3.24.

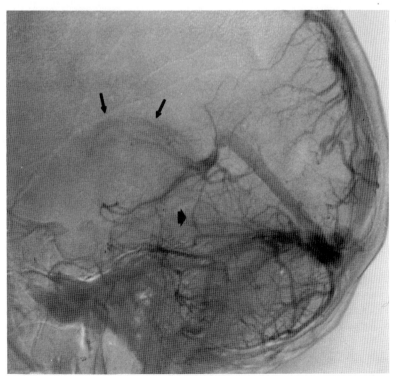

Figure 3.23. Vertebral study, normal venous phase. Note the normal smooth configuration of the choroid plexus stain (*small arrows*), and the normal position of the precentral cerebellar vein (*single arrow*). Compare with Figures 3.22 and 3.25.

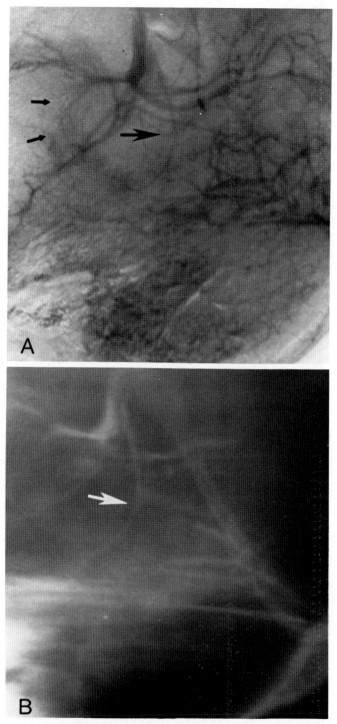

Figure 3.24.   Vertebral venous phase, large pineal mass: *A*, standard view, and *B*, angiotomogram of a patient with a large pineocytoma. Standard view reveals abnormal contour of the internal cerebral vein-vein of Galen complex as seen in Figure 3.21, abnormal (tumor) vessels (*small arrows*), and typical backward shift of the precentral cerebellar vein (*large arrow*). This latter finding is best appreciated on the angiotomogram, *B (arrow)*. Compare with Figures 3.5, 3.22, and 3.23.

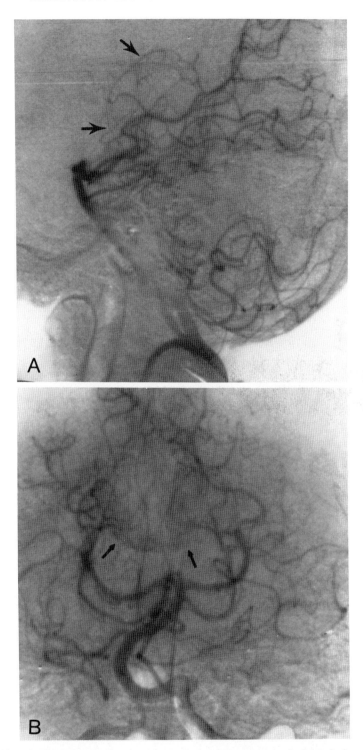

Figure 3.25.   Vertebral angiogram, enhancing mass, pineocytoma: *A*, lateral view in mid-arterial phase shows vessels draped over a mass in the pineal region (*arrows*). Note the typical posterior shift of the superior vermian branches. Compare with Figures 3.15, 3.16 and 3.17). *B*, anteroposterior view shows stretching and spreading of posterior cerebral and superior cerebellar artery branches around a tumor beginning to show abnormal staining (*arrows*). Compare to Figure 3.19, a similar mass without any angiographic tumor staining.

tients to full spinal radiotherapy in view of the late morbidity from that treatment. CSF cytology in cases with proven intraspinal tumors or lesions may be positive in only 25% of the cases (10). Myelography is, therefore, recommended in all patients with pineal region tumors. In patients with negative CSF cytology, the myelogram may prove positive as indicated by the statistics above. Myelography may also be useful in patients with positive cytology. If a focal mass is identified, a higher local dose of radiotherapy may be applied (Fig. 3.26).

SUGGESTED IMAGING PROTOCOL

A recommended strategy for the radiological evaluation of patients suspected of having a pineal region tumor is presented in Figure 3.27. The initial study is a plain and enhanced CT scan. If positive for tumor in the pineal region, cerebral angiography is then recommended to determine the nature of the vascularity of the lesion as well as the displacement of normal arteries and veins in the area. After controlling hydrocephalus with a ventricular shunt, myelography with a water-soluble agent is recommended next, since the discovery of a mass lesion in the spinal canal will provide the surgeon with the option of removing this mass for both diagnostic and therapeutic purposes prior to, or in place of, a brain biopsy. If the mass appears to be confined to the pineal region, a CT-guided stereotaxic biopsy or open biopsy

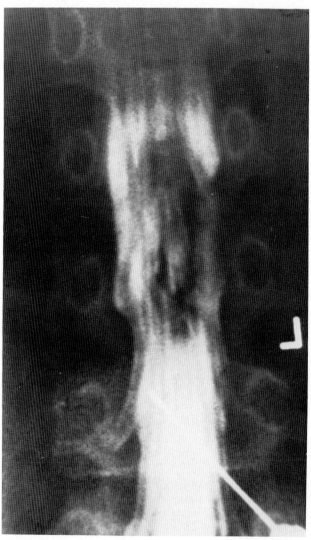

Figure 3.26.   Myelogram. Patient with pineocytoma and cauda equina symptoms. Myelogram shows subarachnoid metastasis.

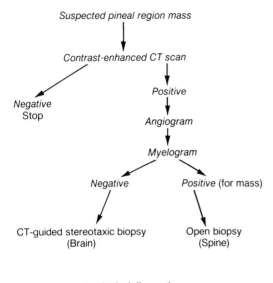

Suspected pineal region mass

↓

Contrast-enhanced CT scan

Negative
Stop

Positive

↓

Angiogram

↓

Myelogram

Negative   *Positive* (for mass)

CT-guided stereotaxic biopsy   Open biopsy
(Brain)   (Spine)

Histological diagnosis

Radiation ℞   Surgical resection

Follow-up: Head CT/myelogram

Figure 3.27.   Radiologic evaluation of pineal lesions.

should be done. Radiotherapy or surgical removal will follow. Follow-up studies for intracranial or intraspinal masses will include CT scan and water-soluble myelogram respectively. Immediately after metrizamide myelography, a cranial CT scan (i.e. a metrizamide cisternogram) may help to rule out intracranial subarachnoid seeding.

SUMMARY

Contrast enhanced CT scan of the head and full column myelography using a water-soluble agent (after controlling increased intracranial pressure) are the screening methods of choice in evaluating patients with tumors of the pineal region. Angiography retains an important role in these patients (1) to document the degree of vascularity of the mass seen on CT scan; (2) to rule out the possibility that the enhancing mass is a benign vascular lesion such as vein of Galen aneurysm, arteriovenous malformation, etc.; (3) to provide the surgeon with a clear image of displaced normal arteries and veins prior to biopsy, and (4) to show the position of cortical veins at the site of the planned surgical approach. While certain CT findings such as a

coarse calcification, a tooth, fat density material, etc. may aid the neuroradiologist in making a histologic prediction, the wide variation in CT scan appearance for many of the tumors of this area make histologic diagnosis imperative. Data now being accumulated regarding the use of CT-guided stereotaxic biopsy methods may demonstrate that needle biopsy of lesions of this area can be performed with much less risk to the patient than was the case with open biopsy methods (see Chapter 12). This new technique, along with microscopic surgical resection methods, may produce better treatment results than have been possible in the past.

References

1. Chang CG, Kageyama N, Kobayashi T, Yoshida J, Negoro M: Pineal tumors: Clinical diagnosis, with special emphasis on the significance of pineal calcification. *Neurosurgery* 8:656–668, 1981.
2. Dupont MG, Gerard JM, Flamant-Durand J, et al: Pathognomonic aspects of germinoma on CT scan. *Neurosurgery* 14:209–211, 1977.
3. Futrell NN, Osborn AG, Cheson BD: Pineal region tumors: Computed tomographic-pathologic spectrum. *AJR* 137:951–956, 1981.
4. Inoue Y, Takeuchi T, Tamaki M, Nin K, Hakuba A, Nishimura S: Sequential CT observations of irradiated intracranial germinomas. *Am J Roentgenol* 132:361–365, 1979.
5. Izquierdo JM, Rougerie J, Lapras C, Sanz F: The so-called ectopic pinealomas. *Childs Brain* 5:505–512, 1979.
6. Neuwelt EA, Glasberg M, Frenkel E, Clark WK: Malignant pinal region tumors. *J Neurosurg* 51:597–607, 1979.
7. Raimondi AJ, Tomita T: Pineal tumors in childhood. *Childs Brain* 9:239–266, 1982.
8. Roda JM, Perez-Higueras A, Oliver B, Alvarez MP, Blazquez MG: Pineal region meningiomas without dural attachment. *Surg Neurol* 17:147–151, 1982.
9. Rozario R, Adelman L, Prager RJ, Stein BM: Meningiomas of the pineal region and third ventricle. *Neurosurgery* 5:489–495, 1979.
10. Sung D, Harisiadis L, Chang CH: Midline pineal tumors and suprasellar germinomas: Highly curable by radiation. *Radiology* 128:745–751, 1978.
11. Takeuchi J, Handa H, Otsuka S, et al: Neuroradiological aspects of suprasellar germinoma. *Neurosurgery* 17:153–159, 1979.
12. Vaquero J, Carrillo R, Casezudo J, Leunda G, Villoria F, Brava G: Cavernous angiomas of the pineal region. Report of two cases. *J Neurosurg* 53(6):833–835, 1980.
13. Zimmerman RA, Bilaniuk LT, Wood JH, Bruce DA, Schut L: Computed tomography of pineal, parapineal, and histologically related tumors. *Radiology* 137:669–677, 1980.
14. Zimmerman RA, Bilaniuk LT: Age-related incidence of pineal calcification detected by computed tomography. *Radiology* 142:659–662, 1982.

CHAPTER 4

Pineal Function in Mammals Including Man

RUSSEL J. REITER, Ph.D.

INTRODUCTION

Within the last decade research on the pineal gland has uncovered some of the functions of this highly active organ of internal secretion. The bulk of these studies indicate a close interaction between the secretory products of the pineal and the neuroendocrine-reproductive axis. Although the bulk of the research effort on the physiology of the pineal gland has been concentrated in this area, the gland also seems to have many other important roles. Indeed, it is this reviewer's opinion that the scientific community has identified only a small number of the interactions of the pineal gland with other organs. The present survey summarizes some of the important biochemical and physiological aspects of this organ.

Central to an understanding of the pineal gland is the knowledge that the activity of the organ is markedly influenced by the photoperiodic environment to which the animal is exposed. In mammals the pineal gland is not capable of direct photoreception; rather, the retina receives information about the light:dark environment which is transferred to the pineal gland over a circuitous series of neurons (92, 93). Some of the proposed neurons involved in connecting the eyes to the pineal gland include retinohypothalamic connections (to the suprachiasmatic nuclei), descending hypothalamo-spinal neurons, and pre- and postganglionic sympathetic neurons (Fig. 4.1). The terminals of the latter cells end in pericapillary spaces or between parenchymal cells within the pineal gland. The system of neurons between the suprachiasmatic nuclei of the hypothalamus and the pineal must remain intact in order for the gland to remain functional. Besides the well-known sympathetic innervation of the mammalian pineal gland, a parasympathetic component also has been described in several species. The functional importance of these fibers remains essentially unknown.

PHARMACOLOGY OF THE MAMMALIAN PINEAL GLAND

Although embryologically the pineal gland is derived from neuroectoderm, it is outside of the blood-brain barrier and therefore accessible to pharmacological agents which are otherwise ineffective in modulating neurons within the central nervous system (6). The functional innervation of the pineal gland in mammals seems to be that derived from the superior cervical ganglia, i.e. postganglionic sympathetic neurons (60).

It is generally conceded that the sympathetic neurons which terminate within the pineal gland release norepinephrine (NE) (196); the release of the catecholamine is believed to occur primarily during the daily dark period. After its release, NE acts on β-adrenergic receptors on pinealocyte membranes resulting in a cascade of biochemical events which eventually result in melatonin production. Melatonin is one of several potential pineal hormones. The sympathetic nerve endings within the pineal gland contain serotonin in addition to NE; the role of this monoamine in neurotransmission at this site remains unknown (6). Besides NE and serotonin, various polypeptides may serve as coneurotransmitters or neuromodulators within the pineal gland (30).

The effects of various sympathomimetic drugs on the mammalian pineal gland have been extensively investigated in both *in vivo* and *in vitro* studies. The specific β-adrenergic agonist, isoproterenol, has been frequently used to investigate pineal indoleamine metabolism; less frequently NE, the natural neurotransmitter, has been employed in such studies (74). Both isoproterenol and NE work postsympathetically within the pineal gland on β-1-adrenergic receptors (99, 195). NE also has α-adrenergic activity; however, within the rat pineal gland the receptors are primarily of the β-type. During the normal daily light:dark cycle the β-adrenergic

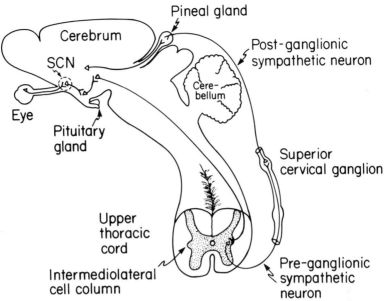

Figure 4.1. Innervation of the mammalian pineal gland. The eyes are connected to the pineal gland by a circuitous series of neurons which involve the ganglion cells of the retinas, cell bodies in the suprachiasmatic nuclei (SCN) and pre- and postganglionic sympathetic neurons. Some fibers may enter the pineal stalk and provide an innervation, of unknown function, to the pinealocytes.

receptors within the pineal gland undergo a change in number related presumably to the degree of previous stimulation. Thus, the binding of radioactive isoproterenol to the rat pineal gland is greater at the end of the light period than at the onset of light (61, 196); this reflects a change in B_{max} or the number of receptors. The nighttime release of NE from the sympathetic neurons within the pineal gland presumably decreases the number of β-receptors within the rat pineal, thus accounting for the lower number of receptors in the early light phase of the light:dark cycle. As support for this idea, isoproterenol administered to rats in the evening provokes a greater increase in N-acetyltransferase (NAT) activity and presumed melatonin production than the same dosage of the drug given in the morning (152). Melatonin is one of the end products of pineal indoleamine metabolism and is a pineal secretory product and hormone (18, 118, 140).

The number of postsynaptic receptors available on the pinealocyte membranes can be modified by manipulation of the photoperiodic conditions to which rats are exposed, or by the sympathetic denervation of the pineal gland in this species. Hence, if rats are maintained in continual light for a period of days or if their superior cervical ganglia are surgically removed,

the response of the pineal gland to exogenously administered β-adrenergic agonists is exaggerated compared to that in otherwise untreated animals (27, 28). Since both these procedures, (i.e., prolonged exposure to light and ganglionectomy), decrease stimulation of the pineal gland and thereby presumably cause an increase in the number of β-receptors on the cell membranes, the gland becomes supersensitive to adrenergically active drugs. The phenomenon of pineal gland supersensitivity can be induced into a subsensitive state by the repeated administration of isoproterenol or NE (29).

Studies similar to those described above for the rat pineal gland have been less successful in other species. For example, in the Syrian hamster, a species extensively used in the definition of the reproductive consequences of the pineal gland (115, 129), neither isoproterenol nor NE have been shown to reliably stimulate the pineal gland after they are exogenously administered. Although a single report did claim that isoproterenol induced a low grade rise in pineal melatonin in this species (163), more extensive investigations have failed to confirm this (77). In the latter study male hamsters were treated with either isoproterenol or NE and pineal melatonin levels were subsequently analyzed. Neither of the compounds greatly influenced the accumulation of melatonin within the pineal gland; in some cases the animals had been kept in continual light for a week or they had been superior cervical ganglionectomized for the same period. Thus, not only were the transmitter and its agonists incapable of stimulating melatonin production under normal conditions, but the pineal did not respond even when, based on the results of experiments with rats, the gland should have been supersensitive.

In the human, as well, the use of isoproterenol thus far has been ineffective in promoting a rise in plasma melatonin levels (170). There is ample evidence that the innervation of the human pineal gland via the central and peripheral autonomic nervous system is similar to that in experimental animals (68, 165, 179). Yet, a dose of isoproterenol which caused a 50% increase in heart rate for 1 hr failed to raise circulating melatonin titers in the human (74). This negative result may relate to the dosage of isoproterenol used or to some yet unrecognized problem. Based on our studies with the hamster (77) as well as the aforementioned observations in the human, we are considering the possibility that there may be a co-neurotransmitter or neuromodulator which normally works in concert with NE in promoting indoleamine metabolism in the pineal gland of the Syrian hamster and human. Examples of compounds which could be involved in such processes include serotonin (28, 66), γ-aminobutyric acid (86), histamine (66), taurine (186), octopamine (66), and DOPA (82).

Drugs which interfere with the action of NE at its receptor level on the pinealocyte membrane also prevent the stimulatory influence of the neurotransmitter on indoleamine metabolism. The most frequently used receptor blocker is propranolol. Typically, its administration to the rat curtails the nighttime rise in pineal melatonin production (190); propranolol blocks β-adrenergic receptors. α-Adrenergic antagonists such as phenoxybenzamine do not interfere with the nocturnal rise in indoleamine metabolism in the rat pineal gland. Likewise, in the Syrian hamster propranolol administration severely limits melatonin production in the pineal gland at night, whereas phentolamine, an α-receptor antagonist, has no capability in this regrad (78). Finally, phenoxybenzamine has a slight inhibitory influence on the rise in pineal melatonin in the hamster pineal; this is speculated to be related to the fact that phenoxybenzamine may possess a real β-adrenergic blocking capacity de-

pending on the concentration of β-receptors per unit area under study and the sympathetic tone of the system at the time of the experiment. There is at least one rodent species, the eastern chipmunk, in which propranolol has been shown to be incapable of suppressing the nocturnal increase in pineal melatonin levels (127).

Limited studies in the human indicate that β-receptor blockers are effective in reducing blood levels of melatonin in this species. Vaughan and colleagues (170) found that propranolol prevented the nocturnal rise in blood melatonin values in one healthy subject, while Hansen et al (43) and Wetterberg (185) confirmed this observation in psychiatric patients. Clearly, it appears that propranolol could be an effective agent in treating hypersecretion of melatonin as well as assisting researchers in uncovering the relationships of melatonin to other hormonal products.

Indole Biochemistry of the Mammalian Pineal Gland

The first step in the synthesis of melatonin is the uptake by the pinealocytes of the amino acid tryptophan. Due to the successive actions of tryptophan hydroxylase and 1-aromatic amino acid decarboxylase, tryptophan is converted to 5-hydroxytryptamine (serotonin) (160). Serotonin is a key intermediate not only in the synthetic pathway for melatonin but other pineal indoleamines as well (Fig. 4.2). The serotonin concentration within the pineal gland exceeds that of any organ in the body (37). Within the pineal, serotonin can be N-acetylated by serotonin NAT using acetyl CoA (183). The product of NAT activity is N-acetylserotonin; this compound is subsequently 0-methylated by the enzyme hydroxyindole-O-methyltransferase (HIOMT) with the resultant formation of N-acetyl-5-methoxytryptamine (melatonin) (5). Although the pineal gland synthesizes melatonin, its production seems not to be confined to this organ. Both the Harderian gland, a compound tubuloalveolor gland which surrounds the eye of some mammals (not present in the human), and the retina may be capable of producing melatonin (36, 96, 130). Inasmuch as melatonin persists in these sites after surgical removal of the pineal gland it is presumed to be produced within these organs (Fig. 4.3). There is presently considerable controversy over the contribution of extra pineal sites of melatonin production to blood levels of the indole. Immu-

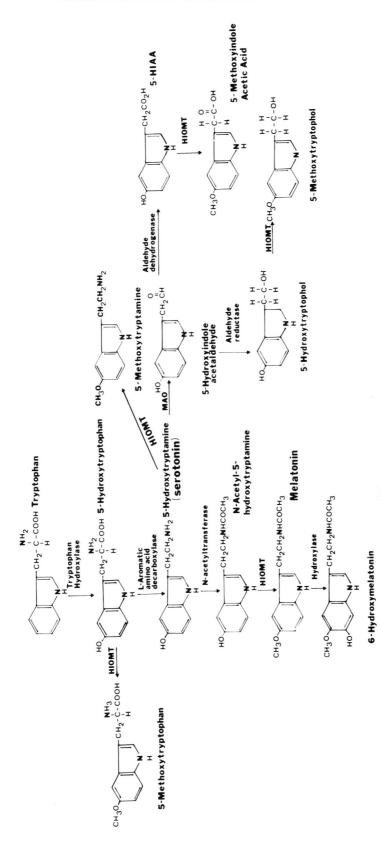

Figure 4.2 Indoleamine metabolism in the mammalian pineal gland. Melatonin is the best known and most extensively investigated pineal hormone. After its synthesis within the pineal gland melatonin is released into the blood vascular system after which it is metabolized in the liver to 6-hydroxymelatonin; this compound is the chief urinary metabolite of melatonin. (HIOMT = hydroxyindole-O-methyltransferase.)

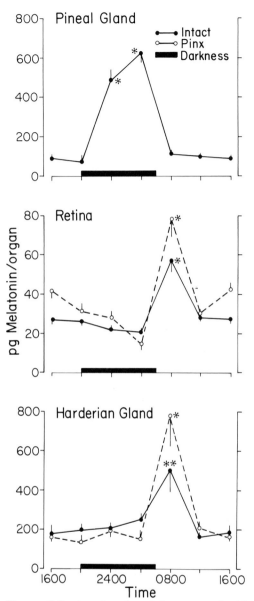

Figure 4.3. Levels of radioimmunoassayable melatonin in the pineal gland, retina, and Harderian gland of adult male rats over a 24-hr period. Pinealectomy (PINX) slightly exaggerated the rhythms in retinal and Harderian gland melatonin. (*$P < 0.001$ or **$P < 0.05$ compared to mean melatonin values measured at other time points during the 24-hr period).

culating melatonin levels in the rat, it was never within the measurable limits of the assay after pinealectomy (75).

Once melatonin is formed within the pineal gland it seems to be immediately released. As a consequence, there is a close correlation between pineal melatonin production and blood levels of the indole (187). This has also contributed to the idea that the pineal gland is primarily responsible for determining blood levels of the constituent. The lack of storage of appreciable quantities of the pineal hormone is somewhat unique among endocrine glands; typically, there are substantial reserves of a hormone in the organ where it is produced.

Pineal melatonin production begins in early postnatal life in those species in which it has been studied. For example, in the rat one of the critical enzymes in melatonin production (NAT) exhibits a nighttime rise when the animals are only 4 days old (26, 55); likewise, the pineal gland in these young animals is already capable of responding to exogenously administered isoproterenol (16, 192). A melatonin rhythm in the pineal gland of the Syrian hamsters has been detected as early as the 15th postnatal day (148). Very young children have not been thoroughly investigated in terms of the onset of the plasma melatonin rhythm, although the day:night variation is clearly detectable in prepubertal children (11). Throughout the young adult life of all animals in which melatonin levels have been measured, they are easily measurable and exhibit clear day:night differences (38). However, in advanced age, both pineal melatonin production and plasma levels of the hormone are diminished, especially at night. When day and night levels of NAT and melatonin were compared in 2-, 12-, and 29-month-old female rats, the oldest animals exhibited markedly depressed nocturnal melatonin while the 1-yr-old rats had indole values half way between those of the young adult and old animals (121). These observations are compatible with findings on pineal melatonin production in the Syrian hamster (137, 143) (Fig. 4.4) and gerbil (64, 137). The decreased pineal melatonin production is reflected in lower blood levels of the constituent as well (122). In humans, also, advanced age is associated with nearly a total elimination of the nocturnal rise in circulating melatonin titers (54). On the whole, accumulated data indicate that the biosynthetic activity of the pineal gland in mammals diminishes with advancing age. The consequences of the reduction in melatonin pro-

noreactive melatonin in the sheep seems not to totally disappear from the blood after pinealectomy (1, 62); conversely, when a highly specific and sensitive gas chromatography-mass spectral (GC-MS) technique was used for detecting cir-

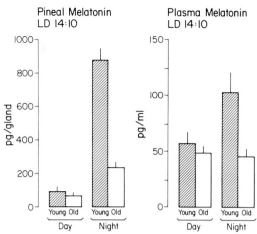

Pineal Melatonin
LD 14:10

Plasma Melatonin
LD 14:10

Figure 4.4. Immunoreactive pineal and plasma melatonin levels in young (4-month old) and old (18-month old) female hamsters. The animals were killed either during the day (at 1600 hr) or at night (0400 hr). The light/dark cycle was 14:10 with lights being on daily from 0600 to 2000 hr. In both the pineal gland and plasma, nocturnal pineal melatonin levels were diminished in the old animals.

duction in old animals, including the human, remain to be uncovered.

Although not specifically discussed until this point, it is obvious from the preceding narrative that pineal melatonin production is highly cyclic. Indeed, the light/dark cycles to which an animal is exposed has profound effects on the ability of the gland to synthesize melatonin. In all species studied to date, melatonin production is clearly higher at night than during the day. A number of other constituents in the melatonin-synthetic pathway as well as the associated enzymes exhibit measurable rhythms. The first pineal rhythm to be discovered was that of serotonin (109). Levels of this compound are highest during the day and fall gradually during darkness when melatonin production is elevated. Whether, in fact, the serotonin rhythm is generated by the cyclic production of melatonin is still open to debate. Following the definition of the cyclic nature of serotonin concentrations within the pineal gland, the NAT (67) and melatonin (81) cycles were described. For both NAT activity (65, 153) and melatonin levels (159, 189) the peaks are reached during the night. Melatonin production increases at night whether the animals are normally nocturnally (39, 97, 98, 163, 187) or diurnally (132, 136, 144) active. These cycles are strictly regulated by the

photoperiodic environment. Extending the light period into the normal dark phase depresses the rhythms, provided the intensity of light is sufficient to have an effect. The rhythms are generated by the release of a neurotransmitter, most likely NE, from the sympathetic nerve endings within the pineal gland during the dark period (194).

The nocturnal pattern of pineal melatonin production varies among species. When Syrian hamsters are maintained under a photoperiodic regimen which provides 14 hr light and 10 hr darkness per 24-hr period, there is a discrete melatonin peak which occurs near the end of the dark period, roughly 8–9 hr after lights out. In this species the rise in pineal melatonin usually does not begin until the animals are in darkness for several hours (97, 98, 163). Increasing the length of the dark phase has a rather minor influence on the pattern of melatonin production (111, 163). Indeed, the exposure of Syrian hamsters to a light/dark cycle of 2:22 does not greatly change either the height or the duration of peak melatonin production; under these circumstances it again occurs during the late dark phase. There is a secondary category of animals in which the pineal melatonin peak occurs near the middle of the dark period; included in this group of animals is the albino rat (59), Richardson's ground squirrel (136), 13-lined ground squirrel (*Spermophilus tridecemlineatus*) (131), eastern chipmunk (127), and Turkish hamster (38). Typically, in these species darkness is associated with a gradual rise in melatonin within the pineal gland with peak levels being reached near the middle of the dark period; thereafter, pineal melatonin production falls until the lights come on. In the final category of animals the melatonin rhythm is essentially a square wave. After the light to dark transition pineal melatonin values increase rapidly, remain elevated during the dark period, and drop just prior to or at the time of lights on. Animals that seem to respond in this manner include the white-footed mouse (*Peromyscus leucopus*) (79, 104), cotton rat (*Sigmodon hispidus*) (88), and Djungarian hamster (*Phodopus sungorus*) (38).

In reference to the above described melatonin patterns it is important to recall that the animals in question were, for the most part, maintained under carefully regulated photoperiodic and temperature conditions of the laboratory where the transitions from light to darkness (and vice versa) were abrupt. Also, during the photophase the light was of uniform intensity and wavelength. These conditions obviously do not duplicate very closely the environmental features to which these animals would be exposed if they were under natural conditions. Thus, the melatonin patterns described above may be determined by the specific environmental circumstances to which these animals were exposed. When Syrian hamsters are kept under natural photoperiodic and temperature conditions throughout the year, the pattern of nocturnal pineal melatonin production is similar to that of animals kept in the laboratory under a seasonally-adjusted photoperiod (15). On the other hand, the nocturnal pattern of pineal melatonin in the 13-lined ground squirrel may be influenced by the previous lighting circumstances to which the animals were exposed (131).

Although it appears clear that pineal levels of melatonin in the human are higher at night than during the day (42, 158), this has been difficult to test directly. On the basis of blood levels of this constituent, however, it is tacitly assumed that the synthesis of melatonin in the human pineal gland is elevated at night compared to daytime levels; this appears to be a highly reliable assumption (191). Typically, circulating titers of melatonin are elevated in the human during darkness (2, 3, 101, 117). Although there is one report to the contrary (157), the pattern of plasma melatonin is generally not considered to be related to the stages of sleep (171, 174, 181). Urinary excretion of melatonin (56, 84) as well as its chief hepatic metabolite, 6-hydroxymelatonin (87), is also higher during the daily dark period. A seasonal variation in human blood levels of melatonin has been proposed (2); however, this possibility is not yet firmly supported with convincing experimental data.

The relative importance of light in influencing pineal and blood levels of melatonin in mammals has been examined in a number of species; the results of these studies indicate there are great variations in the sensitivity of the melatonin-generating system to light during the normal period of darkness. For example, in laboratory born and raised, nocturnal Syrian hamsters an irradiance (intensity) of light as low as 0.186 $\mu W/cm^2$ is effective in totally depressing nighttime pineal levels of melatonin (13, 14). This is in sharp contrast to observations in some other rodent species. In the wild-captured, diurnal eastern chipmunk (127, 132) and the Richardson's ground squirrel (53, 144) an irradiance of

920 $\mu W/cm^2$ is either incapable or slightly suppressive to pineal melatonin levels (Fig. 4.5). This remarkable difference in the responsiveness of the pineal gland to light during the normal dark period was initially thought to be a result of the activity patterns of the animals, i.e. whether they were nocturnal or diurnal. Recent investigations, however, indicate this explanation does not suffice. Rather the current theory is that the sensitivity of the pineal gland to light at night is determined by the previous lighting history of the animal (83, 147). The apparent importance of the lighting history of the animal was recently dramatically demonstrated in an experiment which utilized the 13-lined ground squirrel as the experimental animal (131). Fortuitously, the authors had access to two separate groups of animals from different environmental backgrounds. Half of the animals had been born and raised in captivity and had been exposed during the day to an irradiance of light with a maximal intensity of roughly 300 $\mu W/cm^2$. Con-

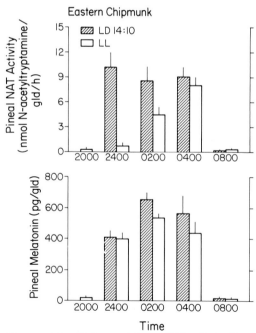

Figure 4.5. Failure of light (920 $\mu W/cm^2$) to curtail the nighttime rise in pineal N-acetyltransferase (NAT) activity and melatonin levels in the eastern chipmunk (*Tamias stratus*). The *hatched bars* are levels in animals killed during the normal period of darkness; *clear bars* are mean values in animals exposed to light during the normal dark period.

versely, the second group of squirrels was captured in the wild where they had been subjected to direct sunlight for at least a portion of each summer day; sunlight may have an irradiance up to at least 36,000 $\mu W/cm^2$ light. The intensity of light required to suppress the nighttime rise in pineal melatonin was far greater in squirrels previously raised under natural photoperiod conditions as compared to laboratory raised animals. This illustrates the remarkable flexibility of the pineal gland in terms of its sensitivity to light at night. It is the current belief that the light irradiance to which animals are exposed prior to experimentation may be critically important in determining sensitivity of their pineal to light during the test period. In the specific experiment cited above (131), there were obviously other differences between the two experimental groups which could also have accounted for the observed differences. The impact of these factors is also being considered.

It has been known for a number of years that human blood melatonin levels are generally not suppressed by normal room light (102, 170). Conversely, if the irradiance of light to which the subjects are exposed is increased, circulating melatonin titers can be lower (76). In the first study concerned with the problem, human subjects were acutely exposed to a light intensity of either 500 or 1500 lux at night. The lower intensity of light failed to alter circulating melatonin values in six subjects while the 1500 lux intensity clearly was effective in suppressing the melatonin concentration in the plasma. In a related study it was shown that the exposure of phase-delayed subjects to sunlight in the morning caused a precipitous decline in blood melatonin concentrations (74). Humans, like the diurnal animals noted above, are typically exposed to bright sunlight during a portion of each day. This presumably decreases the responsivity of their pineal gland to light at night. In other words, if animals (including humans) are normally exposed to bright light during the day (i.e., sunlight), and subsequently exposed to low intensity room light (i.e. 500 lux or about 85 $\mu W/cm^2$) the pineal "interprets" this as darkness and responds accordingly. On the other hand, if the maximal intensity these animals witness is about 200 $\mu W/cm^2$, then their exposure to 500 lux light at night is, indeed, "interpreted" as light and melatonin production is suppressed. Lewy (74) also mentions the possiblity that humans may exhibit a seasonal sensitivity to light.

The extension of light into the normal dark period in humans has recently been shown to have clinical significance in a manic-depressive patient (73).

The abundant research on melatonin has over shadowed the investigation of other pineal indole products which are potential hormonal products of the gland. 5-Methoxytryptophol is produced by the methylation of 5-hydroxytryptophol within the pineal; the enzyme responsible for this conversion is HIOMT (Fig. 4.2). 5-Methoxytryptophol was initially isolated from bovine pineal tissue by McIsaac and colleagues (90) in 1965, but relatively little has been done in determining its physiological consequences.

Wilson and colleagues (188) developed a GC-MS method for measuring 5-methoxytryptophol in the blood and in pineal tissue. With the aid of this technique, they found a strong correlation between serum and pineal levels of this constituent with the pineal concentrations of the methoxyindole being greater than that of melatonin; additionally, the pineal 5-methoxytryptophol varied in a circadian manner with highest levels being associated with the dark phase of the light:dark cycle. In the serum, the indole exhibited what this author referred to as a bimodal rhythm with peaks being observed in both the day and night. The authors did not examine the influence of pinealectomy on the blood levels of this constituent.

5-Methoxytryptophol has also been detected in the blood of humans. In seven subjects, 5-methoxytryptophol was measurable both during the day and night with four of seven individuals exhibiting a significant increase during darkness (94). Again, it could obviously not be definitively stated that the 5-methoxytryptophol detected in the blood of these subjects was derived from the pineal gland. Since assays are available to measure this compound, perhaps this information will be forthcoming in the near future.

Recently, there has been some interest generated in reference to 5-methoxytryptamine. In the pineal, this compound is formed directly from serotonin by an action of HIOMT (Fig. 4.2) (5). The amine has been found in both pineal tissue (91) and in blood (108); however, as with 5-methoxytryptophol, there is still no proof that the 5-methoxytryptamine found in the blood is secreted by the pineal gland. Now that sensitive assays are available for this constituent (35, 52), perhaps more information concerning its metabolism will be forthcoming.

Physiology of the Pineal Gland

Although the bulk of what has been done involves its interactions with the neuroendocrine-reproductive axis, the pineal gland is also functionally related to many other aspects of the organism including thyroid and adrenal physiology (57, 146, 178), central nervous system biochemistry (20, 145), tumor growth (164), temperature regulation (110), behavior (4), and circadian organization (154, 179). Inasmuch as the majority of what is known about pineal function in mammals including man relates to the interrelationships of this organ with reproductive physiology, the emphasis of what follows will be on these findings.

Roughly two decades ago it was discovered that the inhibitory effects of darkness on gonadal function were mediated via the pineal gland. In these early studies it was noted that the exposure of animals to the naturally short days of the winter (25) or to reduced photoperiods in the laboratory (45, 46, 120) caused the reproductive system of these animals to totally involute; indeed, the animals were rendered reproductively incompetent by this treatment (Fig. 4.6). The suppressive influence of darkness on sexual physiology was, however, negated completely if the hamsters had been pinealectomized. These findings constituted the best evidence to that time that the pineal exerts a marked control over the neuroendocrine-repro-

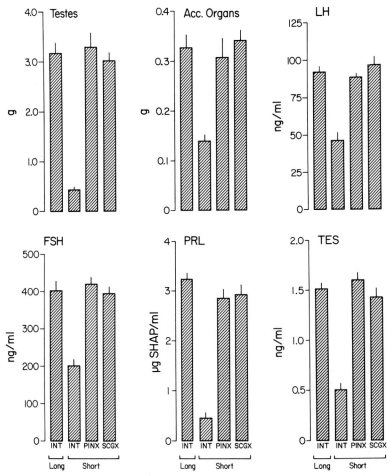

Figure 4.6. Testicular and accessory sex organ weights and plasma levels of luteinizing hormone (LH), follicle-stimulating hormone (FSH), prolactin (PRL), and testosterone (TES) in male hamsters kept under either long (>12.5 hr light/day) or short <12.5 hr light/day) day lengths. The inhibitory effects of short days on an intact animal (INT) are reversed by either pinealectomy (PINX) or by sympathetic denervation of the pineal gland, i.e. superior cervical ganglionectomy (SCGX).

ductive system and established the Syrian hamster as the animal of choice in many subsequent studies. In more recent years studies on other mammals have also contributed substantially to our knowledge of pineal-reproductive interactions. Some of these species include the Djungarian hamster (47, 48), white-footed mouse (80, 103), mole (22), sheep (63), and the white-tailed deer (106). The albino rat has not been particularly useful in assisting investigators in identifying the role of the pineal gland in reproductive physiology. In general, the neuroendocrine-reproductive axis of this species is not especially sensitive to photoperiodic or pineal manipulation. On the other hand, the hypothalamo-pituitary-gonadal axis of the rat can be rendered highly sensitive to the antigonadotrophic activity of the pineal gland with certain perturbations, i.e., rendering the animals surgically anosmic, treating them with androgen (or estrogen) shortly after birth, or reducing their food intake (58, 138). How these findings relate to the normal functioning of the pineal gland in this species remains to be uncovered.

In the case of the Syrian hamster anything less than 12.5 hr of light per 24 hr constitutes a short day (32), and the animals, both males and females, experience pineal-induced gonadal atrophy. The morphological changes associated with short-day exposure are very dramatic. Normally, adult male hamsters kept under long days have testes and accessory sex organs (coagulating glands plus seminal vesicles) weighing about 3200 mg and 350 mg, respectively. If these animals are placed under short-day conditions (46) or if they are surgically blinded (113) the testes regress to about 400 mg while the accessory sex organs assume a weight of about 100 mg. As noted above, the atrophic responses of the reproductive organs in these animals do not occur if the hamsters are pinealectomized (24, 25). The rapidity of the atrophic response is the same whether the animals are exposed to 10 hr or 1 hr of light daily. In other words, the necessary feature of the photoperiod is that the light phase is less than 12.5 hr of light daily. Likewise, whether the short-day lengths are increasing or decreasing in length is unimportant for the response (139); thus, the animal is capable of deciphering only whether it is a long day or a short day and is apparently not influenced by the changing day length. Not only are the reproductive organs of the short-day-exposed animals grossly changed, the microscopic alterations are equally as dramatic. The testes are devoid of spermatozoa, the seminiferous tubules are markedly reduced in cross-sectional area, and the germinal epithelium consists of almost exclusively spermatogonia and Sertoli cells (133). Typically, the epithelial cells lining the accessory sex organs are greatly reduced in height.

In females of the species, short-day exposure results in pineal-induced functional involution of the ovaries and uteri (45). The ovaries, however, may actually be enlarged due to a marked proliferation of the interstitial tissue, although the organs are usually devoid of vesicular follicles and corpora lutea (128). The uteri in these animals are greatly reduced in weight and are histologically atrophic. Finally, normal estrous cyclicity is interrupted. As in males, all these changes are reversed by pinealectomy.

Predictably, associated with the alterations in the morphology of the reproductive organs are changes in the associated hormone levels. The hormonal alterations are different between males and females, however. In males with involuted reproductive organs due to the exposure of the animals to short-day lengths, circulating levels of luteinizing hormone (LH) (10, 161), follicle-stimulating hormone (FSH) (10, 169) and testosterone (10, 116) are normally depressed (Fig. 4.6). Despite the very marked changes in the size and function of the peripheral end organs, the reductions in circulating LH and FSH levels are sometimes only minimal or not changed at all. The hormone which exhibits the most dramatic and reproducible alteration is prolactin (118, 139, 140); a deficiency of this hormone may explain the testicular regression in dark-exposed hamsters since prolactin may be involved in maintaining LH and FSH receptors at the level of the testes (7). Hence, the reduced prolactin levels would provide an explanation for the regressed testes in the presence of ample titers of LH and FSH; without prolactin to maintain the gonadotrophin receptors the testes may well involute. Experimental data certainly supports this supposition. When hamsters with pineal-induced gonadal atrophy were given supplementary luteinizing hormone-releasing hormone (LHRH), which caused the release of LH and FSH from the anterior pituitary, the testes did not grow unless the animals also received intrarenal pituitary transplants which secreted ample amounts of prolactin (23). As with the morphological changes, pinealectomy prevents short-day exposure from altering the gonadotrophin and prolactin levels (Fig. 4.6).

Pituitary reserves of these hormones are typically altered after short-day exposure as well. Whereas all three gondally active hormones, i.e., LH, FSH, and prolactin, are depressed in the pituitary of the male hamster after the animals are maintained under reduced photoperiods for a period of time, again it is prolactin that exhibits the most remarkable and consistent reduction (10, 125). This seems to further emphasize the important role of prolactin in mediating pineal-induced testicular atrophy in this species.

When the hormonal patterns in the male hamster with suppressed reproductive organs were described, it was more or less assumed that in females these constituents would likely be similar; after all, the end organ responses are essentially the same in both species. This, however, is not the case. Indeed, the hormonal patterns change in a completely unexpected, and as of yet not explained, manner. Reproductively competent female Syrian hamsters ovulate every fourth day; on the afternoon before the ova are shed there is an increased release of LH and FSH from the pituitary leading to what is known as the preovulatory gonadotrophin surge in the blood. In animals with pineal mediated ovarian atrophy, rather than being suppressed, the gonadotrophin surge occurs every afternoon (17, 155). Thus, the repressed reproductive organs are actually being exposed to higher than normal levels of LH and FSH; the functional significance of the daily gonadotrophin surge in these animals remains unknown. Interestingly, the elevated LH levels are known to cause a proliferation of the ovarian interstitial tissue (41), a feature which is a prominent aspect of ovaries in hamsters kept under short-day conditions.

Radioimmunoassayable levels of LH and FSH in the pituitary of female hamsters also increase after short-day exposure (123); thus, there are ample hypophyseal reserves of the gonadotrophins to accommodate the daily afternoon release of these secretagogues. Conversely, prolactin concentrations in the pituitary drop coincident with the rise in LH and FSH (123). Relatively little is known of blood titers of prolactin in these animals. Again, pinealectomy reverses the suppressive influence of dark exposure on the hormonal patterns. Indeed, following pineal removal the animals are sexually normal even though they may be under short-day conditions. The conclusion drawn from these findings is that all of the inhibitory effects of reduced photoperiods on the sexual physiology of Syrian hamsters are mediated by the pineal gland.

The reproductive changes induced by short-day exposure in hamsters require a period of time to become manifested. Of some note is that this interval is becoming increasingly prolonged (118). In 1964, Hoffman and Reiter (46) described total gonadal collapse in hamsters exposed to reduced photoperiods for only 4 weeks; in more recent years this interval has become as long as 12 weeks in some experiments with 8–10 weeks being most typical. The reasons for this delayed response of the neuroendocrine-gonadal axis to the activated pineal gland remain unknown; one potential explanation that was considered is that as the animals become more highly inbred they become less responsive to the antigonadotrophic influence of the pineal gland. A test of this possibility proved to be negative, however (116). Hence, the phenomenon remains unexplained.

Once the pineal induces gonadal regression, the reproductive system of dark-exposed hamsters does not remain permanently nonfunctional. Eventually, the neuroendocrine-gonadal axis, by mechanisms that are not understood, becomes refractory to the inhibitory influence of the pineal gland and gonadal regeneration ensues (114, 124); even when the gonads are recrudescing in the dark-exposed animals melatonin production by the pineal gland continues unabated (150). The course of events is as follows: When hamsters are deprived of long days the hypothalamo-pituitary-gonadal system is suppressed by secretory products from the pineal gland and sexual involution ensues within 8–10 weeks. At this point, the gonads begin to recrudesce (even if light deprivation is continued) with full morphological and functional restoration being achieved roughly 8 weeks after the initiation of the regenerative process (124). The entire cycle of degeneration and regeneration, therefore, requires a period of 24–25 weeks. Of course, the hormonal patterns change in accordance with the alternations in the size of the reproductive organs.

In many mammals the information summarized above translates into an important role for the pineal gland in seasonal reproductive events in animals maintained under natural photoperiodic conditions (117) (Fig. 4.7). Most mammals inhabiting the temperate and polar regions of the earth are seasonal in terms of their reproductive capabilities. A number of these species

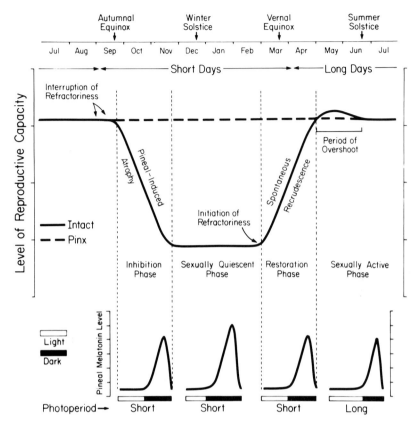

Seasonal Cycle of Reproduction

Figure 4.7.   The seasonal reproductive rhythm in Syrian hamsters maintained under natural photoperiodic and temperature conditions. The annual cycle has been divided into 4 phases: inhibition phase, sexually quiescent phase, restoration phase, and sexually active phase. Pinealectomy (PINX) prevents the winter decline in reproductive competence. At the bottom are shown the pineal melatonin rhythm during the various phases of the annual cycle.

are photoperiodic, i.e., the seasonal characteristics of their sexual cycle are determined by the photoperiod acting via the pineal gland (117, 129, 141, 197). As the day lengths wax and wane the function of the pineal gland changes accordingly and, thereby, determines when animals can and cannot breed. The importance of an annual reproductive cycle is to ensure that the young are delivered at a time of the year that is maximally conducive to their survival, i.e., the spring. Without the pineal gland, photoperiod-dependent species would become continual breeders and would frequently deliver young during the winter months when their survival would be in jeopardy (134). The indiscriminate delivery with the resultant death of the majority

of the young born during the harsh winter months would be detrimental to the survival of the species. In essence, then, whereas the pineal gland may not be necessary for the survival of the individual animal, if the species is to be successfully propagated the pineal must be present to determine when the animals can and cannot breed (117).

This information, although based primarily on data obtained from experiments which utilized the Syrian hamster, is probably applicable to a large number of other species (117, 197). Domestication of laboratory animals has converted them from seasonal to continual breeders because of the controlled long days and warm temperatures of the laboratory animal facilities.

It is this author's opinion that this delayed the discovery of the role of the pineal gland in reproduction. Since some animals seem to be "physiologically pinealectomized" by long photoperiods, surgical pinealectomy under standard laboratory conditions frequently produces no or minimal effects on the reproductive system (117, 118).

The specific impact of the photoperiod, specifically short days or light deprivation, on human sexual physiology has been studied only sparingly. Primarily, only anecdotal information is available. It could obviously be argued that the human, because of the widespread use of artificial light sources, controlled temperature, and improved nutrition has, like the domesticated rodents described above, become a continual as opposed to an intermittent breeder. The most comprehensive studies available on individuals totally deprived of light, i.e., blind human subjects who cannot perceive light, are those of Hollwich (51). Specifically, Hollwich and colleagues (50) report that the urinary excretion of 17-ketosteroid in 225 adult sight-deprived humans was significantly depressed compared to that in sighted, age and sex matched controls. In a later study which included about twice as many subjects as used in the first study, it was again found that 17-ketosteroid excretion is lower in the urine of blind humans than in sighted control subjects (49). In some of these subjects cataract removal, with the restoration of sight and light impinging on the retinas, was followed by a significant rise in 17-ketosteroid excretion. In another study, which admittedly is technically difficult to judge, depressed levels of testosterone were measured in blind men (12). In reference to fertility, Elden (31) claims a great reduction in births in blind married couples.

Finally, whether light deprivation influences pubertal onset in the human is controversial. At least three publications on this subject have appeared in the recent years. One of these claimed that blind females actually reached menarche earlier than sighted girls (193); the study was retrospective and compared institutionalized blinded girls with noninstitutionalized sighted females. These results were seemingly supported by the finding of Magee and colleagues (85) but not those of Thomas and Pizzarello (166). In none of these studies were hormonal patterns or levels determined nor was there any indication of the time of first ovulation. As a consequence, the validity of the findings have been questioned (173). Puberty, as described in these studies, encompasses a 2–3 year period during which ovarian follicular function increases from the time of first breast budding and appearance of sexual hair to the time of initiation of ovulatory cycles. Menarche can occur anytime during this 2–3 year period and does not necessarily signify ovulation. Presumably, during this interval the stimulatory effect of estrogen on the endometrium is mounting; if at some point the pineal would suppress estrogen secretion, withdrawal bleeding could occur. Considering this possibility, a better index of puberty in these individuals would have been ovulation.

In some nonhuman mammals the photoperiod acting via the pineal gland is inextricably linked to seasonal reproduction when animals are maintained under natural environmental conditions. As noted above, however, humans exercise a great deal of control over their environment and, as a consequence, can essentially avoid annual fluctuations in light and temperature. It could be argued that humans too would be seasonal in their reproductive capabilities if they were exposed to the vissicitudes of the environment. There is a modicum of evidence indicating a seasonal fluctuation in sexual competence. A reduction in the incidence of single and, more dramatically, multiple conceptions, i.e. twinning, etc., during the dark winter months was reported in people living near the Arctic Circle (168). The implication is that ovulation was at least partially suppressed at this time of the year. The same group found, with the aid of tissue biopsy, a high incidence of cystic endometrial hyperplasia during the 6-month period containing the greatest amount of darkness (167). The authors attributed the increased incidence of hyperplasia to a greater tendency of anovulatory cycles during the winter months; no hormone levels were reported in these subjects. In a related study, Carletti and colleagues (21) claimed that LH excretion in 11–14-yr-old girls was 10 times higher in the spring when day lengths were increasing than in the fall.

Despite these above mentioned findings, even a cursory review of literature reveals there are a number of studies which shows essentially no effect of the photoperiod on sexual physiology in the human. For example, (69, 70) two short reports concluded that blindness in the human female has no influence on fertility. Likewise, Fatranska and co-workers (33) found that the anterior pituitary gland of blind women responds to synthetic LHRH treatment with the secretion of LH at least as vigorously as does this organ in sighted females.

Unquestionably, the issue of whether light and darkness influence sexuality in the human is controversial. Certainly, judging from plasma melatonin levels, the human pineal is responsive to photoperiodic manipulations. Considering that in a variety of experimental animals melatonin exerts an effect on the pituitary-gonadal axis, it is natural to assume that it would have similar effects in humans. Finally, the failure of some workers to show a relationship between blinding and sexuality may relate to a phenomenon that has already been described in some nonhuman mammals, i.e. refractoriness. It is possible that the hypothalamo-pituitary-gonadal axis in the human may become refractory to the influence of melatonin (or other pineal constituents) in blind humans, such as it does in Syrian hamsters (114, 124). Thus, all of us with interest in this field should be cautious about the interpretation of negative data. One other point should be introduced. Assuming darkness is shown to have an effect on the sexual response of the human, it will still not prove that the pineal gland is involved. Again, however, based on experiments with other pinealectomized mammals this conclusion would seemingly be warranted.

Physiology of Melatonin

Within the last decade, numerous factors have been proposed as potential pineal hormones. In general, two categories of compounds are recognized as being potentially important secretagogues of the pineal gland. Melatonin is by far the most commonly accepted pineal hormone (18, 112, 118, 140); however, some other indoles which have been shown to have physiological effects include 5-methoxytryptophol (44, 89), 5-hydroxytryptophol (175), and most recently 5-methoxytryptophol (105, 151). Although each of these constituents has been shown to be physiologically active; nevertheless, they lack the extensive experimental documentation which support melatonin's candidacy as a pineal hormone.

Besides indoles, polypeptides are often promoted to the status of hormone. In one case the chemical structure of the compound has been identified but the specific composition of other peptidic factors remains to be identified. The structurally elucidated compound is arginine vasotocin (AVT). AVT is a nonpeptide which has, when administered to experimental animals, the capability of altering the release of pituitary hormones related to the reproductive system (100, 176, 177). So-called pineal antigonadotrophin (PAG), a polypeptide, has been isolated primarily due to the efforts of Benson and Ebels (8, 9); however, its specific structure has thus far eluded these workers. Other miscellaneous peptides and compounds have come under consideration as presumed pineal hormones, but supporting evidence is meager.

Clearly, the effects of melatonin on the neuroendocrine axis of the Syrian hamster are similar to those induced by the activated pineal gland. Thus, the morphological changes in the end organs are the same, the hormone alterations are identical, and in both cases the animals are reproductively incompetent (39, 40, 112, 126, 140). Indeed, the seasonal changes in reproductive capability in the hamster which are normally induced by the annual fluctuation in day length can be duplicated in the laboratory by the administration of melatonin (112, 141). In view of this, there is no reason to invoke any other pineal constituent as an antigonadotrophic factor; nevertheless, other factors may still exist.

A unique feature concerning the action of melatonin in terms of its influence on sexual physiology in the Syrian hamster is the requirement for it to be administered at a specific time during the light:dark cycle (135, 162). Hence, the daily injection of melatonin early in the light phase of the light:dark cycle is completely without effect on the reproductive system of this species; conversely, the same dosage of melatonin given daily late in the light phase causes total functional collapse of the reproductive organs. Perhaps even more remarkable is the fact that melatonin given as a continual release subcutaneous reserve not only does not induce gonadal involution but, in fact, prevents darkness (142) or daily melatonin injections (119) from causing involution of the sexual organs. This has been referred to as the counter-antigonadotrophic action of melatonin. Although these observations initially confounded researchers in the field it appears that the myriad of effects of melatonin are explicable by the fact that melatonin has the capability of down-regulating or desensitizing its own receptors (118, 126). The physiological evidence that melatonin is an authentic pineal compound with potent antigona-dotrophic capabilities is now well supported. On this basis it clearly qualifies as a pineal hormone (18, 118, 140, 141).

Besides an extensive literature illustrating the antigonadotrophic capability of melatonin in ex-perimental animals there are indications from some species that melatonin production in the pineal gland may fluctuate in reference to the ovarian cycle in female rodents. These studies have used primarily the rat as the experimental model. It appears that gonadal steroids are sup-pressive to the production of melatonin within the pineal gland (19). Also, the activity of the melatonin-forming enzyme, HIOMT, is lowered when circulating steroids are at the peak (180); the same holds true for pineal melatonin levels (59). Low melatonin production at the time of ovulation implies that the reduction in the amount of available antigonadotrophin at this time may be permissive to ovulatory mecha-nisms. Interestingly, an estrous cycle-linked rhythm in melatonin production was not ob-served in the species that has taught us most about the melatonin-reproductive interactions, i.e. the Syrian hamster (149). In less than defin-itive studies, circulating melatonin levels in the human are reportedly also lowest on the days surrounding ovulation (11, 184).

Melatonin has only been administered a few times to humans for the purposes of testing its effect on the hormones related to reproduction (72). In no case known to this reviewer has melatonin been administered for prolonged pe-riods. This distinction is important, i.e., acute versus long-term administration. Even in Syrian hamsters where melatonin is known to severely limit reproductive capability the indole must be administered for a prolonged period, i.e., a mat-ter of weeks, before any substantial changes are seen in reference to either the reproductive or-gans or the associated hormones. Thus, marked changes in reproductively active hormones in humans after single injections of melatonin should not be expected. As examples of the types of experiments that have been performed to date the work of several authors is cited. Weinberg and colleagues (182) found melatonin to be in-capable of curtailing the rise in serum LH after the administration of LHRH in men; likewise, serum testosterone values were not changed by the administration of melatonin. Similarly, Fed-eleff et al. (34) claim that the administration of melatonin to 3 men (24–30 yr of age) and 3

postmenopausal women (48–52 yr of age) was without detectable influence on basal blood levels of either LH or FSH; like Weinberg and colleagues (182), these workers also found me-latonin to be ineffective in stymieing LH release induced by LHRH. Finally, Norlund and Lerner (95) did find that melatonin was capable of slightly lowering gonadotrophin levels in human subjects. As noted above, the findings in the human may not be particularly compelling be-cause of the short term experimental period. It will probably be sometime yet before melatonin is administered for any prolonged period to hu-mans.

Perhaps the most provocative judgment to date concerning melatonin and reproduction in the human is that proposed by Silman and co-workers (156). These individuals report a marked drop in daytime circulating melatonin levels in human males as they pass through puberty. Thus, males in Tanner stage 1 had much higher morning melatonin values than did individuals in Tanner stage 5; the same relation-ships did not exist in females. Silman and col-leagues (156) proposed that the drop in serum melatonin levels in humans may be a contribu-tory factor to pubertal onset.

The hypothesis of Silman et al (156) is sup-ported by the recent observations of Cohen and co-workers (24). They measured serum immu-noreactive melatonin in 33 male subjects with delayed puberty; 30 of these individuals had simple (idiopathic) pubertal delay while 3 were growth hormone (GH) deficient. Twenty-six age-matched normal subjects served as controls. They found that serum melatonin levels are considerably higher in subjects with either type of delayed puberty; as a result of these observa-tions these workers also tentatively suggest that pubertal onset in the human may be related to pineal production of melatonin. Cohen et al (24) observed that melatonin titers fell during mid to late puberty in the subjects who were suffering from delayed sexual development.

Not all findings support the melatonin-pu-berty interaction hypothesis. For example, Lenko et al (71) have presented data which demonstrates that normal subjects exhibit no noticeable change in either serum or urinary melatonin values before or during puberty. Like-wise, when the major metabolite of melatonin, 6-hydroxymelatonin, was measured in the urine of humans at various pubertal stages, no appar-ent relationships of puberty to melatonin production were found (107). In the final analysis, it appears too early to make any definitive statements between puberty in humans and the importance of pineal melatonin production.

SUMMARY

Quite obviously, knowledge of the pineal gland has progressed rapidly within the last decade. Significant advances have been made in both clarifying the biochemistry of this highly active organ of internal secretion as well as identifying its interactions with other endocrine organs. Yet, it is this reviewer's opinion that these initial studies have uncovered only a small fraction of what the pineal gland is capable of doing. In general, it is known that the light:dark cycle is the primary regulator of pineal indole metabolism; however, a great deal more will soon be forthcoming concerning the role of various light irradiances and wavelengths in determining pineal function. Also, it will be important to discover drugs which may specifically influence pineal indole metabolism, e.g., by regulating the activity of HIOMT. The physiological interactions of the pineal gland with other endocrine structures have been partially described. Although these interrelationships seem, at this point, to involve primarily the reproductive system, it should be emphasized that pineal secretory products influence a large number of other organ systems as well. These latter relationships are the subjects of an increasing number of investigations and will potentially yield valuable information concerning the multifaceted pineal gland. The function of the pineal has been and in some cases continues to be grossly underestimated. An organ with its great synthetic capacity and wide-ranging effects cannot be ignored in clinical medicine despite the fact that most information to date has been derived from studies on nonhuman mammals. To take this approach would be both naive and foolish.

References

1. Arendt J, Forbes JM, Brown WB, Marston A: Effect of pinealectomy on immunossayable melatonin in the sheep. *J Endocrinol* 85:1P–2P, 1980.
2. Arendt J, Wirz-Justice A, Bradtke J: Annual rhythm of serum melatonin in man. *Neurosci Lett* 7:327–330, 1977.
3. Arendt J: Radioimmunoassayable melatonin: Circulating patterns in man and sheep. *Prog Brain Res* 52:249–257, 1979.
4. Armstrong S, Ng KT, Coleman GJ: Influence of the pineal gland on brain-behavior relationship.

In Reiter RJ, (ed): *The Pineal Gland, Vol. 3, Extrareproductive Effects.* Boca Raton, CRC Press, 1982, pp. 81–106.
5. Axelrod J, Weissbach H: Purification and properties of hydroxyindole-*O*-methyltransferase. *J Biol Chem* 236:211–213, 1961.
6. Axelrod J: The pineal gland: A neurochemical transducer. *Science* 184:1341–1348, 1974.
7. Bartke A: Role of prolactin in reproduction in male mammals. *Fed Proc* 39:2577–2581, 1980.
8. Benson B, Ebels I: Other pineal peptides and related substances—Physiological implications for reproductive biology. In Reiter RJ (ed): *The Pineal Gland Vol 2, Reproductive Effects.* Boca Raton, CRC Press, 1981, pp 165–188.
9. Benson B, Ebels I: Pineal peptides. *J Neural Transm* [Suppl 13]:157–173, 1978.
10. Berndtson WE, Desjardins C: Circulating LH and FSH levels and testicular function in hamsters during light deprivation and subsequent photoperiodic stimulation. *Endocrinology* 95:195–205, 1974.
11. Birau N: Melatonin in human serum: Progress in screening investigation and clinic. In Birau N, Schloot W (eds): *Melatonin—Current Status and Perspectives.* New York, Pergamon, 1981, pp 297–326.
12. Bodenheimer S, Winter JSD, Faiman C: Diurnal rhythms of serum gonadotrophins, testosterone, estradiol and cortisol in blind men. *J Clin Endocrinol Metab* 37:472–475, 1973.
13. Brainard GC, Richardson BA, Petterborg LJ, Reiter RJ: The effect of different light intensities on pineal melatonin content. *Brain Res* 233:75–81, 1982.
14. Brainard GC, Richardson BA, King TS, Matthews SA, Reiter RJ: The suppression of pineal melatonin content and *N*-acetyltransferase activity by different light irradiances in the Syrian hamster: A dose-response relationship. *Endocrinology* in press.
15. Brainard GC, Petterborg LJ, Richardson BA, Reiter RJ: Pineal melatonin in Syrian hamsters: Circadian and seasonal rhythms in animals maintained under laboratory and natural conditions. *Neuroendocrinology* 35:342–348, 1982.
16. Brammer M, Binkley S: Pineal glands of immature rats: Rise and fall in *N*-acetyltransferase activity *in vitro*. *J Neurobiol* 12:167–173, 1981.
17. Bridges RS, Goldman BD: Diurnal rhythms in gonadotrophins and progesterone in lactating and photoperiod induced acyclic hamster. *Biol Reprod* 13:613–622, 1975.
18. Cardinali DC: Melatonin. A mammalian pineal hormone. *Endocrine Rev* 2:327–346, 1981.
19. Cardinali DC, Vacas MI: Feedback control of pineal function by reproductive hormones—A neuroendocrine paradigm. *J Neural Transm*, [Suppl 13]:175–204, 1978.
20. Cardinali DC: Molecular biology of melatonin: Assessment of the "microtubule hypothesis of melatonin action." In Birau N, Schloot W (eds): *Melatonin—Current Status and Perspectives.* New York, Pergamon, 1981, pp 247–256.
21. Carletti B, Kehyayan E, Fraschini F: Remarkable seasonal variations of urinary gonadotrophin

excretion in young girls. *Experientia* 20:383, 1964.

22. Charlton HM, Grocock CA, Ostberg A: The effects of pinealectomy and superior cervical ganglionectomy on the testis of the vole, *Microtus agrestis*. *J Reprod Fertil* 48:377–379, 1976.

23. Chen HJ, Reiter RJ: The combination of twice daily luteinizing hormone-releasing factor administration and renal pituitary homografts restores normal reproductive organ size in male hamsters with pineal-mediated gonadal atrophy. *Endocrinology* 106:1382–1385, 1980.

24. Cohen HN, Hoy ID, Annesley TM, Beastall GH, Wallace AM, Spooner R, Thomson JA, Eastwald P, Klee GG: Serum immunoreactive melatonin in boys with delayed puberty. *Clin Endocrinol* 17:517–521, 1982.

25. Czyba JC, Girod G, Durand N: Sur l'antagonisme epiphysohypophysaire et les variations saisonmiere de la spermatogenese chez le hamster dore (*Mesocricetus auratus*). *C R Soc Biol* (*Paris*) 158:742–745, 1964.

26. Deguchi T: Sympathetic regulation of circadian rhythm of serotonin N-acetyltransferase activity in pineal gland of infant rat. *J Neurochem* 38:797–801, 1982.

27. Deguchi T, Axelrod J: Superinduction of serotonin N-acetyltransferase and supersentivity of adenyl cyclase to catecholamines in denervated pineal gland. *Mol Pharmacol* 9:184–190, 1973a.

28. Deguchi T, Axelrod J: Induction and superinduction of serotonin N-acetyltransferase by adrenergic drugs and denervation in the rat pineal organ. *Proc Natl Acad Sci USA* 69:2208–2211, 1972.

29. Deguchi T, Axelrod J: Supersensitivity and subsensitivity of the beta-adrenergic receptor in pineal gland regulated by catecholamine neurotransmitter. *Proc Natl Acad Sci USA* 70:2411–2414, 1973b.

30. Ebadi M, Chan A, Hammad H, Govitrapong P, Swanson S: Serotonin N-acetyltransferase and its regulation by pineal substances. In Reiter RJ (ed): *The Pineal and Its Hormones*. New York, Alan R. Liss, 1982, pp 21–33.

31. Elden CA: Sterility of blind women. *Jap J Fertil Steril* 16:48–50 1971.

32. Elliott J: Circadian rhythms and photoperiodic time measurement in mammals. *Fed Proc* 35:2339–2346, 1976.

33. Fatranska M, Repcekova-Jezova D, Jurcovicova J, Vigas M: LH and testosterone response to LH-RH in blind men. *Horm Metab Res* 10:82–83, 1978.

34. Fedeleff H, Aparicio NJ, Guitelman A, Aebeluk L, Mancini A, Cramer C: Effect of melatonin on the basal and stimulated gonadotrophin levels in normal men and postmenopausal women. *J Clin Endocrinol Metab* 42:1014–1017, 1976.

35. Gefford MR, Puizillout JJ, Delaage MA: A single radioimmunological assay for serotonin, N-acetylserotonin, 5-methoxytryptamine and melatonin. *J Neurochem* 39:1271–1277, 1982.

36. Gern WA, Ralph CL: Melatonin synthesis by the retina. *Science* 204:183–184, 1979.

37. Giarman NJ, Day M: Presence of biogenic amines in the bovine pineal body. *Biochem Pharmacol* 1:235–237, 1959.

38. Goldman B, Hall V, Hollister C, Reppert S, Roychoudhury P, Yellon S, Tamarkin L: Diurnal changes in pineal melatonin content in four rodent species: Relationship to photoperiodism. *Biol Reprod* 24:778–783, 1981.

39. Goldman B, Hall V, Hollister C, Roychoudhury P, Tamarkin L, Westrom W: Effects of melatonin on the reproductive system in intact and pinealectomized male hamsters maintained under various photoperiods. *Endocrinology* 104:82–88, 1979.

40. Goldman BD, Carter DS, Hall VD, Roychoudry P, Yellon SM: Physiology of pineal melatonin in three hamster species. In Klein DC (ed): *Melatonin Rhythm Generating System*. Basel, Karger, 1982, pp 210–231.

41. Greenwald GS: Histologic transformation of the ovary of the lactating hamster. *Endocrinology* 77:641–649, 1965.

42. Greiner AC, Chan AC: Melatonin content of the human pineal gland. *Science* 199:83–84, 1978.

43. Hansen T, Heyden T, Sundberg T, Wetterberg L: Effect of propranolol on serum melatonin. *Lancet* 2:309–310, 1977.

44. Hipkin LJ: Effect of 5-methoxytryptophol and melatonin on uterine weight responses to human chorionic gonadotrophin. *J Endocrinol* 48:287–288, 1970.

45. Hoffman RA, Reiter RJ: Response of some endocrine organs of female hamsters to pinealectomy and light. *Life Sci* 5:1147–1151, 1966.

46. Hoffman RA, Reiter RJ: Pineal gland: Influence on gonads of male hamsters. *Science* 142:1609–1611, 1965.

47. Hoffmann K: Pineal involvement in the photoperiodic control of reproduction and other functions in the Djungarian hamster, *Phodopus sungorus*. In Reiter RJ (ed): *The Pineal Gland Vol. 2, Reproductive Effects*. Boca Raton, CRC Press, 1982, pp 45–82.

48. Hoffmann K: Photoperiod, pineal, melatonin and reproduction in hamsters. *Prog Brain Res* 52:397–415, 1979.

49. Hollwich F, Dieckhues B: Endokrines System und Erblindung. *Deut Med Wschr* 96:363–368, 1971.

50. Hollwich F, Neirmann H, Dieckhues B: Einfluss des Augenlichtes auf die Sexualsteuerung bei Mensch und Tier. *J Neurovisc Rel* [Suppl 10]: 247–255, 1971.

51. Hollwich F: *The Influence of Ocular Light Perception on Metabolism in Man and in Animal*. New York, Springer, 1979.

52. Hooper RJC, Silman RE, Leone RM, Young IM: The development of a plasma assay for 5-methoxytryptamine using gas chromatography-mass spectrometry. In Matthews CD, Seamark RF (eds): *Pineal Function*. New York, Elsevier/North Holland, 1981, pp 1–6.

53. Hurlbut EC, King TS, Richardson BA, Reiter RJ: The effects of the light:dark cycle and sympathetically-active drugs on pineal N-acetyltransferase activity and melatonin content in the Richardson's ground squirrel, *Spermophilus*

richardsonnii. In Reiter RJ (ed): *The Pineal and Its Hormones.* New York, Alan R. Liss, 1982, pp 45–56.

54. Iguchi H, Kato, Iboyashi H: Age-dependent reduction in serum melatonin concentration in healthy human subjects. *J Clin Endocrinol Metab* 55:27–29, 1982.

55. Illnervoa H, Skopkova S: Regulation of the diurnal rhythm in rat pineal serotonin *N*-acetyltransferase activity and serotonin content during ontogenesis. *J Neurochem* 26:1051–1054, 1976.

56. Jimerson DC, Lynch HJ, Post RM, Wurtman RJ, Bunney WE: Urinary melatonin rhythms during sleep deprivation in depressed patients and normals. *Life Sci* 20:1501–1507, 1977.

57. Johnson LY: The pineal gland as a modulator of the adrenal and thyroid axes. In Reiter RJ (ed): *The Pineal Gland Vol. 3 Extra-Reproductive Effects.* Boca Raton, CRC Press, 1982, pp 107–152.

58. Johnson LY, Vaughan MK, Reiter RJ: The pineal and its effects on mammalian reproduction. In Reiter RJ (ed): *The Pineal and Reproduction.* Basel, Karger, 1978, pp 116–156.

59. Johnson LY, Vaughan MK, Richardson BA, Petterborg LJ, Reiter RJ: Variation in pineal melatonin content during the estrous cycle of the rat. *Proc Soc Exp Biol Med* 169:416–419, 1982.

60. Kappers JA: The development, topographical relations and innervation of the epiphysis cerebri in the albino rat. *Z Zellforsch* 52:163–215, 1960.

61. Kebabian JW, Zatz M, Romero JA, Axelrod J: Rapid changes in rat pineal beta-adrenergic receptor. Alterations in 1-(^{3}H) alprenolol binding and adenylate cyclase. *Proc Natl Acad Sci USA* 72:3735–3739, 1975.

62. Kenneway DJ, Frith RG, Phillipou G, Matthews CD and Seamark RF: A specific radioimmunoassay for melatonin in biological tissue and fluid and its validation by gas chromatography-mass spectrometry. *Endocrinology* 101:119–127, 1977.

63. Kenneway DJ, Gilmore TA, Seamark RF: Effect of melatonin feeding on serum prolactin and gonadotrophin levels and the onset of seasonal estrous cyclicity in sheep. *Endocrinology* 110:1766–1772, 1982.

64. King TS, Richardson BA, Reiter RJ: Age-associated changes in pineal serotonin *N*-acetyltransferase activity and melatonin content in the male gerbil. *Endocrinol Res Commun* 8:253–262, 1981.

65. Klein DC, Auerback DA, Namboodiri MAA, Wheler GHT: Indole metabolism in the mammalian pineal gland. In Reiter RJ (ed): *The Pineal Gland Vol. 1 Anatomy and Physiology.* Boca Raton, CRC Press, 1981, pp 199–227.

66. Klein DC, Weller JL: Adrenergic-adenosine 3′,5′-monophosphate regulation of serotonin *N*-acetyltransferase activity and the temporal relationship of serotonin *N*-acetyltansferase activity to synthesis of ^{3}H-*N*-acetylserotonin and ^{3}H-melatonin in the cultured rat pineal gland. *J Pharmacol Exp Ther* 186:516–527, 1973.

67. Klein DC, Weller J: Indole metabolism in the pineal gland: A circadian rhythm in *N*-acetyltransferase. *Science* 169:1093–1095, 1970.

68. Kneisley LW, Moskowitz MH, Lynch HJ: Cervical spinal cord lesions disrupt the rhythm in human melatonin excretion. *J Neural Transm* [Suppl 13]:311–323, 1978.

69. Lehrer S: Fertility and menopause in blind women. *Fertil Steril* 36:396–397, 1981.

70. Lehrer S: Fertility of blind women. *Fertil Steril* 38:751–753, 1982.

71. Lenko HL, Lang U, Aubert ML, Paunier L, Sizonenko PC: Melatonin in plasma and urine before and during puberty. *Pediatr Res* 15:74–79, 1981.

72. Lerner AB, Nordlund JJ: Melatonin: Clinical pharmacology. *J Neural Transm* [Suppl 13]: 339–347, 1978.

73. Lewy AJ, Kern HA, Rosenthal NE, Wehr TA: Bright artificial light treatment of a manic-depressive patient with a seasonal mood cycle. *Am J Psychiatry* 139:1496–1498, 1982.

74. Lewy AJ: Biochemistry and regulation of mammalian melatonin production. In Relkin R (ed): *The Pineal Gland.* New York, Elsevier, 1983, pp. 77–128.

75. Lewy AJ, Tetsuo M, Markey SP, Goodwin FK, Kopin IJ: Pinealectomy abolishes plasma melatonin in the rat. *J Clin Endocrinol Metab* 50:204–205, 1980.

76. Lewy AJ, Wehr TA, Goodwin FK, Newsome DA, Markey SP: Light suppresses melatonin secretion in humans. *Science* 210:1267–1269, 1980.

77. Lipton JS, Petterborg LJ, Steinlechner S, Reiter RJ: *In vivo* responses of the pineal gland of the Syrian hamster to isoproterenol or norepinephrine. In Reiter RJ (ed): *The Pineal and Its Hormones.* New York, Alan R. Liss, 1982, pp 107–115.

78. Lipton JS, Petterborg LJ, Reiter RJ: Influence of propranolol, phenoxybenazmine of phentolamine in the in vivo nocturnal rise of pineal melatonin levels in the Syrian hamster. *Life Sci* 28:2377–2382, 1981.

79. Lynch GR, Sullivan JK, Heath HW, Tamarkin L: Daily melatonin rhythms in photoperiod sensitive and insensitive white-footed mice (*Peromyscus leucopus*). In Reiter RJ (ed): *The Pineal and Its Hormones.* New York, Alan R. Liss, 1982, pp. 67–73.

80. Lynch GR: Effect of simultaneous exposure to differences in photoperiod and temperature on the seasonal molt and reproductive system of the white-footed mouse, *Peromyscus leucopus. Comp Biochem Physiol* 53C:67–68, 1973.

81. Lynch HJ: Diurnal oscillations in pineal melatonin content. *Life Sci* 10:791–795, 1971.

82. Lynch HJ, Wang P, Wurtman RJ: Increase in rat pineal melatonin content following L-DOPA administration. *Life Sci* 12:145–151, 1973.

83. Lynch HL, Rivest RW, Ronsheim PM, Wurtman RJ: Light intensity and the control of melatonin secretion in rats. *Neuroendocrinology* 33:181–186, 1981.

84. Lynch HJ, Wurtman RJ, Moskovitz MA, Archer MC, Ho MH: Daily rhythm in human urinary melatonin. *Science* 187:169–170, 1975.

85. Magee K, Basinska J, Quarrington B, Stancer HC: Blindness and menarche. *Life Sci* 9:7–12,

1970.

86. Mata MM, Schaier BK, Klein DC, Weller JL, Chiou CY: On GABA function and physiology in the pineal gland. *Brain Res* 118:383–397, 1976.

87. Matthews CD, Kenneway DJ, Fellenberg AJG, Phillipou G, Cox LW, Seamark RF: Melatonin in man. In Birau N, Schloot W (ed): *Melatonin—Current Status and Perspectives.* New York, Pergamon, 1981, pp 371–381.

88. Matthews SA, Evans KL, Morgan WW, Petterborg LJ, Rieter RJ: Pineal indoleamine metabolism in the cotton rat, *Sigmodon hispidus*: Studies on norepinephrine, serotonin, *N*-acetyltransferase and melatonin. In Reiter RJ (ed): *The Pineal and Its Hormones.* New York, Alan R. Liss, 1982, pp 35–44.

89. McIsaac WM, Taborsky RG, Farrell G: 5-Methoxytryptophol: Effect on estrus and ovarian weight. *Science* 145:63–64, 1964.

90. McIsaac WM, Farrell G, Toborsky RG, Taylor AN: Indole compounds: Isolation from pineal tissue. *Science* 148:102–103, 1965.

91. Miller FP, Maickel RP: Fluorometric determination of indole derivatives. *Life Sci* 9:747–752, 1970.

92. Moore RY: The retinohypothalamic tract, suprachiasmatic hypothalamic nucleus and central neural mechanisms of circadian rhythm regulation. In Suda M, Hayaishi O, Nakagawa H (eds): *Biological Rhythms and Their Central Mechanisms.* Amsterdam, Elsevier/North Holland, 1979, pp. 343–354.

93. Moore RY: The innervation of the mammalian pineal gland. In Reiter RJ (ed): *The Pineal and Reproduction.* Basel, Karger, 1978, pp 1–29.

94. Mullen PE, Linsell CR, Leone RM, Silman RE, Smith I, Hooper RJC, Finnie M, Parrot J: Melatonin and 5-methoxytryptophol, and 24 hour pattern of secretion in man. In Birau N, Schloot W (eds): *Melatonin—Current Status and Perspectives.* New York, Pergamon, 1981, pp 337–343.

95. Norlund JJ, Lerner AB: Melatonin: Its effect on skin color, pituitary trophic hormones and its toxicity in human subjects. *J Clin Endocrinol Metab* 45:152–158, 1977.

96. Pang SF, Brown GM, Grota LJ, Chambers JW, Rodman RL: Determinations of *N*-acetylserotonin and melatonin activities in the pineal gland, retina, Harderian gland, brain and serum of rats and chickens. *Neuroendocrinology* 23:1–13, 1977.

97. Panke ES, Reiter RJ, Rollag MD, Panke TW: Pineal serotonin *N*-acetyltransferase activity and melatonin concentrations in prepubertal and adult Syrian hamsters exposed to short daily photoperiods. *Endocrinol Res Commun* 5:311–324, 1978.

98. Panke ES, Rollag MD, Reiter RJ: Pineal melatonin concentrations in the Syrian hamster. *Endocrinology* 104:194–197, 1979.

99. Parfitt A, Weller JL, Klein DC: Beta adrenergic-blockers decrease adrenergically stimulated *N*-acetyltransferase activity in pineal glands in organ culture. *Neuropharmacology* 15:353–358, 1976.

100. Pavel S: Arginine vasotocin as a pineal hormone. *J Neural Transm* [Suppl 13]:135–156, 1978.

101. Pelham RW, Vaughan GM, Sandock KL, Vaughan MK: Twenty-four-hour cycle of melatonin-like substance in the plasma of human males. *J Clin Endocrinol Metab* 37:341–346, 1973.

102. Perlow MJ, Reppert SM, Tamarkin L, Wyatt RJ, Klein DC: Photic regulation of the melatonin rhythm: Monkey and man are not the same. *Brain Res* 182:211–216, 1980.

103. Petterborg LJ, Reiter RJ: Effect of photoperiod and pineal indoles on the reproductive system of young female white-footed mice. *J Neural Transm* 55:149–155, 1982.

104. Petterborg LJ, Richardson BA, Reiter RJ: Effect of long or short photoperiod on pineal melatonin content in the white-footed mouse, *Peromyscus leucopus*. *Life Sci* 29:1623–1627, 1981.

105. Pevet P, Haldar-Misra C: Morning injections of large doses of melatonin, but not 5-methoxytryptamine, prevent in the hamster the antigonadotrophic effect of 5-methoxytryptamine administered late in the afternoon. *J Neural Transm* 55:85–94, 1982.

106. Plotka ED, Seal US, Verme LJ: Morphologic and metabolic consequences of pinealectomy in deer. In Reiter RJ (eds): *The Pineal Gland Vol 3, Extra-Reproductive Effects.* Boca Raton, CRC Press, 1982, pp 153–170.

107. Poth M, Tetsuo M, Markey S: Excretion patterns of 6-hydroxymelatonin in pubertal and pre-pubertal children. *Pediatr Res* 15:513–517, 1981.

108. Prozialeck WC, Boehme DH, Vogel WH: The fluorometric determination of 5-methoxytryptamine in mammalian tissues and fluid. *J Neurochem* 30:1471–1477, 1978.

109. Quay WB: Circadian rhythm in rat pineal serotonin and its modulation by estrous cycle and photoperiod. *Gen Comp Endocrinol* 3:473–479, 1963.

110. Ralph CL, Firth BT, Gern WA, Owens DW: The pineal complex and thermoregulation. *Biol Rev* 54:41–72, 197.

111. Reiter RJ: Chronobiological aspects of the pineal gland. In Mayersback HV, Scheving LE, Pauly JE (eds): *Biological Rhythms in Structure and Function.* New York, Alan R. Liss, 1981, pp 223–333.

112. Reiter RJ: The mammalian pineal gland: Structure and function. *Am J Anat* 162:287–313, 1981.

113. Reiter RJ: Morphological studies on the reproductive organs of blinded male hamsters and the effects of pinealectomy or superior cervical ganglionectomy. *Anat Rec* 160:13–24, 1968.

114. Reiter RJ: Evidence for refractoriness of the pituitary-gonadal axis to the pineal gland in golden hamsters and its possible implications in annual reproductive rhythms. *Anat Rec* 173:365–372, 1975.

115. Reiter RJ: Comparative physiology: Pineal gland. *Ann Rev Physiol* 35:305–328, 1973.

116. Reiter RJ, Golovko V: Failure of duration of inbreeding to influence the rate of pineal-induced gonadal regression in short day exposed Syrian hamsters. *Arch Androl* 10:39–44, 1982.

117. Reiter RJ: Circannual reproductive rhythms in mammals related to photoperiod and pineal function: A review. *Chronobiologia* 1:365–395, 1974.

118. Reiter RJ: The pineal and its hormones in the control of reproduction in mammals. *Endocrine Rev* 1:109–131, 1980.

119. Reiter RJ, Rudeen PK, Sackman JW, Vaughan MK, Johnson LY, Little JC: Subcutaneous melatonin implants inhibit reproductive atrophy in male hamsters induced by daily melatonin injections. *Endocrinol Res Comm* 4:35–44, 1977.

120. Reiter RJ, Hester RJ: Interrelationships of the pineal gland, the superior cervical ganglia and the photoperiod in regulation of the endocrine systems of hamsters. *Endocrinology* 79:1168–1170, 1966.

121. Reiter RJ, Craft CM, Johnson JE Jr, King TS, Richardson BA, Vaughan GM, Vaughan MK: Age-associated reduction in nocturnal pineal melatonin levels in female rats. *Endocrinology* 109:1295–1297, 1981.

122. Reiter RJ, Vriend J, Brainard GC, Matthews SA, Craft CM: Reduced pineal and plasma melatonin levels and gonadal atrophy in old hamsters kept under winter photoperiods. *Exp Aging Res* 8:27–30, 1982.

123. Reiter RJ, Johnson LY: Pineal regulation of immunoreactive luteinizing hormone and prolactin in light-deprived female hamsters. *Fertil Steril* 25:958–964, 1974.

124. Reiter RJ: Pineal function in long term blinded male and female golden hamsters. *Gen Comp Endocr* 12:460–468, 1969.

125. Reiter RJ, Johnson LY: Depressant action of the pineal gland, the superior cervical ganglia and the photoperiod on pituitary luteinizing hormone and prolactin in male hamsters. *Horm Res* 5:311–320, 1974.

126. Reiter RJ, Rollag MD, Panke ES, Banks AF: Melatonin: Reproductive effects. *J Neural Transm* [Suppl 13]:209–224, 1978.

127. Reiter RJ, King TS, Richardson BA, Hurlbut EC: Studies on pineal melatonin levels in a diurnal species, the eastern chipmunk (*Tamias striatus*): Effects of light at night, propranolol administration of superior cervical ganglionectomy. *J Neural Transm* 54:275–284, 1982a.

128. Reiter RJ: Changes in the reproductive organs of cold-exposed and light-deprived female hamsters. *J Reprod Fertil* 16:217–222, 1968.

129. Reiter RJ: Interactions of the photoperiod, pineal and seasonal reproduction as exemplified by findings in the hamster. In Reiter RJ (ed): *The Pineal and Reproduction*. Basel, Karger, 1978, pp 169–190.

130. Reiter RJ, Richardson BA, Matthews SA, Lane SJ, Ferguson BN: Rhythms in immunoreactive melatonin in the retina and Harderian gland of rats: Persistence after pinealectomy. *Life Sci* 32:1229–1236, 1983.

131. Reiter RJ, Steinlechner S, Richardson BA, King TS: Differential response of pineal melatonin levels to light at night in laboratory-raised and wild-captured 13-lined ground squirrels (*Spermophilus tridecemlineatus*). *Life Sci*, in press.

132. Reiter RJ, King TS, Richardson BA, Hurlbut EC, Karasek MA, Hansen JT: Failure of room light to inhibit pineal *N*-acetyltransferase activity and melatonin content in a diurnal species, the Eastern chipmunk (*Tamias striatus*). *Neuroendocrinol Lett* 4:1–6, 1982b.

133. Reiter RJ: The effect of pinealectomy, pineal grafts and denervation of the pineal gland on the reproductive organs of male hamsters. *Neuroendocrinology* 2:138–146, 1967.

134. Reiter RJ: Influence of pinealectomy on the breeding capability of hamsters maintained under natural photoperiod and temperature conditions. *Neuroendocrinology* 13:366–370, 1973/74.

135. Reiter RJ, Blask DE, Johnson LY, Rudeen PK, Vaughan MK, Waring PJ: Melatonin inhibition of reproduction in the male hamster: Its dependency on time of day of administration and on an intact and sympathetically innervated pineal gland. *Neuroendocrinology* 22:107–116, 1976.

136. Reiter RJ, Richardson BA, Hurlbut EC: Pineal, retinal and Harderian gland melatonin in a diurnal species, the Richardson's ground squirrel (*Spermophilus richardsonii*). *Neurosci Lett* 22:285–288, 1981.

137. Reiter RJ, Johnson LY, Steger RW, Richardson BA, Petterborg LJ: Pineal biosynthetic activity and neuroendocrine physiology in the aging hamster and gerbil. *Peptides* 1(1):69–77, 1980.

138. Reiter RJ: Reproductive effects of the pineal gland and pineal indoles in the Syrian hamster and the ablino rat. In Reiter RJ (ed): *The Pineal Gland, Vol 2, Reproductive Effects*. Boca Raton, CRC Press, 1982, pp 45–82.

139. Reiter RJ: Reproductive involution in male hamsters exposed to naturally increasing daylengths after the winter solstice. *Proc Soc Exp Biol Med* 163:264–266, 1980.

140. Reiter RJ: The pineal gland: A regulator of regulators. *Prog Psychobiol Physiol Psychol* 9:323–356, 1980.

141. Reiter RJ: Neuroendocrine effects of the pineal gland and of melatonin. In Ganong WF, Martini L (eds): *Frontiers in Neuroendocrinology, Vol 7*. New York, Raven, 1982, pp 278–316.

142. Reiter RJ, Vaughan MK, Blask DE, Johnson LY: Melatonin: Its inhibition of pineal antigonadotrophic activity in male hamsters. *Science* 185:1169–1171, 1974.

143. Reiter RJ, Richardson BA, Johnson LY, Ferguson BN, Dinh DT: Pineal melatonin rhythm: Reduction in aging Syrian hamsters. *Science* 210:1372–1373, 1980.

144. Reiter RJ, Hurlbut EC, Richardson BA, King TS, Wang LCH: Studies on the regulation of pineal melatonin production in the Richardson's ground squirrel (*Spermophilus richardsonii*). In Reiter RJ (ed): *The Pineal and Its Hormones*. New York, Alan R. Liss, 1982, pp 57–65.

145. Reither RJ: Pineal interaction with the central nervous systrem. *Waking Sleeping* 1:253–258, 1977.

146. Relkin R: Pineal-hormonal interactions. In Relkin R (ed): *The Pineal Gland*. New York, Elsevier, 1983, pp 225–246.

147. Rivest RW, Lynch HJ, Ronsheim PM, Wurtman

RJ: Effect of light intensity on regulation of melatonin secretion and drinking behavior in the albino rat. In Birau N, Schloot W (eds): *Melatonin–Current Status and Perspectives.* New York, Pergamon, 1981, pp 119–121.

148. Rollag MD, Stetson MH: Ontogeny of the pineal melatonin rhythm in golden hamsters. *Biol. Reprod* 24:311–314, 1981.

149. Rollag MD, Chen JH, Ferguson BN, Reiter RJ: Pineal melatonin content throughout the hamster estrous cycle. *Proc Soc Exp Biol Med* 160:211–213, 1979.

150. Rollag MD, Panke ES, Reiter RJ: Pineal melatonin content in male hamsters throughout the seasonal reproductive cycle. *Proc Soc Exp Biol Med* 165:330–334, 1980.

151. Rollag MD, Stetson MH: Melatonin injection into Syrian hamsters. In Reiter RJ (ed): *The Pineal and Its Hormones.* New York, Alan R. Liss, 1982, pp 143–151.

152. Romero JA, Alexrod J: Regulation of sensitivity to beta-adrenergic stimulation in induction of pineal *N*-acetyltransferase. *Proc Natl Acad Sci USA* 72:1661–1665, 1975.

153. Rudeen PK, Reiter RJ, Vaughan MK: Pineal serotonin-*N*-acetyltransferase in four mammalian species. *Neurosci Lett* 1:225–229, 1975.

154. Rusak B: Circadian organization in mammals and birds: Role of the pineal gland. In Reiter RJ (ed): *The Pineal Gland, Vol 3 Extra-Reproductive Effects.* Boca Raton, CRC Press, 1982, pp 27–52.

155. Seegal RF, Goldman BD: Effects of photoperiod on cyclicity and serum gonadotrophins in the Syrian hamster. *Biol Reprod* 12:223–231, 1975.

156. Silman RE, Leone RM, Hooper RJL, Preece MA: Melatonin, the pineal gland and human puberty. *Nature* 282:301–303, 1979.

157. Sizonenko PC, Moore DC, Pauneir L, Beaumonoir A, Nahory A: Melatonin secretion in relation to sleep in epileptics. *Prog Brain Res* 52:549–551, 1979.

158. Smith JA, Mee TJ, Padwick DP, Spokes EG: Human post mortem pineal enzyme activity. *Clin Endocrinol* 14:75–81, 1981.

159. Smith JA: The biochemistry and pharmacology of melatonin. In Birau N, Schloot W (eds): *Melatonin—Current Status and Perspectives.* New York, Pergamon, 1981, pp 135–147.

160. Snyder SH, Axelrod J: A sensitive assay for 5-hydroxytryptophan decarboxylase. *Biochem Pharmacol* 13:805–806, 1964.

161. Tamarkin L, Hutchinson JS, Goldman BD: Regulation of serum gonadotropins by photoperiod and testicular hormone in the Syrian hamster. *Endocrinology* 99:1528–1533, 1976.

162. Tamarkin L, Westrom WK, Hamill AI, Goldman BD: Effect of melatonin on the reproductive system of male and female Syrian hamsters: A diurnal rhythm in sensitivity to melatonin. *Endocrinology* 99:1534–1541, 1976.

163. Tarmarkin, L, Reppert SM, Klein DC: Regulation of pineal melatonin in the Syrian hamster. *Endocrinology* 104:385–389, 1979.

164. Tapp E. The pineal gland in malignancy. In Reiter RJ (ed): *The Pineal Gland, Vol 3 Extra-Reproductive Effects.* Boca Raton, CRC Press, 1982, pp 171–188.

165. Tetsuo M, Polinsky RJ, Markey SP, Kopin IJ: Urinary 6-hydroxymelatonin excretion in patients with orthostatic hypotension. *J Clin Endocrinol Metab* 53:607–610, 1981.

166. Thomas JB, Pizzarello PJ: Blindness, biologic rhythms, and menarche. *Obst Gynec* 30:507–509, 1967.

167. Timonen S, Franzas B, Wichman K: Photosensibility of the human pituitary. *Ann Chir Gynaec Fenn* 53:165–172, 1964.

168. Timonen S, Carpen E: Multiple pregnancies and photoperiodicity. *Ann Chir Gynaec Fenn* 57:135–138, 1968.

169. Turek FW, Alvis JD, Elliott JA, Menaker M: Temporal distribution of serum levels of LH and FSH in adult male golden hamsters exposed to long or short days. *Biol Reprod* 14:630–637, 1976.

170. Vaughan GM, Pelham RW, Pang SF, Laughlin LL, Wilson KM, Sandock KL, Vaughan MK, Koslow SH, Reiter RJ: Nocturnal elevation of plasma melatonin and urinary 5-hydroxyindole acetic acid: Attempts at modification by brief changes in environmental lighting and sleep and by autonomic drugs. *J Clin Endocrinol Metab* 42:752–754, 1976.

171. Vaughan GM, Allen JP, Tullis W, Siler-Khodr TM, de la Pena A, Sackman JW: Overnight plasma profiles of melatonin and certain adenohypophyseal hormones in man. *J Clin Endocrinol Metab* 47:566–572, 1978.

172. Vaughan GM, McDonald SA, Bell R, Stevens EA: Melatonin, pituitary function and stress in humans. *Psychoneuroendocrinology* 4:351–362, 1979.

173. Vaughan GM, Meyer CG, Reiter RJ: Evidence for a pineal-induced relationship in the human. In Reiter RJ (ed): *The Pineal and Reproduction.* Basel, Karger, 1978, pp 191–223.

174. Vaughan GM, Allen J, de la Pena A: Rapid melatonin transients. *Waking Sleeping* 3:169–179, 1979.

175. Vaughan MK, Reiter RJ, Vaughan GM, Bigelow L, Altschule MD: Inhibition of compensatory ovarian hypertrophy in the mouse and vole: A comparison of Altschule's pineal extract, pineal indoles, vasopressin, and oxytocin. *Gen Comp Endocrinol* 18:372–377, 1972.

176. Vaughan MK: The pineal gland—A survey of its antigonadotrophic substances and their actions. In McCann SM (ed): *International Review of Physiology, Vol 24 Endocrine Physiology III.* Baltimore, University Park, 1981, pp 41–95.

177. Vaughan MK, Vaughan GM, Klein DC: Arginine vasotocin: Effect on development of reproductive organs. *Science* 186:938–939, 1974.

178. Vriend J: Evidence for pineal gland modulation of the neuroendocrine-thyroid axis. *Neuroendocrinology* 36:67–78, 1983.

179. Wainwright SD: Role of the pineal gland in the vertebrate master biological clock. In Reiter RJ (ed): *The Pineal Gland, Vol 3 Extra-Reproductive Effects.* Boca Raton, CRC Press, 1982, pp 53–80.

180. Wallen EP, Jachim JM: Rhythm function of pineal hydroxyindole-*O*-methyltransferase during the estrous cycle: An analysis. *Biol Reprod* 10:461–466, 1974.

181. Weinberg U, D'Eletto RD, Weitzman ED, Erlich

S, Hollander CS: Circulating melatonin in man: Episodic secretion throughout the light-dark cycle. *J Clin Endocrinol Metab* 48:114–118, 1979.

182. Weinberg U, Weitzman ED, Fukushima DK, Cancel GF, Rosenfeld RS: Melatonin does not suppress the pituitary luteinizing hormone response to luteinizing hormone-releasing hormone in men. *J Clin Endocrinol Metab* 51:161–162, 1980.

183. Weissbach H, Redfield BG, Axelrod J: Biosynthesis of melatonin: Enzymic conversion of serotonin to *N*-acetylserotonin. *Biochim Biophys Acta* 43:352–353, 1960.

184. Wetterberg L, Arendt J, Paunier L, Sizonenko PC, van Donselaar W, Heyden T: Human serum melatonin changes during the menstrual cycle. *J Clin Endocrinol Metab* 42:185–188, 1976.

185. Wetterberg L: Melatonin in humans. Physiological and clinical studies. *J Neural Transm* [Suppl 13]:289–310, 1978.

186. Wheeler GHT, Weller JL, Klein DC: Taurine: Stimulation of pineal *N*-acetyltransferase activity and melatonin production via a β-adrenergic mechanism. *Brain Res* 166:65–74, 1979.

187. Wilkinson M, Ardendt J, Bradtke J, de Ziegler D: Determination of a dark-induced increase in pineal *N*-acetyltransferase activity and simultaneous radioimmunoassay of melatonin in pineal, serum and pituitary tissue of the male rat. *J Endocrinol* 72:243–244, 1977.

188. Wilson BW, Lynch JH, Ozaki Y: 5-methoxytryptophol in rat serum and pineal: Detection, quantitation, and evidence for daily rhythmicity. *Life Sci* 23:1019–1024, 1978.

189. Wurtman RJ, Ozaki Y: Physiological control of melatonin synthesis and secretion: Mechanisms generating rhythms in melatonin, methoxytryptophol, and arginine vasotocin levels and effects of the pineal of endogenous catecholamines, the estrous cycle, and environmental lighting. *J Neural Transm* [Suppl 13], 1978, pp 59–70.

190. Wurtman RJ, Shein HM, Larin F: Mediation by beta-adrenergic receptors of effect of norepinephrine on pineal synthesis of ^{14}C-serotonin and ^{14}C-melatonin. *J Neurochem* 18:1683–1687, 1971.

191. Young IM, Silman RE: Pineal methoxyindoles in the human. In Reiter RJ (ed): *The Pineal Gland, Vol 3, Extra-Reproductive Effects.* 1982, pp 189–218.

192. Yuwiler A, Klein DC, Buda M, Weller JL: Adrenergic control of pineal *N*-acetyltransferase activity: Developmental aspects. *Am J Physiol* 233:E141–E146, 1977.

193. Zacharias L, Wurtman RJ: Blindness and menarche. *Obst Gynec* 33:603–608, 1969.

194. Zatz M: The role of cyclic nucleotides in the pineal gland. *Hdb Exp Pharmacol* 58:691–710, 1982.

195. Zatz M, Kebabian JW, Romero JA, Lefkowitz RJ, Alexrod J: Pineal adrenergic receptor: Correlation of binding of ^{3}H-alprenolol with stimulation of adenylate cyclase. *J Pharmacol Exp Ther* 196:714–722, 1976.

196. Zatz M: Pharmacology of the rat pineal gland. In Reiter RJ (ed): *The Pineal Gland, Vol 1 Anatomy and Biochemistry.* Boca Raton, CRC Press, 1981, pp 229–242.

197. Zucker I, Johnston PG, Frost D: Comparative, physiological and biochronometric.analyses of rodent seasonal reproductive cycles. In Reiter RJ, Follett BK (eds): *Seasonal Reproduction in Higher Vertebrates.* Basel, Karger, 1980, pp 102–133.

CHAPTER 5

Neuro-Ophthalmology of Pineal Tumors

WILLIAM T. SHULTS, M.D.

INTRODUCTION

Eye symptoms are usually a prominent complaint of patients with pineal tumors. The anatomic proximity of the pineal body to the ocular motor and pupillary control centers of the pretectum accounts for this frequent association and for the occurrence of ocular symptoms as one of the earliest manifestations of such neoplasms. Accordingly, an understanding of the variety of ocular complaints, their clinical manifestations, and basic pathophysiology is important in timely diagnosis of such lesions. This chapter will emphasize the common neuro-ophthalmic symptoms and signs of patients with pineal region tumors (Tables 5.1 and 5.2) and the examination techniques most appropriate to define each abnormality at the earliest point in its evolution.

NEURO-OPHTHALMIC SYMPTOMS

Accomodative Deficiency

Impairment of accomodation is often an early symptom of patients with pretectal involvement from pineal tumors. Though usually accompanied by impairment of pupillary reactivity to light, Walsh and Hoyt (45, 46) report accommodation difficulty predating pupillary involvement by a period of weeks. Such patients will note problems with blurring of near work and will necessarily increase their reading distance to compensate. A history of such difficulties in a patient in the pre-presbyopic age group or a rapid loss of accommodation in a presbyopic patient can be a clue to midbrain mischief.

Reading Difficulty

Quite apart from the accommodation problems noted above, the abberations of ocular motility seen in Parinaud's syndrome (see below) can produce marked difficulty with reading.

Though often not expressed succinctly by patients, the impairment of ocular motility producing their reading difficulty is quite distressing to them. Normally, the eyes make a series of conjugate saccades (rapid eye movements) in following a line of print. The superimposed convergent movements often evoked by each saccade in Parinaud's syndrome impede the normally facile ocular scanning needed for reading (26). Though such eye movement problems may intrude into other situations (such as watching moving equipment like conveyor belts), reading is the activity most often cited by patients as evoking the problem.

Diplopia

The particularly distressing symptom of double vision resulting from misalignment of the eyes accompanies palsies of the ocular motor nerves (III, IV, and VI) is sometimes seen in patients with pineal tumors. Depending on which ocular muscles are affected, the images may be separated horizontally, vertically, or obliquely. Involvement of innervation to the superior or inferior oblique muscles produces torsion of one of the pair of vertically separated images. A similar type of diplopia is often seen in patients with skew deviation (vertical divergence of the eyes not explicable on the basis of paresis of an ocular motor nerve), an ocular dysconjugacy sometimes seen in patients with pineal tumors (1, 30, 48).

Gaze Palsy

Though in their pure form, gaze palsies are unaccompanied by diplopia, they can still produce problems for patients. Loss of downward gaze, while not as common as upward gaze palsy in patients with pineal tumors, is a more bothersome impediment because of the frequency of

Table 5.1
Eye Symptoms with Pineal Region Tumors

1) Accommodative deficiency
2) Reading difficulty (secondary to saccadic abnormalities)
3) Diplopia
4) Gaze palsy: upgaze
                downgaze
                pseudo-abducens palsy
5) Field defects: bitemporal hemianopic scotomas

Table 5.2
Eye Signs with Pineal Region Tumors

Most common:
  Pupillary light/near dissociation
  Upgaze palsy
  Convergence/retraction nystagmus
  Papilledema
  Skew deviation
Less common:
  Decreased accommodation
  Convergence paresis
  Downgaze palsy
  Third, fourth, and sixth nerve palsies
  Optic atrophy

needing to read with the eyes in a downward direction. Thus, patients are more likely to report this difficulty to a physician than the more common upward gaze deficiency. However, pilots, or others whose occupations call for upward gaze, will commonly strongly complain of the need to constantly tilt their heads backward to perform their duties. Patients with upgaze paresis may also be noted by other family members to carry their heads with a slight backward tilt and to exhibit mild lid retraction. Though obvious to others, patients may be unaware of such alterations of posture and lid position. Inquiry about such changes in appearance of other family members may gain a positive response even though the patient denies any problems.

Visual Field Disturbance

Downward pressure by a pineal tumor on the aqueduct can produce hydrocephalus with consequent third ventricular enlargement and compression of the posterior chiasmal notch (46). Though distinctly uncommon, such a chain of events can produce bitemporal paracentral scotomas sufficient in magnitude to prompt patients to seek professional attention. Such a field finding in a patient with light-near dissociation of the pupils should prompt consideration of a problem in the midbrain.

NEURO-OPHTHALMIC SIGNS AND EXAMINATION TECHNIQUES

Gaze Palsies

The most prominent neuro-ophthalmic sign of pineal region tumors is vertical gaze palsy (Fig. 5.1). Upgaze palsy is far the more common

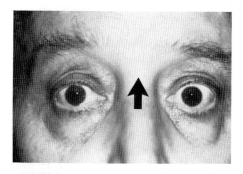
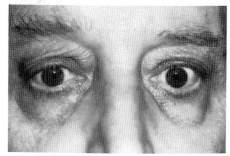
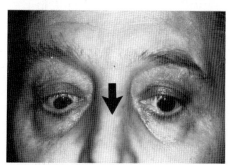

Figure 5.1.   Patient with Sylvian aqueduct syndrome exhibiting intact downgaze, impaired upgaze, lid retraction (Collier's sign) and fixed midposition pupils. Nystagmus retractorius was present with upward saccades. *Arrow* indicates direction of gaze.

gaze disturbance, though downgaze will occassionally be affected late in the course in a few patients (10). In its early evolution, upgaze palsy may only be manifested on attempted upward saccades, the patient being unable to rapidly bring his eyes above the horizontal. At this early stage, smooth pursuit and vertical vestibulo-occular movements may appear to be clinically normal. Bell's phenomenon may be preserved. This brings up an important point in testing techniques. It is best to ask the patient to shift his eyes between two fixed targets placed vertically separated in front of him. Often one target must be placed below the horizontal and the other in primary position as a patient with a complete upgaze palsy will be unable to initiate any vertical movement if the initially viewed target is already placed at the spacial limit of his upgaze capacity. As he attempts to shift his gaze from the lower to the higher target, the eyes will demonstrate the upgaze impairment so characteristic of patients with pineal tumors. The impairment of upgaze so evoked will almost invariably be accompanied by a rapid horizontal wobbling of the eyes, usually with a slight convergence bias superimposed. The eyes may also exhibit mild to moderate retraction into the orbits (nystagmus retractorius) (6, 13, 42) as the attempt at making upward saccades is made.

If the usual method of asking the patient to follow a relatively slowly moving finger in an upward direction is employed, the above-described ocular dyskinesia may be totally absent, the patient making clinically normal vertical pursuit movements. An opportunity will have been missed to detect the subtle early eye movement disturbance of midbrain compression.

Because it evokes a series of upward saccades, the use of a downward-moving optokinetic strip or drum is often employed to elicit the upgaze disturbances produced by pinealomas (42, 48). This is a useful technique, though I have personally found the elicitation of single upward saccades of moderate amplitude to be more useful in permitting the examiner to identify the upgaze palsy and its attendent convergent "wobble." This ocular motor pattern is virtually pathognomonic for midbrain peri-aqueductal involvement.

As gaze palsy worsens, pursuit as well as saccadic function becomes impaired and all vertical eye movement in an upward direction may be lost. As previously mentioned, downward gaze may ultimately be affected as well (46).

As noted above, convergent eye movements often accompany attempts at making vertical upgaze saccades in patients with the so-called Sylvian aqueduct syndrome (7). In general usage, the terms Sylvian aqueduct syndrome, Parinaud's syndrome, Koeber-Salus-Elschnig syndrome, dorsal midbrain syndrome, and peri-aqueductal syndrome are interchangeable and are so used in this chapter. Initially, these movements are noted only with attempted upgaze, but with tumor progression, such bilateral adduction bias may be superimposed upon horizontal as well as vertical saccades resulting in an unusual horizontal dysconjugacy of ocular motility which has been labeled "pseudo-abducens palsy" (10).

In this circumstance, an attempt at making a horizontal saccade in one direction evokes coincident opposed adducting movements of the eyes which are added to the horizontal saccadic movements of the two eyes. Thus the abducting eye is slowed by coincident opposed adductive movement in the opposite direction and the adducting eye overshoots the target because of a coincident adduction saccade in the same direction. The net result is a slowing of the abducting eye evoked by a horizontal eye movement in the direction of the abducting eye, hence the term pseudo-abducens palsy (26). As one might imagine, such a disruption of the normal innervation pattern for conjugate eye movement is often accompanied by major patient complaints of being "unable to see clearly" when reading. Though this complex of disordered ocular motor function has been termed convergence-retraction nystagmus, recent work has suggested that the clinical picture is produced by opposed adducting saccades rather than convergence movements per se (26).

It is important to realize that the distinctive and virtually pathognomonic rapid convergent swimming or wobbling eye movements seen with attempted vertical and horizontal saccades in the Sylvian aqueduct syndrome may be present before the development of any major symptoms or signs of upgaze difficulty. This fact should prompt careful attention to the search for such tell-tale findings when midbrain disease is suspected.

Recent work on the anatomical substrate and neurophysiological correlates of the vertical gaze palsy seen in the Sylvian aqueduct syndrome is briefly reviewed later in this chapter (3, 4, 22, 26, 40, 41).

Palsies of Ocular Motor Nerves and Skew Deviation

The third nerve nuclei are subject to direct involvement by tumor invasion into the zone ventral to the aqueduct. Though an uncommon event in some series (46), in a recent report by Abay and co-workers (1), 10 of 27 youthful patients with pineal tumors had paresis of the oculomotor nerve. Less common, despite an anatomical exit zone at the dorsal midbrain, is trochlear nerve paresis. Though not directly involved by pineal tumors at a nuclear level, the abducens nerves can be indirectly affected because of increased intracranial pressure which results from tumor-induced aqueductal stenosis. Though Posner and Horrax (31) report an incidence of 25% for abducens nerve paresis, more recent series suggest an occurrence rate close to 10% (1, 48), perhaps reflecting earlier diagnosis.

Skew deviation may be one of the neuroophthalmic consequences of tumors in the region of the pineal gland. Defined as a vertical ocular divergence of supranuclear origin, skew deviation may be of several varieties (41) and is occasionally difficult to distinguish from single vertical muscle weakness. Though generally implying brainstem or cerebellar involvement (15, 20), it has no tightly localizing value. Sanders and Bird (34) reported a skew deviation in 3 of 10 patients with pinealoma.

Convergence Palsy

While part of the original triad of signs described by Parinaud (27, 28) (along with vertical gaze paresis and light-near dissociation of the pupils), convergence palsy is an uncommon accompaniment of pinealomas. Patients manifesting a failure of convergence will develop diplopia at near with failure of the eyes to converge on a near target. The preservation of conjugate horizontal eye movements establishes the intact function of the medial rectus muscles. In checking a patient's convergence, it is helpful to instruct him to fixate on his own finger rather than some other target. Such a request will sometimes evoke convergence when the use of other targets fail.

Abnormalities of Lid Position

As mentioned previously, patients with pinealoma may not notice alterations of lid position, particularly when subtle, but lid retraction is an occasional accompaniment of the midbrain dysfunction seen in such patients (8). The normal position of the upper lid in a young child is usually at the corneo-scleral limbus. As aging occurs, the normal lid position descends to cover the limbus by 1–2 mm. Lid retraction is present if one sees sclera between the lid margin and the limbus. Some patients with pineal tumors will exhibit such a sign when their eyes are in primary position or on attempted upgaze.

Even rarer is the occurence of ptosis which receives passing mention in Walsh and Hoyt's text (46), but was not seen by Wray in her extensive review of the Massachusetts General Hospital experience (49). The levator subnucleus is an unpaired midline structure at the caudal end of the third nerve nuclear complex supplying both levator palpebrae muscles. Selective involvement of this structure with consequent midbrain ptosis has been described with vascular and metastatic lesions (14, 43). The mass effect of an expanding posterior third ventricular lesion is probably too gross to selectively involve only this subunit of the oculomotor complex without also involving both third and fourth cranial nerves as well.

Pupillary Abnormalities

Impairment of normal pupillary function is an extremely common finding with tumors in the pineal region. Generally the pupil is neither miotic nor widely dilated, but rather moderately dilated and very poorly reactive or nonreactive to light stimuli. The pupillary response to near is usually clinically normal or nearly so. While meeting the definition of light-near dissociation, such pupils differ from the classical Argyll-Robertson pupil in not exhibiting miosis and in retention of a response to atropine. Seybold et al (38) studied the pupils of eight patients with pineal region tumors using infrared pupillography, a technique which allows precise monitoring and recording of pupil size. With this sensitive technique deficiencies of both light and near response were definable in all but one patient, though the light response was generally the more impaired. One of Lowenstein's patients exhibited alternating contraction anisocoria (23) (pupil in directly stimulated eye exhibits greater degree of constriction than consensual pupil), and since this patient also exhibited the least degree of impairment of pupillary dysfunction, they proposed that such a finding may presage more profound pupillary abnormality.

In 1906, Wilson (48) described three patients (one with a probable colloid cyst of the third ventricle) who exhibited an unusual pupillary abnormality consisting of episodic corectopia (eccentrically placed pupil) which he attributed to midbrain involvement. Seventy years later, similar observations were reported by Selhorst and collegues (37) in a patient with bilateral rostral midbrain infarcts. They proposed central inhibition of iris sphincter tone in the presence of a paralyzed dilator muscle as the most plausible explanation. Such observations would only be made by careful clinicians who are asking the appropriate clinical questions. Though such a pupillary sign has not been reported with pineal tumors it has likely been overlooked amongst the more striking neuro-ophthalmic manifestations.

Walsh and Hoyt (46) report loss of the pupillary light response as the initial sign of a pineal tumor, antedating upgaze disturbance by several weeks. In several other patients, accomodative spasm with induced myopia antedated even the impairment of pupillary light response. Clearly, careful attention to the pupils can prove to be a very helpful adjunct in the early diagnosis of tumor of the pineal region.

The pupils should be examined in a semi-darkened room with just enough light being shined in from below to permit visualization of pupil size, shape and location in the iris. The patient should be instructed to fixate on a distant target to control accomodative constriction. Some assessment of the speed and extent of the pupil reaction to both direct and consensual testing will allow the examiner to pick up alternating contraction anisocoria. The use of a dim light for testing of the light response may extend one's ability to detect light response defects though the clinical validity and reproducibility of this extrapolation from pupillography research remains unproven. Assessment of pupil size in room illumination and at near should also be accomplished. Assessment of the near point of accommodation (minimum distance from patient at which blurring of near target occurs) will assist in detecting early accomodative difficulties.

Funduscopic Abnormalities

Because increased intracranial pressure is an early effect of most pineal tumors, papilledema is a very common physical finding being noted in about half the patients in most series (1, 30,

48). The degree of disc swelling is often profound in patients with pinealomas. Initially asymptomatic, patients with papilledema may experience transient visual obscurations in both eyes lasting for a few seconds. Such episodes may be of highly variable frequency and do not correlate with visual prognosis (9). Occasional patients will develop such profound enlargement of the blind spot that tangent screen examination may yield a pseudo-bitemporal hemianopsia picture. If papilledema is allowed to persist, optic atrophy will eventually occur with attendant loss of both central and peripheral field. As axons die, disc swelling will diminish leaving an atrophic and gliotic nerve head in an eye with profound loss of visual field and acuity.

Space does not permit an elaborate description of the funduscopic abnormalities which evolve during the development of papilledema from its earliest through its most fully developed stage. Miller (24) should be consulted for a discussion of these points.

NEURO-OPHTHALMIC SIGNS OF SUPRASELLAR GERMINOMAS

Germinomas, the commonest form of tumor occurring in the pineal region (32), may also arise in the region of optic chiasm and infundibulum (18, 19). Such tumors are often referred to as "ectopic pinealomas" (17). Diabetes insipidus, hypopituitarism, and visual field defects are the hallmark of such lesions. Given their location, germinomas in the suprasellar region can produce a variety of visual field defects ranging from monocular visual loss to total bilateral blindness though the bitemporal loss so typical of chiasmal involvement is probably the most common (16). Because direct compression and/or invasion of the anterior visual pathway occurs with these tumors, optic atrophy commonly accompanies visual field loss.

A child with vision loss and diabetes insipidus merits careful attention to the region of the anterior third ventricle and infundibulum (35). High resolution thin-section computerized tomography with metrizamide cisternography may be necessary to delineate the anatomy of such lesions. Coronal and sagittal reconstructed images are very helpful in this regard.

Though palsies of the ocular motor nerves are uncommon with ectopic pinealomas, such an event has been reported with invasion of the sella and cavernous sinus by germinoma (39).

PATHOPHYSIOLOGY OF THE SYLVIAN AQUEDUCT SYNDROME

Though the Sylvian aqueduct syndrome was described in the late 1800's and early 1900's (11, 21, 27, 28, 33), it wasn't until the past few years that our understanding of its pertinent anatomy and neurophysiology began to crystallize. The pretectum, defined as a zone located between the thalamus and midbrain (29), has long been known to contain structures mediating vertical eye movements (Fig. 5.2). In addition, it was known that bilateral paramedian pontine reticular formation lesions produced vertical gaze paralysis accompanied by bilateral horizontal gaze paralysis (3). The interrelationship of the various pretectal nuclear groupings and the pon-

tine paramedian reticular formation was unclear, as was the role of the various pretectal nuclei in the production of vertical eye movements. As case studies of finite vascular lesions affecting the midbrain and pretectal region accumulated (2, 4, 5, 25, 40, 44), certain facts became clearer. Structures controlling upgaze were anatomically separate from those controlling downgaze. A unilateral lesion could produce loss of upgaze if it involved the posterior commissure or its nuclei (4, 25, 36, 40), while downgaze paralysis required bilateral lesions.

Büttner-Ennever et al (4), following a careful review of lesion studies in animals and previously reported post mortem studies in humans, concluded that destruction of the rostral interstitial nucleus of the medial longitudinal fascic-

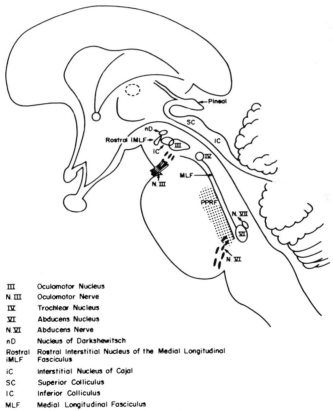

III	Oculomotor Nucleus
N. III	Oculomotor Nerve
IV	Trochlear Nucleus
VI	Abducens Nucleus
N.VI	Abducens Nerve
nD	Nucleus of Darkshewitsch
Rostral iMLF	Rostral Interstitial Nucleus of the Medial Longitudinal Fasciculus
iC	Interstitial Nucleus of Cajal
SC	Superior Colliculus
IC	Inferior Colliculus
MLF	Medial Longitudinal Fasciculus

Figure 5.2. A sagittal section through brainstem shows the relationship of the structures involved in control of vertical eye movements and their relationship to the pineal gland. The shaded area represents the pontine paramedian reticular formation (PPRF). *III*: oculomotor nucleus; *IV*: trochlear nucleus; *VI*: abducens nucleus; *iC*: interstitial nucleus of Cajal; *N VII*: facial nerve; *nD*: nucleus of Darkschewitsch; *sc*: superior colliculus; *ic*: inferior colliculus; *MLF*: Medial longitudinal fasciculus; *rostral iMLF*: rostral interstitial nucleus of the medial longitudinal fasciculus (Modified from Büttner-Ennever, VA: Organization of reticular projections onto oculomotor neurons. *Prog Brain Res* 50:619, 1979).

ulus (riMLF) located dorsomedial to the anterior pole of the red nucleus, rostral to the interstitial nucleus of Cajal, and lateral to the nucleus of Darkschewitsch leads to impairment of vertical saccadic eye movements. This nucleus seemingly participates in the direct premotor control of fast vertical eye movements. It receives input from the pontine paramedian reticular formation (PPRF) and projects primarily to the ipsilateral oculomotor complex. Loss of vertical gaze with bilateral PPRF lesions implies a role for the pontine reticular formation in the genesis of vertical eye movements. The expected connections between the pontine reticular formation and the riMLF have been demonstrated (4), the riMLF being the only part of the midbrain to receive strong input from the PPRF. Lesions in the region of the riMLF affect all types of fast vertical eye movement but spare vestibularly-induced ocular movements implying that signals controlling such movements reach the oculomotor nuclei through another route.

Pierrot-Deseilligny et al (30) came to similar conclusions regarding the importance of the rostral interstitial nucleus of the medial longitudinal fasciculus in Parinaud's syndrome when they reported an electro-oculographic and anatomical analysis of six patients with Parinaud's syndrome resulting from vascular lesions. In patients with upgaze palsy they proposed a lesion of the riMLF efferent tracts exiting the dorsolateral portion of riMLF. Downgaze paralysis, when it occurred in isolation from upgaze palsy, involved bilateral lesions of the mediocaudal portion of the riMLF. Thus the efferent tracts from riMLF mediating upward and downward gaze have clearly separate courses permitting selective involvement.

Ocular electromyography (EMG) and high resolution infrared and DC oculography have contributed in a somewhat conflicting fashion to our understanding of the electrophysiologic events in the Sylvian aqueduct syndrome. Esslen and Papst (12) and later Gay, Brodkey and Miller (13) published EMG recordings which demonstrated excessive tonic activity in the ocular muscles of patients with the Sylvian aqueduct syndrome. Co-firing of medial, lateral, and inferior rectus muscles were demonstrated in Esslen and Papst's patient along with faulty innervation of superior rectus during attempted upgaze. Gay, Brodkey and Miller's recordings from three patients demonstrated co-contrac-

tion of all of the ocular muscles and demonstrated asynchrony of firing more typical of saccades. Though the medial and lateral recti appeared to be firing simultaneously in one patient, use of an expanded time scale revealed a rapid alternation in activity between opposing muscle pairs. Such a finding was not noted in their other two patients. They commented, however, that the EMG activity was more typical of that seen with saccadic eye movements than with convergence or following movements.

Ochs et al (26), using high resolution infrared oculographic recordings demonstrated opposed adducting saccades with slight asynchrony in a patient with convergent-retraction nystagmus. They point out that this finding requires reciprocal innervation of agonist-antagonist pairs rather than synchronous cofiring of opponent pairs of rectus muscles. Such findings support the EMG data from one of Gay, Brodkey and Miller's patients cited above.

SUMMARY

Neuro-ophthalmic signs and symptoms of pineal region tumors, being among the earliest manifestations of such lesions, are of importance to neurosurgeons, neurologists, and ophthalmologists. Use of the simple examination techniques discussed coupled with a familiarity with the eye signs presented will assist the physician charged with the care of such patients to achieve a timely diagnosis and hopefully obtain a better therapeutic result through earlier intervention.

References

1. Abay EO, Laws ER, Grado GL, Bruckman JE, Forbes GS, Gomez MR, Scott M: Pineal tumors in children and adolescents. *J Neurosurg* 55:889–895, 1981.
2. Auerbach SH, DePiero TJ, Romanul F: Sylvian aqueduct syndrome caused by a unilateral midbrain lesion. *Ann Neurol* 11:91–94, 1981.
3. Bender MG: Brain control of conjugate horizontal and vertical eye movements: A survey of the structural and functional correlates. *Brain* 103:23–69, 1980.
4. Büttner-Ennever JA, Büttner U, Cohen B, Baumgartner G: Vertical gaze paralysis and the rostral interstitial nucleus of the medial longitudinal fasciculus. *Brain* 105:125–149, 1982.
5. Christoff N: A clinicopathologic study of vertical eye movements. *Arch Neurol* 31:1–8, 1974.
6. Christoff N, Anderson PJ, Bender MB: Convergence and retractory nystagmus. *Trans Am Neurol Assoc* 85:29–32, 1960.
7. Cogan DG: Convergence nystagmus. *Arch Ophthalmol* 62:295–298, 1959.

8. Collier J: Nuclear ophthalmoplegia with especial reference to retraction of lids and ptosis and to lesions of the posterior commissure. *Brain* 50:488–498, 1927.

9. Corbett JJ, Savino PJ, Thompson HS, Kansu T, Schatz NJ, Orr LS, Hopson D: Visual loss in pseudotumor cerebri: Followup of 57 patients from 5 to 41 years and a profile of 14 patients with permanent severe visual loss. *Arch Neurol* 39:461–474, 1982.

10. Daroff RB, Hoyt WF: Supranuclear disorders of ocular control systems in man: Clinical, anatomical and physiological correlations. In Bach-Y-Rita P, Collins CC (eds): The Control of Eye Movements. New York, Academic Press, 1971, pp 175–235.

11. Elschnig A: Nystagmus retractorius, ein cerebrales herdsymptom. *Med Klin* 9:8–11, 1913.

12. Esslen E, Papst W: Die bedeutung der elektromyographie fur die analyse von motilitatsstorungen der augen. *Bibliotheca Ophthalmologica* 57:1–168, 1961.

13. Gay AJ, Brodkey J, Miller JE: Convergence retraction nystagmus. *Arch Ophthalmol* 70:456–461, 1963.

14. Growdon JH, Winkler GF, Wray SH: Midbrain ptosis—a case with clinicopathologic correlation. *Arch Neurol* 30:179–181, 1974.

15. Hedges III TR, Hoyt WF: Ocular tilt reaction due to an upper brainstem lesion: Paroxysmal skew deviation, torsion and oscillation of the eyes with head tilt. *Ann Neurol* 11:537–540, 1982.

16. Isayama Y, Takahashi T, Inoue M: Ocular findings of suprasellar germinoma: Long-term followup after radiotherapy. *Neurol Opthalmol* 1:53–61, 1980.

17. Izquierdo JM, Rougerie J, Lapras C, Sanz F: The so-called ectopic pinealomas. *Childs Brain* 5:505–512, 1979.

18. Kageyama N: Ectopic pinealoma in the region of the optic chiasm. Report of five cases. *J Neurosurg* 35:755–759, 1971.

19. Kageyama N, Belsky R: Ectopic pinealoma in the chiasmal region. *Neurology* 11:318–327, 1961.

20. Keane JR: Ocular skew deviation. Analysis of 100 cases. *Arch Neurol* 32:185–190, 1975.

21. Koerber HI: Ueber drei falls von retraktronskewegung des bulbus. *Ophthalmol Klin* 7:65–67, 1903.

22. Larmande P, Henin D, Jan M, Elie A, Gouaze A: Abnormal vertical eye movements in the locked-in syndrome. *Ann Neurol* 11:100–102, 1982.

23. Lowenstein O: Alternating contraction anisocoria: Pupillary syndrome of anterior midbrain. *Arch Neurol* 72:742–757, 1954.

24. Miller NR: *Walsh and Hoyt's Clinical Neuro-Ophthalmology*, ed 4, Vol 1. Baltimore, Williams & Wilkins, 1982, pp 175–211.

25. Nashold BS, Gills JP: Ocular signs from brain stimulation and lesions. *Arch Ophthalmol* 77:609–618, 1967.

26. Ochs AL, Stark L, Hoyt WF, D'Amico D: Opposed adducting saccades in convergence-retraction nystagmus—A patient with sylvian aqueduct syndrome. *Brain* 102:497–508, 1979.

27. Parinaud H: Paralysie des mouvements associes

der yeux. *Arch Neurol* 5:149–172, 1883.

28. Parinaud H: Paralysis of the movement of convergence of the eyes. *Brain* 9:330–341, 1886.

29. Pasik P, Pasik T, Bender MB: The pretectal syndrome in monkeys. I. Disturbances of gaze and body posture. *Brain* 92:521–534, 1969.

30. Pierrot-Deseilligny C, Chain F, Gray F, Serdaru M, Escourolle R, Lhermitte F: Parinaud's syndrome-electro-oculographic and anatomical analysis of six vascular cases with deductions about vertical gaze organization in the premotor structures. *Brain* 105:667–697, 1982.

31. Posner M, Horrax G: Eye signs in pineal tumors. *J Neurosurg* 3:15–24, 1946.

32. Russell DS, Rubinstein LJ: *Pathology of Tumors of the Nervous System*, ed 4. Baltimore, Williams & Wilkins, 1977, pp 287–290.

33. Salus R: Uber erworbenc retraktionsbervegungen der augen. *Arch Kinderkeilk* 47:61–76, 1910.

34. Sanders MD, Bird AC: Supranuclear abnormalities of the vertical ocular motor system. *Trans Ophthalmol Soc UK* 90:433–450, 1970.

35. Sano K, Nagai M, Mayanagi Y, Basugi N: Ectopic pinealoma in the chiasmal region in childhood. *Dev Med Child Neurol* 10:258–259, 1968.

36. Seaber JH, Nashold BS: Comparison of ocular motor effect of unilateral stereotaxtic midbrain lesions in man. *Neuro Ophthalmol* 1:95–99, 1980.

37. Selhorst JB, Hoyt WF, Feinsod M. Hosobuchi Y: Midbrain corectopia. *Arch Neurol* 33:193–195, 1976.

38. Seybold ME, Yoss RE, Hollenhorst RW, Moyer NJ: Pupillary abnormalities associated with tumors of the pineal region. *Neurology* 21:232–237, 1971.

39. Simson LR, Lampe I, Abell MR: Suprasellar germinomas. *Cancer* 22:533–544, 1968.

40. Smith JL, Zieper I, Gay AJ, Cogan DG: Nystagmus retractorius. *Arch Ophthalmol* 62:864–867, 1959.

41. Smith JL, David NJ, Klintworth G: Skew deviation. *Neurology* 14:96–105, 1964.

42. Smith MS, Laguna JF: Upward gaze paralysis following unilateral pretectal infarction. *Arch Neurol* 38:127–129, 1981.

43. Stevenson GC, Hoyt WF: Metastasis to the midbrain from mammary carcinoma. *JAMA* 186:160–162, 1963.

44. Trojanowski JQ, Wray SH: Vertical gaze ophthalmoplegia: Selective paralysis of downgaze. *Neurology* 30:605–610, 1971.

45. Walsh FB, Hoyt WF: *Clinical Neuro-Ophthalmology*. Baltimore, Williams & Wilkins, 1969, pp 2240–2246.

46. Walsh FB, Hoyt WF: *Clinical Neuro-Ophthalmology*. Baltimore, Williams & Wilkins, 1969, pp 228–232.

47. Wilson SAK: Ectopia pupillae in certain mesencephalic lesions. *Brain* 29:524–536, 1906.

48. Wray S: The Neuro-Ophthalmic and Neurologic Manifestations of Pinealomas. In Brady LW and DeVita VT (eds): *Schmidek HH, Pineal Tumors*. New York, Masson Publishing USA, Inc, 1977, pp 21–59.

CHAPTER 6

Intracranial Germ Cell Tumors: Natural History and Pathogenesis

MARK T. JENNINGS, M.D., REBECCA GELMAN, Ph.D., and
FRED HOCHBERG, M.D.

INTRODUCTION

Despite recent reviews of "pineal tumors" (110, 182, 215, 223), the neurologic and oncologic clinician often remains uncertain when faced with a patient harboring an intracranial germ cell tumor (GCT). This confusion stems from the frequent failure to clearly distinguish GCT from neoplasms of neuroectodermal origin. In this retrospective study of 389 reported cases of primary intracranial GCT, we characterize their natural history and identify determinants which influence ultimate survival.

Developmental Pathology of Human GCT

Five interrelated neoplasms comprise the family of germinal cell-derived tumors. In relative order of increasing malignant behavior (27), these neoplasms are: germinoma, teratoma (including immature and malignant), embryonal carcinoma, endodermal sinus tumor, and choriocarcinoma (79, 139). Each tumor may represent the malignant correlate of a normal germinal or embryonic stage of development: the primordial germ cell (germinoma), the embryonic differentiated derivative (teratoma) of the pluripotential stem cell of the embryo proper (embryonal carcinoma) as well as the extraembryonic differentiated derivatives which form the yolk sac endoderm (endodermal sinus tumor) and trophoblast (choriocarcinoma) (158, 206).

The cancers of germinal derivation arise in specific midline structures: the gonads, sacrococcygeum, retroperitoneum, mediastinum, and diencephalon. This caudorostral distribution suggests development of these tumors from early embryonal "cell rests" or the malmigration of primordial germ cells (12, 188). Irrespective of site of origin, the histologic appearances of the various GCT are "identical" (63, 64) by light- and electron-microscopic (131, 157, 163) and enzyme- and fluorescent histochemical examination (16, 110).

The Association Betweeen Age and Histologic Pattern of GCT

GCT develop in three principal age periods: infancy (0–3 yr), adolescence-young adulthood (10–30 yr), and middle adult life (Table 6.1). Congenital germinal tumors are characteristically benign teratomas. The subsequently arising GCT of infancy (2 months to 3 yr) present as the malignant endodermal sinus tumor and/or teratoma. By the second and third decades of life, endodermal sinus tumor and embryonal carcinoma, often with teratomatous elements, are prevalent in all locations. In contrast to the typical occurrence of nongerminomatous GCT (nonGE-GCT), i.e., teratoma, embryonal carcinoma, endodermal sinus tumor, before age 30, the majority (60%) of adult GCT are pure germinoma. This correlation of youth with nonGE-GCT remains relatively consistent even among familial cases (162). In Table 6.1 are shown the clinical and histologic features of GCT of gonadal, sacrococcygeal, retroperitoneal mediastinal and diencephalic origin (testis: 27, 28, 73, 88, 139, 140, 176; ovary: 25, 27, 118, 184, 226; sacrococcygeum: 5, 27, 37, 72, 129, 217; retroperitoneum: 27, 58, 154; mediastinum: 27, 48, 135, 149; diencephalon: see text). This table further serves to emphasize that adult GCT are largely restricted to the testes, in contrast to the multiple sites of origin among pediatric cases. The much rarer GCT of the viscera, nasopharynx, and orbit have been recently reviewed (71).

Epidemiologic Observations and Risk Factors

The prevalence of gonadal GCT among the young since World War II has occasioned increasing attention to possible environmental

Table 6.1
Clinical and Histologic Features of Human Germ Cell Tumors[a]

Site of Origin	Peak Age of Occurrence (yr)		Sex Ratio (M:F)	Predominant Histologic Pattern of Malignancy[b]		Mixed Histologic Pattern
Testis	0–3	(2–5%)	1:0	EST, TE	(83+%)	NA
	15–30	(32%)		EC, EST, TE	(62%)	40%
	31+	(65%)		GE	(60%)	40%
Ovary	10–29	(80%)	0:1	TE, EC, EST	(60–80%)	40%
Sacrococcygeum	0–3	(95+%)	1:3	Benign TE	(56–82%)	
				TE, EST, EC		NA
Retroperitoneum	0–3	(33%)	2:1	Benign TE	(90%)	
	11–20	(30%)		TE, EC, EST		
Mediastinum	15–35	(80+%)	4–11:1	TE, EC	(46–67%)	38%
				GE	(32–45%)	
Diencephalon	10–21	(68%)	2:1	GE	(65%)	12%

[a] Associations between sites of origin of primary germ cell tumors and typical age of onset, predominant histologic pattern of malignancy, and the frequency of mixed tumor histology.

[b] GE, germinoma; TE, teratoma; EC, embryonal carcinoma; EST, endodermal sinus tumor; NA, not available.

and genetic risk factors (18, 125, 162, 183). There is no prospective investigation of risk factors for the development of intracranial GCT; the only reported association is with Klinefelter's Syndrome (47, XXY) (2). Available information has emerged from retrospective reviews (51), due to the scarcity of this disease. Among Western series, only 0.4–3.4% of primary intracranial tumors are due to germinally derived neoplasms (99). In Japan the frequency of GCT among primary intracranial neoplasms reaches 4.5% (2.1–9.4%) (7, 110, 179). Similarly testicular GCT with presentation during infancy occur with 5–8 times higher frequency (16%) among the Japanese (176). This may not be strictly a racial susceptibility, as 3.1% of primary intracranial tumors in Taiwan are germinal in origin (185).

ANIMAL MODEL OF TERATOCARCINOGENESIS

Knowledge of the biologic behavior of GCT requires an understanding and clarification of the relationship between normal embryonic cellular proliferation prior to differentiation and malignancy. Animal models have successfully explored this interface, as the morphologic and antigenic features of the primordial germ cell are shared among GCT of human and murine origin (66, 93, 134). Among the contributions of the animal model are the following six important observations.

(a) Germinal origin: Murine teratocarcinoma (more precisely embryonal carcinoma with teratoma) is known to be of germ cell origin (194).

(b) Totipotentiality.

(c) "Reversibility" of malignancy. Inoculation of a single embryonal carcinoma cell into early murine blastocysts can result in a normal adult animal chimeric in all cell lines including the germ cells. The teratocarcinoma cells have been obtained from the highly malignant, well established (200 generations over 8 yr) Strain 129 murine tumor line (OTT 6050). The embryonal carcinoma cell is thus capable of full participation in normal embryogenesis, differentiation and reproduction simultaneous with suppression of its previous neoplastic nature. Mintz and Illmensee (137) conclude that the neoplastic transformation of murine teratocarcinoma has not involved irreversible changes within the genome. Malignancy among these cells is relative to and dependent upon the local milieu (91, 137, 155).

(d) Differentiation antigens: Undifferentiated teratocarcinoma cells share certain antigenic determinants with early embryonic cells of the normal mouse. According to Jacob (93) these antigenic determinants may mediate intercellular communication and facilitate differentiation among stem cells.

(e) In vitro cultivation of teratocarcinoma has revealed that certain malignant and morphologically undifferentiated cell lines already differ in their commitment to disparate paths of tissue differentiation (134, 197).

(*f*) There are teratocarcinoma lines which do not spontaneously differentiate *in vitro*, yet may be induced to do so with ceratin pharmacologic agents such as retinoic acid and dibutyryl cyclic AMP (196, 198).

We believe that the unique neuroendocrinologic milieu of the diencephalon may play a role in the development of germinal malignancies in this region. In order to understand the relationship between normal germ cell embryogenesis, malignant transformation, and the diencephalic origin of intracranial GCT, we reviewed cases of primary GCT of the CNS published in the English language literature between 1950–1981. Although discussed earlier, by 1950 there was general acceptance of the concept of the germinal cell derivation of intracranial germinoma, teratoma, embryonal carcinoma, endodermal sinus tumor, and choriocarcinoma (63, 64, 83, 174). From among 389 reported cases, we have characterized the natural history of intracranial GCT and identified major prognostic variables. We advance specific recommendations regarding therapy and direct attention to peculiarities of the immune response to murine GCT which may have relevance to patient care.

METHODS

Section I: Natural History Study

Of the 711 diencephalic and pineal tumors reviewed, there were 389 histologically confirmed primary intracranial GCT (Table 6.2). These cases were selected from 119 published case reports and series judged to be clinically informative. Excluded were 25 cases in whom the diagnosis of an intracranial tumor could not be established antemortem. Cases acceptable for analysis included.

(*a*) Histologic diagnosis: Confirmation of histologic diagnosis reflected a precise histologic description, accompanying photograph, or among larger series, the specified appreciation of the germinal origin of the tumor. The histologic classification of GCT we employed is modified from that of the Intergroup Testicular Protocol (79) and the World Health Organization (139), whose major subtypes include (in order of increasing malignancy, 27): germinoma, teratoma, embryonal carcinoma, endodermal sinus tumor and choriocarcinoma. We grouped all teratomas together for analysis as reports did not often separate benign, immature, and malignant

forms. Mixed tumors are classified in terms of the most malignant tissue type present, not the predominant cell type. (For example, a mixed endodermal sinus tumor may contain embryonal carcinoma, teratoma, and/or germinomatous elements, though not choriocarcinoma.) Excluded from study were neoplasms which could not otherwise be substantiated as germinal in origin. These included reports in which tumor histology appeared incorrectly identified or not stated. In many of these the nonspecific term "pinealoma" was used to lump a group of tumors. (Accepted as indicating germinoma are "ectopic pinealoma" and "atypical teratoma," terms sanctioned by long custom) (174, 175). An exception exists for the "two-cell pattern of pinealoma" of Sano and Matsutani (180), which is identified and analysed as a germinoma, although its ultimate cell type of origin is considered controversial by these authors. Neoplasms not known to be of germinal cell derivation, such as pineoblastoma, pineocytoma, epidermoid, dermoid, primitive neurectodermal tumors, and hamartomas are outside of the scope of this report.

(*b*) Locus of tumor origin: Clinical, roentgenologic, surgical and pathologic details of each case were examined to precisely identify the site of tumor origin.

(*c*) Age at diagnosis: The age at diagnosis was taken to be the time of diagnosis of an intracranial tumor. Pre- and postdiagnostic intervals (*d*) were calculated from this date.

(*d*) Sex: All case reports were analyzed twice by one of us (MTJ) to ensure uniformity and accuracy.

The natural history of 389 retrospectively analyzed primary intracranial GCT is based upon a population of 253 germinomas (65%), 70 teratomas (18%), 21 embryonal carcinomas (5%), 26 endodermal sinus tumors (7%), and 19 choriocarcinomas (5%).

Section II: Correlation of Patient Characteristics with Survival

Multivariate analysis of patient characteristics was undertaken to identify those clinical and histologic features of greatest prognostic value (Table 6.2). As the therapy of intracranial GCT has evolved over the course of our retrospective analysis, we controlled, for the effect of differing therapies upon survival, by excluding patients: (*a*) who received no treatment despite a diagnosis of an intracranial tumor ($n = 5$); (*b*) those in whom therapy is unknown ($n = 1$); (c) patients treated only surgically ($n = 30$); (d) patients additionally treated with chemotherapy ($n = 19$); and (e) those in whom the duration of survival is unknown ($n = 71$). The remaining 263 patients became the study population of this second section (Section II).

This section reports on 189 germinomas (72%), 35 teratomas (13%), 14 embryonal carcinomas (5%), 15 endodermal sinus tumors (6%), and 10 choriocarcinomas (4%). Despite the difference in population size for this section ($n = 263$ vs 389 for the Section I), the populations of both Sections I and II were alike for distribution by histologic diagnosis, site of tu-

mor origin and dissemination, sex and age at the diagnosis (Table 6.2).

Tests of differences in percentages and distributions used a χ^2 test (170). A step-down procedure is used on Cox proportional hazards models to identify patient characteristics most strongly correlated with survival time (47). Plots of survival curves were made using the modified Kaplan-Meier procedures (106).

RESULTS

Section I: Natural History Study

Intracranial GCT occur in predictable and well-defined locations: 95% appear to originate

Table 6.2
Patient Characteristics[a]

Histologic Diagnosis[b]	Natural History Group (n = 389)		Survival Analysis Group (n = 263)	
	n	(%)	n	(%)
GE	253	(65)	189	(72)
NG-GCT	136	(35)	74	(28)
TE	70	(18)	35	(13)
EC	21	(5)	14	(5)
EST	26	(7)	15	(6)
CC	19	(5)	10	(4)
Site of tumor origin				
Suprasellar	169	(43)	129	(49)
Pineal	210	(54)	129	(49)
Sex				
Male	269	(69)	179	(68)
Female	120	(31)	84	(32)
Age at diagnosis (yr)				
0–6	31	(8)	15	(6)
7–9	33	(9)	23	(9)
10–12	97	(25)	76	(29)
13–15	75	(19)	56	(21)
16–18	56	(14)	32	(12)
19–21	37	(10)	25	(10)
22+	60	(16)	36	(14)
Prodromal interval (months)				
Less than 6	91	(23)	44	(17)
6–24	63	(16)	44	(17)
More than 24	63	(16)	45	(17)
Unknown	174	(45)	130	(49)
Extent of dissemination				
Hypothalamus	44	(11)	29	(11)
Third ventricle	84	(22)	60	(22)
Spinal cord	37	(10)	30	(11)
Noncontiguous site	68	(18)	38	(14)

[a] Comparison between the "Natural History Study" population (Section I) and the "Survival Analysis" population (Section II).
[b] GE, germinoma; NG-GCT, nongerminomatous germ cell tumor; TE, teratoma; EC, embryonal carcinoma; EST, endodermal sinus tumor; CC, choriocarcinoma.

in the midline third ventricular region, along an axis from the suprasellar cistern (43%) to the pineal gland (54%). Involvement of both sites, either simultaneously or sequentially, occurs rarely (6%) as does origin within the third ventricle (3%). Primary presentation within the basal ganglia-thalamus (2.8%), or elsewhere in the ventricular system and adjacent regions (2.6%) is remarkable.

Despite the interrelated nature of the five histologic subtypes of GCT, important distinctions may be made between pure germinomas and the nonGE-GCT.

Locus of Tumor Origin

The site of origin of GCT subtypes is not uniform (Table 6.3). The majority of germinomas (57%) involve the suprasellar region, although some additionally occur in the pineal. In comparison, 68% of nonGE-GCT arise in the pineal. The associations of germinoma with suprasellar origin and any of the nonGE-GCT with pineal involvement are highly correlated ($P <$ 0.0001). There exists as well a strong negative correlation between both suprasellar and pineal involvement ($P <$ 0.0001).

There is histologic specificity among other CNS sites of origin: the GCT arising within the basal ganglia-thalamus are all germinomas (34, 109, 114, 200), whereas those in the lateral ventricle-cerebrum (11, 86, 99, 107, 156, 205), fourth

Table 6.3
Locus of Origin of Primary Intracranial Germ Cell Tumors (n = 389)^a

	Suprasellar	Pineal	Both	Other	
GE	49	38	8	5	100
NG-GCT	18	65	3	14	100
TE	17	61	3	20	
EC	33	67	–	–	
EST	15	81	–	4	
CC	11	68	5	21	
Males	23	61	6	10	100
Females	69	19	6	5	100
Total	37	48	6	8	100

^{a} Percentages characterized by histologic diagnosis and gender. GE, germinoma; NG-GCT, nongerminomatous germ cell tumor; TE, teratoma; EC, embryonal carcinoma; EST, endodermal sinus tumor; CC, choriocarcinoma.

ventricle-cerebellum (11, 195), or those which appear holocranial (205) are all nonGE-GCT.

Sex

For the 269 affected males and 120 females (ratio 2.24:1) (Table 6.4), there is good correlation between gender and histologic subtype (P = 0.01). NonGE-GCT occur more often in males (3.25:1 males-female ratio) than do germinomas (1.88:1).

In addition, the site of tumor origin is correlated with sex (P = 0.0001). Suprasellar GCT were present in 75% of females. In contrast 67% of males had a pineal origin. (This includes patients with multicentric origin.)

Analyzed by histologic subgroup, suprasellar involvement was more notable for females with germinoma (84%) than was pineal localization (22%). Even the rare female nonGE-GCT had suprasellar foci in 50%. On the other hand, the majority of males with germinoma demonstrate pineal origin (59%), although suprasellar tumors are not so uncommon among this group (42%) as among nonGE-GCT (12%). Male nonGE-GCT are predominantly pineal in localization (78%).

Age at Diagnosis

Germ cell tumors of the CNS predominate during the second decade of life (Figs. 6.1–6.6). They range in age from birth to 69 yr. The peak occurrence is in the 10- to 12-yr-old group, with 68% diagnosed between 10–21 yr of age. There are nearly equal numbers of patients both younger and older. The age distribution between the sexes is similar, although more males present between 16–18 yr (18%) than females (8%) (P = 0.06) (Fig. 6.1).

NonGE-GCT (Figs. 6.3–6.6) differ from germinoma (Fig. 6.2) in demonstrating significantly earlier ages of presentation ($P <$ 0.0001). Twenty-four percent of these are diagnosed between 0–9 yr compared with 11% of germinomas. Teratomas and choriocarcinomas are especially remarkable for the number of patients (31% and 36%, respectively) diagnosed during this period.

Duration of Prodromal Period

The prediagnosis symptomatic interval (PDSI) is known for 215 patients (55%); however, this is especially well reported among endodermal sinus tumors and choriocarcinomas

Table 6.4
Relative Percentage Distribution of Presenting Signs and Symptoms among Intracranial Germ Cell Tumors (n = 389)[a]

(M/F)	DI	HP D	VD	SP	HC	Pa	Ob	Py	At	Un-known
GE (130/65)	41	33	33	5	21	14	15	11	9	23
NG-GCT (88/29)	18	19	15	9	47	34	26	21	19	14
TE (43/17)	19	13	11	1	46	33	21	23	23	14
EC (18/1)	43	14	38	5	48	43	24	19	14	10
EST (9/10)	15	15	8	–	50	27	46	27	15	27
CC (18/1)	16	55	16	55	47	37	22	11	17	–

[a] DI, diabetes insipidus; HP D, hypothalamic dysfunction; VD, visual deficits referrable to the optic chiasm; SP, sexual precocity; HC, hydrocephalus; Pa, Parinaud's sign; Ob, obtundation; Py, pyramidal tract deficit; At, ataxia; GE, germinoma; NG-GCT, nongerminomatous germ cell tumor; TE, teratoma; EC, embryonal carcinoma; EST, endodermal sinus tumor; CC, choriocarcinoma.

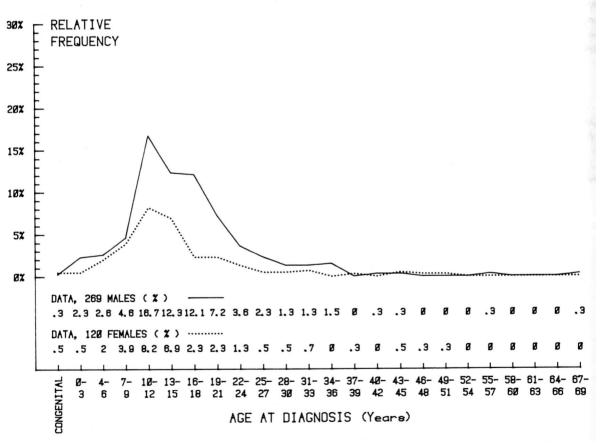

Figure 6.1. Distribution frequency of primary intracranial germ cell tumors by age at diagnosis (in 3-yr groupings). Males: *solid line*: females: *dotted line*.

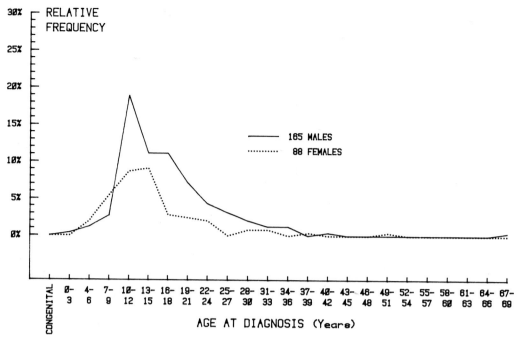

Figure 6.2. Distribution frequency of primary intracranial germinomas by age at diagnosis (in 3-yr groupings).

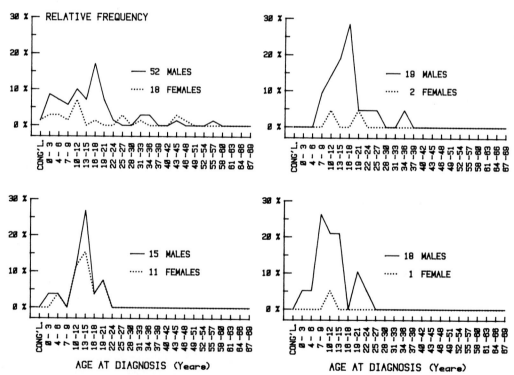

Figure 6.3. (*top left*) Distribution frequency of primary intracranial teratomas by age at diagnosis (in 3-yr groupings).
Figure 6.4. (*top right*) Distribution frequency of primary intracranial embryonal carcinomas by age at diagnosis (in 3-yr groupings).
Figure 6.5. (*bottom left*) Distribution frequency of primary intracranial endodermal sinus tumor by age at diagnosis (in 3-yr groupings).
Figure 6.6. (*bottom right*) Distribution frequency of primary intracranial choriocarcinomas by age at diagnosis (in 3-yr groupings).

(73–79%). With this exception, the population in Table 6.5 was similar to the entire study population in male-female ratio (2.12:1) and histologic subtypes (germinoma 61%, nonGE-GCT 39%).

For germinoma, the PDSI is uniformly distributed from less than 6 months to greater than 24 months. Among the ten cases symptomatic for 5 yr or longer before diagnosis, nine are germinoma (43, 44, 69, 123, 127, 164, 173, 188) and one has germinomatous elements in a mixed tumor (endodermal sinus tumor) (19).

NonGE-GCT behave in a distinctly different fashion, demonstrating much shorter prodromal periods than germinoma ($P = 0.0007$). One-half of embryonal carcinoma, endodermal sinus tumor, and choriocarcinoma patients demonstrate such an abbreviated course, with a minority possessing PDSI longer than 2 yr.

The locus of tumor origin and the patient's sex are major correlates of PDSI (when known), with suprasellar involvement and female sex associated with protracted prediagnosis symptomatic periods ($P = 0.001$ and 0.02, respectively).

Presenting Signs and Symptoms

Details regarding the clinical presentation are available for 312 cases of primary intracranial

Table 6.5
Prediagnosis Symptomatic Interval ($n = 389$)[a]

	Months			
	Less Than 6	6–24	More Than 24	Unknown
GE	17	17	18	48
NG-GCT	35	15	12	38
TE	20	16	17	47
EC	52	10	–	38
EST	54	8	11	27
CC	47	26	5	21
Males	26	17	12	46
Females	18	15	24	43
Suprasellar	13	18	23	46
Pineal	33	15	12	41
Total	23	16	16	45

[a] Analysis of percentage of prodromal interval in terms of histologic diagnosis, gender, and site of origin. GE, germinoma; NG-GCT, nongerminomatous germ cell tumor; TE, teratoma; EC, embryonal carcinoma; EST, endodermal sinus tumor; CC, choriocarcinoma.

GCT (80%) and are better reported for embryonal carcinoma and choriocarcinoma.

Germinomas typically present with the triad of diabetes insipidus, visual field defects referable to the optic chiasm (bitemporal hemianopsia, monocular optic atrophy (5%) with contralateral hemianopsia) and hypothalamic dysfunction. The neuroendocrine features are predominantly secondary deficits, including delay or regression (amenorrhea, atrophic testes in a postpubertal individual) in sexual development (16%), "hypopituitarism" diagnosed clinically and/or serologically (16%), and growth failure (9%). Primary neuroendocrine abnormalities are limited to precocious puberty (31, 34, 109, 112, 113, 115, 124, 173, 185, 200) resulting from tumors in suprasellar ($n = 3$), basal ganglia-thalamus ($n = 5$), and pineal ($n = 4$) locations. Human chorionic gonadotropin (HCG) or luteinizing hormone (LH) levels may be elevated in serum even when the causative tumor appears to be a germinoma without evident choriocarcinomatous elements (34, 102, 108, 109, 113, 144, 146, 208). Nonspecific neurologic deficits include diplopia (10%), seizures (3%), choreoathetosis (2%), ophthalmoplegia (2%), dementia (2%), and psychosis (1%).

NonGE-GCT present with the localizing clinical features of pineal region masses. These include hydrocephalus, failure of upgaze (Parinaud's syndrome), obtundation, pyramidal tract signs, and cerebellar ataxia. Secondary neuroendocrine lesions, such as diabetes insipidus and hypothalamic-pituitary failure are less common.

Choriocarcinoma characteristically occurs in association with sexual precocity (147, 230), typically with elevations in serum and/or CSF HCG and LH (4, 29, 84, 90, 107, 117, 210).

Dissemination of Primary Intracranial GCT

Well localized germ cell tumors of the pineal may expand locally to compress the mesencephalon and brain stem (Table 6.6). Dissemination of GCT occurs both by infiltration of the adjacent hypothalamus or via CSF channels to involve the third ventricle and spinal cord. Surgical or pathologic evidence of hypothalamic infiltration and third ventricular spread may occur with all GCT, however it is especially common with the more malignant EST and CC. Pineal region GCT are far more likely to disseminate into the spinal canal ($P = 0.003$). Spinal cord metastases are seen in relatively greater numbers of GE and EST patients.

Systemic dissemination of intracranial GCT,

Table 6.6
Extent of Dissemination of Intracranial Germ Cell Tumors (n = 389)[a]

	Hypothalamus	Third Ventricle	Spinal Cord	Systemic	Peritoneal	Other
GE	10	16	11	1	2	11
NG-GCT	15	31	7	6	4	23
TE	10	24	3	—	—	9
EC	10	33	5	14	10	33
EST	19	42	23	—	12	42
CC	32	42	5	26	—	37
Males	11	23	11	3	3	17
Females	13	18	7	1	3	18
Total	11	22	10	3	2	14

[a] Comparison of percentages of patterns of dissemination by histologic diagnosis and gender. GE, germinoma; NG-GCT, nongerminomatous germ cell tumor; TE, teratoma; EC, embryonal carcinoma; EST, endodermal sinus tumor; CC, choriocarcinoma.

especially to lung and bone, occurs in only 3% (choriocarcinoma: 76, 84, 105, 147, 230; embryonal carcinoma: 177, 212; germinoma: 20, 124, 212; also reported in 172).

Extension of tumor via ventriculoperitoneal shunt to the abdomen and pelvis developed in 10% of the 106 patients stated to have been shunted (34, 114, 124, 145, 178, 206, 224, 227; also reported by 78).

Significant correlations are demonstrable in the relationships between (a) combined neoplastic involvement of the hypothalamus and third ventricle ($P = 0.0005$); (b) third ventricle and dissemination to a site noncontiguous to the primary tumor ($P = 0.001$); and (c) spinal cord involvement and extension to a site noncontiguous to the original tumor ($P = 0.02$). There is no significant difference in the patterns of dissemination between the sexes.

Section II: Multivariate Analysis of Patient Characteristics Correlated with Survival

This section reports a study population composed of the 263 patients (Figs. 6.7–6.12). Most patients evaluated had a treatment plan involving antemortem histologic diagnosis and conventional radiation therapy. There were 203 patients in whom surgical biopsy or resection of the primary GCT was performed, followed by radiation treatment. (There were 44 postoperative deaths within this group before or during radiotherapy.) In 10 patients the histologic diagnosis was achieved through CSF cytologic examination or by biopsy of a metastasis. These

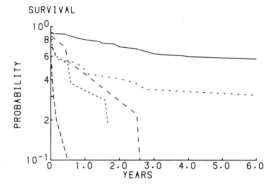

CATEGORY		ALIVE	DEAD	TOTAL	QUARTILE
——	G	122	67	189	1.4
- - -	T	11	24	35	0.0
— —	EC	4	10	14	0.4
- - - -	EST	4	11	15	0.1
— - -	CC	0	10	10	0.0

Figure 6.7. Kaplan-Meier survival curves and quartile survival periods for each of the primary intracranial germ cell tumors. Abbreviations: germinoma, G; teratoma, T; embryonal carcinoma, EC; endodermal sinus tumor, EST; choriocarcinoma, CC.

patients received radiation therapy. Forty-two cases were irradiated with the histologic diagnosis being made at the time of later surgery, postmortem examination, or by unspecified means. Finally, the eight patients who died prior to treatment, during the evaluation of a known brain tumor proven to be GCT, were also included. One hundred and twenty-two patients

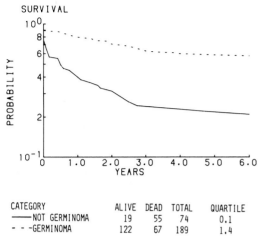

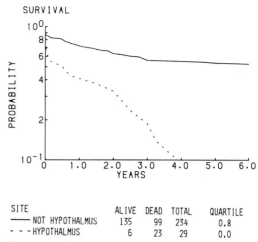

CATEGORY	ALIVE	DEAD	TOTAL	QUARTILE
——NOT GERMINOMA	19	55	74	0.1
- - -GERMINOMA	122	67	189	1.4

Figure 6.8. Kaplan-Meier survival curves and quartile survival periods for primary intracranial germinomas and nongerminoma germ cell tumors.

SITE	ALIVE	DEAD	TOTAL	QUARTILE
——NOT HYPOTHALMUS	135	99	234	0.8
- - - HYPOTHALMUS	6	23	29	0.0

Figure 6.10. Kaplan-Meier survival curves and quartile survival periods for primary intracranial germ cell tumors with and without dissemination to the hypothalamus.

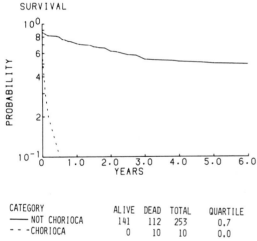

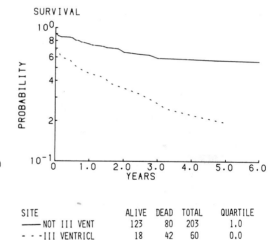

CATEGORY	ALIVE	DEAD	TOTAL	QUARTILE
—— NOT CHORIOCA	141	112	253	0.7
- - -CHORIOCA	0	10	10	0.0

Figure 6.9. Kaplan-Meier survival curves and quartile survival periods for primary intracranial choriocarcinoma and other germ cell tumors.

SITE	ALIVE	DEAD	TOTAL	QUARTILE
——NOT III VENT	123	80	203	1.0
- - -III VENTRICL	18	42	60	0.0

Figure 6.11. Kaplan-Meier survival curves and quartile survival periods for primary intracranial germ cell tumors with and without dissemination to the third ventricle.

(46%) were known to be have died at time of original reporting.

As shown in Table 6.2, the marginal distributions of the various patient characteristics among the 263 patients analyzed for survival are very similar to those of the natural history study population of 389 patients. All the two-way correlations are also similar.

Histologic diagnosis demonstrates the greatest level of significance in its impact upon survival (Fig. 6.7). Germinoma is associated with significantly longer survival than other histo-

logic categories ($P < 0.0001$) (Fig. 6.8). Conversely, choriocarcinoma exhibits a singularly dismal prognosis ($P = 0.009$) (Fig. 6.9). No significant differences in survival were evident among teratoma (including all types), embryonal carcinoma, or endodermal sinus tumor (Fig. 6.7).

The extent of dissemination also figures highly as a predictive variable in survival. Surgical, cytologic, or pathologic evidence of neoplastic involvement of the hypothalamus ($P =$

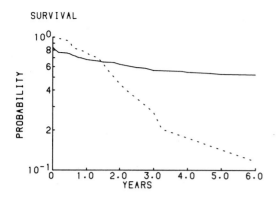

SITE	ALIVE	DEAD	TOTAL	QUARTILE
——— NOT SPINAL CORD	133	100	233	0.5
- - - SPINAL CORD	8	22	30	1.1

Figure 6.12. Kaplan-Meier survival curves and quartile survival periods for primary intracranial germ cell tumors with and without dissemination to the spinal cord.

0.0002), third ventricle ($P = 0.02$), and spinal cord ($P = 0.01$) are significantly ominous associations (Figs. 6.10–6.12).

The next variable which would have been added to the Cox models (47) is the age of onset (10–12-yr group) which was associated with a slightly better prognosis than other groups ($P = 0.1$). The following variables did not reach statistical significance in the Cox models: site of tumor origin, sex, other age groups, or the pre-diagnosis symptomatic interval.

Since medians cannot be reliably estimated when only 46% of the population has died, survival quartiles are reported in Figures 6.7 to 6.12. The median is the time by which half of the patients can be expected to have died; the quartile is the time by which a quarter of the patients can be expected to have died.

Section III

REVIEW OF SPECIFIC SEROLOGIC BIOMARKERS

Immunocytochemical techniques have related elevated serum and CSF levels of alpha fetoprotein (AFP) and HCG with the presence of these peptides on the cell surface of certain intracranial GCT (148). AFP is an accepted biomarker of embryonal carcinoma and endodermal sinus tumor. The presence of HCG indicates secretory syncytiotrophoblastic tissue (98, 139). Inappropriately high CSF levels imply local tumor synthesis (126).

Among primary intracranial GCT, there is good though not absolute correlation between CSF and serum biomarkers with the histologic category. The association is strongest for HCG secretion by syncytiotrophoblast among choriocarcinomas (4, 9, 29, 65, 76, 84, 107, 117, 210), and is less strong for germinoma (9, 34, 102, 108, 113, 144, 146, 208, also 189), embryonal carcinoma (4, 102, 148), and endodermal sinus tumor (4). Increases in LH above physiologic levels have been reported in intracranial germinoma (42, 109, 117, 208), embryonal carcinoma (102), and choriocarcinoma (90, 107). Such elevations of LH may be due to cross reactivity with HCG in the radioimmunoassay, a not uncommon finding with testicular GCT (60). AFP levels have been found elevated in intracranial germinoma (9), teratoma (34), embryonal carcinoma (4, 9, 148), endodermal sinus tumor (4, 8, 121, 224, 229), and choriocarcinoma (9).

In practical terms, elevation of HCG and/or AFP in serum of CSF is suggestive of a NG-GCT. Intracranial germinomas also secrete HCG; this is a property shared with testicular germinomas, 7–8% of which do so. It remains controversial whether HCG production by a germinoma alters its prognosis (23, 139). Certainly the presence of these biomarkers among testicular GCT is considered a grave prognostic sign (68, 203). This may well be true among intracranial germinal malignancies as well (9). In the future these markers will be increasingly used for diagnosis, staging and identification of recurrent disease.

Section IV

REVIEW OF THERAPY FOR PRIMARY INTRACRANIAL GCT

We identify histologic diagnosis as the major determinant of survival among neuropathologically examined intracranial GCT. The distinction of germinally derived neoplasia from that of neurectodermal origin is equally compelling as recent technical advances make biopsy feasible and provide the indication for efficacious chemotherapeutic intervention which is specific for GCT.

The lack of a consistent therapeutic approach is explainable by the rarity of this neoplasm, the paucity of data which allow stratification of GCT patient populations and the proclivity of these tumors to arise in areas previously considered surgically inaccessible. The treatment of pineal tumors has reflected the neurosurgical skill available, thus favoring surgical intervention in larger centers and empiric irradiation elsewhere. In recent years these have become interrelated diagnostic and therapeutic approaches.

SURGICAL INTERVENTION

The core of the controversy is the feasibility of the safe tissue diagnosis of intracranial GCT. The surgical management of pineal tumors has carried a 25–70% operative mortality risk. Surgery therefore has been advocated for "benign" lesions and those progressing despite radiotherapy (182). An intermediate position has been suggested by Griffin et al (74) and Handa and Yamashita (81) who support the empiric irradiation of a germinoma suspected on radiologic, cytologic, and serologic (absent HCG and AFP) grounds. Surgical excision is considered following failure of tumor regression.

The substitution of therapeutic response for histologic diagnosis has been questioned for two reasons. Chapman and Linggood (35) emphasize that radiation response is not in and of itself diagnostic of tumor type. These workers note with recent advances in microsurgical technique and the computerized tomographic (CT) guided stereotactic biopsy available in major centers, that the tissue diagnosis of a pineal tumor may be achieved with a safety not anticipated 6 yr ago. Seventy-one patients with pineal masses (many children with GCT) have been operated upon in recent series with the single fatality a patient with metastatic disease (35, 144, 180, 220).

RADIATION THERAPY

The knowledge gained through tissue diagnosis may be applied to the more selective radiotherapy of pineal region tumors with differing malignant potential. Despite germinoma's reputation of "radiosensitivity", conventional radiotherapy doses of 5000–5500 R have not achieved appreciably better survival rates for this neoplasm compared with empirically treated pineal tumors (75% and 79% 5 yr survival rates, respectively) (180, 199). However these dosages are probably excessive for pure germinoma and likely to produce late neurotoxicity in a pediatric population. Takeuchi et al (208) have pointed out that as "little" as 1500 R may effect appreciable diminution of germinomas on serial CT scans. Radiotherapy with 2500–3000 R has achieved 90% 10 yr survival

rates for stage I testicular germinoma in combination with surgery (62, 82, 97). More conservative dosage regimens eventually will be safely attainable only among histologically defined, surgically debulked, and closely monitored germinomas (100).

Histologic diagnosis influences other radiotherapeutic decisions such as prophylactic irradiation of the neuraxis. Spinal meningeal seeding rates of 7–57% have been reported for pineal region tumors. Known risk factors for this type of dissemination include germinoma (14% in one series), extensive pineal tumors, and those with hypothalamic infiltration (199, 208, 223).

CHEMOTHERAPY

Most importantly histologic diagnosis provides the major indication for early adjunctive chemotherapy of GCT (see "Discussion"). Synergistically cytotoxic agents including vinblastine (V), actinomycin-D (A), bleomycin (B), adriamycin, cyclophosphamide, and cis-platinum have been used with advantage among extraneural GCT. The "VAB" drug protocols achieved complete remission rates of 60–80% against testicular germinal tumors (22, 55, 62, 97). Extended to higher risk nongonadal GCT patients, a VAB-based drug trial yielded response in 56% (19% complete, 37% partial remission) (59). Systemic delivery of these agents across the blood-brain barrier has significantly lengthened survival in cases of single GCT metastases to the brain (126).

These data have encouraged neurologists, neurosurgeons, and oncologists to apply similar chemotherapeutic protocols in the treatment of primary intracranial GCT (Table 6.7).

DISCUSSION

Natural History of Primary Intracranial Germ Cell Tumors

This review of 389 histologically defined primary intracranial GCT enables us to: (*a*) characterize the natural history of these tumors; (*b*) identify high risk patients to create a rationale for aggressive intervention; (*c*) generate hypotheses to explain the relationships between neoplastic embryonal tissue, the neuroendocrinologic environment of the diencephalon, and the immunologic response to such tumors; and (*d*) create a basis upon which to build pharmacologic and immunologic modulators of human GCT.

Table 6.7
Reported Experience with Chemotherapeutic Control of Intracranial Germ Cell Tumors[a]

Tumor	Chemotherapy[b]	Survival/Fate	Reference
Germinoma	MTX, CyP, ActD	13 days/dead	(228)
	MTX, CyP, ActD	114 months/alive	(20)
	BCNU	1 month/dead	(89)
	CyP	12 months/alive	(4)
	Vbl, Pbz, CCNU	4 months/alive	(4)
	c-Pl, Ble, Vbl	12 months/alive	(144)
	c-Pl, Ble, Vbl	9 weeks/alive	(146)
	Vcr, NM	38 months/alive	(114)
	c-Pl, Ble, Vbl	8 months/dead	(108)
Embryonal carcinoma	Ble	4 months/dead	(177)
	Ble	11 months/dead	(10)
	Cyp, ActD, Vcr	9 months/alive	(133)
Endodermal sinus tu-mor	CyP, ActD, Vcr	12 months/alive	(160)
	Pbz, Vcr, DHGC	9 months/dead	(224)
	Cyp, ActD, c-Pl, Chl, Vbl, Ble		(224)
	MTX, Ble, Vcr	8 months/dead	(8)
Choriocarcinoma	Ble	1 month/dead	(84)
	MTX, BCNU, Vcr	30 months/alive	(4)
	MTX, ActD, Ble, Vbl	20 months/alive	(77)
	MTX, ActD	48 months/alive	(107)
	MTX	20 months/alive	(107)
	MTX	3 months/dead	(107)

[a] Stated in terms of histologic diagnosis, agents used, and survival.

[b] MTX, methotrexate; CyP, cyclophosphamide; ActD, actinomycin D; BCNU, 1,3bis(2-chloroethyl)1-nitrosourea; CCNU, 1-(2-chloroethyl)-3-cyclohexyl-1-nitrosourea; Vbl, vinblastine; Vcr, vincristine; Pbz, procarbazine; Ble, bleomycin; NM, nitrogen mustard; DHGC, dianhydrogalactictol; c-Pl, cis-Platinum; Chl, chlorambucil.

NATURAL HISTORY

Intracranial germ cell tumors represent a homogenous entity with predictable clinical and histologic characteristics. Three factors most influence the natural history and provide insight into the pathogenesis of CNS germinal neoplasms. These are histologic diagnosis, age of onset, and the site of origin.

Germ cell tumors of the CNS are histologically indistinguishable from those of gonadal or somatic origin. Germinoma is the most common germ cell tumor arising within the cranium- a predominance which is also the case for testicular GCT. This is unexpected as GCT arising at other sites overwhelmingly demonstrate nonGE-GCT (Table 6.1), especially during the adolescent years.

Intracranial GCT, occurring more often in males, show an abrupt increase in frequency with the onset of puberty. More than two-thirds of patients are diagnosed during the second decade of life. The exceptions to this pattern occur among the nonGE-GCT which present at an earlier age ($P < 0.0001$), and with a greater male predominance ($P = 0.01$). Despite the frequency of nonGE-GCT during infancy and childhood, puberty remains a strong association with choriocarcinoma, whose secretion of gonadotropin may induce sexual precocity.

The site specificity of GCT is striking. These tumors are oriented along either extreme of an axis from the suprasellar cistern to the pineal. Germinomas preferentially arise in the suprasellar region in contrast nonGE-GCT prefer pineal localization ($P < 0.0001$). The site predilection is affected by sex. Females characteristically evidence suprasellar GCT; males show pineal origin ($P = 0.0001$). Only 5% arise elsewhere in the CNS. Other locations such as the lateral or fourth ventricles are limited to nonGE-GCT among infants or older adults.

Site is a major determinant of the clinical presentation of GCT. Germinomas of the parasellar region present with diabetes insipidus, visual field defects, and hypothalamic-pituitary insufficiency. NonGE-GCT typically of pineal origin present with rapidly progressive hydrocephalus and brainstem compression. Less clear is the origin of protracted prodromal periods which occur with germinoma ($P = 0.0007$), females ($P = 0.02$) and suprasellar localization ($P = 0.001$).

The patterns of GCT dissemination relate to both histologic subtype and locus of origin. Not uncommonly GCT infiltrate the hypothalamus, invade the third ventricle, or involve other areas of the CNS. This infiltration is more likely among the progressively more malignant nonGE-GCT. These malignancies may also yield systemic metastases, and peritoneal seeding via ventriculoperitoneal shunts. Spinal subarachnoid dissemination is most common for GCT of pineal origin ($P = 0.003$). In general, dissemination to one site implies dissemination elsewhere. Such associations exist between tumor invasion of the hypothalamus and third ventricle ($P = 0.0005$), third ventricle and dissemination elsewhere within the neuraxis ($P = 0.001$), and spinal subarachnoid involvement with extension to another site within the CNS ($P = 0.02$).

THE PROGNOSTIC DETERMINANTS OF SURVIVAL

Multivariate analysis has allowed us to delineate clinical and histologic variables which affect survival. There are two factors which bear most upon prognosis: the histologic diagnosis and the extent of tumor dissemination.

Germinoma posesses a good prognosis (75–79% 5-yr survival rates) (180, 199) as it is effectively treated by the combination of surgical biopsy/resection and conventional radiotherapy (4000–5500 R) in our review. NonGE-GCT demonstrate a dismal prognosis despite such treatment ($P < 0.0001$) (Figs. 6.7 and 6.8). This is especially true for choriocarcinoma ($P = 0.009$) (Fig. 6.9).

Prognosis is also dependent upon the extent of tumor dissemination within the neuraxis and to systemic organs. Survival is seriously endangered by neoplastic involvement of the hypothalamus ($P = 0.0002$), third ventricle ($P = 0.02$), and spinal cord ($P = 0.01$) (Figs. 6.10–6.12).

Recognition of these prognostic determinants underscores the need for histologic diagnosis and determination of the extent of disease dissemination as a basis for rational therapy. Our first conclusion is that nonGE-GCT represent as *a priori* threat of sufficient magnitude to warrant adjunctive chemotherapy in addition to surgery and conventional radiotherapy. A tissue diagnosis is critical information in the rational treatment of suprasellar and pineal tumors. Given the dramatic improvements in neurosurgical technique and chemotherapeutic specificity (above), we must question the empiric irradiation of these neoplasms.

Second is the threat posed by GCT dissemination within the neuraxis. Extension to one site escalates the probability of extension elsewhere. We believe that neoplastic involvement of the hypothalamus, third ventricle, and/or spinal cord warrants neuroaxis irradiation and systemic chemotherapeutic attempts at disease control.

Accurate staging of disease extent requires serologic, cytologic, and roentgenologic approaches: (a) The most sensitive indicator of hypothalamic infiltration by GCT is the neuroendocrinologic evaluation of the hypothalamic-pituitary axis (75). (b) Investigation of hypothalamic and third ventricular disease should be supplemented with CT scanning, and if necessary gas or iodopamidol cisternography. (c) Serial CSF cytologic examinations may allow the preemptive treatment of spinal cord metastases prior to their appearance at myelography. (d) The identification and localization of HCG, LH, and AFP secretion may be made by comparison of CSF and serum levels. Unfortunately our data are insufficient to isolate the prognostic significance of these biomarkers. Their presence is regarded as a grave prognostic sign and reflects the generally poorer prognosis of tumors with nongerminomatous elements as well as a specific effect of gonadotropin secretion (9, 68, 203). (e) The possibility of systemic dissemination of embryonal carcinoma and choriocarcinoma at time of presentation, or soon after should be borne in mind. We feel that full staging is obligatory at initial presentation and advocate reevaluation (CT scan, chest X-ray, CSF cytology, CSF and serum biomarker levels) routinely at 3 monthly intervals for the first year (or longer for NG-GCT). The great majority of disease recurrences develop within the first 3–6 months following surgery and radiotherapy (unpublished data).

PATHOGENESIS OF INTRACRANIAL GERM CELL TUMORS

Germ cell tumors comprise a family of neoplastic embryonal tissue types. A fundamental biologic character of these appears to be a hierarchical order of neoplasia: Germinoma, teratoma (immature, malignant), embryonal carcinoma, endodermal sinus tumor, and choriocarcinoma (27). Thus, the neoplastic correlate of the primordial germ cell, the germinoma, is the most radiosensitive and potentially curable (82, 208).

Our review of the natural history of intracranial GCT suggests that these tumors emerge from pluripotent tissue (malmigrated germ cells, embryonic "cell rests", localized hamartomtous or dysplastic cells) (75,188) present during early development. Relevant evidence for this includes the embryonal character of the neoplasms, the sharply defined age of onset, the skewed sex distribution, and the protracted prodrome of many germinomas. The stimuli for their emergence may include the attraction of peregrine germ cells to certain hormonally unique regions of the CNS and/or the age related appearance of endogenous biochemical factors which permit the presence of undifferentiated cells and activate the neoplastic potential of those rests. Rephrased, what local factor(s) allow the suprasellar and pineal regions to serve as sanctuaries for undifferentiated germinal cells?

The predictability of site of origin and natural history of GCT has much to do with the specific and unique neuroendocrinologic environment of the diencephalon. Knowledge of the neuroembryogenesis of this region reveals the ontogenetic, synaptic, and functional interrelationship between the hypothalamus adjacent to the suprasellar cistern and the pineal. Both the ventral hypothalamus and epiphysis are identifiable by Streeter's Stage XV (35–38 days). In the early postneurulation stages, the diencephalic-mesencephalic border (which roughly corresponds to the axis between the suprasellar cistern and the pineal) appears to develop precociously in comparison to the remainder of the rostral neural tube (168). The early maturation of these diencephalic structures (14, 46) coincides with the major migration phase of the human germ cells, in transit from the hindgut-allantois region (posterior yolk sac) to the germinal ridges (101, 225). It is possible to envision malmigrated embryonic germ cells as the origin of GCT in the sacrococcygeum, retroperitoneum, and mediastinum (188). The frequent occurrence of GCT in diencephalic foci suggests that preco-cious development or other local factors may play a major role in either drawing germ cells to these locations or altering their normal patterns of development. Normally in fetuses older than 60 days (Streeter's Stage XXIII, 35 mm), extragenital germ cells disappear (101, 225).

Within the mature diencephalon the hypothalamus and the pineal are directly involved in the regulation of a major neurophysiologic function. There exists a synaptic connection between the hypothalamic suprachiasmatic nucleus, which lies adjacent to the suprasellar cistern, and the pineal. The suprachiasmatic nucleus is entrained to the pineal in the establishment of the circadian rhythm. This is accomplished by the accessory optic tract, linking the optic chiasm to the suprachiasmatic nucleus (171), and a direct connection via the lateral hypothalamus to the intermediolateral cell column of the upper thoracic spinal cord. These neurons provide the sympathetic innervation of the pineal through the superior cervical ganglion (181).

The functional purpose of this entrainment may be the regulation of gonadotrophic activity. Within the suprachiasmatic and the preoptic nuclei lie the follicle stimulating hormone and luteinizing hormone releasing hormone secretory neurons of the hypothalamus (26). Antagonism of this system is provided by the pineal through an antigonadotrophic substance other than melatonin or vasotocin arginine (17, 53). An additional role for the pineal in the neuroendocrinologic regulation of neoplastic growth has also been suggested (120).

Germ cell tumors of the CNS arise within/adjacent to the diencephalic centers for the regulation of gonadotrophic activity. Gonadotropins are implicated in the pathogenesis of CNS germinal tumors not only in determining their site of origin but also as carcinogenic inducers. Our review suggests that the neuroendocrinologic events of puberty are an "activating" influence in the expression of malignant behavior among intracranial GCT. Supporting evidence for an inductive or transforming role of gonadotropins (steroidal sex hormones or the gonadotropin-releasing hormones) on germinal tumors includes: (a) The association of GCT with increased gonadotropin secretion in cases of cryptorchidism, testicular feminization, and gonadal dysgenesis (2, 125, 140, 183, 221). (b) The increased incidence of GCT during infancy and adolescence, periods of changing gonadotropin exposure. (*c*) Elevated gonadotropin levels which may persist after unilateral orchidectomy in cases of testicular GCT. These elevations are unrelated to GCT metastases and are not detected in extracts of the primary tumor or the metastases (80). (*d*) In tissue culture, androsterone accelerates the growth of certain testicular tumors (140). (*e*) The observation that gonadotropin secreting GCT are associated with a worse prognosis (68, 139, 203). This may be the result of LH-Releasing Hormone induction of more malignant HCG-secreting trophoblastic tissue elements within a GCT (30, 142). The presence and functional role of sex steroid, gonadotropin, and gonadotropin-releasing hormone membrane receptors is yet to be shown for intracranial GCT.

Basic to our understanding of the origin of germinal malignancies is the elucidation of the mechanism by which unnecessary germinally derived, undifferentiated tissue is eliminated (206). We are uncertain as to how undifferentiated germ cells and their derivatives become immunogenic to the host. Lymphocytic infiltration characterizes germinoma, yet the nature and significance of this response is uncertain (132, 140, 143). Primordial germinal malignancies may employ several embryonic "defenses" to avoid immune attack, such as antigenic modulation: (*a*) The nonexpression of histocompatibility antigens—the determinants of cellular recognition—is a property of undifferentiated embryonal cells such as murine teratocarcinoma (66, 93) and human choriocarcinoma (213). The absence of histocompatibility antigen complex expression is the mechanism by which teratocarcinoma evades cell-mediated immunity (218). (*b*) Another form of antigenic modulation may be the "nonpermissiveness" of undifferentiated murine teratocarcinoma and early embryonic cells for certain DNA and retroviruses. These cells do not demonstrate viral antigens when infected. This is related to the capacity of the preimplantation blastocyst to methylate the segment of viral genome incorporated into its own and so prevent its translation and transcription. Such may be an important method of gene regulation in the differentiation of the early embryo (94).

Local secretion of immunosuppressive hormones such as progesterone accomplishes significant inhibition of the T lymphocyte immune response. Progesterone synthesis by syncytiotrophoblastic tissue occurs in pregnancy as well as in germinal malignancies (23, 187).

THE CONTROL OF GERMINAL TUMOR DIFFERENTIATION

Various systemic and local hormonal and immunologic factors may "control" the development or differentiation of germ cell tumors. Evidence for this "control," often reversible, comes from the murine teratocarcinoma which may be modulated *in vivo* and *in vitro* by retinoic acid. Using an animal model, tumor growth may be slowed and the survival time prolonged (198). Similar growth inhibitory effects of retinoids have been shown *in vitro* for human cancers, including those of neurectodermal origin (186). Differentiation of human choriocarcinoma, as shown by morphologic and cytochemical (increased HCG secretion) changes, has been achieved with retinoic acid (116). The growth inhibition has been related to expansion of total cellular ATP nucleotide pools (165).

In contrast to the improvement found in the animal model, it is paradoxic that differentiation among human germinomas to any other GCT than a benign teratoma is accompanied by a disastrous change in prognosis (27). The clinical experience to date would predict an unfavorable outcome for the pharmacologic induction of differentiation of human GCT should gonadotropoin secretion by the tumor be enhanced. A more fruitful avenue of research might be the prevention of differentiation among these tumors by the blockade of gonadotropin (or sex steroidal) secretion and uptake.

Immunologic "control" of differentiation may involve T-lymphocytes. The course and nature of *in vivo* differentiation of murine teratocarcinoma appears mediated through the reversible modulation of tumor histocompatibility antigen expression by T-lymphocytes. Resistive mouse strains are capable of inducing tumor expression of these recognition antigens, thus rendering the teratocarcinoma susceptible to cell-mediated immune attack (151, 152). Histocompatibility antigen expression appeared to occur in the absence of other signs of differentiation. Expression of these recognition determinants had been taken as a marker of teratocarcinoma and embryonal cellular differentiation (93).

The unique predominance of pure germinomas among those human GT arising in the testes or ventral hypothalamus-suprasellar cistern may be related to the "immunologically privileged" character of these two sites. The association of nonGE-GCT with the pineal gland, which lacks a blood-brain barrier (166), may have its basis in local accessibility to the immune system, which induces differentiation among GCT rests (reviews for and against the immunologic sanctity of the CNS in 6, 145).

Intracranial GCT of the human represent a definable disease which is influenced directly not only by the inherent biologic characteristics of neoplastic germinal-embryonal tissues but also by the neuroendocrinologic environment and immunologic response of the host. Research into this entity is important for the understanding of the interface between embryology and malignancy.

SUMMARY

The natural history of primary intracranial germ cell tumors (GCT) is defined from the published experience with 389 histologically examined cases. These developmental tumors do not differ histologically from GCT of the gonadal or somatic origin. The relative distribution is 65% germinoma, 18% teratoma, 5% embryonal carcinoma, 7% endodermal sinus tumor, and 5% choriocarcinoma. Intracranial GCT display an extraordinary specificity in site of origin—95% arise along a midline axis from the suprasellar cistern (44%) to the pineal (54%). Histologic subtype and site of origin are highly correlated ($P < 0.0001$). The majority of germinomas (57%) arise in the suprasellar cistern while most nonGE-GCT preferentially involve the pineal. A similar correlation is seen with gender ($P = 0.0001$) as most females (75%) exhibit suprasellar tumors in contrast to the male predilection (67%) for pineal origin. The age distribution is unimodal, centering at an abrupt surge in frequency in the early pubertal years. Sixty-eight percent are diagnosed between 10–21 yr of age. NonGE-GCT demonstrate earlier onset than germinomas ($P < 0.0001$). Prolonged prediagnosis prodromal periods (longer than 2 yr) are common to germinoma ($P = 0.0007$), suprasellar origin ($P = 0.001$), and females ($P = 0.02$). Parasellar germinomas typically present with the triad of diabetes insipidus, visual field defects, and hypothalamic-pituitary failure. NonGE-GCT present as posterior third ventricular masses with hydrocephalus and midbrain compression. Precocious puberty may be seen in nearly all types of GCT though appears relatively specific to choriocarcinoma, and is usually associated with elevated gonadotropin levels. GCT may infiltrate the hypothalamus (11%), or disseminate via CSF channels to involve the third ventricle (22%) and spinal cord (10%). Extraneural metastasis by hematogenous (3%) or ventriculoperitoneal shunt (2%) routes is exceptional.

Two patient characteristics have been identified as of significant prognostic importance among a subpopulation ($n = 263$) of patients who received radiotherapy typically following surgical biopsy and/or resection. Histologic diagnosis is most important, as germinoma displays significantly greater survival than other GCT ($P < 0.0001$). Choriocarcinoma is singularly dismal in prognosis ($P = 0.009$). No significant differences exist between teratoma, embryonal, carcinoma, or endodermal sinus tumor, all of which do poorly. Staging of extent of disease emphasized the ominous character of hypothalamic ($P = 0.002$), third ventricular ($P = 0.02$), or spinal cord ($P = 0.01$) involvement. Specific recommendations regarding the necessity of histologic diagnosis, staging of disease, and appropriate therapeutic intervention are advanced.

Insight into the pathogenesis of these embryonal malignancies may be gained from the appreciation that these tumors preferentially arise within or adjacent to the positive (suprasellar cistern-suprachiasmatic nucleus) and negative (pineal) regulatory centers for puberty within the diencephalon. The abrupt rise in age-distribution at 10–12 yr suggests that the neuroendocrine events of puberty are an "activating" influence in the malignant expression of these embryonal tumors. Further avenues of research suggested both by this patient population and the teratocarcinoma animal model are discussed.

Acknowledgments. The authors wish to express their gratitude to Dr. Raymond D. Adams for his helpful comments, and to V. D. L. Jennings and B. Kennedy for their assistance with the graphics.

References

1. Abell MR, Fayos JV, Lampe I: Pathology-Radiation Therapy Conference—Parapituitary germinoma. *Univ Mich Med Ctr J* 32:250–251, 1966.
2. Ahagon A, Yoshida Y, Kusano K, et al: Suprasellar germinoma in association with Klinefelter's syndrome. *J Neurosurg* 58:136–138, 1983.

3. Albrechtsen E, Klee JG, Møller JE: Primary intracranial germ cell tumours, including five cases of endodermal sinus tumour. *Acta Pathol Microbiol Scand* [A80 Suppl]233:32–38, 1972.

4. Allen JC, Nisselbaum J, Epstein F, Rosen G, Schwartz MK: Alphafetoprotein and human chorionic gonadotropin determination in cerebrospinal fluid. *J Neurosurg* 51:368–374, 1979.

5. Altman RP, Randolph JG, Lilly JR: Sacrococcygeal teratoma: American Academy of Pediatrics Surgical Section Survey-1973. *J Pediatr Surg* 9:389–398, 1974.

6. Appuzzo MLJ, Mitchell MS: Immunologic aspects of intrinsic glial tumors. *J Neurosurg* 55:1–18, 1981.

7. Araki C, Matsumoto S: Statistical reevaluation of pinealoma and related tumors in Japan. *J Neurosurg* 30:146–149, 1969.

8. Arita N, Bitoh S, Ushio Y, Hayakawa T, Hasegawa H, Fujiwara M, Ozaki K, Par-khen L, Mori T: Primary pineal endodermal sinus tumor with elevated serum and CSF alphafetoprotein levels. *J Neurosurg* 53:244–248, 1980.

9. Arita N, Ushio Y, Hayakawa T, Uozumi T, Watanabe M, Mori T, Mogami H: Serum levels of alpha-fetoprotein, human chorionic gonadotropin and carcinoembryonic antigen in patients with primary intracranial germ cell tumors. *Oncodev Biol Med* 1:235–240, 1980.

10. Arita N, Ushio Y, Abekura M, Koshino K, Hayakawa T: Embryonal carcinoma with teratomatous elements in the region of the pineal gland. *Surg Neurol* 9:198–203, 1978.

11. Arseni C, Danaila L, Nicola L, et al: Intracranial teratomas. *Acta Neurochirurg* (Wien) 20:37–51, 1969.

12. Askanazy M: Die teratome nach ihrem ban, ihrem verlauf, ihrer genese und im vergleich zum experimentellen teratoid. *Verhandl d. Deutsch path Gesellesch* 11:39–82, 1907.

13. Baker GS, Rucher CW: Metastatic pinealoma involving the optic chiasm. *J Neurosurg* 7:377–378, 1950.

14. Bartlemez GW, Dekaban AS: The early development of the human brain. *Contribut Embryol* 37:13–32, 1962.

15. Bebin J: Seminar in neuropathology: Part III Germinoma (atypical pineal teratoma, ectopic pinealoma). *Mississippi State Med Assoc* 15:329–330, 1974.

16. Beeley JM, Daly JT, Timperley WR, et al: Ectopic pinealoma an unusual clinical presentation and a histochemical comparison with seminoma of the testis. *J Neurol Neurosurg Psychiatr* 36:864–873, 1973.

17. Benson B: Current status of pineal peptides. *Neuroendocrinology* 24:241–258, 1977.

18. Berg JW, Baylor SM: The epidemiologic pathology of ovarian cancer. *Human Pathol* 4:537–547, 1973.

19. Bestle J: Extragonadal endodermal sinus tumor originating in the region of the pineal gland. *Acta Pathol Microbiol Scand* 74:214–222, 1968.

20. Borden IV S, Weber AL, Toch R, Wang CC: Pineal germinoma. Long term survival despite hematogenous metastases. *Am J Dis Child* 126:214–216, 1973.

21. Borit A: Embryonal carcinoma of the pineal region. *J Pathol* 97:165–168, 1969.

22. Bosl GJ, Lange PH, Fraley EE, et al: Vinblastine, bleomycin and cis-diamminedichloroplatinum in the treatment of advanced testicular carcinoma. Possible importance of longer induction and shorter maintenance schedules. *Amer J Medic* 68:492–496, 1980.

23. Bosman FT, Giard RWM, Nieuwenhuijen AC, et al: Human chorionic gonadotropin and alphafetoprotein in testicular germ cell tumors: A retrospective immunohistochemical study. *Histopathology* 4:673–684, 1980.

24. Bradfield JS, Perez CA: Pineal tumors and ectopic pinealomas. Analysis of treatment and failures. *Radiology* 103:399–406, 1972.

25. Breen JL, Maxson WS: Ovarian tumors in children and adolescents. *Clin Obstet Gynec* 20:607–623, 1977.

26. Brodal A: *Neurologic Anatomy*, (ed 3). New York, Oxford University Press, 1981, p 747.

27. Brodeur GM, Howarth CB, Pratt CB, Caces J, Hustu HO: Malignant germ cell tumors in 57 children and adolescents. *Cancer* 48:1890–1898, 1981.

28. Brosman S, Gondos B: Testicular teratoms in children. In JH Johnston, WE Goodwin (eds): *Reviews in Pediatric Urology*. Amsterdam, Excerpta Medica, 1974, p 131.

29. Bruton OC, Martz DC, Gerard ES: Precocious puberty due to secreting chorionepithelioma (teratoma) of the brain. *J Pediat* 59:719–725, 1961.

30. Butzow R: Luteinizing hormone-releasing factor increases release of human chorionic gonadotropin in isolated cell columns of normal and malignant trophoblasts. *Int J Cancer* 29:9–11, 1982.

31. Camins MB, Mount LA: Primary suprasellar atypical teratoma. *Brain* 97:447–456, 1974.

32. Camins MB, Takeuchi J: Normotopic plus heterotopic atypical teratomas. *Childs Brain* 4:157–160, 1978.

33. Carrillo R, Coy JR, del Pozo JM, Garcia-Uria J, Herrero J: Dissemination with malignant changes from a pineal tumor through the corpus callosum after total removal. *Childs Brain* 3:230–237, 1977.

34. Chang CG, Kageyama, N, Kobayashi T, Yoshida J, Negoro M: Pineal tumors: Clinical diagnosis, with special emphasis on the significance of pineal calcification. *Neurosurgery* 8:656–668, 1981.

35. Chapman PH, Linggood RM: The management of pineal area tumors: A recent reappraisal. *Cancer* 46:1253–1257, 1980.

36. Chen HP: Intracranial teratoma of a newborn. *J Neuropathol Exper Neurol* 17:599–603, 1958.

37. Chretien PB, Milam JD, Foote FW, et al: Embryonal adenocarcinoma sacrococcygeal region. *Cancer* 26:522–535, 1970.

38. Christie SBM, Ross EJ: Ectopic pinealoma with adipsia and hypernatremia. *Br Med J* 2:669–670, 1968.

39. Clinicopathologic Conference: Pineal germinoma with endocrine manifestations. *Calif Medic* 106:196–202, 1967.

40. Clinicopathologic Conference: Case report of the

Massachusetts General Hospital #25-1971. *N Engl J Med* 284:1427–1434, 1971.

41. Clinicopathologic Conference: Case report of the Massachusetts General Hospital #41-1974. *N Engl J Med* 291:837–843, 1974.

42. Clinicopathologic Conference: Case report of the Massachusetts General Hospital #38-1975. *N Engl J Med* 293:653–660, 1975.

43. Clinicopathologic Conference: Panhypopituitarism due to ectopic pinealoma. *Stanford Med Bull* 13:56–61, 1955.

44. Cohen DN, Steinberg M, Buchwald R: Suprasellar germinomas: Diagnostic confusion with optic gliomas. *J Neurosurg* 41:490–493, 1974.

45. Cole H: Tumours in the region of the pineal. *Clin Radiol* 22:110–117, 1971.

46. Cooper ERA: The development of the thalamus. *Acta Anat* 9:201–225, 1950.

47. Cox DR: Regression models and life tables. *J Royal Statist Soc* Series B 34:187–202, 1972.

48. Cox JD: Primary malignant germinal tumors of the mediastinum. *Cancer* 36:1162–1168, 1975.

49. Cox JN: Hypothalamic syndrome cause by "pinealoma" occupying the 3rd ventricle. *Arch Dis Childhood* 49:75–76, 1974.

50. Cravioto H, Dart D: The ultrastructure of "pinealoma". *J Neuropathol Exp Neurol* 32:552–565, 1973.

51. Dayan AD, Marshall AHE, Miller AA, Pick FJ, Rankin NE: Atypical teratomas of the pineal and hypothalamus. *J Pathol Bacteriol* 92:1–28, 1966.

52. Dupont MG, Gerard JM, Flamant-Durand J, et al: Pathognomonic aspects of germinoma on CT scan. *Neuroradiology* 14:209–211, 1977.

53. Ebels I, Benson B: A survey of the evidence that unidentified pineal substances affect the reproductive system in mammals. *Prog Reprod Biol* 4:51–57, 1978.

54. Eberts TH, Ransburg RC: Primary intracranial endodermal sinus tumor. *J Neurosurg* 50:246–252, 1979.

55. Einhorn LH: Testicular cancer as a model for a curable neoplasm. The Richard and Hilda Rosenthal Foundation Award Lecture. *Cancer Res* 41:3275–3280, 1981.

56. El-Mahdi AM, Philips E, Lott S: The role of radiation therapy in pinealoma. *Radiology* 103:407–412, 1972.

57. Engel E: Pinealoma metastasizing within the central nervous system. *J Oslo City Hosp* 19:62–67, 1969.

58. Engel RM, Elkins RC, Fletcher BD: Retroperitoneal teratoma. *Cancer* 22:1068–1073, 1968.

59. Feun LG, Samson MK, Stephens RL: Vinblastine, bleomycin, cis-diammine-dichloroplatinum in disseminated extragonadal germ cell tumors. *Cancer* 45:2543–2549, 1980.

60. Fossa SD, Klepp O, Barth E, et al: Endocrinological studies in patients with metastatic malignant testicular germ cell tumors. *Int J Androl* 3:487–501, 1980.

61. Fowler FD, Alexander Jr. E, David Jr. CH: Pinealoma with metastases in the CNS: A rationale for treatment. *J Neurol* 13:271–288, 1974.

62. Fraley EE, Lange PH, Kennedy BJ: Germ cell testicular cancer in adults. *N Engl J Med*

301:1370–1377, 1420–1426, 1979.

63. Friedman NB: Germinoma of the pineal. Its identity with germinoma ("seminoma") of the testis. *Cancer Res* 7:363–368, 1947.

64. Friedman NB: Comparative morphogenesis of extragenital and gonadal teratoid tumors. *Cancer* 4:256–276, 1951.

65. Fujii T, Itakura T, Hayashi S, Komai N, Nakamine H, Saito K: Primary pineal choriocarcinoma with hemorrhage monitored by computerized tomography. Case Report. *J Neurosurg* 55:484–487, 1981.

66. Gachelin G: The cell surface antigens of mouse embryonal carcinoma cells. *Biochim Biophys Acta* 516:27–60, 1978.

67. Gale G: Malignant mediastinal germ cell tumors. *Med Ped Oncol* 9:375–380, 1981.

68. Germa-Lluch JR, Begent RH, Bagshawe KD: Tumour-marker levels and prognosis in malignant teratoma of the testis. *Br J Cancer* 42:850–855, 1980.

69. Ghatak NR, Hirano A, Zimmerman HM: Intrasellar germinomas: A form of ectopic pinealoma. *J Neurosurg* 31:670–675, 1969.

70. Ghoshhajra K, Baghai-Naiini P, Hahn HS, et al: Spontaneous rupture of pineal teratoma. *Neuroradiology* 17:215–217, 1979.

71. Gonzales-Cruzzi F: Extragonadal Teratomas: In *Atlas of Tumor Pathology*, 2nd series, Fasc. 18. Washington DC, Armed Forces Institute of Pathology, 1982.

72. Gonzalez-Crussi F, Winkler RF, Mirkin DC: Sacrococcygeal teratomas in infants and children. *Arch Pathol Lab Med* 102:420–425, 1978.

73. Graham S, Gibson R, West D, et al: Epidemiology of cancer of the testis in upstate New York. *J Natl Cancer Inst* 58:1255–1261, 1977.

74. Griffin BR, Griffin TW, Tong DYK, Russell AH, Kurtz J, Laramore GE, Groudine M: Pineal region tumors: Results of radiation therapy and indications for elective spinal irradiation. *Int J Rad Oncol Biol Phys* 7:605–608, 1981.

75. Grote E, Lorenz R, Vuia O: Clinical and endocrinological findings in ectopic pinealoma and spongioblastoma of the hypothalamus. *Acta Neurochir* 53:89–98, 1980.

76. Guiffre R, DiLorenzo N: Evolution of a primary intrasellar germinomatous teratoma into a choriocarcinoma. *J Neurosurg* 42:602–604, 1975.

77. Haase J, Neilsen K: Value of tumor markers in the treatment of endodermal sinus tumors and choriocarcinomas in the pineal region. *Neurosurgery* 5:485–488, 1979.

78. Haimovic IC, Sharer L, Hyman RA, Beresford R: Metastasis of intra-cranial germinoma through a ventriculoperitoneal shunt. *Cancer* 48:1033–1036, 1981.

79. Hajdu SI: Pathology of germ cell tumors of the testis. *Sem Oncol* 6:14–25, 1979.

80. Hamburger C: Gonadotropins, androgens and oestrogens in cases of malignant tumours of the testis. In Wolstenholme GEW, O'Connor M (eds): *Hormone Production in Endocrine Tumours*. Boston, Little, Brown and Co, 1958, p 200.

81. Handa H, Yamashita J. Summary: Current treat-

ment of pineal tumors. *Surg Neurol* 16:279, 1981.

82. Hanks GE, Herring DF, Kramer S: Patterns of care outcome studies: Results of the national practice in seminoma of the testis. *Int J Rad Oncol Biol Phys* 7:1413–1417, 1981.

83. Harris W, Cairns H: Diagnosis and treatment of pineal tumors. *Lancet* 1:3–9, 1932.

84. Hasegawa H, Ushio Y, Hori M, et al: Primary intracranial choriocarcinoma in the pineal regions: A case report. *Med J Osaka Univ* 25:63–71, 1974.

85. Hayashi S, Nishii T, Osaki A, et al: Akinetic mutism associated with pineal teratoma. *Brain Nerve* (Tokyo) 24:119–125, 1972.

86. Hirsch LF, Rorke LB, Schmidek HH: Unusual cause of relapsin hydrocephalus. Congenital intracranial teratoma. *Arch Neurol* 34:505–507, 1977.

87. Ho K-L, Rassekh ZS: Endodermal sinus tumor of the pineal region. Case report and review of the literature. *Cancer* 44:1081–1086, 1979.

88. Houser R, Izant Jr. RJ, Persky L: Testicular germ cell tumors in children. *Amer J Surg* 110:876–892, 1965.

89. Huckman MS, Robeson GM, Norton T: Radiology of suprasellar ectopic pinealoma. *Acta Radiol Suppl* 347:515–527, 1975.

90. Hutchinson JSM, Brooks RV, Barratt TM, Newman CGH, Prunty FTG: Sexual precocity due to an intracranial tumour causing unusual testicular secretion of testosterone. *Arch Dis Child* 44:732–737, 1969.

91. Illmensee K, Mintz B: Totipotentiality and normal differentiation of single teratocarcinoma cells cloned by injection into blastocysts. *Proc Natl Acad Sci USA* 73:549–553, 1976.

92. Iraci G: Ectopic pinealoma. Report of a case and remarks on the treatment. *Acta Neurochir* (Wien) 38:293–303, 1977.

93. Jacob F: The Leeuwenhoek Lecture 1977: Mouse teratocarcinoma and mouse embryo. *Proc Roy Soc London B* 201:249–270, 1978.

94. Jahner D, Stuhlmann H, Stewart CI, et al: De novo methylation of retroviral genomes during mouse embryogenesis. *Nature* 298:623–628, 1982.

95. James W, Dudley HR: Teratoma in the region of the pineal body. Report of a case. *J Neurosurg* 14:235–241, 1957.

96. Jamieson KG: Excision of pineal tumors. *J Neurosurg* 35:550–553, 1971.

97. Javadpour N, Bergman S: Recent advances in testicular cancer. *Curr Problems Surg* XV:5–53, 1978.

98. Javadpour N: The value of biologic markers in diagnosis and treatment of testicular cancer. *Sem Oncol* 6:37–47, 1979.

99. Jellinger K: Primary intracranial germ cell tumours. *Acta Neuropathol* 25:291–306, 1973.

100. Jenkins RDT, Simpson WJK, Keen CW: Pineal and suprasellar germinomas: Results of radiation treatment. *J Neurosurg* 48:99–107, 1978.

101. Jirasek J: *Development of the Genital System and Male Pseudohermaphrotism.* Baltimore, *Johns Hopkins Press* 1971, pp 3–10.

102. Jordan RM, Kendall JW, McClung M, et al: Concentration of human chorionic gonadotropin in the cerebrospinal fluid of patients with germinal cell hypothalamic tumors. *Pediatrics* 65:121–124, 1980.

103. Kabashima K, Harada M, Morabayashi T: A case of ectopic pinealoma: Study on course and autopsy. *Brain Nerve* 29:453–458, 1977.

104. Kageyama N: Ectopic pinealoma in the region of the optic chiasm. Report of five cases. *J Neurosurg* 35:755–759, 1971.

105. Kageyama N, Belsky R: Ectopic pinealoma in the chiasmal region. *Neurology* 11:318–327, 1961.

106. Kaplan EL, Meier P: Nonparametric estimation from incomplete observations. *J Amer Stat Assoc* 53:457–481, 1958.

107. Kawakami Y, Yamada O, Tabuchi K, Ohmoto T, Nishimoto A: Primary intracranial choriocarcinoma. *J Neurosurg* 53:369–374, 1980.

108. Kirshner JJ, Ginsberg SJ, Fitzpatrick AV, Comis RL: Treatment of a primary intracranial germ cell tumor with systemic chemotherapy. *Med Ped Oncol* 9:361–365, 1981.

109. Kobayashi T, Kageyama N, Kida Y, Yoshida J, Shibuya N, Okamura K: Unilateral germinomas involving the basal ganglia and thalamus. *J Neurosurg* 55:55–62, 1981.

110. Koide O, Watanabe Y, Sato K: A pathological survey of intracranial germinoma and pinealoma in Japan. *Cancer* 45:2119–2130, 1980.

111. Komatsu K, Kiratsuka H, Inaba Y: Pathologic study of four cases with tumors in the region of the pineal body. *Brain Nerve* 23:917–926, 1971.

112. Komrower GM: Precocious puberty in association with pineal seminoma. *Arch Dis Childhood* 49:822, 1974.

113. Kubo O, Yamasaki N, Kamijo Y, Amano K, Kitamura K, Demura R: Human chorionic gonadotropin produced by ectopic pinealoma in a girl with precocious puberty. *J Neurosurg* 47:101–105, 1977.

114. Kun LE, Tang TT, Sty JR, Camitta BM: Primary cerebral germinoma and ventriculoperitoneal shunt metastasis. *Cancer* 48:213–216, 1981.

115. Kunicki A: Operative experiences in 8 cases of pineal tumors. *J Neurosurg* 17:815–823, 1960.

116. Kuramoto H, Hamano M, Suzuki M, et al: Study of so called "cellular effect" methotrexate on choriocarcinoma and its mode of manifestation. *Nippon-Sanka-Fujinka-Gakkai-Zasshi* 34:187–195, 1982.

117. Kurisaka M, Moriyasu N, Kitajima K: Immunohistochemical studies of brain tumors associated with precocious puberty, preliminary report of correlation between tumor secreting hormone and leydig cells in precocious puberty. *Neurologica Med Chirurg* 19:675–682, 1979.

118. Kurman RT, Norris HJ: Endodermal sinus tumor of the ovary: A clinical and pathologic analysis of 71 cases. *Cancer* 38:2404–2419, 1976.

119. Kurumado K, Mori W: Virus like particles in human pinealoma. *Acta Neuropathol* 35:273–276, 1976.

120. Lapin V, Ebels I: The role of the pineal gland in neuroendocrine control mechanisms of neoplastic growth. *J Neural Transm* 50:275–282, 1981.

121. Lee SH, Sundararasan N, Jereb B, et al: Endodermal sinus tumor of the pineal region: A case

report. *Neurosurgery* 3:407–411, 1978.

122. Lehman RAW, Torres-Reyes E: Cystic intracranial teratoma in an infant: Case report. *J Neurosurg* 33:334–338, 1970.

123. Lewis I, Baxter DW, Stratford JG: Atypical teratomas of the pineal. *Can Med Assoc J* 89:103–110, 1963.

124. Lin S-R, Crane MD, Lin ZS, et al: Characteristics of calcification in tumors of the pineal gland. *Radiology* 126:721–726, 1978.

125. Lingeman CH: Etiology of cancer of the human ovary: A review. *J Natl Cancer Inst* 53:1603–1618, 1974.

126. Logothetis CJ, Samuels ML, Trindade A: The management of brain metastases in germ cell tumors. *Cancer* 49:12–18, 1982.

127. Loken AC: On relation of atypical pinealomas to teratoid tumors. *Acta Pathol Microbiol Scand* 40:417–424, 1957.

128. Luccarelli G: Ectopic pinealomas of the optic nerve and chiasm. Report of two personal cases. *Acta Neurochir* (Wien) 27:205–221, 1972.

129. Mahour G, Wooley M, Trivedi S, et al: Sacrococcygeal teratoma: A 33 year experience. *J Pediatr Surg* 10:183–188, 1975.

130. Maier JG, Dejong D: Pineal body tumors. *Am J Roentgenol* 99:826–832, 1967.

131. Markesbery WR, Brooks WH, Milsow L, Mortara RH: Ultrastructural study of the pineal germinoma *in vivo* and *in vitro*. *Cancer* 37:327–337, 1976.

132. Marshall AHE, Dayan AD: An immune reaction in man against seminomas, dysgerminomas, pinealomas, and the mediastinal tumors of similar histological appearance? *Lancet* 2:1102–1104, 1964.

133. Marshall LF, Rorke LB, Schut L: Teratocarcinoma of the brain—A treatable disease? *Childs Brain* 5:96–102, 1979.

134. Martin GR: Teratocarcinomas as a model system for the study of embryogenesis and neoplasia: A review. *Cell* 5:229–243, 1975.

135. Martini N, Golbey RB, Hajdu SI, et al: Primary mediastinal germ cell tumors. *Cancer* 33:763–769, 1974.

136. Mincer F, Meltzer J, Botstein C: Pinealoma. A report of twelve irradiated cases. *Cancer* 37:2713–2718, 1976.

137. Mintz B, Illmensee K: Normal genetically mosaic mice produced from malignant teratocarcinoma cells. *Proc Natl Acad Sci USA* 72:3585–3589, 1975.

138. Misugi K, Liss L, Bradel EJ, et al: Electron microscopic study of an ectopic pinealoma. *Acta Neuropathol* 9:346–356, 1967.

139. Mostofi FK: Pathology of germ cell tumors of testis. *Cancer* 45:1735–1754, 1980.

140. Mostofi FK, Price EB Jr: Tumors of the male genital system. *Atlas of Tumor Pathology*, 2nd Series. *Washington DC Armed Forces Inst Pathol*, Fasc. 8, 1973.

141. Murovic J, Ongley JP, Parker JC, Page LK: Manifestations and therapeutic considerations in pineal yolk-sac tumors. Case report. *J Neurosurg* 55:303–307, 1981.

142. Nakano T: Studies on influence of synthetic LH-RH and dbcAMP on normal chorionic villi and BeWo cells. *Nippon-Sanka-Fujunka-Gakka-Zasshi* 33:2105–2114, 1981.

143. Neuwelt EA, Smith RG: Presence of lymphocyte membrane surface markers on "small cells" in a pineal germinoma. *Ann Neurol* 6:133–136, 1979.

144. Neuwelt EA, Glasberg M, Frenkel E, Clark WK: Malignant pineal region tumors. *J Neurosurg* 51:597–607, 1979.

145. Neuwelt EA, Clark WK: Unique aspects of central nervous system immunology. *Neurosurgery* 3:419–430, 1978.

146. Neuwelt EA, Frenkel EP, Smith RG: Suprasellar germinoma (ectopic pinealoma): Aspects of immunologic characterization and successful chemotherapeutic responses in recurrent disease. *Neurosurgery* 7:352–358, 1980.

147. Nishiyama RH, Batsakis JG, Weaver DK, Simrall JH: Germinal neoplasms of the central nervous system. *Arch Surg* 93:342–347, 1966.

148. Norgaard-Pedersen B, Landholm J, Albrechtsen R, et al: Alpha-fetoprotein and human chorionic gonadotropin in a patient with a primary intracranial germ cell tumor. *Cancer* 41:2315–2320, 1978.

149. Oberman HA, Libcke JH: Malignant germinal neoplasms of the mediastinum. *Cancer* 17:498–507, 1964.

150. Ojikuta NA: The pathology and clinical history of pineal teratoma. *West Africa Med J* 17:130–135, 1968.

151. Ostrand-Rosenberg S, Cohan VL: H-2 negative teratocarcinoma cells become H-2 positive when passaged in genetically resistant host mice. *J Immunol* 126:2190–2193, 1981.

152. Ostrand-Rosenberg S, Cohn A: H-2 antigen expression on teratocarcinoma cells passaged in genetically resistant mice is regulated by lymphoid cells. *Proc Natl Acad Sci USA* 78:7106–7110, 1981.

153. Page LK: The infratentorial-supracerebellar exposure of tumors in the pineal area. *Neurosurgery* 1:36–40, 1977.

154. Palumbo LT, Cross KR, Smith AN, et al: Primary teratomas of the lateral retroperitoneal spaces. *Surgery* 26:149–159, 1949.

155. Papaioannou VE, McBurney MW, Gardner RL, et al: Fate of teratocarcinoma cells injected into early mouse embryos. *Nature* 258:70–73, 1975.

156. Partlow WR, Taybi T: Teratomas in infants and children. *Am J Roentogen* 112:155–166, 1971.

157. Pierce GB: Ultrastructure of human testicular tumors. *Cancer* 19:1963–1983, 1966.

158. Pierce GB, Abell MR: Embryonal carcinoma of the testis. *Pathol Ann* 5:27–60, 1970.

159. Preissig SH, Smith MT, Huntington HW: Rhabdomyosarcoma arising in a pineal teratoma. *Cancer* 44:281–284, 1979.

160. Prioleau G, Wilson CB: Endodermal sinus tumor of the pineal region. A case report. *Cancer* 38:2489–2493, 1976.

161. Puschett JB, Goldberg M: Endocrinopathy associated with pineal tumor. *Ann Intern Med* 69:203–219, 1968.

162. Raghavan D, Jelikovsky T, Fox RM: Father-son testicular malignancy. Does anticipation occur?

Cancer 45:1005–1009, 1980.

163. Ramsey HJ: Ultrastructure of a pineal tumor. *Cancer* 18:1014–1025, 1965.

164. Rand RW, Lemmen LJ: Tumors of the posterior portion of the third ventricle. *J Neurosurg* 10:1–18, 1953.

165. Rapaport E, Schroeder EW, Black PH: Retinoic acid-promoted expansion of total cellular ATP pools in 3T3 cells can mediate its stimulatory and growth inhibitory effects. *J Cell Physiol* 110:318–322, 1982.

166. Rapoport SI: *Blood-Brain Barrier in Physiology and Medicine.* New York, Raven Press, 1976, pp 77–78.

167. Reid WS, Clark WK: Comparison of the infratentorial and transtentorial approaches to the pineal region. *Neurosurgery* 3:1–8, 1978.

168. Rhines R, Windle WR: Early development of fasciculus longitudinalis medialis and associated secondary neurons in the rat, cat and man. *J Comp Neurol* 75:165–189, 1941.

169. Robinson RG: A second brain tumour and irradiation. *J Neurol Neurosurg Psychiat* 41:1005–1012, 1978.

170. Roussas GG: *A First Course in Mathematical Statistics.* Reading, MA, Addison-Wesley, 1973, pp 306–308.

171. Roussy G, Mosinger M: L'hypothalamus chez l'homme et chez le chien. *Revue Neurol* (Paris) 63:1–35, 1935.

172. Rubery ED, Wheeler TK: Metastases outside the central nervous system from a presumed pineal germinoma. *J Neurosurg* 53:562–565, 1980.

173. Rubin P, Kramer S: Ectopic pinealoma: A radiocurable neuro-endocrinologic entity. *Radiology* 85:512–523, 1965.

174. Russell DS: The pinealoma: Its relationship to teratoma. *J Path Bact* 56:145–150, 1944.

175. Russell DS: "Ectopic pinealoma": Its kinship to atypical teratomas of the pineal gland. *J Pathol Bacteriol* 68:125–129, 1954.

176. Sakashita S, Loyanagi T, Tsuji I, et al: Congenital anomalies in children with testicular germ cell tumors. *J Urol* 124:889–891, 1980.

177. Sakata K, Yamada H, Sakai N, Hosono Y, Kawasako T, Sasaoka I: Extraneural metastasis of pineal tumor. *Surg Neurol* 3:49–54, 1975.

178. Salazar OM, Castro-Vita H, Bakos RS, Feldstein ML, Keller B, Rubin P: Radiation therapy for tumors of the pineal region. *Int J Rad Oncol Biol Phys* 5:491–499, 1979.

179. Sano K: Pinealoma in children. *Childs Brain* 2:67–72, 1976.

180. Sano K, Matsutani M: Pinealoma (germinoma) treated by direct surgery and postoperative irradiation. *Childs Brain* 8:81–97, 1981.

181. Saper CB, Loewy AB, Swanson LW, et al: Direct hypothalamic-autonomic connections. *Brain Res* 117:305–312, 1976.

182. Schmidek, HH (ed): Ch. 5: Surgical management of pineal region tumors. *Pineal Tumors.* New York, Masson Publishing USA, Inc, NY. 1977, pp 1–138.

183. Schottenfeld D, Warshauer ME, Sherlock S, et al: The epidemiology of testicular cancer in young adults. *Am J Epidemiol* 112:232–246, 1980.

184. Scully RE: Tumors of ovary and maldeveloped gonads. In *Atlas of Tumor Pathology.* Washington DC, *Armed Forces Inst of Pathol,* Fasc. 16, 1979.

185. Shih CJ: Intracranial tumors in Taiwan. A cooperative study of 1,200 cases with special reference to the intracranial tumors of childhood. *J Formosan Med Assoc* 76:515–528, 1977.

186. Sidell N: Retinoic acid-induced growth inhibition and morphologic differentiation of human neuroblastoma cells in vitro. *J Natl Cancer Inst* 68:589–596, 1981.

187. Siiteri PK, Febres F, Clemens LE, et al: Progesterone and the maintenance of pregnancy. Is progesterone nature's immunosuppressant? *Ann NY Acad Sci* 286:384–387, 1977.

188. Simson LR, Lampe I, Abell MR: Suprasellar germinomas. *Cancer* 22:533–544, 1968.

189. Sklar CA, Grumback M, Kaplan SL, et al: Hormonal and metabolic abnormalities associated with central nervous system germinoma in children and adolescents and the effect of therapy: Report of 10 patients. *J Clin Endocrinol Metab* 52:9–16, 1981.

190. Sohn AP, Pittman JG: Multiple hypothalamic disorders produced by a suprasellar germinoma. *Rocky Mtn Med J* 68:23–27, 1971.

191. Sones Jr. PJ, Hoffman JC, Jr: Angiography of tumors involving the posterior third ventricle. *Amer J Roentgenol* 124:241–249, 1975.

192. Spiegel AM, Di Chiro G, Gorden P, Ommaya AK, Kolins J, Pomeroy TC: Diagnosis of radiosensitive hypothalamic tumors without craniotomy. *Ann Int Med* 85:290–293, 1976.

193. Stein BM: The infratentorial supracerebellar approach to pineal lesions. *J Neurosurg* 35:197–202, 1971.

194. Stevens LC: Origin of testicular teratomas from primordial germ cells in mice. *J Natl Cancer Inst* 38:549–552, 1967.

195. Strang RR, Tovi D, Schiano G: Teratomas of the posterior cranial fossa. *Zbl Neurochir* 20:359–372, 1960.

196. Strickland, S, Mahdavi V: Induction of differentiation in teratocarcinoma stem cells by retinoic acid. *Cell* 15:393–403, 1978.

197. Strickland S: Mouse teratocarcinoma cells: Prospects for study of embryogenesis and neoplasia. *Cell* 24:277–278, 1981.

198. Strickland S, Sawey MJ: Studies on the effect of retinoids on the differentiation of teratocarcinoma stem cells in vitro and in vivo. *Develop Biol* 78:76–85, 1980.

199. Sung D, Harisiadis L, Chang CH: Midline pineal tumors and suprasellar germinomas: Highly curable by radiation. *Radiology* 128:745–751, 1978.

200. Suzuki J, Iwabuchi T: Surgical removal of pineal tumors (pinealomas and teratomas). *J Neurosurg* 23:565–571, 1965.

201. Suzuki J, Hori S: Evaluation of radiotherapy of tumors in the pineal region by ventriculographic studies with iodized oil. *J Neurosurg* 30:595–603, 1969.

202. Swischuk LE, Byan RN: Double midline intracranial atypical teratomas. *Am J Roentgenol* 122:517–524, 1974.

203. Szymendera JJ, Zborzic J, Sikorowa L, et al: Evaluation of five tumor markers (AFP, CEA, hCG, hPL, and SP1) in monitoring therapy and follow-up of patients with testicular germ cell tumors. *Oncology* 40:1–10, 1983.

204. Tabuchi K, Tanigawa M, Baba Y, et al: Primary intracranial choriocarcinoma in the pineal region, a case report and review of the literature. *Acta Med Okayama* 27:125–132, 1973.

205. Takaku A, Mita R, Suzuki J: Intracranial teratomas in early infancy. *J Neurosurg* 38:265–268, 1973.

206. Takei Y, Pearl GS: Ultrastructural study of intracranial yolk sac tumor: With special reference to the oncologic phylogeny of germ cell tumors. *Cancer* 48:2038–2046, 1981.

207. Takei Y, Mirra SS, Miles ML: Primary intracranial yolk sac tumor: Report of three cases and an ultrastructural study. *J Neuropathol Exp Neurol* (Abstract) 36:633, 1977.

208. Takeuchi J, Handa H, Nagata I: Suprasellar germinoma. *J Neurosurg* 49:41–48, 1978.

209. Takeuchi J, Handa H, Otsuka S, et al: Neuroradiological aspects of suprasellar germinoma. *Neurology* 17:153–159, 1979.

210. Takeuchi J, Mori K, Moritake K, et al: Teratomas in the suprasellar region, report of 5 cases. *Surg Neurol* 3:247–255, 1975.

211. Takeuchi J, Handa H, Oda Y, Uchida Y: Alphafetoprotein in intracranial malignant teratoma. *Surg Neurol* 12:400–404, 1979.

212. Tompkins VN, Haymaker W, Campbell EH: Metastatic pineal tumors. A clinico-pathologic report of two cases. *J Neurosurg* 7:159–169, 1950.

213. Travers PJ, Arklie JL, Trowsdale J, et al: Lack of expression of HLA-ABC antigens in choriocarcinoma and other human tumor cell lines. *Natl Cancer Inst Monograph* 60:175–180, 1982.

214. Tsuchida T, Tanaka R, Kobayashi K, et al: A case of two cell pattern pinealoma developed 15 years after removal of pineal teratoma. *Brain Nerve* 28:893–899, 1976.

215. Ueki K, Tanaka R: Treatments and prognoses of pineal tumors—experience of 110 cases. *Neurologia Medico-chirurgica* 20:1–26, 1980.

216. Utz DC, Baucemi MF: Extragonadal testicular tumors. *J Urol* 105:271–274, 1971.

217. Valdiserri RO, Yunis EJ: Sacrococcygeal teratoma. A review of 68 cases. *Cancer* 48:217–221, 1981.

218. VanHaelen CPV, Fisher RI, Appello E, et al: Lack of histocompatibility antigens on a murine ovarian teratocarcinoma. *Cancer Res* 41:3186–3191, 1981.

219. Vejjajiva A, Sitprija V, Shuangshoti S: Chronic sustained hypernatremia and hypovolemia in hypothalamic tumor: A physiologic study. *Neurology* 19:161–166, 1969.

220. Ventureyra ECG: Pineal region: Surgical management of tumours and vascular malformations. *Surg Neurol* 16:77–84, 1981.

221. Volpe R, Knowlton T, Foster AD, et al: Testicular feminization: A study of two cases, one with a seminoma. *Can Med Assoc J* 98:438–445, 1968.

222. Wakai S, Segawa H, Kitahara S, Asano T, Sano K, Ogihara R, Tomita S: Teratoma in the pineal region in two brothers. Case reports. *J Neurosurg* 53:239–243, 1980.

223. Wara WM, Jenkin RDT, Evans A, Ertel I, Hittle R, Ortega J, Wilson CB, Hammond D: Tumors of the pineal and suprasellar region: Childrens cancer study group treatment results 1960–1975. *Cancer* 43:698–701, 1979.

224. Wilson ER, Takei Y, Bikoff WT, O'Brien M, Tindall GT: Abdominal metastases of primary intracranial yolk sac tumors through ventriculoperitoneal shunts: Report of three cases. *Neurosurgery* 5:356–364, 1979.

225. Witschi E: Migration of germ cells of human embryos from the yolk sac to the primitive gonadal folds. *Contrib Emryol Carnegie Inst* 209:67–80, 1948.

226. Wollner N, Exelby PR, Woodruff JM, et al: Malignant ovarian tumors in childhood: Prognosis in relation to initial therapy. *Cancer* 37:1953–1964, 1976.

227. Wood BP, Haller JO, Berdon WE, Lin SR: Shunt metastases of pineal tumors presenting as pelvic mass. *Pediatr Radiol* 8:108–109, 1979.

228. Wurtman RJ, Kammer H: Melatonin synthesis by an ectopic pinealoma. *N Engl J Med* 274:1233–1237, 1966.

229. Yoshiki T, Itoh T, Shirai T, Noro T, Tomino Y, Hamajima I, Takeda T: Primary intracranial yolk sac tumor. Immunofluorescent demonstration of alpha-fetoprotein synthesis. *Cancer* 37:2343–2348, 1976.

230. Zondek H, Kaatz A, Unger H; Precocious puberty and chorionepithelioma of the pineal gland with report of a case. *J Endocrinol* 10:12–16, 1953b.

CHAPTER 7

The Surgery of Pineal Lesions— Historical Perspective

GERHARD PENDL, M.D.

The surgical removal of pineal lesions was and still is considered to be both dangerous and tedious. In 1932, Cushing (9) made the statement that he had "never succeeded in exposing a pineal tumor sufficiently well to justify an attempt to remove it." In 1945, Dandy (14) said that pineal tumors "are perhaps the most dangerous of all intracranial tumors to attack surgically." Torkildsen (75), in 1948, wrote that "attempts at the removal of neoplasms in the regions of the pineal gland and the third ventricle of the brain are associated with such a grave mortality rate that, if possible, such operations should be avoided." He recommended, as do other neurosurgeons (8, 15, 27, 33, 52, 67, 68, 71, 77), that the correct surgical measures are procedures to relieve the intracranial pressure. In 1968, Poppen and Marino (54) stated that "tumors of the pineal are troublesome to remove because of their inaccessible location" and preferred conservative treatment with ventriculoatrial shunting followed by radiation therapy, a statement reiterated by Camins and Schlesinger (6) in 1978.

Even as recently as 1981, Abay et al (1) stated that "direct surgical removal of pineal tumors, in the hands of an experienced surgeon, may be curative in some pineal neoplasms, but must be measured against the results of a more conservative initial approach consisting of CSF shunting and radiation therapy." They admit that a direct surgical attack may be indicated in a patient who does not respond to radiation or whose disease continues to progress.

Not until neuroradiologic diagnostic techniques were sufficiently well developed and lesions of the pineal region, including the tectum and posterior part of the third ventricle, precisely located, could a direct surgical attack be made in the area. It took painstaking clinical research to define the neurological symptoms related to the pineal and midbrain area. Noth-

nagel (44), in 1889, drew attention to the diagnosis of diseases of the corpora quadrigemina, noting that hydrocephalus and the resultant increased intracranial pressure from compression of the aqueduct of Sylvius were typical for tumors in the pineal area. Prus (57), the following year, published his results on experimental electrical stimulation of the quadrigeminal plate. In 1901, Ferrier and Turner (17) discovered that experimental lesions of the corpora quadrigemina influenced eye movements in monkeys. Obstructive hydrocephalus was diagnosed by occlusion of the aqueduct of Sylvius (73). Orton (46), in 1908, differentiated chronic inflammatory processes from pericanalicular gliosis as two causes of aqeuductal stenosis.

Cushing (10) called attention to a third cause of aqueductal stenosis, periaqueductal tumors. In 1904 he performed a bitemporal decompression in a 28-yr-old patient with clinical evidence of a quadrigeminal tumor; some weeks later an autopsy revealed a glioma of the quadrigeminal region. According to Thomson (73), tumors of the pineal gland were first described as a pineal teratoma by Weigert (78) in 1875 in a 14-yr-old boy, but were clinically not defined as an entity until the turn of the century. Gutzeit (22) (1896), Marburg (39) (1908), Frankl-Hochwart (21) (1909), and Pellizzi (50) (1910) suggested a diagnosis of pineal tumor in the setting of precocious puberty, or other hormonal and metabolic disturbances; especially if associated with intracranial hypertension and paralysis of upward or downward gaze and convergence, as described by Parinaud (49) in 1879.

It was Horsley (29) (1905) who first attempted to remove a pineal tumor by direct surgical attack. Howell (30) presented this case to the Royal Society of Medicine in 1910 where he reported that the "operation was performed over the cerebellum for the relief of pressure." In another case in 1909, he mentioned that "the patient died after an operation in the posterior fossa, designed to relieve intracranial tension." In this discussion of Howell's paper, Horsley is quoted as follows: "With regard to the side of the question in which he felt a special interest—namely, the possibility of doing anything surgically—he was bound to confess that the surgical results so far were far from favorable. He thought this might be due to the fact that in each case he had approached the lesion subtentorially. In the next case with which he had to deal, he would certainly go supratentorially splitting the tentorium from the ventroposterior position and exposing the dura in that manner". He suggested that all future decompression operations, or all operations for the removal of these tumors, should be supratentorial instead of infratentorial.

Marburg (39) (1908) reported Eiselsberg's palliative surgical approach to a pineal tumor via the cerebellar route. The patient did not survive. Attempted palliation via occipital decompression was reported by Bailey and Jelliffe (4) in 1910 and also by Pappenheim (48) in 1906.

Pussep (58) was probably the first to reach a pineal tumor by direct surgical approach in 1910. In the case of a 10-yr-old boy, he exposed the tumor through a temporal flap by transecting the transverse sinus and splitting the tentorium. He was able to resect parts of a cystic tumor in the quadrigeminal cistern; however, the child died on the third postoperative day (Fig. 7.1).

In his neurosurgical textbook, Krause (35) suggested in 1911 an infratentorial and supracerebellar route for surgical exploration of the upper vermis and quadrigeminal region. In 1913 he presented a 10-yr-old boy to the Medical Society in Berlin, from whom, 6 weeks prior, he had resected a 4 cm pineal tumor. This was achieved in the sitting position using an infratentorial-supracerebellar approach (Fig. 7.2) (45). As was pointed out by Zülch (80), this was the first report of a successful extirpation of a tumor from the pineal region. The completely removed tumor was histologically diagnosed as a "fibrosarcoma." There was no neurological deficit at the time of the presentation, with the exception of Argyll-Robinson pupils and dysdiadochokinesis in the left hand. Krause (36) reported again in 1926 that he was able to decompress pineal tumors in an additional two cases. All the patient's deficits improved considerably postoperatively.

Concurrently, Rorschach (64) (1913) reported

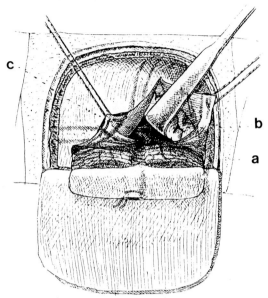

Figure 7.1. Pussep's occipital approach to the pineal region: (*a*) cerebellum; (*b*) retracted occipital pole; (*c*) exposed tumor. (Used with permission from Pussep L: Die Operative Entfernung einer Zyste der Glandula pinealis. *Neurolog Centralbl* 33:560–563, 1914. © Springer-Verlag)

an exploration of the posterior fossa by Brunner (5) in 1911. A quadrigeminal tumor of walnut size was diagnosed and later verified by dissection; however, it was not found during surgery and the 27-yr-old male patient died during the second stage of the surgical procedure. One year later, Brunner decided to approach a pineal tumor in a cousin of the first case, also 27 yr of age, by transcallosal route. Because of severe venous hemorrhage and difficulties in exposure, the tumor was not reached and the operation abandoned. The patient had tolerated the procedure well, but sensory defects remained.

Although this approach later became the pineal approach of choice by many neurosurgeons, Brunner experimented on cadavers with an infratentorial-supracerebellar route in order to avoid the deep veins that had given him so much trouble in the above case. He then proposed this latter approach for extirpation of pineal tumors. In 1920, Tandler and Ranzi (72) suggested modifying Brunner's operation by cutting the tentorium along the sinus rectus so as to expose the entire mesencephalic roof, a technique that was advocated later by Naffziger (41) for treatment of obstructive hydrocephalus.

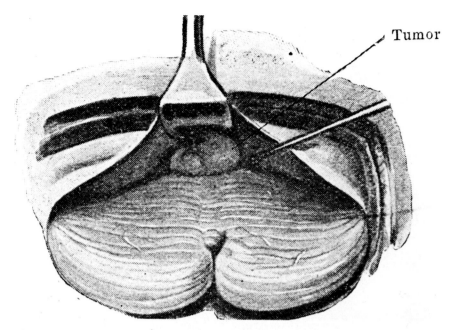

Tumor

Figure 7.2. First successful infratentorial supracerebellar exposure of a pineal tumor by Krause in 1913. (Used with permission from Oppenheim H, Krause F: Operativer Erfolg bei Geschwülsten der Sehhügel- und Vierhügelgegend. *Berl Klin Wschr* 50:2316–2322, 1913. © Springer-Verlag)

A decompression with temporary improvement but subsequent death was achieved in Schloffer's case of a 21-yr-old patient with a suspected quadrigeminal tumor, as reported by Elschnig (16) in 1913. Also in 1913, Roman (63), published an account of a posterior third ventricular tumor, possibly an ependymoma (80).

Nassetti (42) (1913) suggested resection of the longitudinal sinus, falx and sinus rectus followed by transection of the posterior part of the corpus callosum as a potential approach to the pineal. The mutilating results in animals and cadavers obviated its use in patients (Fig. 7.3).

In 1915, Dandy (12) published his experimental operation for removal of the pineal gland in dogs. None of the 12 animals survived the parieto-occipital approach through a midline transection of the posterior half of the corpus callosum. Postmortem examination revealed hemorrhage from the great vein of Galen. Better results were achieved by a more frontal approach to avoid this vein (Fig. 7.4). Nevertheless, he suggested a similar approach for removal of pineal tumors in humans. In 1921, he published his first experiences with three cases of pineal tumors via this approach. He used a very long parieto-occipital bone flap up to the superior longitudinal sinus on the right. The dura was opened and reflected over the longitudinal sinus, the bridging veins were ligated and divided. The cerebral hemisphere was then retracted laterally and the falx exposed; the posterior half of the exposed corpus callosum was then carefully incised in the midline for a distance of 3–4 cm. By further retraction of the hemisphere, the tumor was brought into full view: "under the splenium of the corpus callosum the vena magna Galeni will always be brought into full view at its entrance into the sinus rectus. In one of the cases reported here, the tumor lay anterior to the great vein of Galen and between it and the corpus callosum. In the other case, about one-half cm of the great vein of Galen was free between the upper margin of the tumor and the beginning of the sinus rectus, an amount sufficient to permit double ligation and division of the vein between the ligatures. . . ." (Fig. 7.5). Survival time of these three patients was not long. In the case of a huge tuberculoma, Dandy's patient died 8 months after the extirpation. He had approached this lesion from the left side because a deforming operation had been previously performed on the right. Postoperatively the patient had no speech disturbance, although he was left with a right hemiparesis for several days. By 1936, Dandy (11) was able to report removal of

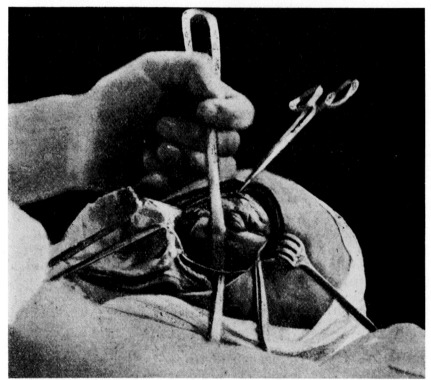

Figure 7.3. Photograph of Nassetti's attempt to expose the pineal region in a cadaver by lifting up the left occipital lobe and transecting the corpus callosum. (Used with permission from Nassetti F: Dell' operabilita delle vie di accesso ai tumori della ghiandola pineale. *Il Policlinico Sez Chir* 20:497–501, 1913.)

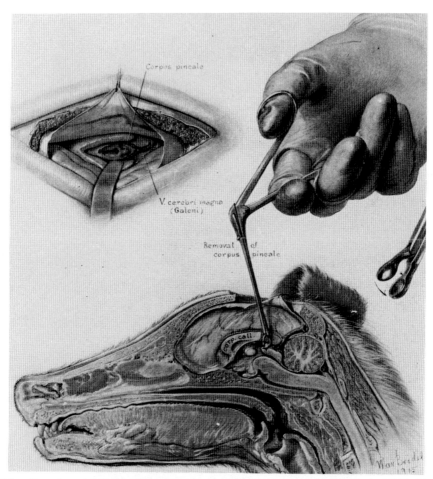

Figure 7.4. Experimental transcallosal pinealectomy in young dogs by Dandy in 1912. (Used with permission from Dandy WE: Extirpation of the pineal body. *J Exp Med* 22:237–247, 1915.)

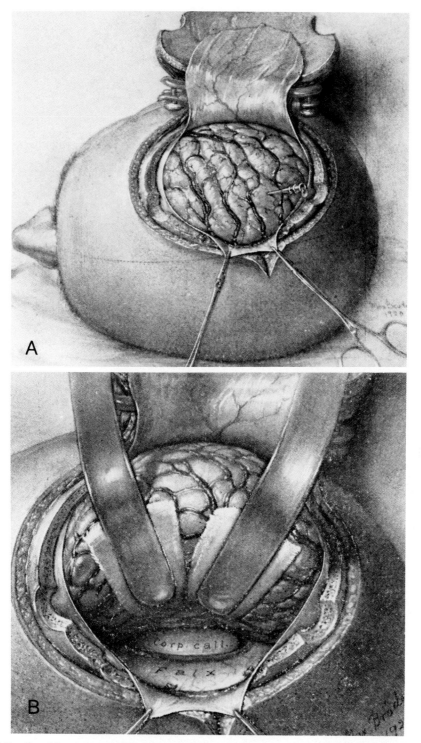

Figure 7.5. Dandy's approach for removal of pineal tumors in 1921 showing the parieto-occipital paramedian opening (*A*) and consecutive steps by retraction of the right hemisphere exposing the corpus callosum and the falx (*B*), dividing of the corpus callosum longitudinally exposing the tumor (*C*), and enucleation of the encapsulated tumor and presentation of the roof of the third ventricle after removal of the tumor leaving the deep veins intact (*D*). (Used with permission from Dandy WE: An operation for the removal of pineal tumors. *Surg Gyn Obst* 33:113–119, 1921.)

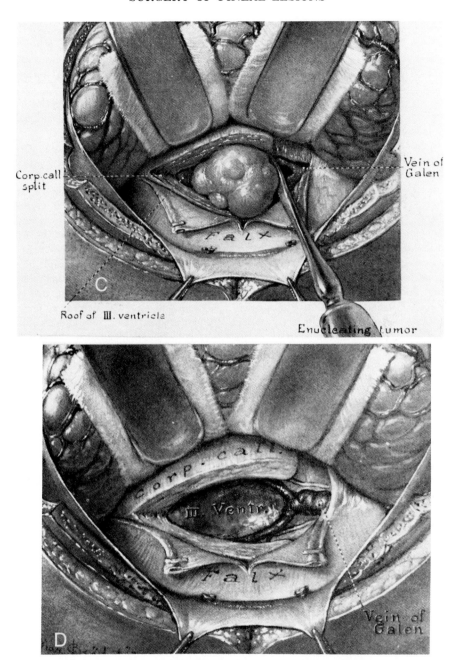

Figure 7.5. *C* and *D*.

ten pineal tumors by this approach, the most favored for a long period.

In 1937, Kahn (32) reported the removal of a large cystic tumor from the pineal area by Sachs in 1926. The tumor was considered by Sachs to be a form of cholesteatoma; it was not established that it actually was of pineal origin (80).

Horrax (26), as well as Camins and Schlesin-

ger (6), gave credit to Peet for the first successful total removal of a pineal tumor. As reported by Allen and Lovell (2), as well as Kahn (32), Peet removed a firm fibrous tumor from the pineal area via a right parieto-occipital transcallosal approach in a 13-yr-old boy in 1927. The tumor was 1.5 cm in diameter and was totally excised. A single course of radiation therapy was given in the same year. The same patient was seen by Smith (69) in 1951. He was in excellent health working as a painter 31 yr after surgery.

The second successful removal of a pineal tumor must be credited to Foerster (20). In 1928, he published his experience with exposure of the quadrigeminal plate and pineal area in three cases. He always used an occipital approach as already suggested by Tandler and Ranzi (72) (Fig. 7.6). A large occipital craniotomy, close to the superior longitudinal sinus and the right transverse sinus, exposed the occipital lobe; the dura was opened and reflected as well over the sagittal and transverse sinuses; the bridging veins were ligated and transected. The posterior horn of the lateral ventricle was punctured by a cannula with sufficient decompression to allow retraction of the occipital lobe from the falx and tentorium. The splenium corporis callosi was thus exposed. For better access to the quadrigeminal area, the tentorium along the sinus rectus could be cut and reflected laterally, and a few centimeters of the splenium split. If the tumor on the left was not sufficiently exposed, the falx could be incised to better visualize the opposite side.

Foerster's first case, a 25-yr-old man, was operated on in 1927 with a total removal of a glioma and subsequent full recovery. The second reported case, operated on initially in 1923 with only a partial evacuation of a cystic tumor, required a second approach. However, the well-exposed tumor could not be removed from dense adhesions to the midbrain and the patient died on the second postoperative day. In the third case, the clinical signs indicated a pineal tumor; the whole quadrigeminal area was exposed, but no tumor and also no pineal gland was found. Neurological and endocrinological deficits improved, as reported in 1932 (20).

Van Wagenen (76) successfully introduced an entirely different approach to pineal tumor surgery. In 1931, he used the dilated right lateral ventricle for exposure of a "spongioblastic type" tumor in a 34-yr-old woman who had previously undergone subtemporal decompression and radiation therapy (Figs. 7.7 and 7.8). The operation began with a right parieto-occipital bone flap. A reversed L-shaped incision 6–7 cm long was made in the cortex extending from the posterior end of the superior temporal lobe gyrus upward and slightly backward. The ventricle was entered at the atrium and its thinned median wall was divided with electrocautery, thus exposing a bluish bulge. The tumor was adherent to the venous tributaries and proved to be of 3–3.5 cm in diameter, red in color, soft, and apparently not actually invading brain tissue (Fig. 7.8). The tumor was entirely removed except for a small bit adherent to the large adjoining veins. The postoperative course was uneventful and "she remained entirely free from symptoms of hydrocephalus for 15 months following surgery."

Harris and Cairns (23) (1930) tried to remove

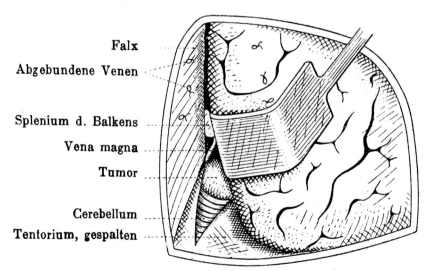

Falx
Abgebundene Venen
Splenium d. Balkens
Vena magna
Tumor
Cerebellum
Tentorium, gespalten

Figure 7.6. Foerster's right occipital transtentorial exposure of a pineal tumor with successful extirpation in 1927. (Used with permission from Foerster O: Das operative Vorgehen bei Tumoren der Vierhügelgegend. *Wiener Klin Wschr.* 41:986–990, 1928. © Springer-Verlag)

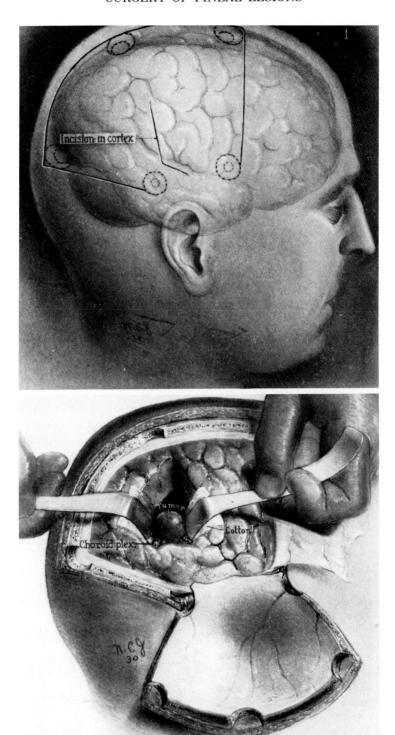

Figure 7.7. Site and extension of the cortical incision of Van Wagenen's transventricular approach to pineal tumors after removal of the medial wall of the ventricle over the tumor. (Used with permission from Van Wagenen WP: A surgical approach for the removal of certain pineal tumors. *Surg Gyn Obst* 53:216–220, 1931.)

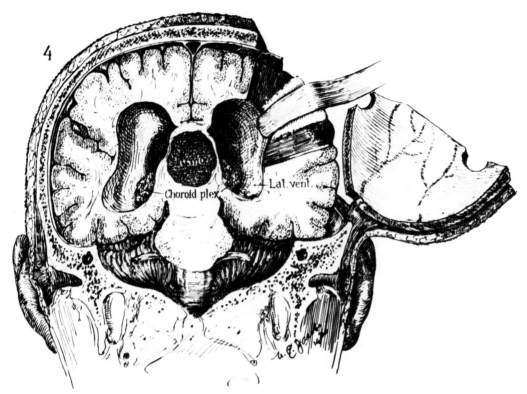

Figure 7.8. Reconstructed drawing of frontal section showing relationship of tumor to the lateral ventricle of Van Wagenen's approach. (Used with permission from Van Wagenen WP: A surgical approach for the removal of certain pineal tumors. *Surg Gyn Obst* 53:216–220, 1931.)

a pineal tumor through a posterior fossa craniotomy, but apparently achieved only a decompression in their 20-yr-old patient. Five months later the tumor could be extirpated by a right parietal transcallosal approach and was diagnosed as a "pinealoma." He was given radiation treatment postoperatively and a further radiation series the following year.

Pratt and Brooks (56) who claimed to be the first to have successfully extirpated a pineal tumor in 1934, reported on their case in 1938. They used a suboccipital approach similar to Foerster's approach reported in 1928 and suggested by Tandler and Ranzi (72) in 1920. This suboccipital approach was later exactly described and repeatedly used with success. Tönnies (74) successfully removed pineal tumors in two boys, 5 and 13 yr old, in 1935 using the parieto-occipital transcallosal approach, which had then become the standard surgical technique.

Horrax (26) (1937) added another possibility for better access to the pineal area. In cases of

large tumors impossible to remove via a transventricular approach, he advocated partial resection of the occipital lobe (Fig. 7.9). However, in 1950 (27), he emphasized the importance and far greater safety of the conservative treatment of these tumors by decompression and roentgen therapy rather than radical tumor extirpation. This became the pineal tumor treatment of choice by many neurosurgeons before and after, primarily because the mortality rate remained so high with such surgery: Dandy (14) (1945) reported a mortality of 20% in 20 patients, Rand and Lemmen (51) (1953) had a mortality rate of 70%, and Ringertz et al (62) (1954) reported a mortality rate of 58.8% among 51 patients from the Olivecrona Clinic.

After having reported in 1954 on five cases of third ventricular meningiomas removed by transcallosal/transventricular approach and an additional sixth case in which a meningioma of the pineal region was removed by an occipital approach, Heppner (25) (1959) described nine patients with tumors of the pineal region oper-

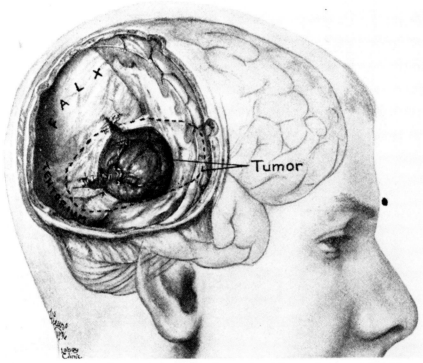

Figure 7.9. Horrax's complete exposure of a large pineal tumor by an occipital bone flap and resection of the occipital lobe in 1934. (Used with permission from Horrax G: Extirpation of a large pinealoma from a patient with pubertas praecox: A new operative approach. *Arch Neurol Psychiat* 37:385–397. © 1937, American Medical Association)

ated via the posterior approach in a sitting position as described and suggested earlier by Tandler and Ranzi. Although it was not until 1960 that Poppen (55) described this technique with modification (Fig. 7.10), he is sometimes given credit for having developed the approach.

Baggenstoss and Love (3) (1939) suggested a combined approach: At the first operation parts of the tumor should be removed by the transcallosal approach; in the second operation the remainder of the tumor should be removed by a suboccipital approach.

In 1956, Zapletal (79) published his experience with an infratentorial-supracerebellar approach to the quadrigeminal area in four patients; an approach he propounded after intense anatomical studies. It was not until his manuscript was completed that Zapletal discovered the earlier

publications of this approach (especially that by Krause). This was then perhaps the first modern revival of the oldest and most successful approach to the pineal area. Nonetheless, this route was used only occasionally (3, 14, 40, 54), until Stein (70) in 1971 published his first series of six cases attacked via a similar exposure with modern equipment and the operating microscope (Fig. 7.11). Stein boasted no operative mortality and negligible morbidity.

In the past 10–15 yr, the old infratentorial-supracerebellar route has been favored by many; whereas others favor the occipital transtentorial or transcallosal approach (7, 31, 34, 38, 43, 47, 51, 59, 61, 65). In recent years, all three approaches using microsurgical technique have been used successfully with a minimum of morbidity and mortality.

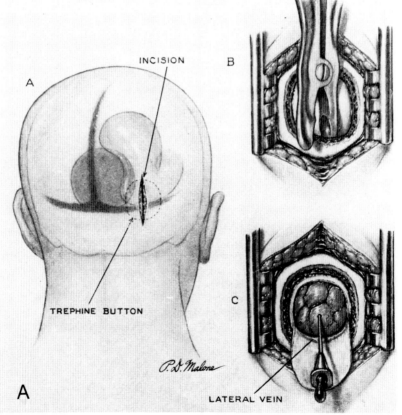

Figure 7.10. Site of the skin incision and removal of bone in Poppen's right occipital approach to pineal tumors. Ventricular catheter enables lifting of the occipital lobe, removal of a wedge of tentorium exposes the tumor. (Used with permission from Poppen JL: The right occipital approach to a pinealoma. *J Neurosurg* 25:706–710, 1966.)

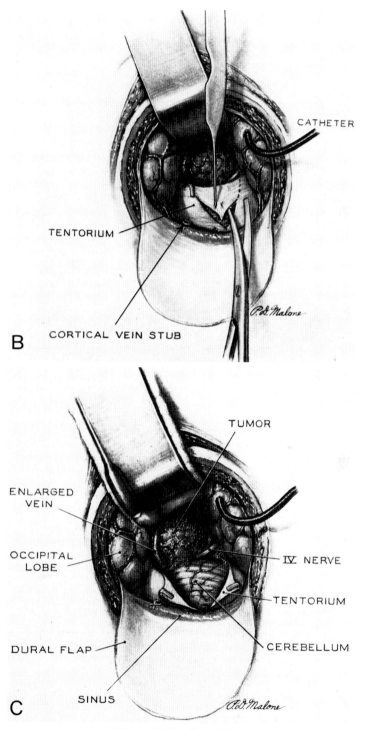

Figure 7.10. *B* and *C*.

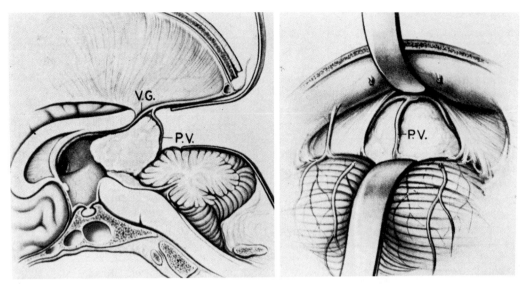

Figure 7.11. Reconstructed drawing of Stein's infratentorial supracerebellar exposure of pineal tumors since 1968 using Krause's approach utilizing microsurgical technique. (Used with permission from Stein BM: The infratentorial supracerebellar approach to pineal lesions. *J Neurosurg* 35:197–202, 1971.)

References

1. Abay EO, Laws ER, Grado GL, Bruckman JE, Forbes GS, Gomez MR, Scott M: Pineal tumors in children and adolescents. *J Neurosurg* 55:889–895, 1981.
2. Allen SS, Lovell HW: Tumors of the third ventricle. *Arch Neurol Psychiat* 28:990–1006, 1932.
3. Baggenstoss AH, Love JG: Pinealomas. *Arch Neurol Psychiat* 41:1187–1206, 1939.
4. Bailey P, Jelliffe SE: Tumors of the pineal body. *Arch Int Med* 8:851–880, 1911.
5. Brunner C, Rorschach H: Über einen Fall von Tumor der Glandula pinealis cerebri. *Cor Blatt Schweiz. Arzte* 642–643, 1911.
6. Camins MB, Schlesinger EB: Treatment of tumours of the posterior part of the third ventricle and the pineal region: A long term follow-up. *Acta Neurochir* 40:131–143, 1978.
7. Copty M, Bedard F, Turcotte JF: Successful removal of an entirely calcified aneurysm of the vein of Galen. *Surg Neurol* 14:396–400, 1980.
8. Cummins FM, Taveras JN, Schlesinger EB: Treatment of gliomas of the third ventricle and pinealomas. *Neurology* 10:1031–1036, 1960.
9. Cushing H: Intracranial tumors: Notes upon a series of two thousand verified cases with surgical mortality pertaining thereto. Springfield, IL Charles C Thomas, 1932.
10. Cushing H: The establishment of cerebral hernia as a decompressive measure for inaccessible brain tumors. *Surg Gyn Obst* 1:297–314, 1905.
11. Dandy WE: Operative experiences in cases of pineal tumors. *Arch Surg* 33:19–46, 1936.
12. Dandy WE: Extirpation of the pineal body. *J Exp Med* 22:237–247, 1915.
13. Dandy WE: An operation for removal of pineal

tumors. *Surg Gyn Obst* 33:113–119, 1921.
14. Dandy WE: Surgery of the brain. In *Lewis' Practice of Surgery*, Vol. 12. Hagerstown, MD, WF. Prior, 1945.
15. DeGirolami U, Schmidek H: Clinicopathological study of 53 tumors of the pineal region. *J Neurosurg* 39:455–462, 1973.
16. Elschning A: Nystagmus retractorius, ein cerebrales Herdsymptom. *Med Klin* 9:8–11, 1913.
17. Ferrier D, Turner WA: Experimental lesions of the corpora quadrigemina in monkeys. *Brain* 24:27–46, 1901.
18. Foerster O: Ein Fall von Vierhügeltumor, durch Operation entfernt. *Arch Psychiat* 84:515–516, 1928.
19. Foerster O: Das operative Vorgehen bei Tumoren der Vierhügelgegend. *Wiener Klin Wschr* 41:986–990, 1928.
20. Foerster O: Über das operative Vorgehen bei Operationen der Vierhügelgegend. *Zbl Ges Neurol Psychiat* 61:457–459, 1932.
21. Frankl-Hochwart L: Über Diagnose der Zirbeldrüsentumoren. *Dtsch Z Nervenh* 37:455–465, 1909.
22. Gutzeit R: Ein Teratom der Zirbeldrüse. Thesis, E. Erlatis, Königsberg, 1896.
23. Harris W, Cairns H: Diagnosis and treatment of pineal tumors. *Lancet* 1:3–9, 1932.
24. Heppner F: Über Meningeome des 3. Ventrikels. *Acta Neurochir* 4:55–67, 1956.
25. Heppner F: Zur Operationstechnik bei Pinealomen. *Zbl Neurochir* 19:219–224, 1959.
26. Horrax G: Extirpation of a large pinealoma from a patient with pubertas parecox: A new operative approach. *Arch Neurol Psychiat* 37:385–397, 1937.
27. Horrax G: Treatment of tumors of the pineal body. Experience in a series of twenty-two cases. *Arch*

Neurol Psychiat 64:227–242, 1950.

28. Horrax G: The diagnosis and treatment of pineal tumors. *Radiology* 52:186–192, 1959.

29. Horsley V: Discussion of paper by CMH Howell on tumors of the pineal body. *Proc R Soc Med* 3:77–78, 1910.

30. Howell CMH: Tumours of the pineal gland. *Proc R Soc Med* 3:64–77, 1910.

31. Isamat F: Tumours of the posterior part of the third ventricle: Neurosurgical criteria. In *Advances and Technical Standards in Neurosurgery*, Vol 6. Wien-New York, Springer-Verlag, 1979, pp 171–184.

32. Kahn EA: Surgical treatment of pineal tumors. *Arch Neurol Psychiat* 38:833–842, 1937.

33. Katsura S, Suzuki J, Wada I: A statistical study of brain tumors in the neurosurgical clinics in Japan. *J Neurosurg* 16:570–580, 1959.

34. Kobayashi S, Sugita K, Tanaka Y, Kyoshima K: Infratentorial approach to the pineal region in the prone position: Concorde position. *J Neurosurg* 58:141–143, 1983.

35. Krause F: *Chirurgie des Gehirns und Rückenmarks*, Vol. 1. Berlin-Wien, Urban and Schwarzenberg, 1911.

36. Krause F: Operative Freilegung der Vierhügel, nebst Beobachtungen über Hirndruck und Dekompression. *Zbl Chirurgie* 53:2812–2819, 1926.

37. Kundert JG: Pinealom und Tumoren des III. Ventrikels. Katamnestische Untersuchungen von 20 neurochirurgisch behandelten Patienten. Schweiz. *Arch Neurol Psychiat* 92:296–333, 1963.

38. Lazar ML, Clark K: Direct surgical management of masses in the region of the vein of Galen. *Surg Neurol* 2:17–22, 1974.

39. Marburg O: Die adipositas cerebralis. Ein Beitrag zur Pathologie der Zirbeldrüse. *Wiener Med Wschr* 28:2617–2622, 1908.

40. Matson DD: Neurosurgery of infancy and childhood. Springfield, IL, Charles C Thomas, 1969.

41. Naffziger HC: Brain surgery with special reference to exposure of the brain stem and posterior fossa, the principle of intracranial decompression, and the relief of impactions in the posterior fossa. *Surg Gyn Obst* 46:240–248, 1928.

42. Nassetti F: Dell' operabilita delle vie di accesso ai tumori della ghiandola pineale. *II Policlinico Sez Chir* 20:497–501, 1913.

43. Neuwelt EA, Glasberg M, Frenkel E, Clark WK: Malignant pineal region tumors. *J Neurosurg* 51:597–607, 1979.

44. Nothnagel H: The diagnosis of diseases of the corpora quadrigemina. *Brain* 1889;12:21–35.

45. Oppenheim H, Krause F: Operative Erfolg bei Geschwülsten der Sehhügel- und Vierhügelgegend. *Berl Klin Wschr* 50:2316–2322, 1913.

46. Orton ST: A pathological study of a case of hydrocephalus. *Am J Insan* 65:229–278, 1908.

47. Page LK: The infratentorial-supracerebellar exposure of tumors in the pineal area. *Neurosurgery* 1:36–40, 1977.

48. Pappenheim AM: Über Geschwülste der Corpora pineale. *Virchows Arch Path Anat* 200:122–141, 1910.

49. Parinaud H: De la neurite optique dans les affections cérébrales. *Ann d'Ocul* 82:5–47, 1879.

50. Pellizzi GB: La syndrome epifi saria "macrogenitosomia precoc." *Riv Ital Neuropat* 3:193–250, 1910.

51. Pendl G: Infratentoria approach to mesencephalic tumors. In Koos W TH, Böck F, Spetzler RF, (eds): *Clinical Microneurosurgery*. Stuttgart, Thieme Verlag, 1976, 143–150.

52. Pia HW: Klinik, Differenzialdiagnose und Behandlung der Vierhügelgeschwülste. *Dtsch Z Nervenh* 172:12–32, 1954.

53. Poppen JL: The right occipital approach to a pinealoma. *J Neurosurg* 25:706–710, 1966.

54. Poppen JL, Marino R Jr: Pinealomas and tumors of the posterior portion of the third ventricle. *J Neurosurg* 28:357–364, 1968.

55. Poppen JL: *An Atlas of Neurosurgical Techniques*. Philadelphia, W. B. Saunders, 1960.

56. Pratt DW, Brooks EF: Successful excision of a tumor of the pineal gland. *Canad Med Assn J* 39:240–243, 1938.

57. Prus J: Untersuchungen über elektrische Reizung der Vierhügel. *Wiener Klin Wschr* 12:1124–1130, 1899.

58. Pussep L: Die operative Entfernung einer Zyste der Glandula pinealis. *Neurol Centralbl* 33:560–563, 1914.

59. Raimondi AJ, Tomita T: Pineal tumors in childhood. *Childs Brain* 9:239–266, 1982.

60. Rand RW, Lemmen LJ: Tumors of the posterior portion of the third ventricle. *J Neurosurg* 10:1–18, 1953.

61. Reid WS, Clark WK: Comparison of the infratentorial and transtentorial approaches to the pineal region. *Neurosurgery* 3:1–8, 1978.

62. Ringertz N, Nordenstam H, Flyger G: Tumors of the pineal region. *J Neuropathol Exp Neurol* 13:540–561, 1954.

63. Roman B: Zur Kenntnis des Neuroepithelioma gliomatosum. *Virchows Arch Path Anat* 211:126–140, 1913.

64. Rorschach H: Zur Pathologie und Operabilität der Tumoren der Zirbeldrüse. *Bruns Beitr* 83:451–474, 1913.

65. Rozario R, Adelman L, Prager RJ, Stein BM: Meningiomas of the pineal region and third ventricle. *Neurosurgery* 5:489–495, 1979.

66. Rydygier RV: Erfahrungen über die Dekompressiv-Trepanation und der Balkenstich nach Anton v. Bramann beim Gehirndruck. *Dtsch Z Chir* 117:344–474, 1912.

67. Schürmann K: Die Neurochirurgie der intrakraniellen Tumoren der Mittellinie. *Radiologe* 5:459–473, 1965.

68. Skrzypczak J: Zur Symptomatologie, Diagnostik und Therapie der Vierhügeltumoren. *Neurochirurgia* 10:128–142, 1967.

69. Smith RA: Pineal tumors. *Univ of Mich Med Bull* 27:33–43, 1961.

70. Stein BM: The infratentorial supracerebellar approach to pineal lesions. *J Neurosurg* 35:197–202, 1971.

71. Suzuki J. Iwabuchi T: Surgical removal of pineal tumors (pinealomas and teratomas). *J Neurosurg* 23:565–571, 1965.

72. Tandler J, Ranzi E: Chirurgische Anatomie und Operationstechnik des Zentralnervensystems. In

Kirschner M, Normann O (eds): *Die Chirurgie.* Berlin, Springer Verlag, 1920.

73. Thomson AF: Surgery of the third ventricle. In Walker AE (ed): *A History of Neurological Surgery.* New York, Hafner Publishing Co, 1967, pp 136–141.

74. Tönnies W: Behandlung der Geschwülste im hinteren Teil des 3.Ventrikels. *Langenbecks Arch Klin Chir* 183:426–429, 1935.

75. Torkildsen A: Should extirpation be attempted in cases of neoplasms in or near the third ventricle of the brain? Experiences with a palliative method. *J Neurosurg* 5:249–275, 1948.

76. Van Wagenen WP: A surgical approach for the removal of certain pineal tumors. *Surg Gyn Obst* 53:216–220, 1931.

77. Weber G: Tumoren der Glandula pinealis und ektopische Pinealocytome. *Schweiz Arch Neurol Neurochir Psychiat* 91:473–509, 1963.

78. Weigert C: Zur Lehre von den Tumoren der Hirnanhänge. *Virchows Arch Path Anat* 65:212–219, 1875.

79. Zapletal B: Ein neuer operativer Zugang zum Gebiet der Incisura tentorii. *Zbl Neurochir* 16:64–69, 1956.

80. Zülch KJ: Reflections on the surgery of the pineal gland (A glimpse into the past). *Neurosurg Rev* 4:152–162, 1981.

CHAPTER 8

Microsurgical Anatomy of the Pineal Region

GERHARD PENDL, M.D.

INTRODUCTION

Since microsurgical techniques have renewed the debate as to the feasibility of direct management of pineal lesions, it has become necessary to provide a more detailed anatomical knowledge of this region (32, 38, 39, 40, 45, 46, 55, 58, 67, 68). Knowledge of the vascular structures and their microtopographic relationships, and knowledge of the finer anatomical structures for microsurgical dissection must be provided, not only in order to select the proper approach to this region, but also to avoid further morbidity. This study is based on the results obtained from 26 cadaver brains studied under microsurgical operating conditions, as well as 6 human brains fixed in formalin, whose vascular systems were previously injected with acrylate. Further results are based on studies of 32 cases of surgically treated lesions in the pineal and midbrain region.

TOPOGRAPHY

From the strictly anatomical point of view, the midbrain with the pineal body is part of the brainstem (Fig. 8.1). The pineal body lies above it within the quadrigeminal cistern. The midbrain measures in its sagittal superior-inferior length 12–18 mm over the quadrigeminal plate, 16–18 mm in the aqueduct area, and 9–10 mm at the base of the peduncles of the brain (49). It is bounded rostrally by the prosencephalon, the telencephalon, and diencephalon, and caudally by the rhombencephalon and the pons. Important landmarks in the pineal region are formed by the structures of the third ventricle. The inferior border of the third ventricle consists of the midbrain with the cerebral peduncles. The posterior border of the third ventricle consists of the pineal body with its pineal and suprapineal recesses, the posterior commissure and habenular commissure, the tectum, and the aqueduct. The posterior part of the roof of the third ventricle consists of the velum interpositum and the choroid plexus.

Spatz (53) places the anterior boundary of the midbrain caudal to the posterior commissure, the thalamus, the pulvinar of the thalamus, and caudal to the hypothalamus with the subthalamic and mammillary bodies. The caudal limit is bordered ventrally by the anterior edge of the pons and dorsally by the trochlear nerve (Fig. 8.1).

Most authors associate the pineal body with the diencephalon. Some, however, e.g. Pernkopf (41), assign it to the midbrain. The pineal body (Figs. 8.2 and 8.3) has an average length of 7 mm ($\pm$2 mm) and the dimensions of its oval shape in a transverse section are 7.7 mm ($\pm$2 mm) in transverse diameter, and 3 mm ($\pm$1.5 mm) in vertical diameter.

It is generally accepted that, in normal anatomy, the position of the pineal body is located in the midline. Detailed measurements with computerized tomography, however, may indicate some degree of pineal shift in a normal CT scan. The range of percentage shift of the pineal body was defined as a mean value of 18% with a standard deviation of 0.6%, i.e. the pineal body can be expected to be shifted 2.6% or less of the calvarian diameter from the midline (17). This deviation, however, causes no interference during microsurgical exposure.

Topographically, the midbrain lies in the tentorial notch with the rostrally lying basal ganglia forming almost a right angle. Plaut (42) states that the width of the tentorial notch varies, independent of the size of the cranium in a breadth of between 39–61 mm. But Klintworth (25) states that the size (surface of the notch opening) is unaltered in regard to the ontogenetic development in relation to the stage of skull size in infants and children. Thirty-five fresh cadavers in the 40–70-yr-old range were measured from the posterior of the sella in a straight line to where the great vein of Galen

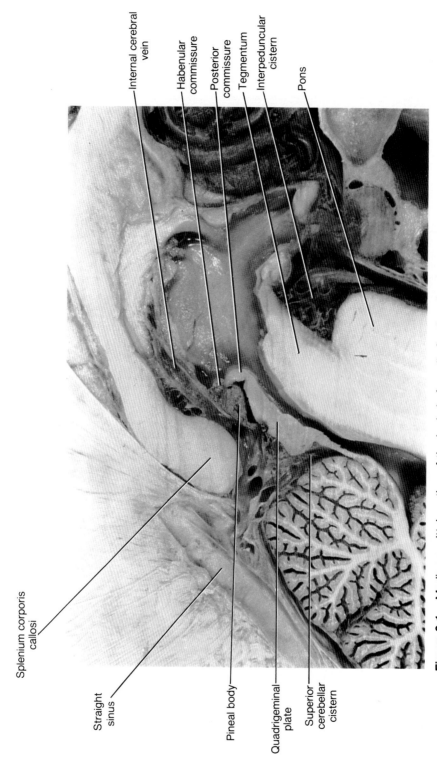

Figure 8.1. Median sagittal section of the brain in formalin fixation showing the upper brain stem and pineal region with the third ventricle.

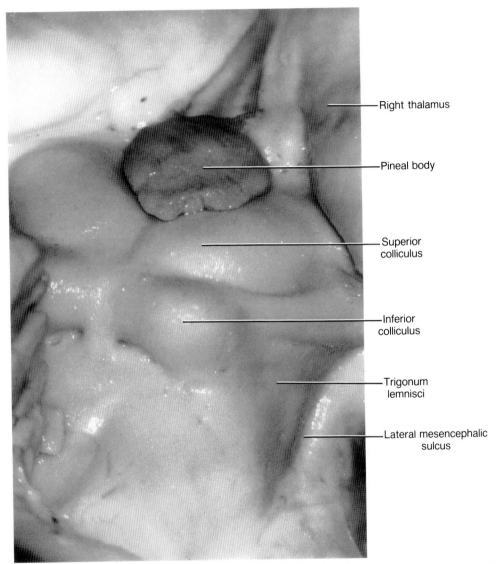

Figure 8.2. The quadrigeminal plate in a formalin-fixed brain after removal of the splenium and the right cerebellar hemisphere. View from the right and occipital.

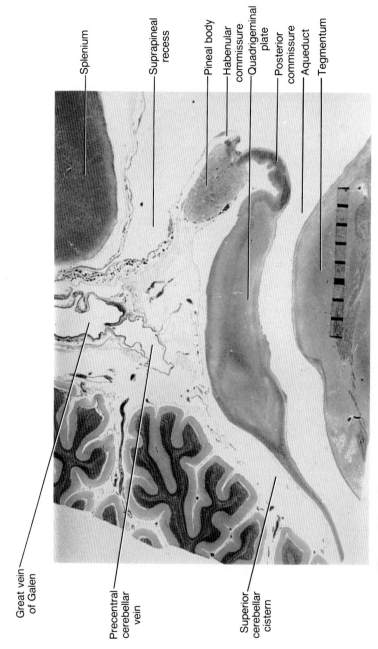

Figure 8.3. Histological slice of the pineal region in H + E staining, midsagittal section. Note the size relationship according to the millimeter marker. (By courtesy of J. Lang, M.D., Professor of Anatomy, Würzburg, Germany.)

Splenium

Suprapineal recess

Pineal body

Habenular commissure

Quadrigeminal plate

Posterior commissure

Aqueduct

Tegmentum

Great vein of Galen

Precentral cerebellar vein

Superior cerebellar cistern

discharges at the high end of the roof of the tentorium. The length varied from 40–72 mm, and the width ranged from 22–40 mm. The measurements agree with Plaut (42) and Klintworth's (25) size relationships.

On the basis of clinical and morphological findings, neurosurgery has devised another topographical relationship. In this relationship the pineal body and its tumors, the invading tumors of the midbrain, and those of the inferior part of the third ventricle are grouped together into the so-called tumors of the pineal region (72). Thus Ringertz et al (47) define the pineal region as that region limited dorsally by the splenium of the corpus callosum and the tela choroidea ventrally by quadrigeminal plate, rostrally by the posterior point of the third ventricle, and caudally by the vermis of the cerebellum. Olivecrona (35) uses the same definition of pineal tumors but adds that ventriculogram findings should show a common deformation protruding into the posterior part of the third ventricle. Thus, Olivecrona includes tumors of the quadrigeminal plate and even those of the basal ganglia into the topographical definition. Even Stein et al (56) include third ventricular masses in their description of pineal tumors. Cushing (9), Koos and Miller (26) also group pineal region and midbrain tumors together topographically. Other authors (8, 12) do the same on the basis of radiological diagnosis.

THE CISTERNS OF THE MIDBRAIN

The midbrain is surrounded by cisterns as a protection against the sharp edges of the tentorial notch (27, 53). Here the veins and arteries are embedded in the very firm arachnoid septa. The quadrigeminal cistern bathing the superior and inferior colliculi extends anteriorly to the pineal body and the trigonum of the habenula; it then continues anteriorly over these structures into the cistern of the tela choroidea of the third ventricle. The quadrigeminal cistern empties laterally into the alae (29, 64). Dorsally, there is a connection to the dorsal cistern of the corpus callosum along the great vein of the Galen between the splenium of the corpus callosum and the culmen of the vermis of the cerebellum. Caudally, the quadrigeminal cistern is bounded by the anterior medullary velum, the anterior cerebellum, and the superior vermis; this CSF space between the medullary velum and the vermis is called the superior cistern of the cerebellum. On both sides, anterobasally

wrapping itself around the tegmentum and the crura cerebri, is the ambient cistern contiguous to the pulvinar of the thalamus. In it, accompanied by the edge of the tentorium, lie the large arteries (posterior cerebral artery and its branches, superior cerebellar artery). The former courses to the midbrain and the brainstem ganglia, the latter, to the cerebellum and terminates near the basal vein of Rosenthal. Dorsally the trochlear nerves traverse anteriorly around the crura cerebri. Basally, the ambient cistern connects with the crural cistern (peripeduncular cistern) around the crura cerebri with the intercrural cistern (interpeducular cistern) between the crura cerebri, anteriorly into the chiasmatic cistern, and inferiorly into the pontine cistern. The transition between the intercrural cistern to the ambient cistern before and around the crura cerebri is also called the crural cistern or the prepeduncular cistern (3, 29, 30, 50, 69) (Fig. 8.3).

VESSELS IN THE MIDBRAIN AREA

Wackenheim and Braun (69) correctly emphasized that exact knowledge of the angiology of the midbrain, based on angiography, makes even the tentative interpretation of vessels in that area no longer seem so problematic. It is our opinion, however, that tumor diagnosis and prognosis based on angiography is inferior to a diagnosis based on computerized tomography, brain scan, and ventriculogram. Fundamentally, the vascular course in the midbrain itself determines the choice of operative approach to the area surrounding the quadrigeminal body. It should be noted that the normal anatomy of the mesencephalic veins and arteries, already quite varied themselves, may be further fundamentally altered in angioarchitecture and vascular course by pathological conditions (2, 34, 36, 62, 71).

The purpose of this article is to study the principal vessels the surgeon always encounters in the midbrain region. The pertinent literature on the usefulness of angiograms of the mesencephalic vascular systems should be reviewed (4, 5, 13, 37, 52, 57, and Chapter 3 of this volume). Wackenheim and Braun (61) compare and critically review the different nomenclatures. Wollenschlager et al (66) can also be reviewed in reference to the small vessels supplying the parenchyma. These vessels arise predominantly from the posterior cerebral artery and its connection between the basilar artery and the communicating artery and its anastomoses.

Figure 8.4 shows the common course of the arteries and veins schematically. Additionally it should be noted that the basal vein of Rosenthal runs anterior to the posterior cerebral artery and that both lie superior to the tentorial notch. The superior cerebellar artery and the trochlear nerve lie inferior to the tentorial notch, while the trochlear nerve lies between the posterior cerebral artery and superior cerebellar artery, crossing the latter in its course (Figs. 8.5 and 8.6).

ARTERIES OF THE MIDBRAIN

As the terminal branch of the basilar artery, the posterior cerebral artery winds obliquely and occipitally around the cerebral peduncle in the ambient cistern. Duvernoy (13) states that only a few small perforating branches directly supply the cerebral peduncles and the rest of the midbrain. These small vessels supplying the parenchyma, which Wollenschlager et al (66) call an internal or direct system, all arise from the posterior communicating artery, whereby the posterior thalamoperforating arteries are only partial suppliers; the latter send out small branches to the red nucleus, substantia nigra, and to the anterior part of the crura cerebri (63). The medial peduncular arteries, short and long branches of the posterior cerebral artery, supply the different tissue sections of the mesencephalon individually. This redundancy of vascular supply systems and anastomosis formation (51) explain the rather rare occurrence of infarcts in the mesencephalic area and the remarkable tolerance of the midbrain to direct surgical intervention (38, 39). Above and posterior to the quadrigeminal plate, the two posterior cerebral arteries, supplying mainly the occipital lobes, approach each other. Small branches of the posterior communicating artery and branches of the quadrigeminal artery and the anterior choroidal artery supply the crura cerebri. The anterior choroidal artery also has an anastomosis with the quadrigeminal artery and the medial posterior choroidal artery. In two-thirds of the brains examined, the pineal artery branches off the medial posterior choroidal artery and supplies the pineal body from both sides, penetrating into the lateral portion of the pineal body (67).

Superior Cerebellar Artery

Somewhat inferior to the pontomesencephalic sulcus, the superior cerebellar artery first arises

from the basilar artery and courses to the pontomesencephalic sulcus. Here it arrives at the lateral and anterior edge of the cerebellum and continues along it in the inferior area of the ambient cistern in the direction of the quadrigeminal cistern. With its median branch (ramus vermis) it sends out a branch to the inferior colliculi in that area, thus becoming, together with the main trunk itself, laterally visible proximal to the superior vermis above the superior cerebellar hemisphere. In the results of this study, the author determined two main trunks in 40 cases (71%), 3 main trunks in 7 instances (12%); ramification from the basilar artery was found in a simple form of 41 cases (73%) (Fig. 8.7), and a two-part ramification in 13 instances (23%) (Fig. 8.8). Two of these cases of two-part branching were found bilaterally in one brain, and twice unilaterally from the posterior cerebral artery. The vascular ramification to the cerebellar hemisphere (medial and lateral branches) arose from the pontine segment in only 6 cases (11%), and in 50 cases (89%) from the segment in the ambient cistern from the point where it crosses the lateral mesencephalic sulcus.

The superior vermian branch arose from the segment of the ambient cistern in 44 cases (79%), and in 12 cases (21%) from the segment in the quadrigeminal area. In all 44 cases the function of the vermian artery of supplying the inferior colliculi could be demonstrated, whereas anastomoses with branches of the quadrigeminal arteries was not always proven (Figs. 8.6, 8.10, and 8.11).

Posterior Cerebral Artery

The posterior cerebral artery originates in the peduncular cistern (Figs. 8.7 and 8.8) as a paired terminal branch of the basilar artery, and occasionally as a branch of the internal carotid. It then passes over the anterior and lateral surface of the crura cerebri in the ambient cistern accompanying the basal vein of Rosenthal closely against the hippocampal gyrus, and runs to the lateral mesencaphalic sulcus. It is here the artery first divides into two or three main branches and continues in a lateral direction away from the cisternal region to the temporal and occipital lobes (Figs. 8.5 and 8.13). The following variations in form and branching of the posterior cerebral artery were observed in our 56 separate examinations: in 36 cases (64%) it originated bilaterally from the basilar artery with a medium-sized posterior communicating artery; in 8

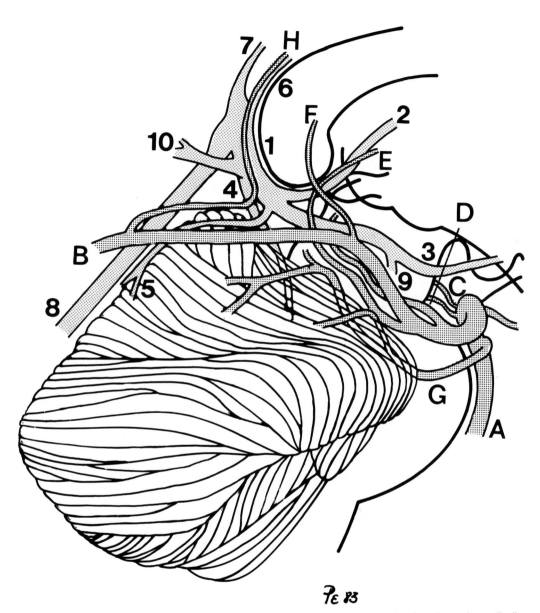

Figure 8.4. Common course of arteries and veins of the midbrain and pineal region schematically: A, basilar artery; B, posterior cerebral artery; C, posterior thalamoperforating arteries; D, quadrigeminal artery; E, medial posterior choroidal artery; F, lateral posterior choroidal artery; G, superior cerebellar artery; H, posterior pericallosal artery; 1, great vein of Galen; 2, internal cerebral vein; 3, basal vein of Rosenthal; 4, precentral cerebellar vein; 5, superior cerebellar vein; 6, posterior pericallosal vein; 7, inferior sagittal sinus; 8, straight sinus; 9, mesencephalic vein; 10, internal occipital vein.

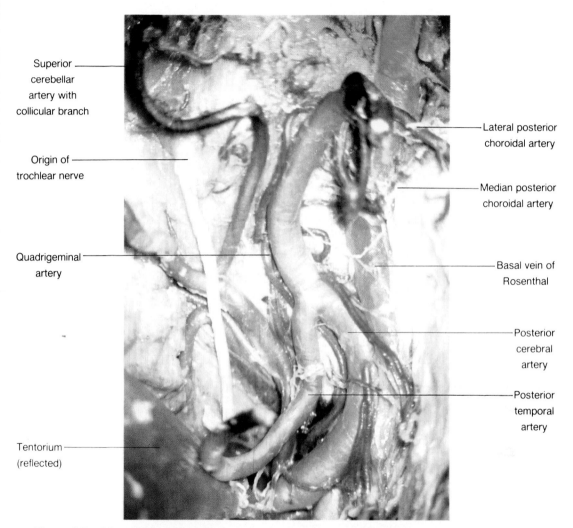

Superior cerebellar artery with collicular branch

Origin of trochlear nerve

Quadrigeminal artery

Tentorium (reflected)

Lateral posterior choroidal artery

Median posterior choroidal artery

Basal vein of Rosenthal

Posterior cerebral artery

Posterior temporal artery

Figure 8.5.   View of the right ambient cistern from lateral, the occipital lobe has been removed, also the tentorium has been turned laterally. (Kallocryl-M-injection).

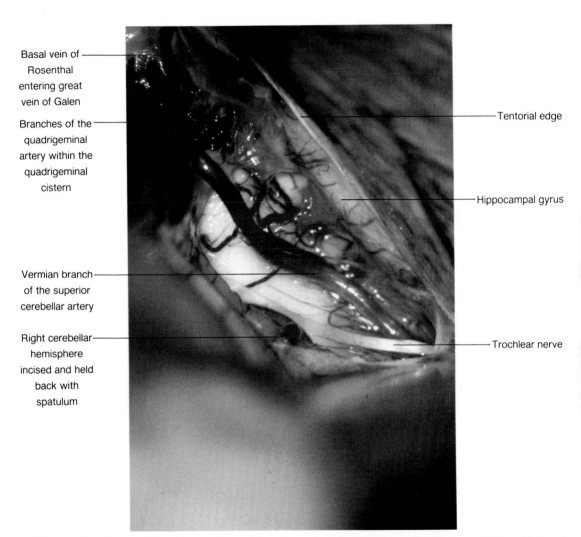

Basal vein of Rosenthal entering great vein of Galen

Branches of the quadrigeminal artery within the quadrigeminal cistern

Vermian branch of the superior cerebellar artery

Right cerebellar hemisphere incised and held back with spatulum

Tentorial edge

Hippocampal gyrus

Trochlear nerve

Figure 8.6. View of the right ambient cistern from an infratentorial approach in a patient with a hamartoma in the midbrain.

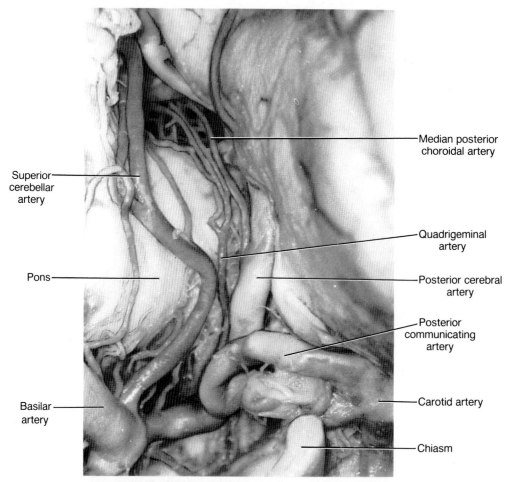

Superior
cerebellar
artery

Pons

Basilar
artery

Median posterior
choroidal artery

Quadrigeminal
artery

Posterior cerebral
artery

Posterior
communicating
artery

Carotid artery

Chiasm

Figure 8.7. View of the right ambient cistern from slightly below with the arteries running around the cerebral peduncle towards the quadrigeminal cistern. The temporal lobe of the formalin-fixed brain is pulled upwards slightly.

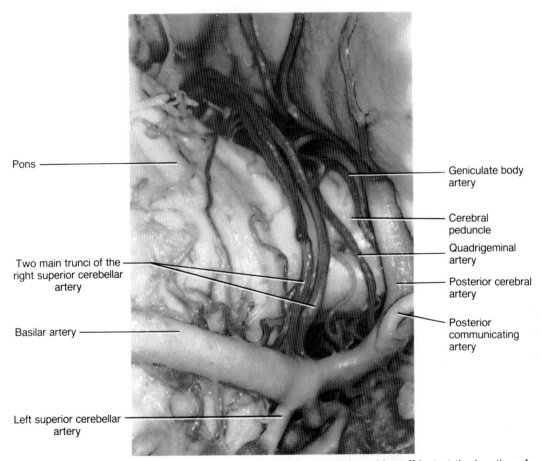

Figure 8.8. Two main trunks of the superior cerebellar artery, branching off just at the junction of the pons with the midbrain. View from the right and below in a formalin-fixed brain.

cases (14%) it arose directly from the internal carotid artery with a bilateral medium-sized anastomoses to the basilar artery; and in 4 cases (7%) it arose from the basilar artery on one side and from the internal carotid artery on the other side with variable communicating vessels in between. In two cases the posterior communicating artery was unilaterally absent, and the posterior cerebral artery originated bilaterally from the basilar artery. In four cases (7%) a marked difference in the lumen size of both posterior communicating arteries and a corresponding size difference in origin from the basilar artery were observed. In only two cases the posterior cerebrals originated from the basilar artery unilaterally and jointly with the superior cerebellar artery (4%). Perforating branches of the posterior cerebral artery to the interpeduncular region as well as peduncular branches and circumflexing mesencephalic branches were observed in all 56 cases (Fig. 8.9).

Quadrigeminal Artery

This artery is the first large branch of the posterior cerebral artery after the origin of the posterior communicating artery and principally supplies the superior colliculi. It more commonly also lies beneath the posterior cerebral artery in the crural cistern and diverges from the same course only in the ambient cistern or usually after the lateral mesencephalic sulcus (Figs. 8.5–8.7 and 8.9–8.11). The quadrigeminal artery, in the majority of cases, thus lies anterior to the oculomotor nerve, and separation occurs at the level of the inferior collicular brachium, the inferior branch going to the intercollicular sulcus. The superior branch winds around the superior colliculus and divides up into many branchlets. The quadrigeminal artery with its fine branches supplies the crus cerebri and the trigeminal lemniscus. It then forms anastomoses with branches of the medial posterior choroidal artery and branches off the medial superior cerebellar artery (13). It was recognizable in all 56 examined cases, and had, in 24 cases (43%), a simple main branch which branched first at the quadrigeminal plate, and in 32 cases (57%) it was double, each segment arising individually from the posterior cerebral artery. The branches themselves in 40 cases (71%) were still located in the interpeduncular segment of the posterior cerebral artery before the junction of the posterior communicating artery, and in 16 cases

(29%) the branching occurred after the junction of the posterior communicating artery.

Medial Posterior Choroidal Artery

This artery branches off the posterior cerebral artery shortly after the quadrigeminal artery (Figs. 8.7, 8.9–8.11, and 8.13). It proceeds inferior to the medial geniculate body and, covered by the pulvinar, it continues in a pronounced loop lateral to the pineal body, anteriolaterally to the tela choroidea of the third ventricle. With its ramifications the medial posterior choroidal artery supplies the crus cerebri, the medial geniculate body, and superior parts of the midbrain. Many branches also reach to the extended capillary network above the quadrigeminal bodies, but they only supply the superior colliculi. The shapes of the loop formation and ramifications of these vessels are highly variable and their differentiation during an operative approach to the tentorial notch is anything but easy.

Geniculate Body Artery

This especially variably formed artery runs as a single vessel or in multiple branches to the medial and lateral geniculate bodies, giving off branches to the midbrain and to the region of the pineal body and to the superior aspect of the thalamus (Fig. 8.12). In 42 cases (75%) 3–5 branches arose from the posterior cerebral artery in the ambient segment, and in 14 cases (25%) branches of this artery arose from the quadrigeminal artery.

Lateral Posterior Choroidal Artery

This branch of the posterior cerebral artery in the ambient or quadrigeminal region goes in the choroidal fissure rostrally and laterally to the plexus of the temporal horn (Fig. 8.14). Some branches draw off to the pulvinar and the thalamus. The artery was definitely identifiable in all 56 cases. In 40 cases (72%) it was seen as a simple main branch, and in 16 cases (28%) as a double main branch each with an individual junction. In 44 cases (79%) the junctions were located in the ambient segment, in 8 cases (14%) they were located above the quadrigeminal cistern in the hemisphere region, and in 4 cases (7%) the junction was recognizable in the interpeduncular segment. In all cases with junctions

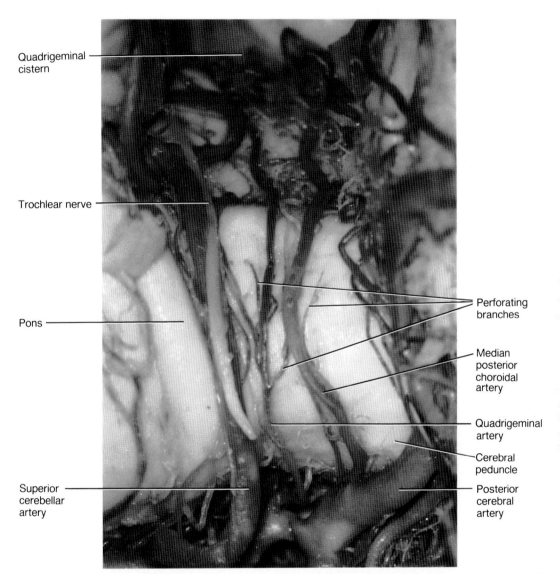

Figure 8.9. View of the right ambient cistern in a formalin-fixed brain, the trochlear nerve well preserved crossing the superior cerebellar artery. Note the perforating small branches to the parenchyma of the midbrain.

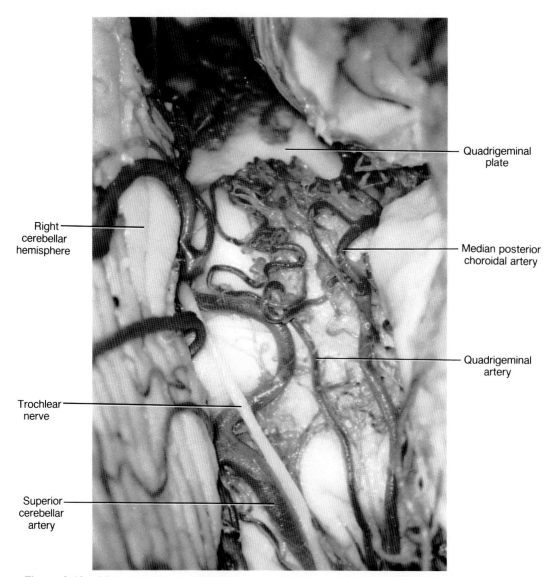

Quadrigeminal plate

Right cerebellar hemisphere

Median posterior choroidal artery

Quadrigeminal artery

Trochlear nerve

Superior cerebellar artery

Figure 8.10. View into the quadrigeminal cistern from the right, the occipital lobe of the formalin-fixed brain has been removed. Loops of the quadrigeminal artery supplying the upper colliculi.

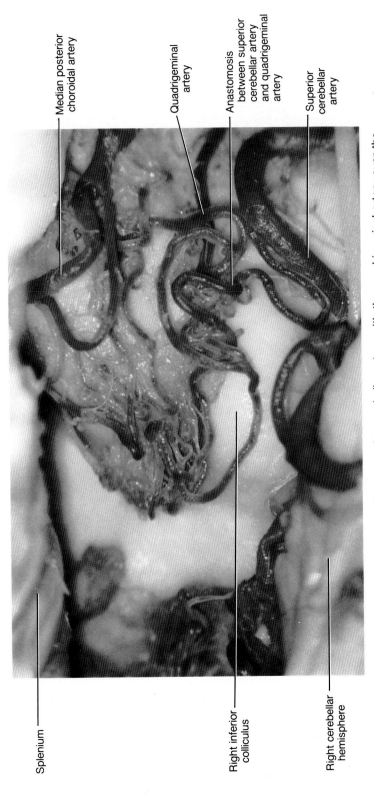

Figure 8.11. Anastomosis of the superior cerebellar artery with the quadrigeminal artery over the quadrigeminal plate in a formalin-fixed brain.

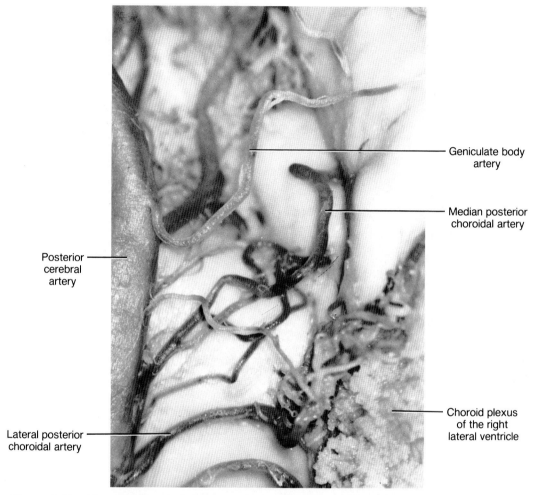

Geniculate body artery

Median posterior choroidal artery

Posterior cerebral artery

Choroid plexus of the right lateral ventricle

Lateral posterior choroidal artery

Figure 8.12. View into the quadrigeminal cistern after removal of the occipital lobe in a formalin-fixed brain. Note the marked geniculate body artery.

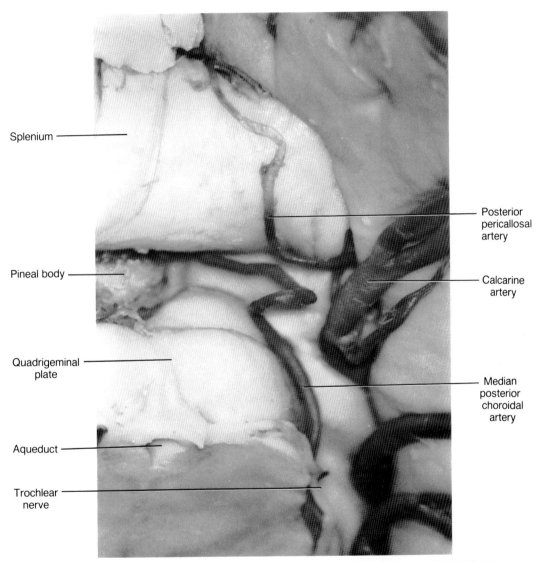

Splenium

Pineal body

Quadrigeminal
plate

Aqueduct

Trochlear
nerve

Posterior
pericallosal
artery

Calcarine
artery

Median
posterior
choroidal
artery

Figure 8.13.   View into the right pineal region after removal of the cerebellum and pons.

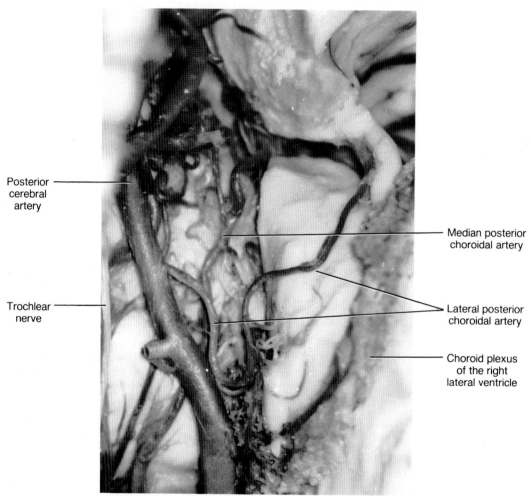

Posterior cerebral artery

Trochlear nerve

Median posterior choroidal artery

Lateral posterior choroidal artery

Choroid plexus of the right lateral ventricle

Figure 8.14.   Demonstration of the lateral posterior choroidal artery after removal of the right parietal and temporal lobe in a formalin-fixed brain.

in the hemisphere region with a single main branch, the artery traversed the lateral region of the quadrigeminal cistern as a large loop. In all the other cases the artery did not reach the quadrigeminal area.

Posterior Pericallosal Artery

This artery represents an anastomosis to the anterior pericallosal artery. Branching off later from the posterior cerebral artery, the posterior pericallosal artery proceeds superior to the quadrigeminal plate close to midline and with a loop anteriorly into the lateral quadrigeminal cistern bends further on around the splenium of the corpus callosum, and has an anastomosis with the anterior pericallosal artery (30). The vessel was observed to have many variations (Fig. 8.13). In 38 cases (68%) it was seen arising from the posterior cerebral artery in the parietal-occipital region after the branching off the calcarinal artery. In 10 cases (18%) it arose from the lateral posterior choroidal artery which originates here from the parietal segment. In 8 cases (18%) the artery was identified as a branch of the anterior pericallosal artery (Fig. 8.15).

Posterior Temporal Artery and the Calcarinal Artery

The posterior temporal artery and the calcarinal artery (forming a loop) (Fig. 8.13) were not observed in the cistern because they immediately disappear into the sulci of the temporal and occipital lobes after arising from the posterior cerebral artery in the ambient and quadrigeminal segment. In the ambient segment, in 8 cases (14%), they were located above the quadrigeminal cistern in the hemisphere region, and in 4 cases (7%) the junction was recognizable in the interpeduncular segment. In all cases with junctions in the hemisphere region with a single main branch, the temporal artery traversed the lateral region of the quadrigeminal cistern as a large loop. In all the other cases the artery did not reach the quadrigeminal area.

THE VEINS OF THE MIDBRAIN

The deep venous structures of the great vein of Galen and its tributaries form a roof-like dense venous network above the pineal body and the quadrigeminal plate. Their vulnerability during pineal region surgery was the main cause of the pessimistic attitude towards lesion in the pineal region. Clear cut representations and identifications of the veins as well as results for evaluation were obtained in 22 cases of cadaver brains studied. Figure 8.16, an injected specimen, shows the venous system of the midbrain-quadrigeminal region as the mainstream flow to the great vein of Galen and to the straight sinus. The basal vein of Rosenthal bounds the superior lateral region of the midbrain. It courses in the ambient cistern parallel to the posterior cerebral artery and flows into the great vein of Galen next to the pineal body. The lateral mesencephalic vein courses in and about the lateral mesencephalic sulcus rostrally upwards and flows into the basal vein of Rosenthal and also anastomoses to the petrosal vein. The solitary precentral cerebellar vein arises from the anterior

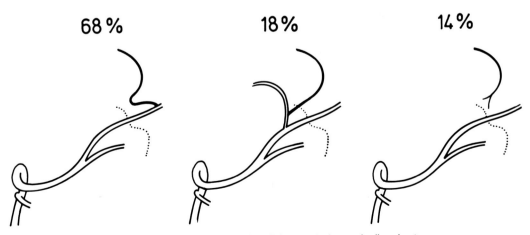

Figure 8.15.   Variations or origin of the posterior pericallosal artery.

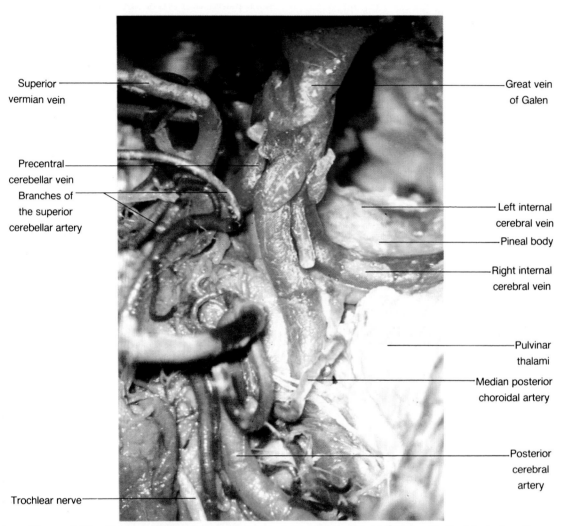

Figure 8.16. Kallocryl-M-injection preparation of the great vein of Galen with its tributaries, the splenium of the corpus callosum has been removed as well as the hemispheres and the tentorium with the straight sinus. View from the right.

region of the fourth ventricle, courses upwards and rostrally in the precentral cerebellar fissure and again somewhat occipitally in the quadrigeminal cistern before the vermis, and finally empties into the great vein of Galen shortly before the junction into the straight sinus. This vein seldom occurs as a pair (48). The smaller and paired precentral lateral veins flow somewhat laterally to it, to the vena magna of Galen. The superior vermian vein originates in the cerebellar hemisphere, courses over the culmen, and empties into the great vein of Galen somewhat before the precentral vein (59). The paired internal cerebral veins course from rostral under the splenium and over the pineal gland and empty in the great vein of Galen. The basal vein of Rosenthal flows in from a lateral inferior direction (22, 65).

Pineal Veins

The pineal veins were extensively studied by Tamaki et al in 1973 (58). Since then, their importance in the angiographic anatomy and pathology as well as their diagnostic importance in the early and specific recognition of pineal lesions has become less important since the introduction of computerized tomography. These veins can originate as far away as the trigonum habenulae and the dorsal aspect of the pineal body. A ventral group originates at the junction of the superior colliculi to the base of the pineal body and forms a single trunk with the superior group in the quadrigeminal cistern. They empty directly into the great vein of Galen. They have little or no importance during microsurgical exposure of pineal lesions. The various nomenclatures given to these pineal veins in literature are listed by Yamamoto and Kageyama (67), who classified them into five types according to the mode of drainage into either the internal cerebral veins, the great vein of Galen, or the precentral cerebellar vein.

Great Vein of Galen

This vein arises from the junction of the paired internal cerebral veins, is adjacent to the splenium of the corpus callosum, and empties into the foremost part of the straight sinus (Figs. 8.16 and 8.19) in the area of the superior posterior sharp border of the tentorial incisure. On the basis of 131 cadaver studies, Browder et al (6) determined that its length varies from 1.5–4

cm. In the current series, the junction of the vein into the straight sinus was acutely angled in 15 cases and square, angled, or flat in 7 cases studied.

Internal Cerebral Veins

This paired vein arises from the transverse fissure cistern and forms the great vein of Galen. It was always located above and lateral to the pineal gland before its junction to the great vein of Galen. In our study no variations in its positions were observed (Fig. 8.16).

Basal Vein of Rosenthal

This vein is formed in the region of the optic tract and runs closely along the optic tract, around the peduncle, and nestles in the ambient cistern close to the basal ganglia (Figs. 8.5 and 8.16). This segment in the region of the cerebral peduncle could only be seen by extreme retraction of the temporal lobe of the cadaver brain. During a temporal surgical approach, this segment is concealed by the parahippocampal gyrus and the uncinate gyrus in the ala of the ambient cistern. In its dorsal segment, after it crosses the lateral mesencephalic sulcus, it junctions with the lateral mesencephalic vein, which is an anastomosis to the superior petrosal sinus. This anastomosis was not always observed in our study. The further laterodorsal course of the basal vein to the great vein of Galen is crossed somewhat rostrally by several branches of the posterior cerebral artery (medial and lateral posterior quadrigeminal arteries, geniculate body artery) (Fig. 8.5). Occasionally a branch of the medial posterior choroidal artery can also be observed basal to this vein. In 12 cases (54%) the basal vein was seen to flow directly into the great vein of Galen, in 8 cases (36%) it emptied into the internal cerebral vein, and in only 2 cases (9%) it emptied bilaterally, symmetrically, and directly into the straight sinus (Fig. 8.17).

Internal Occipital Vein

In all 22 cases a relatively large-lumen internal occipital vein, approximately ⅔ the size of the internal cerebral vein, was observed. In 17 cases this vein ran on the basal medial surface of the occipital lobe obliquely, occipitally, and directly into the great vein of Galen. The main branch is formed 0.5–1 cm before the junction

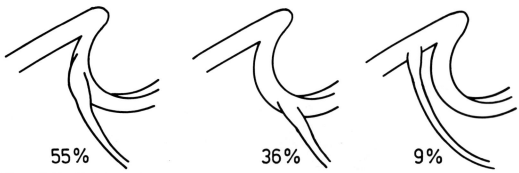

Figure 8.17.   Variations of draining of the basal vein of Rosenthal with the great vein of Galen and straight sinus.

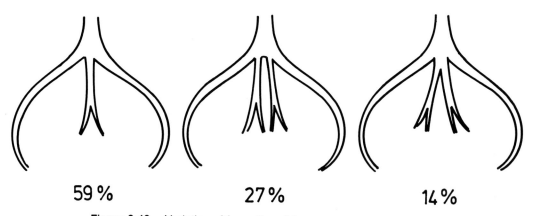

Figure 8.18.   Variation of formation of the precentral cerebellar vein.

from numerous joining branches (Fig. 8.23). In 2 cases it emptied into the basal vein, and in 3 cases it had 2 or more terminal branches.

Precentral Cerebellar Vein

This vein runs from the precentral cerebellar fissure between the lingular and the central lobe, anterior to the vermis, through the quadrigeminal cistern to the great vein of Galen. This vein was observed unpaired in 13 cases (59%) and paired in 6 cases (27%). In 3 cases (14%) it junctioned with a paired vein shortly before emptying into the great vein of Galen. All drained into the upper third of the great vein of Galen (Figs. 8.16, 8.18, and 8.19). Coagulation of this vein in the infratentorial approach to the pineal region causes no further morbidity (38, 46, 54).

Superior Cerebellar Vein

This vein, also called the superior vermian vein, shows many variations. It runs rostrally on the dorsal surface of the cerebellar hemisphere and on the surface of the vermis (Fig. 8.16). In 15 cases (68%) it emptied directly into the great vein of Galen underneath the junction of the precentral cerebellar vein. In 2 cases (9%) it emptied into the basal vein of Rosenthal, and in 5 cases (23%) directly into the straight sinus (Fig. 8.20).

Posterior Pericallosal Vein

This small vein runs over the splenium corpora callosa and drains into the great vein of Galen shortly before the junction in the straight sinus (Fig. 8.4). In 11 cases (50%) this vein was

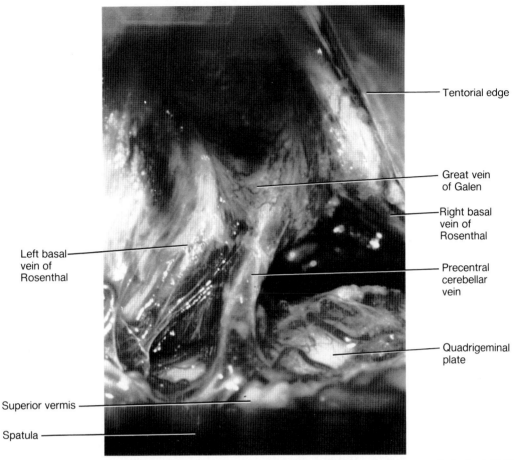

Tentorial edge

Great vein of Galen

Right basal vein of Rosenthal

Left basal vein of Rosenthal

Precentral cerebellar vein

Quadrigeminal plate

Superior vermis

Spatula

Figure 8.19. Preserved precentral cerebellar vein in a clinical case of a pineal tumor. Note the tumor cavity above the quadrigeminal plate.

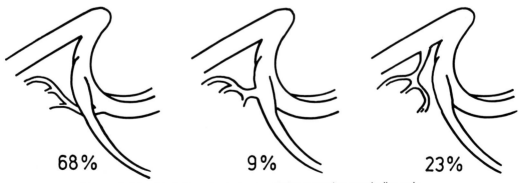

68%   9%   23%

Figure 8.20. Variations in drainage of the superior cerebellar vein.

doubled and had a variable lumen. In 4 cases (18%) it was a single vein, and in the rest of the cases (7%) it was not present at all.

Inferior Sagittal Sinus

Located in the inferior border of the falx, it drains directly into the straight sinus together with the great vein of Galen. Out of a total of 26 cadaver brains studied, this sinus was totally missing in 2 cases (8%), and in the other 24 specimens it had a variable lumen.

Mesencephalic Vein

This vein is the most frequent and most important anastomosis between the system of the great vein of Galen and the superior petrosal sinus, and lies in the lateral mesencephalic sulcus. A prominent mesencephalic vein was observed in only 10 cases (45%). In five cases (23%) the vein was delicately branched, and in seven cases (32%) remained undetermined for technical reasons (Fig. 8.4).

ANATOMICAL EVALUATION OF THE APPROACHES TO THE PINEAL REGION USING MICROSURGICAL TECHNIQUES

Since the first surgical attempt to remove pinealomas, the discussion as to the optimal approach has not ceased. As early as 1935 McLean (31) compared the different surgical approaches without criticism or preferences to any single one. Baggenstoss and Love (1) determined that all the approaches known in 1939 were unsatisfactory. Some authors are of the opinion that tumors in the pineal and midbrain region, per se, are inoperable lesions because of the important and vulnerable surrounding structures (11). Divided opinions exist as to whether pure pineal lesions, i.e., tumors of various histological origin above the quadrigeminal plate, are an indication for surgery. High mortality as well as morbidity in the operated cases made many surgeons skeptical as to the possibility of radical surgical removal. Thus the problems involved in the surgical approach to benign lesions located in deep areas has met with skepticism. Also Olivecrona (35), among others, stressed the vulnerability of the deep venous structures located above the quadrigeminal plate, foremost the great vein of Galen. Caron et al (7), however, reported on a well tolerated ligature of the great

vein of Galen in four exceptional cases. In 16 cases of pineal tumors reported by Hammock et al (18) the ligature of the great vein of Galen was also tolerated.

There are five possible surgical approaches to the pineal region:

Transcallosal approach by Dandy-Foerster;
Resection of the occipital lobe by Horrax;
Transventricular approach by VanWagenen;
Occipital-transtentorial approach by Heppner-Poppen;
Infratentorial-supracerebellar approach by Krause-Brunner.

Since the various surgical approaches reported in the literature incorporate many personal and individualistic characteristics developed mainly by macrosurgical techniques, we have attempted to compare and evaluate all these various approaches using microsurgical techniques in fresh cadavers as to their possibilities and as limits. The resection of the occipital lobe is not included in this study. The microsurgical techniques and the microtopographical anatomical details are compared as well.

Transcallosal Approach by Dandy-Foerster

This approach, preferred by most neurosurgeons, was successfully introduced by Dandy in 1921 and has been extensively described (10, 14, 23). The approach by Dandy-Foerster entails a rather large paramedian parieto-occipital osteoplastic craniotomy up to the sagittal sinus (Fig. 8.21), the dura mater is flapped toward the sinus and the bridging veins are sacrificed. After evacuation of the CSF from the hydrocephalic enlarged lateral ventricle, the hemisphere in most of the cases is gently pushed laterally with retractors away from the falx. When the splenium corporis callosi is reached, it is divided for a length of 2–4 cm. The bridging internal occipital vein, running either towards the great vein of Galen or towards the basal vein of Rosenthal, has to be sacrificed. To get a better view of the quadrigeminal area, the tentorium is incised along the straight sinus from the tentorial edge, a distance of about 2 cm. It may also be necessary to vertically incise the inferior sagittal sinus and the lower part of the falx in order to obtain a better view towards the opposite side. The deep venous structures are now exposed, but they still hinder the approach to the quadrigeminal plate and pineal body. Figures 8.22 through 8.24 demonstrate the operating field in a microsurgical preparation in a fresh cadaver.

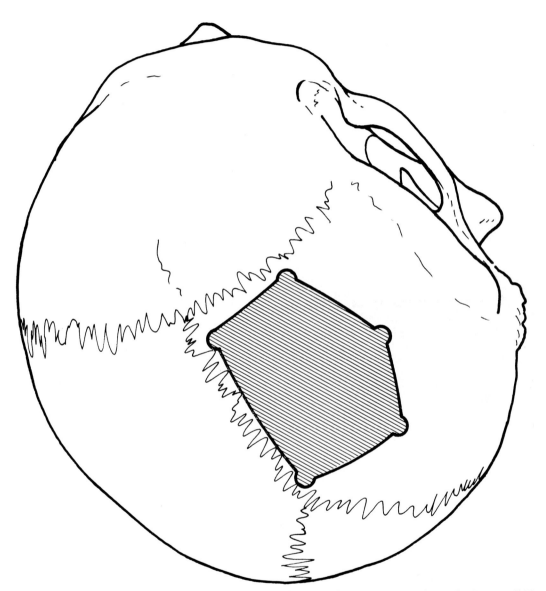

Figure 8.21. Projection of the skull with the bone flap area for the position of view for Figures 8.22 through 8.24.

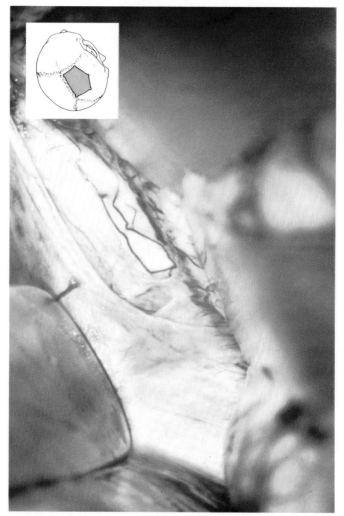

Figure 8.22A. Transcallosal approach by Dandy-Foerster showing the splenium, falx, and tentorial edge after retraction of the right hemisphere.

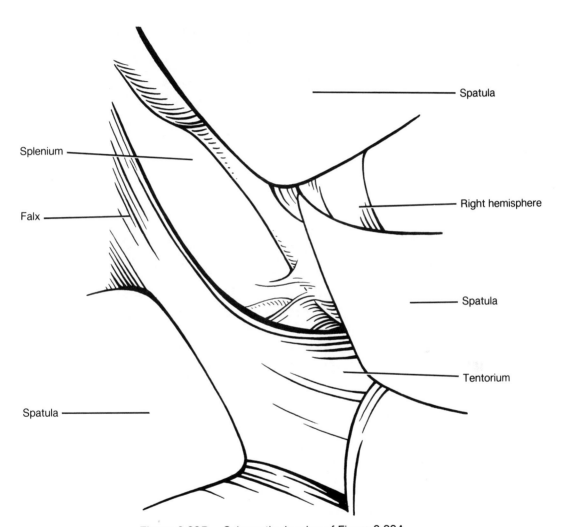

Figure 8.22B. Schematic drawing of Figure 8.22A.

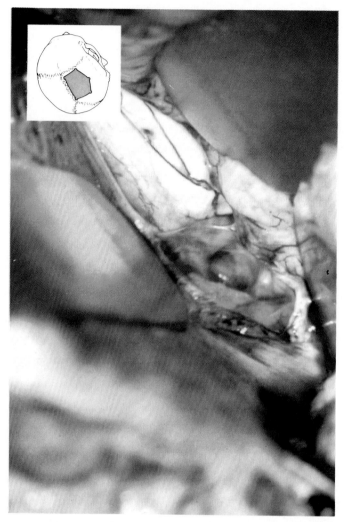

Figure 8.23A.   The tentorial edge is incised to expose part of the pineal region.

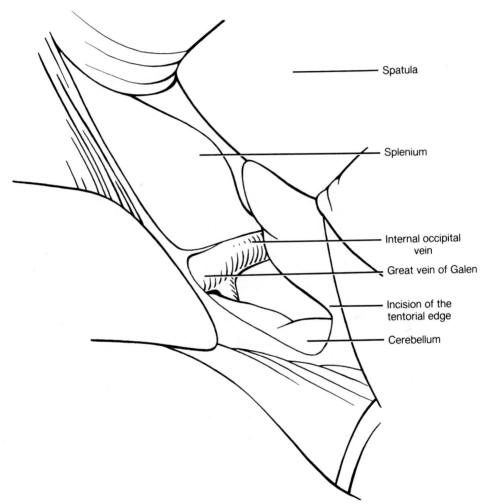

Spatula

Splenium

Internal occipital
vein

Great vein of Galen

Incision of the
tentorial edge

Cerebellum

Figure 8.23*B.*   Schematic drawing of Figure 8.23*A.*

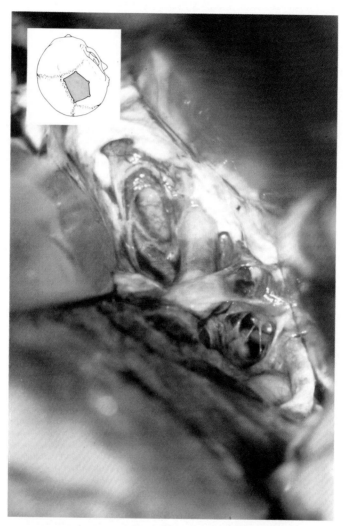

Figure 8.24A.   Exposure of the pineal region by the transcallosal approach; the splenium had also been transsected; the pineal body is partly covered by the deep venous structures.

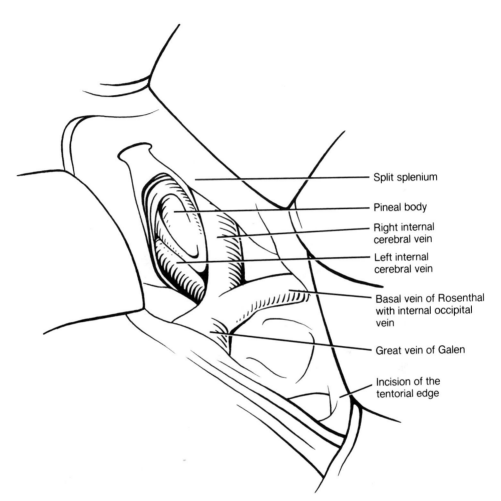

— Split splenium

— Pineal body

— Right internal cerebral vein

— Left internal cerebral vein

— Basal vein of Rosenthal with internal occipital vein

— Great vein of Galen

— Incision of the tentorial edge

Figure 8.24B. Schematic drawing of Figure 8.24A.

Transventricular Approach by Van Wagenen

This approach, published by Van Wagenen in 1931 (60), uses the hydrocephalic enlarged lateral ventricle as an access. After an L-shaped cortical incision in the superior temporal gyrus towards the parietal region of the trigonal area of the lateral ventricle, the ventricle is reached just behind the choroid plexus. The expansive lesion can be clearly localized under the thinned wall of the ventricle. The medial aspect of the ventricular wall is incised and the tumor is enucleated easily, sparing the deep lying structures, especially in more laterally located tumors. Figure 8.25 shows the location of the opening in the skull above the angular region. By dissecting the trigone, the quadrigeminal plate is accessible within a few millimeters, thus the great vein of Galen lies posteriorly, and the internal cerebral veins more apically, and the basal vein of Rosenthal is situated towards the base. Figures 8.26 and 8.27 demonstrate the surgical approach in an anatomical preparation in a fresh cadaver.

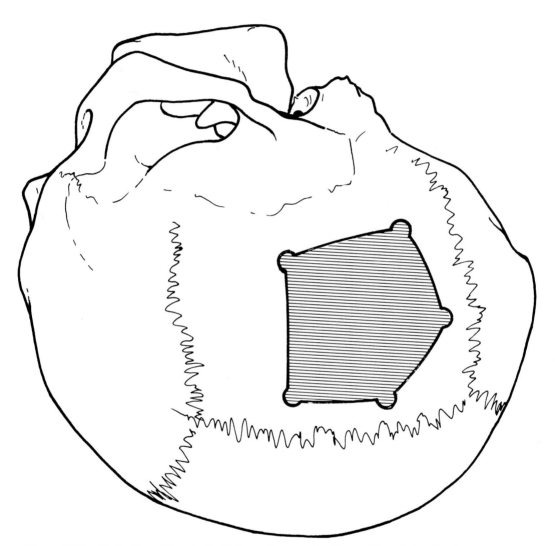

Figure 8.25. Projection of the skull with bone flap area for the position of view for Figures 8.26 and 8.27.

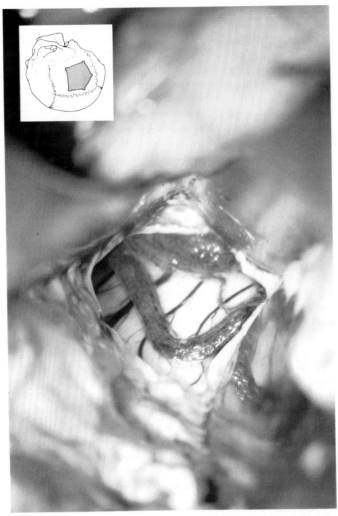

Figure 8.26A.   Exposure of the trigone of the right lateral ventricle in the transventricular approach by Van Wagenen (60).

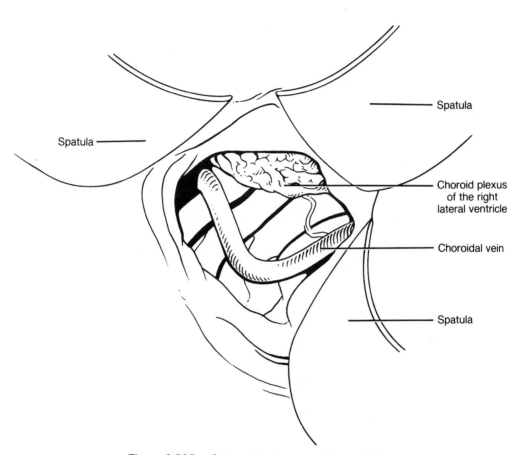

Figure 8.26B.   Schematic drawing of Figure 8.26A.

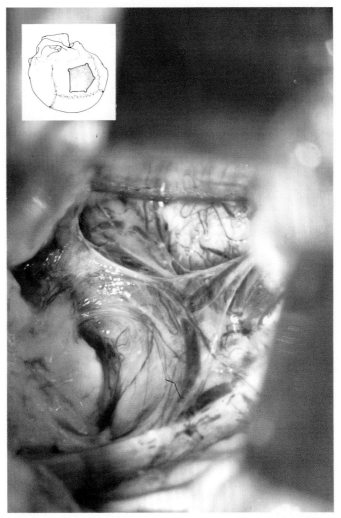

Figure 8.27A. Exposition of the pineal area without a space occupying lesion by the transventricular approach from the right.

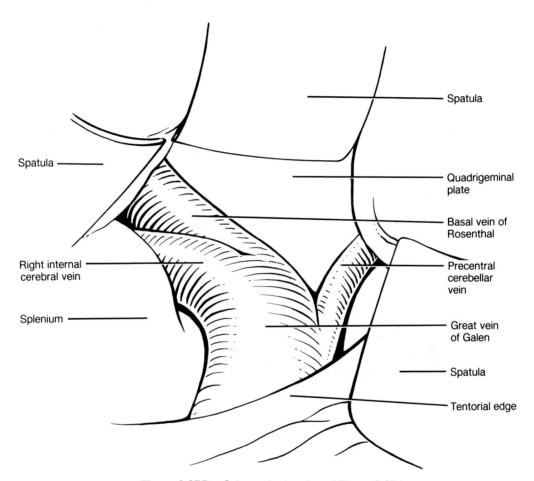

Figure 8.27B.   Schematic drawing of Figure 8.27A.

Occipital-Transtentorial Approach by Heppner-Poppen

This approach, later described by Poppen (43, 44), is technically difficult because the approach is much too narrow. To achieve a better view many authors (15, 28, 33) prefer the approach proposed by Heppner. This approach is performed with the patient in a sitting position. An osteoplastic trepanation is made in the occipital pole area, with enlargement to the contralateral side above the sagittal sinus and down to the confluens sinus. Fig. 8.28 shows the site of the craniotomy. After the dura has been opened crosswise, to spare the bridging veins to the sagittal sinus as well as to the transverse sinus, the posterior horn of the lateral ventricle is punctured and CSF aspirated to reduce ventricular pressure and to obtain more space. The occipital lobe is then lifted up laterally and thus access to the pineal region is obtained in the angle along the straight sinus between the falx and the tentorium. When the splenium corporis callosi is reached, the tentorial edge must be incised lateral to the straight sinus and paramedian for a length of at least 2 cm. A good view of the pineal region and the quadrigeminal plate is obtained without the hindering deep venous structures, which are now positioned above the approach. It is also possible to save the internal occipital vein using this approach. Figures 8.29 through 8.31 show the approach in anatomical preparation in a fresh cadaver.

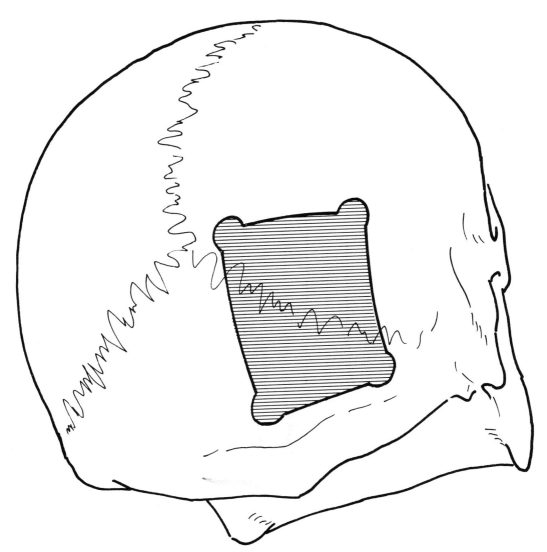

Figure 8.28.   Projection of the skull with bone flap area for the position of view for Figures 8.29 through 8.31.

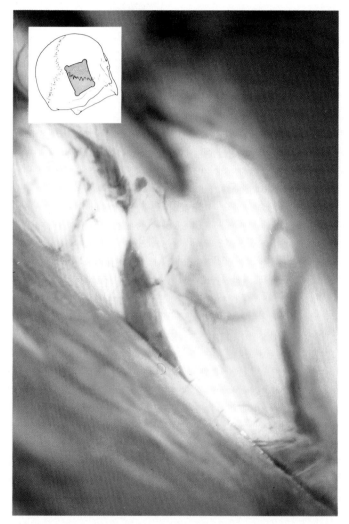

Figure 8.29A. Exposure of the splenium and tentorial edge in the suboccipital-transtentorial approach by Heppner-Poppen. The occipital lobe is lifted upwards and laterally.

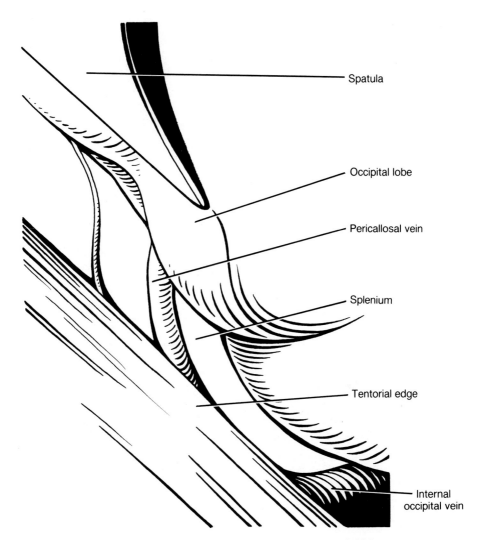

Spatula

Occipital lobe

Pericallosal vein

Splenium

Tentorial edge

Internal occipital vein

Figure 8.29B. Schematic drawing of Figure 8.29A.

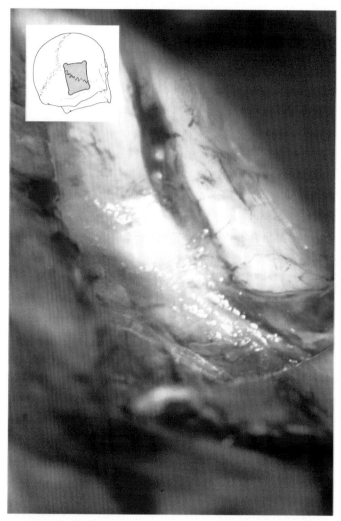

Figure 8.30A. The edge of the tentorium has been incised and reflected lateraly, the pineal area is beginning to be exposed.

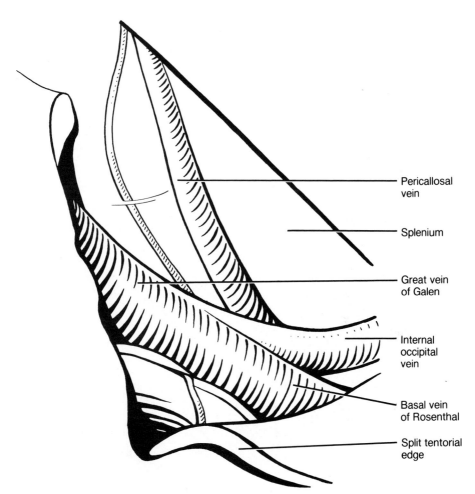

Figure 8.30B.   Schematic drawing of Figure 8.30A.

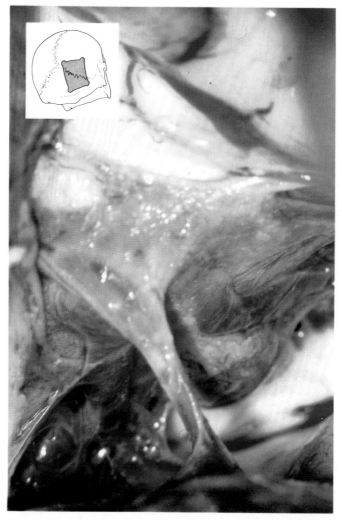

Figure 8.31*A*.   Exposure of the pineal region by the Heppner-Poppen approach.

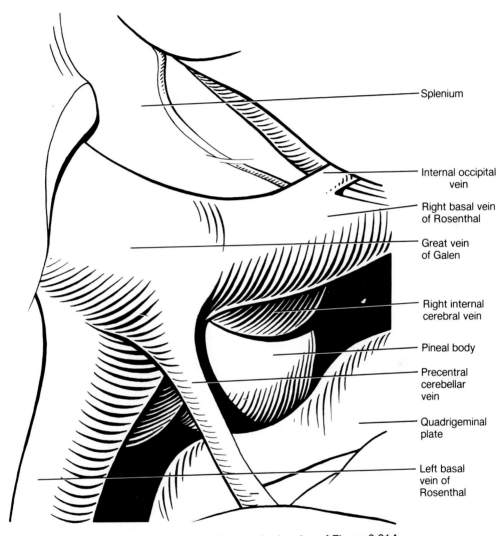

Splenium

Internal occipital
vein

Right basal vein
of Rosenthal

Great vein
of Galen

Right internal
cerebral vein

Pineal body

Precentral
cerebellar
vein

Quadrigeminal
plate

Left basal
vein of
Rosenthal

Figure 8.31B. Schematic drawing of Figure 8.31A.

Infratentorial-Supracerebellar Approach by Krause-Brunner

Special credit must be given to Stein (54) and Zapletal (70) for reviving this surgical approach to the pineal region. In this approach, a suboccipital craniectomy with extension well above the transverse sinus bilaterally is performed with the patient in a sitting position. It is possible to spare the arch of the atlas (Fig. 8.32). After the dura is opened in a Y-shape and the bridging veins from the cerebellar hemispheres and vermis to the tentorium are sacrificed, the cerebellum sinks well down and reveals a wide enough gap under the tentorium to the quadrigeminal cistern. Almost no further pressure with a retractor is necessary. The dense arachnoid of the quadrigeminal cisterns must be parted with a sharp incision in order not to tear the venous structures. After the dissection, the quadrigeminal plate is sufficiently exposed. Splitting the upper vermis will occasionally improve the view (16). The deeper venous structures are well exposed above the surgical field, occasionally only the precentral cerebellar vein must be sacrificed. Figs. 8.33 and 8.34 show this approach stepwise in a microsurgical preparation in a fresh cadaver.

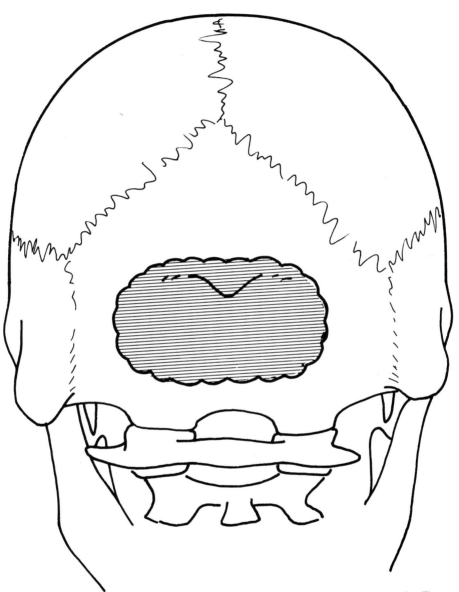

Figure 8.32.   Projection of the skull with trephination area for the position of view for Figures 8.33 and 8.34.

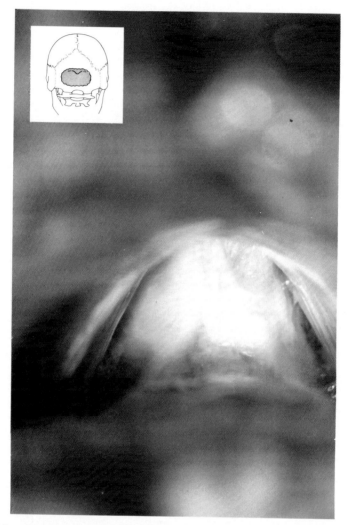

Figure 8.33A. View into the infratentorial space towards the dense folds of the quadrigeminal cistern in the infratentorial-supracerebellar approach by Krause-Brunner.

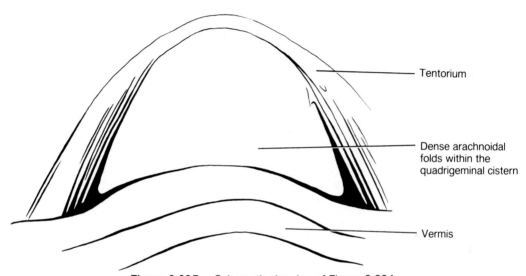

Figure 8.33B.   Schematic drawing of Figure 8.33A.

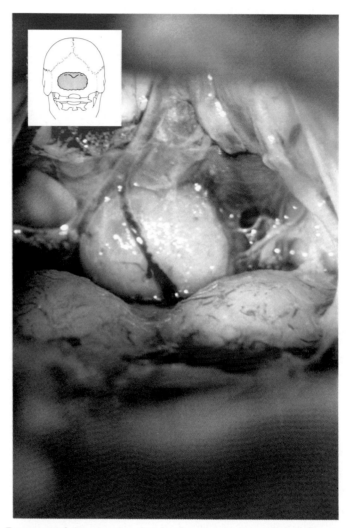

Figure 8.34A. Exposure of the pineal region by the approach by Krause-Brunner, the deep veins well above the surgical field.

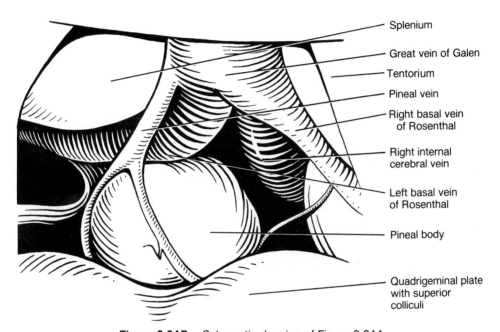

Splenium

Great vein of Galen

Tentorium

Pineal vein

Right basal vein
of Rosenthal

Right internal
cerebral vein

Left basal vein
of Rosenthal

Pineal body

Quadrigeminal plate
with superior
colliculi

Figure 8.34B.   Schematic drawing of Figure 8.34A.

SUMMARY

Surgically, the angioarchitecture of the pineal region is characterized by the microtopography of the parenchymal structures. Most important is the vascular course of the deep veins. The various surgical approaches to the pineal area must take notice of these structures. Anatomical considerations in regard to the vascular architecture conclude that, especially with small lesions with an intact deep venous system of the great vein of Galen and its tributaries, approaches from the occipital route should be more valuable, i.e., the occipital transtentorial approach by Heppner-Poppen and the infratentorial supracerebellar approach by Krause-Brunner. The less gratifying approach seems to be the classical transcallosal route by Dandy, which for many years was preferred but burdened with greater surgical risk than the other two mentioned approaches. The microtopographic study seems to support this attitude as does the surgical experience in the last 10 yr.

References

1. Baggenstoss AH, Love JG: Pinealomas. *Arch Neurol Psychiat* 41:1187–1206, 1939.
2. Baker Jr, HL: The venous angiogram: A frequently overlooked phase of carotid angiography. *Clin Neurosurg* 10:130–150, 1964.
3. Betz H: Das Pneumotomogramm der Cisterna laminae quadrigeminae. *Radiologe* 8:366–368, 1968.
4. Bradac GB, Holdorff B, Simon RS: Aspects of the venous drainage of the pons and the mesencephalon. *Neuroradiology* 3:102–108, 1971.
5. Braun JP, Wackenheim A: Phlébographie mésencéphalique dans les tumeurs du tronc cérébral. *Acta Radiol* 13:45–53, 1972.
6. Browder J, Kaplan H, Krieger AJ: Anatomical features of the straight sinus and its tributaries. Clinical correlations. *J Neurosurg* 44:55–61, 1976.
7. Caron JP, Nick J, Contamin F, Singer B, Comoy J, Keravel Y: Tolerance de la ligature et de la thrombose aseptique des veines cérébrales profondes chez l'homme. *Ann Med Interne* 128:899–906, 1977.
8. Clar HE, Bock WJ, Grote W, Lohr E: *Atlas der Enzephalotomographie*. Stuttgart, Thieme Verlag, 1976.
9. Cushing H: *Intrakranielle Tumoren*. Berlin, Springer Verlag, 1935.
10. Dandy WE: An operation for the removal of pineal tumors. *Surg Gyn Obst* 33:113–119, 1921.
11. Davis L: *The Principles of Neurological Survey*. Philadelphia, Lea & Febiger, 1946.
12. DeGirolami U: Pathology of tumors of the pineal region. In HH Schmidek (ed): *Pineal Tumors*, Masson Publishers, New York-Paris-Barcelona-Mailand, 1977, pp 1–19.
13. Duvernoy HM: *Human brainstem vessels*. Berlin-Heidelberg-New York, Springer Verlag, 1978.
14. Foerster O: Das operative Vorgehen bei Tumoren der Vierhügelgegend. *Wiener Klin Wschr* 41:986–990, 1928.
15. Glasauer FE: An operative approach to pineal tumors. *Acta Neurochir* 22:177–180, 1970.
16. Goldhahn WE, Goldhahn G: *Hirntumore*. Leipzig, JA Barth Verlag, 1978.
17. Hahn FJY, Rim K, Schapiro RL: The moral range and position of the pineal gland on computed tomography. *Radiology* 119:599–600, 1976.
18. Hammock MK, Milhorat TH, Earle K, DiChiro G: Vein of Galen ligation in the primate. *J Neurosurg* 34:77–83, 1971.
19. Heppner F: Über Meningeome des 3. Ventrikels. *Acta Neurochir* 4:55–67, 1956.
20. Heppner F: Zur Operationstechnik bei Pinealomen. *Zbl Neurochir* 19:219–224, 1959.
21. Horrax G: Extirpation of a large pinealoma from a patient with pubertas praecox: A new operation approach. *Arch Neurol Psychiat* 37:385–397, 1937.
22. Huang YP, Wolf BS: The veins of the posterior fossa—superior or Galenic draining group. *Am J Roentgenol* 95:808–821, 1965.
23. Kempe LG: *Operative Neurosurgery*. Berlin-Heidelberg-New York, Springer Verlag, 1968.
24. Klintworth GK: The ontogeny and growth of the human tentorium cerebelli. *Anat Rec* 158:433–441, 1967.
25. Klintworth GK: The comparative anatomy and phylogeny of the tentorium cerebelli. *Anat Rec* 160:635–641, 1968.
26. Koos WTH, Miller MH: *Intracranial Tumors of Infants and Children*. Stuttgart, Thieme Verlag, 1971.
27. Lang J: Die äusseren Liquorräume des Gehirns. *Acta Anat* 86:267–299, 1973.
28. Lazar ML, Clark K: Direct surgical management of masses in the region of the vein of Galen. *Surg Neurol* 2:17–22, 1974.
29. Liliequist B: The subarachnoid cisterns. An anatomic and roentgenologic study. *Acta Radiol* [Suppl]183:1–108, 1959.
30. Marx P, Kleihues P, Zülch KJ: Normale und pathologische Anatomie des Mittelhirns. *Radiologe* 8:335–347, 1968.
31. McLean AJ: Pineal teratomas. With report of a case of operative removal. *Surg Gynec Obstet* 61:523–533, 1935.
32. Messina AV, Potts DG, Sigel RM, Liebeskind AL: Computed tomography: Evaluation of the posterior third ventricle. *Radiology* 119:581–592, 1976.
33. Negrin Jr, J: A new approach in the surgical treatment of tumors of the pineal region. The posterior coroneal flap. *Am J Surg* 80:581–583, 1950.
34. Newton THH, Potts DG (eds). *Radiology of the Skull and Brain*, Vol. 2/3. St. Louis, Mosby, 1974.
35. Olivecrona H: The surgical treatment of intracranial tumors. In *Handbuch der Neurochirurgie*, Vol IV/4. Berlin-Heidelberg-New York, Springer Verlag, 1967, pp 48–68.
36. Pachtman H, Hilal SK, Wood EH: The posterior choroidal arteries. *Radiology* 112:343–352, 1974.

37. Peeters FLM: The vertebral angiogram in patients with tumors in or near the midline. *Neuroradiology* 5:53–58, 1973.

38. Pendl G: Mikrotopographische Untersuchungen über die operativen Zugänge zur Mittelhirn-Pinealis-Region. Thesis, University of Vienna Medical Faculty, 1981.

39. Pendl G: Infratentorial approach to mesencephalic tumors. In Koos WTh, Böck F, Spetzler RF (eds): *Clinical Microneurosurgery.* Stuttgart, Thieme Verlag, 1976, pp. 143–150.

40. Pendl G, Koos W, Witzmann A: Surgical approach to pineal tumours in childhood. *Z Kinderchir* 34:203–204, 1981.

41. Pernkopf E: Topographische Anatomie des Menschen. München-Berlin-Wien, Urban and Schwarzenberg, 1960.

42. Plaut HF: Size of the tentorial incisura related to cerebral herniation. *Acta Radiolog* 1:916–998, 1963.

43. Poppen JL: The right occipital approach to a pinealoma. *J Neurosurg* 25:706–710, 1966.

44. Poppen JL: *An atlas of Neurosurgical Techniques.* Philadelphia, W.B. Saunders, 1960.

45. Quest DO, Kleriga E: Microsurgical anatomy of the pineal region. *Neurosurgery* 6:385–390, 1980.

46. Rhoton AL, Yamamoto I, Peace DA: Microsurgery of the third ventricle: Part 2. Operative approaches. *Neurosurgery* 8:357–373, 1981.

47. Ringertz N, Nordenstam H, Flyger G: Tumors of the pineal region. *J Neuropathol Exp Neurol* 13:540–561, 1954.

48. Saxena RC, Beg MAQ, Das AC: The straight sinus. *J Neurosurg* 41:724–727, 1974.

49. Schaltenbrand G, Bailey P: *Introduction to stereotaxis with an Atlas of the Human Brain.* Stuttgart, Thieme Verlag, 1959.

50. Schindler E: Enzaphalographische Befunde bei Tumoren der Pinealisregion. *Radiologe* 16:405–411, 1976.

51. Seeger W: *Atlas of Topographical Anatomy of the Brain and Surrounding Structures.* Wien-New York, Springer Verlag, 1978.

52. Sones Jr, PJ, Hoffman Jr, JC: Angiography of tumors involving the posterior third ventricle. *Am J Roentgenol* 124:241–249, 1975.

53. Spatz H: Anatomie des Mittelhirns. In Bumke O, Foerster O (eds): *Handbuch der Neurologie*, Vol I/1. Berlin, Springer Verlag, pp 474–540.

54. Stein BM: The infratentorial supracerebellar approach to pineal lesions. *J Neurosurg* 35:197–202, 1971.

55. Stein BM: Surgical treatment of pineal tumors. *Clin Neurosurg* 26:490–510, 1979.

56. Stein BM, Fraser RAR, Tenner MS: Tumours of the third ventricle in children. *J Neurol Neurosurg Psychiat* 35:776–778, 1972.

57. Takahashi M: *Atlas of Vertebral Angiography.* München-Berlin-Wien, Urban and Schwarzenberg, 1974.

58. Tamaki N, Fujiwara K, Matsumoto S, Takeda H: Veins draining the pineal body. An anatomical and neuroradiological study of "pineal veins." *J Neurosurg* 39:448–454, 1973.

59. Tschabitscher M: Die Venen des menschlichen Kleinhirns. *Acta Anat* 105:344–366, 1979.

60. Van Wagenen WP: A surgical approach for the removal of certain pineal tumors. *Surg Gyn Obst* 53:216–220, 1931.

61. Wackenheim A, Braun JP: *Angiography of the Mesencephalon.* Berlin-Heidelberg-New York, Springer Verlag, 1970.

62. Waddington MM: *Atlas of Cerebral Angiography with Anatomic Correlation.* Boston, Little, Brown and Co, 1974.

63. Weber G: Midbrain tumours. In Vinken PJ, Bruyn GW (eds): *Handbook of Clinical Neurology,* Vol 17/II. Amsterdam, North Holland Publishing Co, 1974, 620–647.

64. Wende S, Ciba K: Die pneumographische Darstellung des Mittelhirns und seiner Nachbarschaft. *Radiologe* 8:347–354, 1968.

65. Wilner HI, Crockett J, Gilroy J: The Galenic venous system: A selective radiographic study. *Am J Roentgenol* 115:1–13, 1972.

66. Wollschlager PB, Wollschlager G, Meyer PG: Die postmortale Angiographie des Mesencephalon und seiner direkten Umgebung. *Radiologe* 8:377–381, 1968.

67. Yamamoto I, Kageyama N: Microsurgical anatomy of the pineal region. *J Neurosurg* 53:205–221, 1980.

68. Yamamoto I, Rhoton AL, Peace DA: Microsurgery of the third ventricle: Part 1. Microsurgical anatomy. *Neurosurgery* 8:334–356, 1981.

69. Yasargil MG, Kasdaglis K, Jain KK, Weber HP: Anatomical observation of the subarachnoid cisterns of the brain during surgery. *J Neurosurg* 44:298–302, 1976.

70. Zapletal B: Ein neuer operativer Zugang zum Gebiet der Incisura tentorii. *Zbl Neurochir* 16:64–69, 1956.

71. Zeal AA, Rhoton AL: Microsurgical anatomy of the posterior cerebral artery. *J Neurosurg* 4:534–559, 1978.

72. Zülch KJ: Die Pathologie und Biologie der Tumoren des dritten Ventrikels. *Acta Neurochir* 9:277–296, 1961.

CHAPTER 9

Pre- and Postoperative Management of Pineal Region Tumors and the Occipital Transtentorial Approach

EDWARD A. NEUWELT, M.D. and H. HUNT BATJER, M.D.

INDICATIONS

With the use of the operating microscope, a variety of malignant as well as benign lesions of the pineal region can be excised safely. In cases in which complete excision is impossible, obtaining tissue for a histological diagnosis has been extremely helpful in planning appropriate postoperative radiotherapy and chemotherapy. Reducing tumor bulk may also be beneficial, as has been shown to be the case in medulloblastoma. As adjunctive modes of therapy for malignant pineal tumors become available, such as chemotherapy and possibly immunotherapy, we believe that the burden will be on the neurosurgeon to provide a tissue diagnosis. Thus, in our opinion, surgical excision or biopsy should be the primary therapeutic modality in most patients with pineal tumors in order to provide a more rational approach to their care.

CONTRAINDICATIONS

The usual studies should be performed to ensure that the patient has adequate myocardial, pulmonary, renal, and hepatic function to withstand a major operation. Due to the propensity of tumors in this region to seed via CSF pathways, special situations are created by the patient who presents with a positive CSF cytology, by the patient who has both a spinal tumor and a pineal tumor, or by the patient who has both a pineal and an "ectopic" (i.e., suprasellar) tumor. In addition, the literature contains reports of at least eight cases of extraneural metastases from hematogenous dissemination of malignant pineal tumors. Even in those patients who present with demonstrable local or systemic metastases, we do not believe that surgery is contraindicated; craniotomy is still sometimes advisable in selected cases to establish a tissue diagnosis.

PREOPERATIVE PREPARATION OF PATIENT

The CT scan is the diagnostic procedure of choice in the patient presenting with elevated intracranial pressure (ICP) and/or components of Parinaud's syndrome. The use of metrizamide CT cisternography and/or ventriculography can also provide valuable information in defining the extent of tumor involvement in adjacent regions and cisterns. Cerebral angiography is indicated to detect vascular tumors, such as meningiomas, and to rule out a vascular lesion, such as a vein of Galen aneurysm.

Endocrine dysfunction is a frequent complication of pineal tumors. Precocious puberty in males with pineal lesions is well described, but these patients may also have other abnormalities which will greatly influence their operative and postoperative care. Of particular importance are diabetes insipidus and anterior pituitary insufficiencies. The presence of these disorders, particularly diabetes insipidus, often reflects either extension of the tumor from the pineal region to the hypothalamus or an "ectopic pinealoma" in the hypothalamus. "Ectopic pinealomas" are sometimes not apparent radiographically (9, 11). The pathogenesis of anterior pituitary dysfunction in these patients is not clear.

Routine screening tests that should be done preoperatively include urine-specific gravity, urine and serum osmolalities, as well as anterior pituitary function studies. ACTH deficiency with resultant adrenocortical insufficiency is potentially life-threatening in these patients who are to undergo major diagnostic and operative procedures.

Patients who are threatened by symptomatic hydrocephalus should undergo ventricular shunting. This should be inserted in the left occipital or right frontal region to stay away from the surgical approach. The use of a cell filter in the shunting device may be of value, since one patient in our nonoperative series developed massive intraperitoneal seeding, presumably through the shunt catheter. Although this case appears to be unique, since most extraneural metastases from pineal tumors are hematogenous, the potential for dissemination via the peritoneal catheter remains, and this risk must be weighed against the increased risk of shunt malfunction with a filter. We generally wait 7–10 days after insertion of a VP shunt before approaching the tumor directly to minimize the risk of a postoperative subdural hematoma following the definitive operation.

The incidence of meningeal seeding with malignant pineal tumors may be as high as 57%. CSF should be obtained for cytology by lumbar puncture if ICP is not elevated. When hydrocephalus is severe enough to require shunting, CSF may be obtained at the time of shunting.

When tumor markers are present, they are a valuable means of following patients for postoperative recurrence. With pineal tumors, CSF tumor marker levels are often greater than serum levels. The beta chain of human chorionic gonadotropin (HCG) is the most common marker secreted by germinomatous tumors. Carcinoembryonic antigen (CEA) and alpha fetoprotein (AFP) have also been reported to be secreted by germ cell tumors. Melatonin (12) and luteinizing hormone-releasing hormone (LHRH) are of potential but not proven value. We suggest that both CSF and serum be sent preoperatively for HCG, AFP, and CEA (9–11).

Complete myelography should be considered preoperatively or postoperatively to detect asymptomatic meningeal implants. The presence of such metastases makes postoperative craniospinal irradiation essential.

We advocate liberal dosages of corticosteroids (i.e. 10–20 mg dexamethasone/day) for 24–48 hr prior to surgery. On the afternoon prior to surgery, we place a right atrial catheter and confirm its position radiographically. This catheter provides access for aspirating potential air emboli and for monitoring central venous pressure intraoperatively and postoperatively.

SURGICAL TECHNIQUE

Currently there are two major techniques advocated for exploration of the pineal region— the transtentorial (9, 15), and the infratentorial

supracerebellar (18). We prefer to use the Jamieson modification (6) of Poppen's (13) occipital transtentorial approach. Stein (18) (see also Chapter 10) supports an infratentorial supracerebellar approach.

In using the transtentorial approach, the patient is placed in the semisitting position. The head is flexed and stabilized in three-point fixation with a Mayfield head-holder. Children under 2 yr of age are taped to a cerebellar head rest in the semisitting position or positioned prone. A right occipital scalp flap is hinged inferiorly (Fig. 9.1A) and fashioned so that a generous bone flap can be removed exposing the sagittal sinus medially and the torcula herophili and transverse sinus inferiorly. The craniotomy is generous laterally and superiorly to prevent entrapping the occipital lobe with the retractor. The dura is opened in a stellate fashion. The occipital lobe is then retracted superiorly and laterally, exposing the tentorium, falx, and straight sinus (Fig. 9.1B). It is rare to be hampered by bridging veins between the occipital lobe and the sagittal sinus, but veins are frequently noted from the inferior aspect of the occipital lobe to the transverse sinus. The tentorium is then incised about 1.0 cm from the torcular herophili, and the incision extended just lateral to the straight sinus anteriorly up to the tentorial incisura. The medial edge of the divided tentorium is retracted with sutures, exposing the dense arachnoid covering the deep venous system. The thickened milky-appearing arachnoid is then opened sharply starting inferiorly. The resulting exposure (Fig. 9.1C) demonstrates the quadrigeminal plate, superior vermis, splenium, and the major veins draining into the straight sinus (i.e., the internal cerebral veins, the basilar veins of Rosenthal, the vein of Galen, and the precentral cerebellar vein). Aside from the precentral cerebellar vein, which is routinely sacrificed in the exposure of pineal lesions, compromise of the other veins can result in major morbidity and mortality. Indeed, the greatest risk in surgically exposing the pineal region is damaging the vein of Galen, basilar veins of Rosenthal, or internal cerebral veins.

Careful microdissection is required to dissect the major draining veins from the tumor capsule. With the use of the operating microscope, safe dissection has been possible with avoidance of the major veins in all our cases. In some cases, well-encapsulated tumors can be removed without prior internal decompression. If necessary, the capsule is opened sharply, and the tumor is debulked with tumor forceps, suction, and any

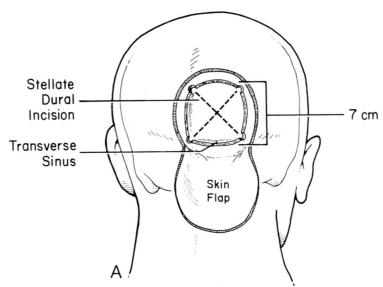

Stellate
Dural
Incision

Transverse
Sinus

7 cm

Skin
Flap

A

Figure 9.1. Occipital transtentorial approach to pineal region tumors. *A*, skin flap, bone flap and dural incision. A large bone flap and dural incision is important to prevent injury to the occipital lobe. *B*, retraction of occipital lobe superolaterally and section of the tentorium just lateral to the straight sinus from the torcula to the incisura. *C*, exposure of the pineal tumor and the surrounding large, draining venous system.

available automated dissection device, such as the Cavitron ultrasonic surgical aspirator. After complete tumor resection, the entire third ventricle can be visualized, as the posterior wall is now open.

POSTOPERATIVE CARE

After reversal of anesthesia, all patients are monitored closely in an ICU setting. Patients without shunts should be watched closely for the development of increased ICP due to acute hydrocephalus from postoperative swelling or clot. In addition, the potential for a convexity subdural or epidural hematoma should be kept in mind, especially in those patients with severe hydrocephalus.

We recommend postoperative radiotherapy in all patients with malignant pineal region lesions regardless of whether or not complete excision was possible. The lowest incidence of recurrence in the literature seems to occur following 5,000–5,500 rads (19, 20). This is delivered as 4,000 rads to whole head with a 1,000–1,500-rad boost to the tumor bed. The radiotherapy of pineal lesions is discussed in detail in Chapter 16.

In the face of negative myelography and CSF cytology, there is controversy regarding prophylactic spinal axis irradiation. As was stated earlier, the incidence of meningeal seeding may be

as high as 57%, and opinions differ as to which histological types have the highest propensity for seeding. Periodic myelography with or without CT scanning with metrizamide with follow-up CSF cytology might be an alternative to prophylactic spinal irradiation, particularly in children in whom craniospinal irradiation is accompanied by mental retardation, growth retardation, and a compromise of the bone marrow reserve.

A recent addition to the therapeutic approach to pineal region tumors is chemotherapy (3, 4, 9–11), as described in Chapter 19. The pineal gland has no blood-brain barrier (14), and this may improve the sensitivity of nonglial pineal tumors to chemotherapy. A few reports have been published showing objective regression of the primary or metastatic pineal tumor after combination chemotherapy.

In patients whose tumors secrete tumor markers, follow-up should include periodic serum and CSF: HCG, CEA, and AFP levels. Elevations in the levels of theses markers may herald preclinical and radiographically nondetectable recurrence. Shunted patients whose CSF pathways are opened after complete tumor removal should undergo removal of their shunt prior to undergoing radiotherapy to avoid the risk of shunt metastases.

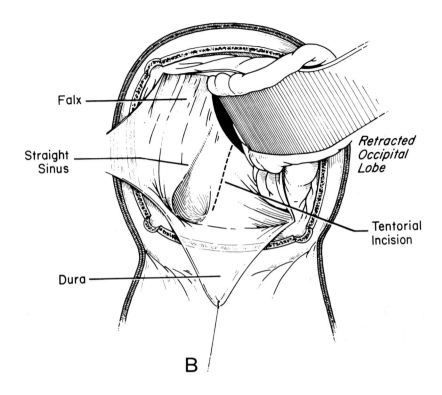

Falx

Straight
Sinus

*Retracted
Occipital
Lobe*

Tentorial
Incision

Dura

B

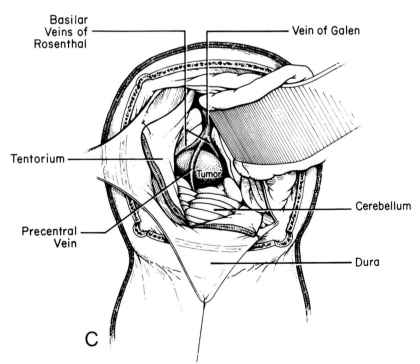

Basilar
Veins of
Rosenthal

Vein of Galen

Tentorium

Tumor

Cerebellum

Precentral
Vein

Dura

C

Figure 9.1. *B* and *C*.

PITFALLS IN SURGERY AND POSTOPERATIVE CARE

The most important pitfall in pineal surgery is a lack of knowledge of the microsurgical pineal region anatomy and microsurgical technique regardless which surgical approach is chosen. Indeed, experience with an approach is generally more important than which surgical approach is chosen. The surgical approach to the pineal in many centers is still associated with an unacceptable morbidity and mortality. Before undertaking this surgical approach, firsthand observation of its successful use is very helpful. The dissection of the thickened arachnoid from the major veins around the pineal tumor is particularly hazardous.

A significant percentage of our patients have emerged from occipital transtentorial surgery with either transient or permanent visual field defects. These problems have been minimized. in our more recent cases by gentle retraction of the occipital pole and by generous removal of bone superiorly and laterally. This complication is not seen following a suboccipital, supracerebellar approach. On the other hand, if the tumor mass is unexpectedly above the internal cerebral veins, resection is straight-forward via the occipital transtentorial approach and is difficult and dangerous via the suboccipital supracerebellar approach.

Patients with exquisitely radiosensitive or chemotherapeutically sensitive tumors, such as germinomas, may be best served by a conservative but definitive diagnostic approach. For instance, consider a young patient in whom CSF cytology shows definite malignant cells suggestive of germinoma. The patient may even have an elevated CSF and/or serum level of HCG. The use of chemotherapy and/or radiotherapy is probably the initial therapy of choice in such a patient. Following this, if a small, localized tumor burden remains, it can be removed surgically, as is done with localized residual tumor in testicular cancer.

Failure to adequately assess the presence of meningeal seeding by cytology and melography may make certain patients vulnerable to spinal recurrence of disease in the face of complete local remission. For instance, one of our patients, initially treated at another hospital, developed high cervical metastases with quadriplegia and pulmonary compromise following shunting and only cranial irradiation. Aggressive follow-up evaluation is probably the best prevention against such unfortunate occurrences.

Acknowledgments. Portions of this chapter have been derived from Reference 10 and are included with permission.

References

1. Borden S IV, Weber AL, Toch R, Wang CC: Pineal germinoma. *Am J Dis Child* 126:214–216, 1973.
2. Dandy WE: Surgery of the brain. In *Lewis' Practice of Surgery*, Vol 12. Hagerstown, Md, W. F. Prior, 1945.
3. deTribolet N, Barrelet L: Successful chemotherapy of pinealoma. *Lancet* 12:1228–1229, 1977.
4. Donat JF, Okazaki H, Gomez MR, Reagan TJ, Baker HL, Laws ER: Pineal tumors. *Arch Neurol* 35:736–740, 1978.
5. Einhorn LH: Combination chemotherapy of disseminated testicular carcinoma with cis-diamminedichloroplatinum, vinblastine, and bleomycin (PVB): An update. *Proc Amer Assoc Clin Oncolog*, Wash. DC, April 1978.
6. Jamieson KG: Excision of pineal tumors. *J Neurosurg* 35:550–553, 1971.
7. Jenkin RDT, Simpson WJK, Keen CW: Pineal and suprasellar germinomas. *J Neurosurg* 48:99–107, 1978.
8. Neuwelt EA, Smith RG: Presence of lymphocyte membrane surface markers on "small cells" in a pineal germinoma. *Ann Neurol* 6:133–136, 1979.
9. Neuwelt EA, Glasberg M, Frenkel E, Clark WK: Malignant pineal region tumors. *J Neurosurg* 51:597–607, 1979.
10. Neuwelt EA, Batjer H: Surgical management of pineal region tumors. *Contemp Neurosurg* 4(1):1–5, 1983.
11. Neuwelt EA, Frenkel EP, Smith RG: Suprasellar germinoma (ectopic pinealoma): Aspects of immunologic characterization and successful chemotherapeutic responses in recurrent disease. *Neurosurgery* 7:352–358, 1980.
12. Neuwelt EA, Lewy A: Disappearance of plasma melatonin after removal of a neoplastic pineal gland. *N Eng J Med* 308:1132–1135, 1983.
13. Poppen JL: The right occipital approach to a pinealoma. *J Neurosurg* 25:706–710, 1966.
14. Rapoport SI: *Blood-Brain Barrier in Physiology and Medicine.* New York, Raven Press, 1976, pp 77–78.
15. Reid WS, Clark WK: Comparison of the infratentorial and transtentorial approaches to the pineal region. *Neurosurgery* 3:1–8, 1978.
16. Schmidek HH, Sweet WH (eds): *Current Techniques in Operative Neurosurgery.* New York, Grune & Stratton, 1977.
17. Schmidek, HH: Brady, LW, De Vita VT (eds): *Pineal Tumors.* New York, Masson Publishing USA, Inc, 1977, pp 1–138.
18. Stein BM: The infratentorial supracerebellar approach to pineal lesions. *J Neurosurg* 35:197–202, 1971.
19. Sung D, Harisiadis L, Chang CH: Midline pineal tumors and suprasellar germinomas: Highly curable by radiation. *Radiology* 128:745–751, 1978.
20. Wara WM, Fellows CF, Sheline GE, Wilson CB, Townsend JJ: Radiation therapy for pineal tumors and suprasellar germinomas. *Radiology* 124:221–223, 1977.

CHAPTER 10

The Suboccipital, Supracerebellar Approach to the Pineal Region

BENNETT M. STEIN, M.D.

Many surgical approaches to the pineal region have been described (Fig. 10.1) (2–5). It appears that Krause (1) was the first to successfully describe a posterior fossa approach, which he utilized in three cases. His terminology makes it impossible to determine what type of tumors he encountered. However, one was benign and was resected. The difficulty of this approach was not minimized by Krause and has been further highlighted by the modest difficulty that is cur-

rently encountered in spite of the refinements of microneurosurgery.

Pineal tumors occur in one of the most inaccessible areas of the brain and lie about equidistant from all points of the skull from which they can be approached (Fig. 10.2). For the most part, these tumors lie infratentorial, albeit often extending anterior to the junction of the tentorium and falx. Logic suggests that these centrally located tumors, which are primarily posterior

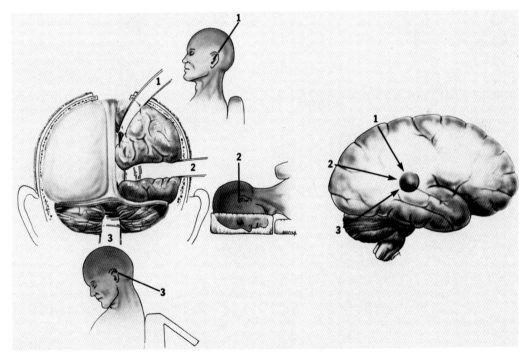

Figure 10.1. Drawing to indicate the three basic approaches to the pineal region. (*1*) Classic approach of Dandy, parafalx accomplished by retracting the parietal lobe and removing a portion of the posterior corpus callosum if necessary. (*2*) Occipital lobe approach of Popen and Horrax in which the occipital lobe is retracted away from the falx or away from the tentorium and the pineal region approached in an eccentric fashion from the right side. (*3*) The posterior fossa approach of Krause performed under the tentorium and over the cerebellum. The optimum position of the patient for these operative approaches is indicated in this diagram. (From Stein BM: *Surgical Neurology.* 11:331–337, 1979.)

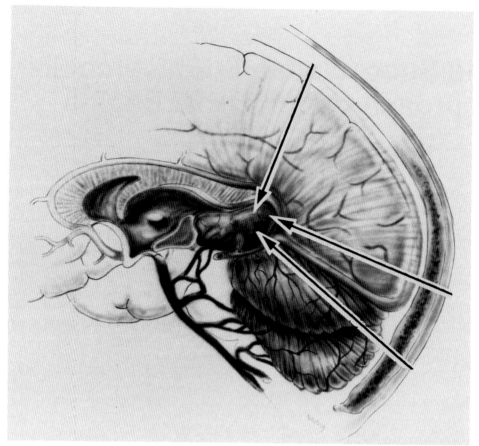

Figure 10.2.   Drawing of a sagittal representation of the brain and a pineal tumor. The approaches are diagrammed by *arrows* which demonstrate that the three approaches are equidistant from skull to tumor. (From Rozario R, Stein BM, Ackelman, Prager: *Neurosurgery.* 5:489–495, 1979.)

fossa in location, be approached by a central and high posterior fossa exposure. Other exposures for this region utilize a supratentorial exposure which is somewhat eccentric, requiring in many cases a sectioning of the tentorium when the occipital approach is used, or division of the bridging veins between the parietal lobe and sagittal sinus when the para falx-parietal approach is used (2, 3). While these latter approaches may provide reasonable exposure of the pineal region, they are, after all, eccentric, and being supratentorial reach the tumor at its superior aspect where it is invariably covered by a network of important veins, including the vein of Galen, internal cerebral veins, and laterally, the veins of Rosenthal. It is primarily for these anatomical reasons that I have adopted the posterior fossa approach (5).

The distance from the posterior fossa to the pineal region being equal to that of the other exposures, exposure is further improved by gravity. When performed in the sitting position, gravity, affecting the cerebellum, provides additional exposure and there is no need of forceful retraction (Fig. 10.3). The sitting position also relaxes the venous system and the congestion in the region of the pineal tumor. The position and gravity also assist in the removal of the tumor since most of these tumors are attached to the tela choroidea in the region of the vein of Galen and the internal cerebral veins. As the weight of the tumor is released by internal gutting, it is possible to carry out a microsurgical dissection and incision between the tumor capsule and these important deep venous structures. I believe the disadvantages of the sitting position, including, air embolism and cerebral cortical collapse (in the presence of hydrocephalus), are far outstripped by the advantages of this midline approach directly to the tumor.

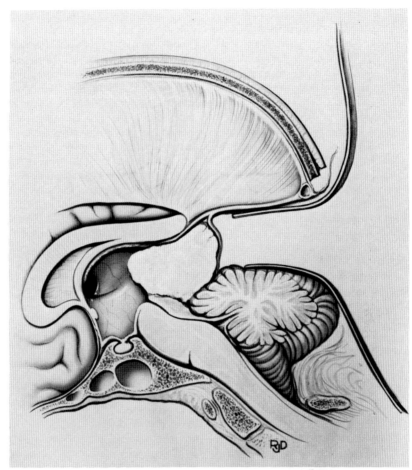

Figure 10.3.   Drawing of a sagittal representation of the brain and a pineal tumor indicating placement of retractors, one elevating the tentorium and torcular region, and the other gently depressing the cerebellum with the patient in the sitting position. (From Stein BM: *Journal of Neurosurgery.* 35:197–202, 1971.)

I have had only one opportunity out of 65 operations on pineal region tumors to utilize the occipital exposure carried out in the sitting position. I found it difficult to retract the occipital lobe, against gravity, and to follow the upward curve of the tentorium. Furthermore, this patient developed an unresolved hemianopsia. This is a recognized complication of the supratentorial occipital approach to the pineal region. This complication has not been observed in the infratentorial approach to pineal tumors. In fact, there has been no morbidity that can be related directly to the use of the posterior fossa exposure (Table 10.1). Any complications, in the realm of mortality or morbidity, are related to work on the tumor, specifically the vascularity of the tumor which may be difficult to control by any route.

Table 10.1

Total cases operated	65
Mortality	2
Morbidity	2[a]

[a] One unrecognized fracture C-spine postoperative quadriplegia and one unrecognized extensive spinal seeding of tumor with postoperative quadriparesis.

The suboccipital supracerebellar approach requires astute preparation, especially in the positioning of the patient. We have modified the position and the size of the craniectomy, while most of the other aspects of the operation remain unchanged.

It is essential to fix the head and to position

the patient with a maximum degree of flexion and forward tilt. This allows the surgeon to work over the shoulders of the patient toward the region of the tentorial incisura, much as one would do if the patient were in a prone position and the surgeon were working over the back. The position is not one of a military flexed posture, but rather having the patient's entire body in a C-shape or flowing curve to the vertex of the skull. In addition to flexion, by using the pinvise headholder, the patient's shoulders are brought forward assisted by a sandbag behind. Care is taken not to overflex the patient and compromise the endotracheal tube. Other precautions taken as a routine in a sitting position include: the use of leg wraps, Doppler monitoring, and a central venous catheter. Once the patient's position is established, the headpiece of the operating table is turned down so that it may be utilized as an armrest. In addition, padded armrests can be clamped to the side of the operating table to support the surgeon's forearms.

A long midline incision has been used in all cases and the muscles are stripped from the suboccipital region including their area of attachment along the superior nuchal line. The craniectomy must be wide, but its dorsoventral extent does not have to be larger than approximately 2½–3 inches. The lateral sinuses and the torcula should be exposed to allow some upward retraction on these structures when the dura is opened. The foramen magnum need not be reached by the craniectomy. In fact, in most of our recent cases, the craniectomy falls short, by a few centimeters, of the foramen magnum. In order to reduce the intracranial tension, and therefore the tension of the dura of the posterior fossa, if the patient has not been previously shunted, ventricular drainage is established at the time of the primary operation. Rarely has it been necessary to use dehydrating agents. The over-decompression that is accomplished is often enough to create subdural collections of air or fluid.

Whenever feasible, it is appropriate to reduce the ventricular size and pressure gradually by preoperative shunting removed by a week or two from the primary operative procedure. If there is still some tension in the posterior fossa, a small nick in the cisterna magna, even though it is on the "wrong" side of the obstruction, often suffices to relax the posterior fossa contents. The dura must then be opened widely in a cruciate fashion. The initial limbs of this incision should not be too far from the midline and should reach upward to the lateral sinuses. They are brought down in a V to the midline at the lower border of the craniectomy (Fig. 10.4).

In younger individuals, there may be a prominent suboccipital sinus or a falx overlying the vermis and care must be taken not to lose control of this important area. Upon opening the dura and retracting the dural flaps, the cerebellum is already sagging because of its weight and the effect of gravity. If the dura is opened, right up to the margins of the lateral sinuses, the veins bridging the cerebellum to the tentorium will be readily visible. Methodically, they are cauterized and divided in order to maximize exposure. It is most distressing to have one of these veins tear loose as work is being commenced or carried out on the pineal tumor. This has not lead to cerebellar infarction to the best of my knowledge. Once the dorsal surface of the cerebellum is freed from the tentorium the operating microscope is brought into the field and appropriate retraction applied. There are two basic retractors utilized: (a) a narrow one that extends from the torcula region to the incisura to elevate the central portion of the tentorium a few millimeters; (b) another medium retractor blade is brought in a gentle S-curve over the cerebellum to the most anterior part of the cerebellar vermis. This must be so positioned as not to interfere with the motion of the surgeon's hands. This retractor, with the assistance of gravity, gently retracts the surface of the cerebellum to allow additional exposure of the pineal region. The surface of the cerebellum is covered by protective material which can be easily removed at the end of the operation without creating bleeding.

At this point, the surgeon has gained an initial exposure of the pineal region (Fig. 10.5). Invariably the arachnoid over the area of the tumor will be thickened, obscuring the actual nature and configuration of the tumor. Utilizing the operating microscope and long microsurgical instruments, this thickened arachnoid is then opened by sharp dissection, care being taken to coagulate and divide the precentral cerebellar vein which further frees up the anterior lobe of the cerebellum, which can be retracted further downward exposing more of the area of the tumor. Laterally the dissection is continued, care being taken not to damage the veins of Rosenthal, which lie behind the thickened arachnoid. A few small arterial twigs from the superior cerebellar arteries and the medial and lateral posterior choroidal arteries may be encountered. These arteries have no importance; they can be cauterized and divided with impunity. This dissection should accomplish an excellent exposure of the posterior face of the tumor.

It should be realized that the trajectory of the surgeon's instruments at this point are directed toward the vein of Galen and the roof of the third ventricle. This is because of the slant of the tentorium and the extreme forward flexion of the head. Once the cerebellum has been adequately retracted to expose the tumor, then the operating microscope should be angled in a more ventral direction so that the tumor is encountered in a trajectory appropriate to its maximum diameter toward the anterior portion of the third ventricle rather than the roof (Fig. 10.6).

Even with a maximum area of tumor exposed, it may still be difficult to determine the nature of the tumor at this point. However, certain characteristics of some of the more unique pineal tumors may be appreciated at this point. Benign, encapsulated teratomas generally have a firm, avascular capsule that is greyish-yellow. Upon opening the capsule one may encounter sebaceous or grumous material associated with the dermoid or epidermoid component of a teratoma. Cartilage, calcium, and bone may also be encountered and recognized.

At the other extreme are the poorly encapsulated pineoblastoma and pineocytomas. These may have little or no capsule with their substance resembling a medulloblastoma. The germinomas tend to be partially encapsulated with soft, sometimes fibrous or calcified material in the interior. Rarely a germinoma may contain a gross cyst with dark yellow fluid. The astrocytomas generally have a yellowish-grey capsule and an interior varying in consistency but usually soft. Some of the astrocytomas may bear a resemblance to those seen in the cerebellum, especially when associated with a cyst. Although soft, some Grade I astrocytomas are encapsulated, distinguishable from the surrounding brain, and can be totally removed. The greatest vascularity has been noted in the pineocytoma, pineoblastoma, and the glioblastoma. Some of these tumors, may be extremely vascular and it is difficult to control the bleeding in a confined area. In such cases, no attempt at gross removal of the tumor should be made.

When tumors are encapsulated, the surrounding structures from which they can be dissected include:

(a) Superiorly, the tela choroidea containing the internal cerebral veins and the vein of Galen. Often, tumors are quite separable while receiving their blood supply and giving venous drainage to these structures. Meningiomas which we have encountered have had this area as their prime attachment. After debulking the interior of the tumor, the capsule may be dissected freely from these structures with care taken not to enter the large veins over the dorsal surface of the tumor.

(b) Laterally, the encapsulated tumors are related to the walls of the third ventricle and the medial thalamic regions, including the pulvinar and medial thalamic nuclei. Some of the tumors may have modest attachment to these structures, which can be separated with the bipolar cautery, scissors, and dissectors.

(c) Inferiorly, the most treacherous and difficult dissection is in the interface of encapsulated tumors with the dorsal midbrain. The midbrain, including the collicular region and the fourth cranial nerve, generally are markedly compressed by large encapsulated tumors. This also is a somewhat obscure area for the surgeon approaching these tumors through the posterior fossa. However, by gently retracting the tumor upward a plane can be developed between these structures and the intervening adhesions, which are separated by bipolar cautery and sharp dissection.

As the tumor is gutted and the capsule surrounded and dissected free, large portions of the tumor may come away freely from the third ventricle, leaving an opening into the posterior third ventricle (Fig. 10.7). It is important in considering total removal of the tumor at this juncture to prevent blood from getting into the third ventricle. This may cause a postoperative obstruction of the CSF passage, and a distressful hydrocephalus. In most cases of benign tumors, the attachments are modest and can be quite easily separated. In some tumors, especially the more malignant variety, there will be subependymal extensions of the tumor and here it may be impossible to remove the tumor from these areas, especially in the walls of the third ventricle. We have not found a major blood supply from the choroid plexus or significant attachment of benign encapsulated tumors to the choroid plexus. In terms of malignant tumors, the invasive nature of these tumors precludes a cap-

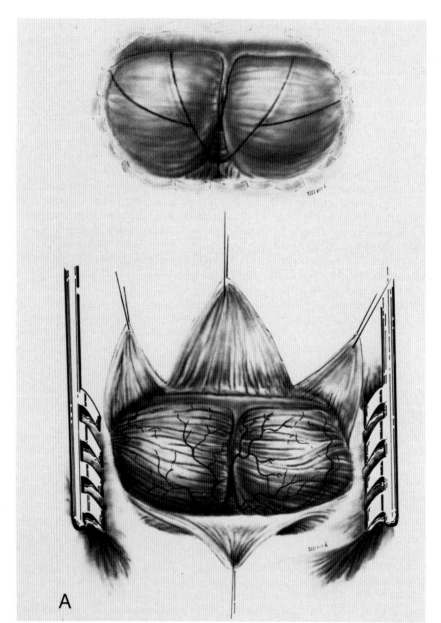

Figure 10.4. *A*, drawing showing (*upper*) the proposed incision of the dura of the posterior fossa, and in the *lower drawing*, the actual opening of the dura in cruciate fashion to gain maximum exposure of the superior surface of the cerebellum and transverse sinuses. (From Stein BM: *Surgical Neurology.* 11:331–337, 1979.)

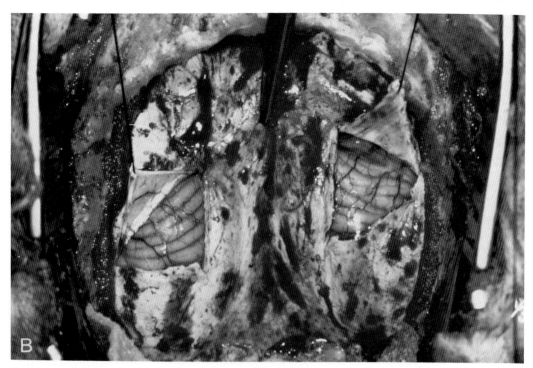

Figure 10.4. *B,* operative photograph showing the bilateral opening of the dura with creation of dural flaps. The patient is in the sitting position with dural flap on the right folding along the transverse sinus.

sular dissection, and in these instances it is surmised that the tumor invades subependymally into the walls of the third ventricle and into the dorsal surface of the midbrain. This is especially true of the astrocytomas, especially of higher grades which may, in fact, arise from the dorsal midbrain and grow in an exophytic fashion upward into the pineal region. It is impossible in these cases to tell if the cell of origin has been in the midbrain or in the pineal gland, known to contain astrocytes.

Upon removal of the maximum amount of tumor, a good thorough decompression of malignant tumors that are not highly vascular or only a biopsy in those malignant tumors which are vascular and presumably a total resection of the benign encapsulated tumors, one has accomplished maximal surgical therapy. In only 1 out of 65 tumors have we encountered a major problem with hemostasis and an anticipated postoperative hemorrhage. This was a patient who had a malignant pineocytoma which was very vascular on the preoperative angiogram. From the instant that the patient had been put to sleep, difficulties were encountered in control-

ling the blood pressure. We suspected that the tumor might have been secreting catecholamines or perhaps there was an unrecognized pheochromocytoma. With great effort some control was established over the blood pressure and at surgery, after taking only a few small biopsies, we could predict the degree of difficulty in obtaining hemostasis by the level of the blood pressure. The blood pressure was kept in the range of 100–110 mm Hg systolic and hemostasis could be obtained, but when it went out of control to levels of 200 mm Hg systolic, great difficulty was experienced in obtaining hemostasis. Therefore, after backing out of this difficult situation and alerting the anesthesiologist to keep the blood pressure under control, we were chagrined to find uncontrolled blood pressure levels as this patient reached the recovery room. The expected occurred with a massive hemorrhage into the tumor at this point. Other than this patient, we had one similar episode unrelated to blood pressure elevation which was associated with a pineocytoma where there was a massive postoperative hemorrhage. There was one other patient with a delayed hemorrhage

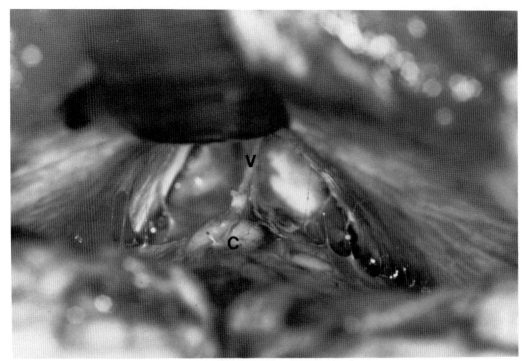

Figure 10.5. Initial exposure of the incisura region. The precentral cerebellar vein and overlying arachnoid is marked *V*. The retractor against the tentorium and straight sinus can be seen in the *upper left* portion of the photograph. The cerebellar vermis is marked *C*.

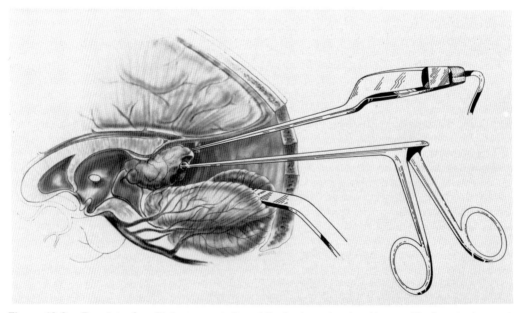

Figure 10.6. Drawing of sagittal representation of the brain and a pineal tumor. The long instruments used to work on the tumor are directed toward the anterior portion of the third ventricle through the center of the tumor rather than dorsal toward the roof of the third ventricle. The bipolar cautery is depicted cauterizing the precentral cerebellar vein. (From Stein BM, Post K: *Current Concepts in Oncology.* 1982, Profession Communications Association, Chicago.)

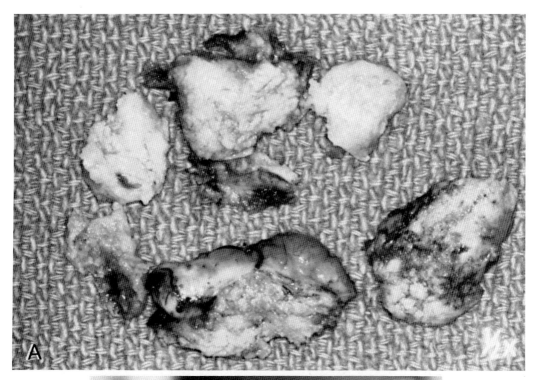

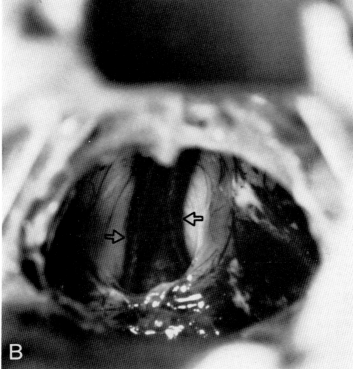

Figure 10.7. *A*, fragments of tumor (meningioma) removed from the pineal region. Additional tumor was removed by the Cavitron. *B*, operative photograph viewing the roof of the third ventricle and the tela choroidea (*arrows*). The opening into the posterior third ventricle created by a gross total removal of a meningioma is in the foreground of the photograph. The patient was in the sitting position for this operation.

into a glioblastoma, this hemorrhage occurring 1 week postoperatively. Therefore, attention to blood pressure and hemostasis is critical.

In those instances where the patient has had hydrocephalus due to the tumor obstruction and the tumor is removed at the time of surgery, there is a potential for CSF flow from the third ventricle out the area of tumor removal over the surface of the cerebellum into the cisterna magna. This route is assisted by placing a small ventricular catheter between the third ventricle and the cisterna magna, insuring that the cisterna magna is opened to the subdural space postoperatively so that a cistern-like tract is formed over the dorsal surface of the cerebellum to decompress the third ventricle. There is no way at the time of surgery to visualize the upper end of the aqueduct to insure that it is patent following removal of the tumor. One may assume that swelling will occur around this area after a prolonged dissection in the region so that at least temporarily the aqueduct may be expected to be nonfunctional.

If the dural opening has been done with care, and the craniectomy is of a modest size, as recommended previously, it may be possible to close the dura or close it with the assistance of a small fascial or dural graft. I believe this is essential in benign tumors where one hopes to reestablish CSF pathways. In the malignant tumors, where radiation will be carried out and in the face of a difficult dural closure, we have often placed a large sheet of compressed Gelfoam (Upjohn Company, Kalamazoo, MI) over the dura, and any potential bleeding sites in the dural edges must be cauterized. The muscles of the midline incision and fascia are brought together with a potentially weak area prone to CSF leakage at the upper margin of the wound where the muscles have been stripped from the bone and the craniectomy performed over the lateral sinuses. Here closure may only consist of the deep fascia and scalp. In most of these instances, however, the patients are either decompressed by tumor removal, have had a previous shunt, or remain on ventricular drainage following operation. These methods of decompression avoid CSF leaks in an otherwise tenuous wound.

In terms of postoperative ventricular drain-

age, few of our patients are managed by this technique at the present time. Most patients have either received a shunt prior to the definitive surgery or the amount of tumor removed reestablishes CSF pathways internally and precludes the need for postoperative ventricular drainage. If ventricular drainage is used, then one has the opportunity of analyzing the fluid for biological markers, cytology, and frequent cultures to insure that ventriculitis is not impending. We have routinely carried our patients on postoperative antibiotics for 48 hr. Decadron (Merck Sharp & Dohme, West Point, PA), is also used in high doses for the immediate and subsequent 1–2 weeks postoperative period. Many of these patients develop aseptic meningitis or the so-called posterior fossa syndrome which is significantly alleviated by the continuance of Decadron. The patient is kept in a 45° upright head position following the operation with a cervical collar to ease tension on the wound.

The postoperative management of these patients consists of the management of any aseptic or septic meningitides, three evaluations of the CSF in the postoperative period for cytological examination, as well as routine studies and evaluation of the biological markers. We now routinely perform myelograms on those tumors which have a propensity to seed irregardless of the CSF cytology postoperative. As yet we have not accumulated sufficient data to establish whether or not cytological examination on three different occasions or myelography is more definitive in recognizing seeding in the spinal canal.

References

1. Krause F: Operative Freilegung der Vierhügel, nebst Beobachtungen über Hirndruck and Dekompression. *Zbl Chirurgie* 53:2812–2819, 1926.
2. Reid WS, Clark WK: Comparison of the infratentorial and transtentorial approaches to the pineal region. *Neurosurgery* 3:1–8, 1978.
3. Schmidek, HH: Brady, LW, De Vita VT (eds): *Pineal Tumors.* New York, Masson Publishing USA, Inc, 1977, pp 1–138.
4. Stein BM: Surgical treatment of pineal tumors. *Clinical Neurosurg* 26:490–510, 1979.
5. Stein BM: Supracerebellar approach for pineal region neoplasms. In Schmidek HH, Sweet WH (eds): *Operative Neurosurgical Techniques,* Vol 1. New York, Grune & Stratton, 1982.

CHAPTER 11

Transcallosal Approach to Pineal Tumors and the Hospital for Sick Children Series of Pineal Region Tumors

HAROLD J. HOFFMAN, M.D., F.R.C.S.(C)

INTRODUCTION

The transcallosal approach for removal of pineal tumors was originally described by Dandy (5) in 1921. When Russell and Sachs (20) in 1943 reviewed the 32 patients whose pineal tumors were treated by direct attack on the tumor up to that point in time, they found that only 3 of these patients survived the immediate postoperative period; an operative mortality of 90%. Torkildsen (27) in 1948 wrote a paper entitled "Should Extirpation be Attempted in Cases of Neoplasms in or Near the Third Ventricle of the Brain?" His answer was a decisive no. Instead, he advocated a diversionary ventriculocisternostomy followed by radiotherapy.

Despite these pessimistic reports, surgeons continued to attempt removal of pineal tumors. Suzuki and Iwabuchi (26) in 1965 reported on 17 patients with pineal tumors whom they treated using Van Wagenen's (32) approach in 3 and Dandy's approach in 14, with an operative mortality of 17.6%. Davidoff (6), however, in his address on pineal tumors in 1967 stated "and the direct surgical attack on these tumors was in the past and still is by and large a harmful procedure". He concluded with the statement "the radical surgical treatment of tumors originating in the pineal region, after 50 yr more or less of bold, aggressive efforts on the part of several generations of neurosurgeons to extirpate them, is even to this day dismally unsuccessful."

CLINICAL EXPERIENCE AT THE HOSPITAL FOR SICK CHILDREN

Sixty-one patients with pineal region tumors were managed at the Hospital for Sick Children during the period 1950–1982. During this same period, 1,184 children with brain tumors were treated at our institution. Pineal region neoplasms comprised 5.2% of the brain tumors seen in our pediatric population. Forty of these occurred in boys and 21 in girls (Table 11.1). The patients ranged in age from the neonatal period to 16 yr of age (Table 11.2). The vast majority presented with a rapid history of less than 3 months duration with 38 of the 61 having a history of less than 1 month.

The most common feature of presentation was raised intracranial pressure, as evidenced by a bulging fontanelle in the infant and papilledema in the older child. Forty-two patients presented with papilledema and 4 with an enlarged head and bulging fontanelle. Parinaud's sign was common and was evident in 21 of 61 patients. Twenty-four patients had ataxia. Seven patients presented with diabetes insipidus; 5 of these were subsequently found to have germinomas and 2 had unverified tumors. Sexual precocity was seen in 2 boys with choriocarcinomas, both of whom were found to have high levels of gonadotrophins in the urine. Delayed sexual maturity was seen in only 1 patient.

Fatal intracranial hemorrhage was the presentation in 1 patient with a mixed pineocytoma-pineoblastoma. In 2 patients, fatal hemorrhage occurred after a shunting procedure. One of these patients had a benign teratoma and the other a choriocarcinoma. In a fourth patient, massive but nonfatal intraventricular hemorrhage occurred 2 weeks after an uneventful transcallosal biopsy of a choriocarcinoma.

Fifty-nine of the 61 patients had hydrocephalus at the time of first presentation. It is of interest that in 7 of these 59 patients, the initial

Table 11.1
Hospital for Sick Children—Pathology of 61 Pineal Region Neoplasms, 1950–1982

	Male	Female	Total
Germ cell tumors			
Germinoma	14	1	15
Choriocarcinoma	3	0	3
Benign teratoma	2	0	2
Germinoma and ter-atoma	2	1	3
Dermoid and endo-dermal sinus tumor	1	0	1
Total	22	2	24
Pineal parenchymal tumors			
Pineocytoma	1	0	1
Pineoblastoma	5	6	11
Pineoblastoma-pi-neocytoma	0	1	1
Pineoblastoma-gan-glioglioma	1	0	1
Total	7	7	14
Supporting tissue origin			
Astrocytoma Grade 1–2	2	3	5
Astrocytoma Grade 3–4	2	1	3
Total	4	4	8
Unverified	7	8	15
TOTAL	40	21	61

Table 11.2
Pineal Region Neoplasms—Age of Presentation

	Number of Cases	Age in Years	
		Range	Mean
Germ cell tumors			
Germinoma	15	2–14	9.8
Choriocarcinoma	3	9–15	11.7
Teratoma	2	5–16	10.5
Germinoma and teratoma	3	6–13	9.0
Dermoid and en-dodermal sinus tumor	1	—	13.0
Pineal parenchymal tumors			
Pineocytoma	1	—	10.0
Pineoblastoma	9	0.08–8	2.1
Pineoblastoma-pi-neocytoma	1	—	0.9
Pineoblastoma-ganglioglioma	1	—	0.9
Supporting tissue origin			
Astrocytoma Grade 1–2	5	5–12	8.6
Astrocytoma Grade 3–4	3	2–8	5.7
Unverified	15	2–14	9.3

diagnosis was aqueductal stenosis, made on the basis of radiologic studies. One of our patients was regarded as a case of aqueductal stenosis for 9 yr before his tumor was finally diagnosed on CT scan. It was biopsied then and found to be a Grade 1–2 astrocytoma. Our 1 patient with a pineocytoma was treated as a case of aqueductal stenosis for 7 yr before his tumor became apparent on CT scan and was subsequently biopsied. One patient with a germinoma was regarded as a case of aqueductal stenosis for 1 yr before final diagnosis. Two patients with pineoblastoma were also managed in this fashion; one for 1 yr, and one for 3 months. Two patients with unverified pineal region tumors were initially regarded as having aqueductal stenosis, one for 1 yr and one for 4 yr.

Tumor markers were looked for in 10 patients. Gonadotrophins were found in the urine in 2 patients with choriocarcinomas. Elevated serum and CSF HCG were found in a third patient with a choriocarcinoma. In the other 7 patients tested, the results were negative.

Calcification of the pineal region on plain skull X-ray was noted in 16 of the 24 germ cell tumors and in 2 of the unverified tumors. We did not see calcification in pineal parenchymal tumors or in pineal astrocytomas.

On angiography, the internal cerebral veins were typically elevated with pineal region tumors, but we found them pushed down in one of the germinomas. Tumor vascularity on angiogram was common with germ cell tumors, with 10 of our 15 germ cell tumors showing such vascularity.

On CT scan, the germ cell tumors were typically of high density and showed intense contrast enhancement (Fig. 11.1).

Pathology

The final pathological breakdown of 46 tumors among the 61 patients was made possible using surgical material, autopsy material and serum, CSF and urine markers (Table 11.1). Twenty-four of the tumors were germ cell in origin with 15 germinomas, 3 choriocarcinomas, 2 benign teratomas, 3 a mixture of germinoma and teratoma, and 1 a mixture of dermoid and endodermal sinus tumor. Only 2 of these 24 patients were female; 1 had a mixed germinoma and teratoma in the pineal region and the other had a germinoma in the pineal and suprasellar regions. The 15 patients with germinomas ranged in age from 2–14 yr with a median age of 9 yr (Table 11.2).

There were 14 pineal parenchymal tumors. Seven of these occurred in boys and 7 in girls. The most common pineal parenchymal tumor was a pineoblastoma which was seen in 11 patients, 5 of whom were boys and 6 were girls. One of the pineoblastomas had portions of retinoblastoma within it, similar to the case described by Herrick and Rubinstein (9). Another pineoblastoma showed neuronal differentiation. Among the 11 patients with pineoblastomas, 5 were under one yr of age, 4 between 1 and 2 yr of age, and only 2 were older than 2—one being 5 yr of age and the other 8 yr of age.

There were 8 astrocytomas, 5 of which were low grade. Four of the astrocytomas occurred in boys and 4 in girls.

The low-grade astrocytomas occurred in children between 5–12 yr of age with a median age of 8.6 yr and the high grade astrocytomas in children between 2–8 yr of age with a median age of 5.7 yr.

We had 15 unverified tumors. These patients ranged in age from 2–14 yr with a median age of 9.3 yr. Seven were boys and 8 were girls.

Method of Management

Prior to 1967, the traditional approach to a pineal region tumor at our institution was a diversionary CSF shunt and radiotherapy. During the period 1950–1966, 20 pineal region tumors were seen at the Hospital for Sick Children. Of these, 9 were treated in this traditional fashion. However, 6 patients were treated by direct surgery on their tumor. In 5 of these, a transventricular approach was used as suggested by Van Wagenen (32). In one patient with a pineal germinoma, a posterior fossa approach was used unsuccessfully. Of the 6 patients treated by direct surgery, 4 died either at the time of surgery or shortly thereafter. Of the 2 survivors, one had a low-grade astrocytoma and this patient is alive and well 31 yr after her initial treatment. She has never received radiotherapy. The other patient was an infant with a pineoblastoma who was irradiated after his surgical procedure and survived for 6 yr before

succumbing to a ganglioglioma at the site of his original pineoblastoma.

We were stimulated by the article by Suzuki and Iwabuchi (26) in 1965 who reported using Dandy's approach on a large series of pineal tumors with minimal morbidity and mortality. Following upon this article, we were presented with a 13-yr-old boy with a small tumor in the pineal region who did not have hydrocephalus and presented with diabetes insipidus and headache. We elected to remove his tumor using Dandy's approach. This was carried out uneventfully. The tumor proved to be a germinoma and this patient is alive and well 16 yr later.

During the period 1967–1974, 14 patients with pineal region tumors were seen in our institution. Eleven of these had direct surgery on their pineal region mass. Although the majority of these tumors were operated on by microsurgical technique, this was not uniform during this period of time. Nine of the patients were approached by a transcallosal route, 1 by a transtentorial route, and 1 by a transventricular route. Three of the patients died either during surgery or shortly thereafter for an operative mortality of 27.3%.

During the interval 1975–1982 27 patients with pineal region tumors were seen at our institution. Twenty-three of these had direct surgery on their tumor and the microscope was used in every case. A transcallosal route was used in 22 patients, and an infratentorial supracerebellar route was used in 1. There was 1 operative death, an incidence of 4.3%.

Our last operative death was in 1977. Since then, we have surgically treated 13 patients with pineal region masses without mortality.

The Posterior Transcallosal Approach

We have found this approach best suited for tumors which expand anteriorly into the third ventricle as well as those extending upward into the corpus callosum (Fig. 11.2).

The patient is positioned supine with the body and head flexed and the head in the pin-fixation headrest in anatomical position (Fig. 11.3). A right parietal bone flap is turned extending to the midline medially and extending 4 cm laterally (Fig. 11.4). The length of the bone flap is determined by the preoperative angiogram which shows the draining parasagittal veins. The position of these veins will determine where the parietal lobe will be retracted. The bone flap never reaches as far anteriorly as motor strip

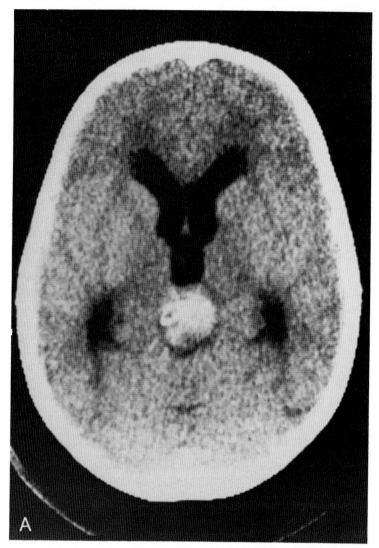

Figure 11.1. *A*, unenhanced CT scan of calcified radiodense pineal germinoma.

and never goes back to lambdoid suture. The medial cut is made just to the left of midline thus, exposing sagittal sinus in the operative field.

The dura is then reflected. The dural reflection is started out laterally and extended upwards anteriorly and posteriorly, depending on the course of the draining parasagittal veins. Every effort is made not to compromise any of these veins during opening of the dura. The dural incision is carried up to the sagittal sinus anteriorly and posteriorly, allowing the dura to be reflected to the left. It should not be necessary to take any draining veins because one can usually go safely between the draining veins and thus preserve them.

The patient is given mannitol in a dose of 2 g/kg during the opening of the bone flap and we have frequently used a diversionary CSF shunt preoperatively, so that the brain is slack. The parietal lobe is gently retracted away from the falx, and the corpus callosum exposed, care being taken not to damage the anterior cerebral arteries. The parietal lobe and the falx are kept retracted by self-retaining brain retractors. The microscope is now used to make an incision in

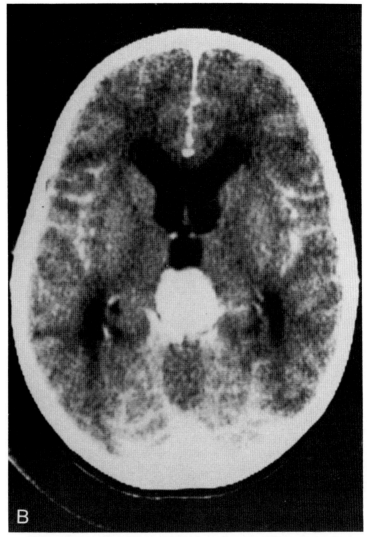

Figure 11.1. *B,* enhanced CT scan of same patient as 11.1*A.*

corpus callosum 1 cm in length just in front of splenium. During the callosal incision, care should be taken not to divide the splenium of the corpus callosum because this carries the risk of producing a homonymous hemianopia.

In the case of most pineal region tumors, the internal cerebral veins will be situated over the dome of the tumor (Fig. 11.4). These veins are venae communicantes and can both be retracted to one side off of the dome of the tumor. Once this is done, the tumor can be dissected from surrounding structures. In the case of a large tumor, we have found it very useful to debulk it

with the ultrasonic aspirator. Furthermore, this device allows for histologic examination of all removed tumor tissue, which is particularly important in the pineal region where so many tumors have mixed histology. In the case of a benign tumor such as a teratoma or dermoid, it should be possible to totally remove the tumor. In the case of infiltrating tumors such as germinomas, pineoblastomas, and astrocytomas, a subtotal resection is usually carried out.

When the tumor surrounds the internal cerebral veins, care must be taken to preserve these veins. We have on occasion seen a germinoma

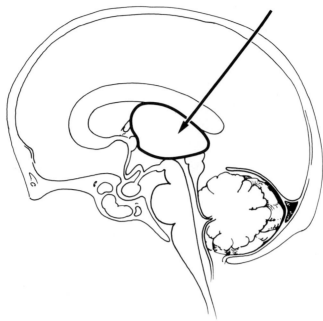

Figure 11.2. Transcallosal approach—ideal for pineal neoplasms extending anteriorly in third ventricle.

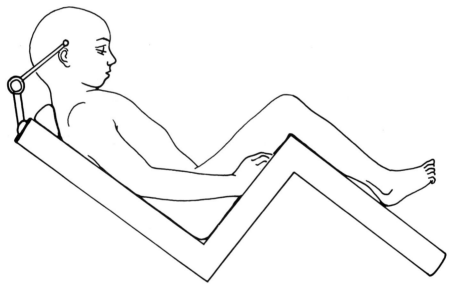

Figure 11.3. Patient positioned for transcallosal approach.

actually depress the internal cerebral veins so that as the corpus callosum is divided, one comes down directly on the tumor. This is more characteristic of glial tumors, but is never seen with the large benign teratomas and dermoids in this region. When the internal cerebral veins are not visualized after incision of the corpus callosum, and the angiogram shows that the veins have not been elevated by the tumor, great care must be taken not to damage these veins during tumor removal. We have not had to sacrifice internal cerebral veins in any of the cases that we have approached transcallosally.

The collicular plate and brainstem are not

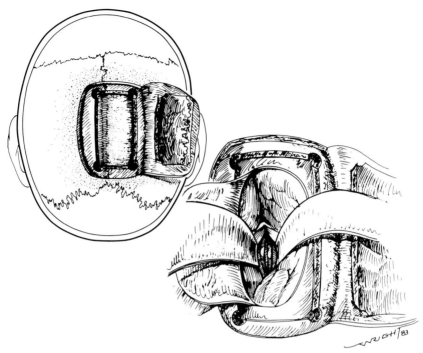

Figure 11.4. Position of bone flap for transcallosal approach to pineal tumor. Following callosal incision, the internal cerebral veins can usually be seen capping the tumor.

well visualized in the transcallosal approach until the tumor has been removed. Brainstem function is therefore carefully monitored as the tumor is removed because there can be serious disturbances in vital signs with traction on tumors which infiltrate collicular plate.

Diversionary CSF Shunting in Pineal Region Tumors

Hydrocephalus due to obstruction of the aqueduct and posterior third ventricle is a common finding in the patient with a pineal region tumor. It was apparent on initial presentation in 59 of our 61 patients with pineal region tumors. Frequently, the patient's symptoms and signs are related predominantly to the attendant hydrocephalus rather than to the tumor itself. For this reason, a diversionary CSF shunt was inserted shortly after admission in virtually all of the treated patients including the ones who went on to direct surgery on their tumor.

Six patients had a diversionary shunt only. These patients were critically ill and most were treated during the period 1950–1966. Following shunting, these patients failed to improve and in two, fatal intracranial hemorrhage occurred

after the shunting procedure. Between 1975 and 1982, only 1 patient was treated solely by shunting. This was an infant who was regarded as having aqueductal stenosis. Her initial CT scan did not show the pineal region tumor. The child did poorly and in her final admission, 1 yr later, she was found to have an enormous pineal region mass which the parents did not want treated and which proved to be a pineoblastoma at postmortem.

A total of 13 patients were treated with diversionary CSF shunt followed by radiotherapy. In addition, 1 patient was treated with radiotherapy alone without a diversionary shunt. The majority of these were treated during the years 1950–1966. However, during the past 15 yr, a further 5 patients have been treated in this fashion, usually because of parental decision not to have the tumor operated upon.

Of the 9 patients treated with radiotherapy and a diversionary shunt during the years 1950–1966, 5 are still alive. One of these had an elevated gonadotrophin level in urine and presented with precocious puberty. Presumably, this patient had a choriocarcinoma. The other 4 survivors have unverified tumors. During the years 1967–1982, 3 of 5 patients so treated are still alive. Thus, of the 14 patients treated with radiation with or without a diversionary shunt, 8 are alive.

Diversionary CSF shunting is not without risk. Two of our patients developed fatal intracranial hemorrhage following diversionary shunting. Furthermore, there is risk of systemic metastases. In our own series of patients, we had 2 children with systemic metastases, both of whom had ventriculoperitoneal shunts. One of these patients had a mixed dermoid and endodermal sinus tumor with metastatic spread of the endodermal sinus component. The other child had a pineoblastoma that was never operated upon. The child was managed with a diversionary ventriculoperitoneal shunt and radiotherapy. The tumor spread into the peritoneal cavity and the child died of the systemic metastases.

Systemic metastases from pineal neoplasms have been commented upon in the literature. In 1975, Sakata et al (21) reported on an 8-yr-old boy with a pineal mixed germ cell tumor consisting of teratoma, malignant ependymoma, and embryonal carcinoma in whom a VP shunt had been inserted, and who died with systemic metastases. They reviewed the literature up to that date and found 7 other patients with pineal region tumors who developed systemic metastases. All of these patients had germ cell tumors with 5 having choriocarcinoma in a portion of the tumor, 1 having germinoma, and 1 a malignant teratoma. Of these 7 patients with systemic metastases, only 1 had a systemic shunt and this was a patient with a ventriculoatrial shunt. In 1979, Wilson et al (32) reported on 3 patients with endodermal sinus tumors and VP shunts, all of whom metastasized to their peritoneal cavity through the shunt. In 1980, Rubery and Wheeler (19) reported on a young man with an unverified pineal region mass and a ventriculoatrial shunt who developed systemic metastases.

Recognition that pineal germ cell tumors can metastasize through a diversionary CSF shunt is readily apparent from our own data as well as the data in the literature. In an effort to prevent such metastases, we began to incorporate a millipore filter in the shunting system of these patients in 1974. Because of problems with the filter, such as fracturing as well as blockage of the filter and the need for many of these patients for a permanent diversionary shunt, millipore filters have only been incorporated in 6 of 25 shunted patients treated since 1974. In the 6 patients with millipore filters, we have not seen systemic metastases.

We are now using a versapore filter, which is malleable, and will not fracture. It has a built-in bypass system so that if the filter should clog, the filter can be safely bypassed on the presumption that by this time the radiotherapy would have destroyed any CSF-borne cells.

Radiotherapy and Pineal Region Tumors

Radiotherapy is obviously an effective method of management for certain pineal tumors (Table 11.3). Forty-two of our 61 patients received radiotherapy. Of interest is the fact that 2 of our patients with low-grade astrocytomas and our 1 patient with a pineocytoma are alive and well and have not received radiotherapy. Furthermore, 1 of the patients with a low-grade astrocytoma was treated 31 yr ago and has shown no evidence of clinical recurrence of her tumor. Another 2 of our patients with low-grade astrocytomas were treated with delayed local irradiation after evidence of further growth of the tumor following primary resection. All of the other patients who received radiotherapy were treated in the immediate postoperative period.

Nineteen of 42 patients received local irradiation to their tumor only. This was true in 2 patients with germinomas, 10 patients with unverified tumors, and the above-mentioned patients with astrocytomas. Twelve patients had local and whole head irradiation, including 7 patients with germinomas and 3 with unverified tumors. Prophylactic spinal irradiation in addition to local and whole head radiotherapy was used in an effort to prevent spinal metastases in 4 patients with germinomas and 3 with pineoblastomas.

Ten patients developed spinal metastases (Table 11.3). None of them had received prophylactic spinal radiotherapy. Thus, of 31 pineal region tumors receiving either local irradiation or local and whole head irradiation, 10 developed spinal metastases, an incidence of 32%. Metastases occurred in 3 patients with germinomas, in 5 patients with pineoblastoma, in 1 patient with a high-grade astrocytoma, and in 1 patient with an unverified tumor. Following subsequent therapy, 3 of these patients remain alive. Two with germinomas have survived for 8 and 4 yr, and 1 patient with an unverified tumor is alive 1 yr after treatment of her spinal cord secondary tumor.

Jenkin et al (12) indicated that the risk of

Table 11.3
Hospital for Sick Children—Radiotherapy of Pineal Region Neoplasms, 1950–1982

Tumor Type	No.	Local Irradiation Only	Local & Whole Head Irradiation Only	Local Whole Head & Spinal Irradiation	No Radiotherapy	Spinal Metastases (No Spinal Radiotherapy)
Germinoma	15	2	7 (3)*	4	2	3*
Choriocarcinoma	3	1	1	–	1	–
Teratoma	2	–	–	1	1	–
Germinoma and teratoma	3	–	–	2	1	–
Dermoid & endodermal sinus tumor	1	–	–	1†	–	–
Pineocytoma	1	–	–	–	1	–
Pineoblastoma	11	2 (1)*†	1*	3	5 (2)*	4*
Pineoblastoma-pineocytoma	1	–	–	–	1	–
Pineoblastoma-ganglioglioma	1	1*	–	–	–	1*
Astrocytoma Grade 1–2	5	2	–	–	3	–
Astrocytoma Grade 3–4	3	1*	–	–	2	1*
Unverified	15	10*	3	–	2	1*
Total	61	19	12	11	19	10

* Spinal metastases.
† Systemic metastases.

meningeal seeding in patients with pineal or suprasellar germinomas was 10–15%. Rao et al (15) feel that the low rate of meningeal seeding together with the risk of growth deformity in a child after irradiation of the spine would suggest that no spinal irradiation be given. The study by Wara et al (30) concluded that spinal metastases occurred in 8% of their pineal tumors and that therefore prophylactic spinal radiotherapy was not warranted. However, these authors include a large number of unverified tumors in their series. We know from our own series that metastases to the spinal cord are not seen in patients with teratomas and low-grade astrocytomas, whereas they are particularly common with germinomas and pineoblastomas.

We would therefore strongly advise spinal irradiation where a proven germinoma, malignant germ cell tumor, or pineoblastoma are found.

The blind conservatism which was favored in the past is obviously not without inherent problems. Radiotherapy is not a benign form of treatment. In our own series of patients, we have seen several serious consequences of such treatment. Four patients have gross evidence of cerebral atrophy on CT scans and in addition, one of these patients has marked calcification of both cerebral hemispheres (Fig. 11.5). This latter patient had systemic methotrexate in addition to radiotherapy following spinal recurrence. In addition to his seizure problem, he has an IQ below 40. Two patients have died as a result of radiation damage. One of these was found to have a severe vasculitis and necrosis of brain at postmortem. Endocrine consequences of radiotherapy are common. Six of our survivors are deficient in cortisone and are on replacement therapy, 5 require treatment for diabetes insipidus, 5 are hypothyroid, and 5 are deficient in growth hormone and show a short stature. Eleven of our survivors are significantly impaired mentally and 5 have IQ ratings below 70.

Results of Management

Thirty-two of our 61 patients are alive. Eight died as the direct result of surgery. Six patients died with no therapy other than a shunt. One patient died without any treatment. Two patients died of radiation damage. Twelve patients died of their tumor despite therapy (Table 11.4).

The 32 survivors were judged according to

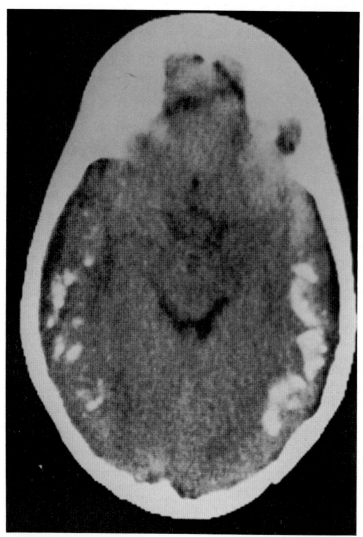

Figure 11.5.   Unenhanced CT scan of patient with germinoma who developed spinal metastases and was treated with systemic methotrexate as well as radiotherapy. Note extensive calcification in cerebral cortex.

Table 11.4
Hospital for Sick Children—Results of Management of 61 Pineal Region Neoplasms

	1950–1966	1967–1974	1975–1982	Total
Number of cases	20	14	27	61
Direct surgery ± radiation	6	1	23	40
Operative deaths	4 (66.7%)	3 (27.3%)	1 (4.3%)	8 (20%)
Subsequent deaths—tumor, radiation	1	3	4	8
Survivors—direct surgery	1	5	18	24
Shunt only	5	0	1	6
Survivors	0	0	0	0
Radiotherapy ± shunt	9	3	2	14
Survivors	5	1	2	8
No treatment	0	0	1	1
Survivors	0	0	0	0
Total survivors	6 (30%)	6 (42.9%)	20 (74.1%)	32 (52.5%)

functional criteria. The quality of survival was divided into 3 categories. Good patients had no functional impairment, were attending regular school, and conducting a normal social life in unsheltered conditions. Moderately disabled patients were physically or mentally handicapped, but capable of independent life. Many of these attended special schools or worked in sheltered conditions. Severely disabled patients required care for daily life.

Of the 32 surviving patients, 15 had made a good recovery, 15 are moderately disabled, and 2 are severely disabled.

DISCUSSION

Without surgical verification, it becomes virtually impossible to assess the results of management. Many authors have drawn conclusions about the management of germinomas without histologic evidence that the patients that they treated did indeed have a germinoma. We have reviewed six large series of pineal region neoplasms which have detailed the type of histology seen in their patients (Table 11.5). We restricted out perusal to these six series, because each of them had more then 30 pineal region tumors in their series. We added our own series of cases to these six series and found that overall, germ cell tumors account for some 59.1% of pineal region tumors. The germinomas account for 39.0% of pineal region tumors. The pineal parenchymal tumors, largely consisting of pineoblastomas, account for 14.1% of pineal region tumors, and

the gliomas account for 26.0% of pineal region tumors.

Of particular interest is the fact that 11.1% of pineal region tumors are benign teratomas, 23% are relatively benign gliomas, 1.9% are pineocytomas, and 0.8% are meningiomas. Consequently, over 36% of pineal region neoplasms are benign and should not be treated with radiotherapy. Without a histologic diagnosis, this decision cannot be made.

The proponents of stereotactic biopsy state that such a biopsy might lead to proper therapy. However, mixed tumors are common in the pineal region accounting for some 3% of pineal region tumors. Furthermore, there is increasing evidence that radiotherapy for malignant brain tumors is more effective after gross total removal rather than biopsy.

At the present time, there is no hesitation in the minds of most neurosurgeons that histologic evidence is necessary before the administration of radiation for most tumors occurring intracranially. There are certain regions however, where there has been a good deal of hesitation about obtaining tissue for biopsy. These areas include the brainstem, the basal ganglia, and the pineal region. In recent years, several proponents have come forward advocating biopsy or resection of brainstem and thalamic tumors (1, 3, 10, 13, 17, 28, 30). The pineal region has been avoided by neurosurgeons because of the fear of a very high operative mortality. Numerous authors have shown that this fear is no longer justified (4, 11,

Table 11.5
Six Series of Pineal Region Neoplasms*

	Ringertz et al 1954	DiGirolami and Schmidek 1973	Camins and Schlesinger 1978	Donat et al 1978	Sano and Matsutani 1981	Stein 1982	HSC 1982	Total	%
Germinoma	27	10	13	10	58	11	15	144	39
Benign teratoma	7	3	5	5	15	4	2	41	11.1
Malignant teratoma	1	–	–	7	–	–	–	8	2.2
Choriocarcinoma	–	–	2	–	2	–	3	7	2.0
Embryonal carcinoma	–	–	–	1	2	–	–	3	0.8
Mixed germ cell	3	–	–	2	–	–	4	9	2.4
Epidermoid	–	–	1	1	3	1	–	6	1.6
Subtotal								218	59.1
Pineocytoma	–	3	–	–	–	3	1	7	1.9
Pineoblastoma	12	5	–	7	6	2	11	43	11.7
Mixed pineoblastoma	–	–	–	–	–	–	2	2	0.5
Subtotal								52	14.1
Astrocytoma/other gliomata	11	7	31	1	20	10	5	85	23
Malignant astrocytoma	1	3	2	1	–	1	3	11	3.0
Subtotal								96	26
Meningioma	–	–	1	–	–	2	–	3	0.8
Subtotal								3	0.8
TOTAL	62	31	54	56	106	34	46	369	100

* References: Ringertz et al (18); DeGirolami and Schmidek (7); Camins and Schlesinger (2); Donat et al (8); Sano and Matsutani (22); and Stein (25).

14, 15, 23–25). At the Hospital for Sick Children, our overall operative mortality was 20% in a series of 40 pineal region tumors directly operated upon during the years 1950–1982. However, this operative mortality has steadily fallen during this period of time, so that of 23 tumors operated on between 1975 and 1982, there was only 1 operative death; an operative mortality of 4.3%. There have been no operative deaths in the 13 patients whose tumors were directly operated upon since 1977.

SUMMARY

Direct surgery on a pineal region mass can be carried out safely and is justified in that the pineal region harbors many benign tumors which would not benefit from radiotherapy. Furthermore, this region contains some highly malignant tumors that need more than just local radiotherapy. In order to discern between these various groups of tumors, histologic proof of the nature of the entire tumor is necessary.

We have found the posterior transcallosal approach to the pineal region a safe and satisfactory approach to tumors in this region and have found this approach particularly advantageous when the tumor extends upwards and forwards into the third ventricle.

Direct surgery on pineal tumors can now be carried out confidently and safely and in many cases, radical if not total removal of the neoplasm can be achieved.

Acknowledgment. Portions of this chapter have been previously published (Hoffman HJ, Yoshida M, Becker LE, Hendrick EB, Humphreys RP: Pineal region tumors in Childhood. Experience at The Hospital for Sick Children. *Concepts Pediatr Neurosurg* 4:360–386, 1983).

References

1. Baghai P, Vries JK, Bechtel PC: Retromastoid approach for biopsy of brain stem tumors. *Neurosurgery* 10:574–579, 1982.
2. Camins MB, Schlesinger EB: Treatment of tumours of the posterior part of the third ventricle and the pineal region: A long term follow-up. *Acta Neurochir* 40:131–143, 1978.
3. Chandler WF, Farhar SM, Pauli FJ: Intrathalamic epidermoid tumor. Case report. *J Neurosurg* 43:614–617, 1975.
4. Chapman PH, Linggood RM: The management of pineal area tumors: A recent reappraisal. *Cancer* 46:1253–1257, 1980.
5. Dandy WE: An operation for the removal of pineal tumors. *Surg Gyn Obst* 33:113–119, 1921.
6. Davidoff LM: Some considerations in the therapy of pineal tumors. *Bull NY Acad Med* 43:537–561, 1967.
7. DeGirolami U, Schmidek H: Clinicopathological study of 53 tumors of the pineal region. *J Neurosurg* 39:455–462, 1973.
8. Donat JF, Okazaki H, Gomez MR, Reagan TJ, Baker HL, Laws ER: Pineal tumors. *Arch Neurol* 35:736–740, 1978.
9. Herrick MK, Rubinstein LJ: The cytological differentiating potential of pineal parenchymal neoplasms (true pinealomas). *Brain* 102:289–320, 1979.
10. Hoffman HJ, Becker L, Craven MA: A clinically and pathologically distinct group of benign brainstem gliomas. *Neurosurgery* 7:243–284, 1980.
11. Jamieson KG: Excision of pineal tumors. *J Neurosurg* 35:550–553, 1971.
12. Jenkin RDT, Simpson WJK, Keen CW: Pineal and suprasellar germinomas. *J Neurosurg* 48:99–107, 1978.
13. Kobayashi T, Kageyama N, Kida Y, Yoshida J, Shibuya N, Okamura K: Unilateral germinomas involving the basal ganglia and thalamus. *J Neurosurg* 55:55–62, 1981.
14. Page LK: The infratentorial-supracerebellar exposure of tumors in the pineal area. *Neurosurgery* 1:36–40, 1977.
15. Rao YTR, Medini E, Haselow RE, Jones TK, Levitt SH: Pineal and ectopic pineal tumors: The role of radiation therapy. *Cancer* 48:708–713, 1981.
16. Reid WS, Clark WK: Comparison of the infratentorial and transtentorial approaches to the pineal region. *Neurosurgery* 3:1–8, 1978.
17. Reigel DH, Scarff TB, Woodford JE: Biopsy of pediatric brainstem tumors. *Childs Brain* 5:329–340, 1979.
18. Ringertz N, Nordenstam H, Flyger G: Tumors of the pineal region. *J Neuropathol Exp Neurol* 13:540–561, 1954.
19. Rubery ED, Wheeler TK: Metastases outside the central nervous system from a presumed pineal germinoma. *J Neurosurg* 53:562–565, 1980.
20. Russell WD, Sachs E: Pinealoma. A clinicopathologic study of 7 cases with a review of literature. *Arch Path* 35:869–888, 1943.
21. Sakata K, Yamada H, Sakai N, Hosono Y, Kawasako T, Sasaoka I: Extraneural metastasis of pineal tumor. *Surg Neurol* 3:49–54, 1975.
22. Sano K, Matsutani M: Pinealoma (germinoma) treated by direct surgery and postoperative irradiation. *Childs Brain* 8:81–97, 1981.
23. Schaefer M, Lapras C, Thomalske G, Grau H, Schober R: Sarcoidosis of the pineal gland. *J Neurosurg* 47:630–632, 1977.
24. Sonntag VKH, Waggener JO, Kaplan AM: Surgical removal of a hemangioma of the pineal region in a 4 week old infant. *Neurosurgery* 8:586–588, 1981.
25. Stein BM: Pineal region tumors. In *Pediatric Neurosurgery, Surgery of the Developing Nervous System*, Section of Pediatric Neurosurgery, AANS (ed). New York, Grune & Stratton, 1982, pp 469–485.
26. Suzuki J, Iwabuchi T: Surgical removal of pineal tumors (pinealomas and teratomas). *J Neurosurg* 23:565–571, 1965.
27. Torkildsen A: Should extirpation be attempted in cases of neoplasm in or near the third ventricle of the brain. Experiences with a palliative method. *J Neurosurg* 5:249–275, 1948.
28. Van Wagenen WP: A surgical approach for the removal of certain pineal tumors. *Surg Gyn Obst* 53:216–220, 1931.
29. Wald SL, Fogelson H, McLaurin RL: Cystic thalamic gliomas. *Childs Brain* 9:381–393, 1982.
30. Wara WM, Jenkin RDT, Evans A, Ertel I, Hittle R, Ortega J, Wilson CB, Hammond D: Tumors of the pineal and suprasellar region: Childrens cancer study group treatment results 1960–1975. *Cancer* 43:698–701, 1979.
31. Weaver EN, Coulon RA: Excision of a brainstem epidermoid cyst. Case report. *J Neurosurg* 51:254–257, 1979.
32. Wilson ER, Takei Y, Bikoff WT, O'Brien M, Tindall GT: Abdominal metastases of primary intracranial yolk sac tumors through ventriculoperitoneal shunts: Report of three cases. *Neurosurgery* 5:356–364, 1979.

CHAPTER 12

Stereotactic Techniques in the Diagnosis and Treatment of Pineal Region Tumors

RICHARD P. MOSER, M.D. and ERIK-OLOF BACKLUND, M.D.

INTRODUCTION

The marked diversity of pathological lesions arising in the pineal region (11) supports the increasing need to obtain a definitive tissue diagnosis. The progressive advances in multimodality therapy, including microsurgery, improved irradiation techniques, and combination chemotherapy are applied more effectively when tailored to the specific pathology. In the pre-CT era, radiographic studies rarely allowed for anything more than the outlining of a mass lesion. Contrast ventriculography could not distinguish between a non-neoplastic cyst and an astrocytoma (Fig. 12.1). This limitation illustrates the difficulty of interpreting the results of previous retrospective series in which the majority of patients treated had neither a tissue diagnosis nor a CT scan to confirm the clinical impression of a pineal region tumor (1, 29).

Computerized tomography now offers a much improved definition of the pathological process (36), although the actual histology can rarely be ascertained with certitude (8, 14). The utilization of computerized tomography, angiography, biochemical markers, and the clinical presentation all contribute to the establishment of the correct diagnosis (4). Prior to the widespread application of microsurgical techniques, exploration of the pineal region had proved hazardous even in the best of hands (10). More recently, several experienced neurosurgeons have reported satisfactory results in the microsurgical exploration of the pineal region (7, 17, 26, 32).

Stereotactic needle biopsy has been used predominantly in European centers as an alternative to either open surgical exploration or blind radiation therapy (13, 19, 25, 27). Their published series have demonstrated both a high degree of efficacy in establishing the diagnosis while avoiding some of the risk associated with direct surgical visualization of the pineal region.

In this chapter we will describe the technique of CT/stereotactic biopsy at the M.D. Anderson Hospital and Tumor Institute and review the results obtained at several major centers. The use of, and indications for, stereotactic radiosurgery and interstitial brachytherapy will be discussed.

STEREOTACTIC INSTRUMENTATION

Stereotaxy is based on the fundamental concept that the brain remains relatively stationary within the rigid intracranial compartment. Any anatomical structure or pathologic lesion within the brain can be defined spatially in terms of its x, y, and z position with respect to an external coordinate system (the stereotactic frame) secured to the skull. With the target point precisely defined within the intracranial volume, an electrode, probe, or biopsy instrument can be directed to it without the need for direct visual identification of the desired target. Therefore, the disruption of surrounding neural tissue is minimized while still allowing the neurosurgeon safe access to nearly all regions of the brain. Horsley and Clark (16) in 1908 devised a prototype stereotactic apparatus for use in animal experimentation. In 1947 Speigel and co-workers (31) first used a stereotactic instrument, which they called a stereoencephalotome, for intracerebral ablative procedures in functional neurosurgery. Since that time several stereotactic instruments have been developed and used with success in many neurosurgical centers throughout the world.

The most significant impetus for the development of new stereotactic instrumentation was the introduction of computerized tomography.

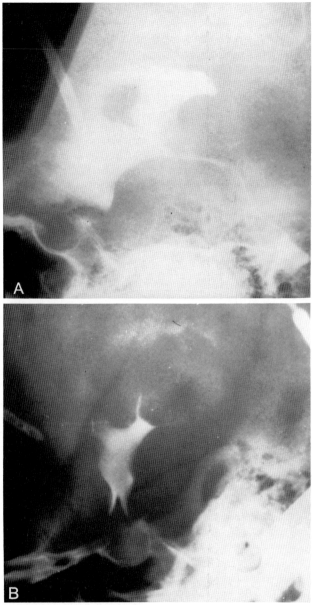

Figure 12.1. A, ventriculogram in a 9-yr-old girl with obstructive hydrocephalus secondary to pineal mass which at the time of stereotactic biopsy was found to be a Grade II astrocytoma. B, ventriculogram of a pineal region mass lesion in a 17-yr-old female, which was revealed to be a non-neoplastic pineal region cyst.

Prior to the CT era, stereotactic localization of the intracranial target depended on the identification of specific landmarks, either bony or internal anatomical structures outlined with contrast ventriculography. Using AP and lateral radiographs, the visualized reference points were then correlated with the stereotactic atlas in order to determine the specific target coordinates for the desired subcortical structures. The application of such stereotactic localization for diagnostic procedures in cases of central nervous system neoplasia is limited due to the difficulty of precise target localization which could no longer be based on a reference atlas. Rarely could plain radiographs be employed and ventriculography, while revealing mass effect in certain areas, would have difficulty in pinpointing the actual lesion itself. Where distinct tumor vascularity was present, angiography done in the stereotactic frame could be used for specific target location. In addition, tumor localization was further defined using intraoperative EEG and impedance probe monitoring in an effort to distinguish tumor tissue from the surrounding edematous brain (30).

Computerized tomography now makes possible the visualization of a brain tumor without regard to mass effect or abnormal vascularity. Small lesions, less than a centimeter in diameter, can still be appreciated and thereby require biopsy in order to determine etiology. Early attempts at CT stereotaxis involved a clumsy and inherently error-prone method of indirect determination of the stereotactic coordinates. The location of the lesion on CT was transferred to the usual AP and lateral stereotactic radiographs, and from there the stereotactic coordinates for the lesion determined. In order to realize the full benefit of CT visualization for stereotactic localization, the coordinates must be obtained directly from the CT images. This requires that the stereotactic instrument itself be modified in order to become CT compatible. The material used to secure the stereotactic base ring to the skull must be radiolucent, if included in the scan image, or the fixation to the skull must be done in such a way that the apparatus is not included in the desired CT image. The CT-compatible Leksell frame has been made with new material allowing for use in CT. In contrast, the Riechert-Mundinger frame achieves CT compatibility by maintaining a low profile on the supporting posts of the base ring thereby allowing the base ring to be applied to the head in such a way that it is positioned either above or below the target slice desired. The problem here is that one needs to select the plane in which to secure the frame making sure that the target area is not included in it. This may create some difficulty if it is desired to also visualize adjacent structures. In addition, if multiple lesions are present and target coordinates are desired for each, it may not be feasible to position the base ring in any given plane which would exclude artifacts involving one of the desired targets. Nonetheless, it should be realized that many different systems have been developed and used successfully to meet the particular needs of the surgeon(s) involved.

The CT scan obtained with the compatible stereotactic frame in place still remains a two-dimension image. Successful CT/stereotactic localization requires that sufficient information be incorporated in each scan in order to determine all three target coordinates. Various localization schemes have been developed depending on the stereotactic apparatus used (3, 5, 6, 18, 28). A set of markers is generally fixed to the base ring and included in each scan. The "fiducial" system as employed by the Brown-Roberts-Wells (BRW) frame (6) and the Todd-Wells as modified by Kelly et al (18) allows for the mathematical rotation and translation of the plane through which the target area has been scanned into a position parallel with the base ring. The fiducial bars do not require alignment or fixation of the stereotactic apparatus to the scanner itself. While this has been viewed by its proponents as an advantage, in practice, we have found that securing the head allows not only for motion-free scanning but also excellent three-dimensional reconstruction capabilities. The type of mathematical computations required, while readily accomplished, can be avoided by simply positioning the base ring in a secure manner parallel with the CT images obtained (3, 5). Depending on the scanner used, the target coordinates can be obtained directly from the CT computer console using the interactive cursor. At the Karolinska Hospital in Stockholm, the University Clinic in Freiburg, and the M.D. Anderson Hospital and Tumor Institute in Houston, the GE 8800 scanner has been used quite successfully for this purpose. Alternatively, when localization markers are included in each scan, the stereotactic coordinates can be read directly from the CT films brought into the operating room.

PINEAL REGION BIOPSY

Computed tomography more clearly defines the mass lesion present in the pineal region, though the exact histology can rarely be determined without a tissue specimen (Fig. 12.2). For stereotactic biopsy in the pineal region, four-vessel angiography is felt to be essential due to the confluence of major vascular structures. We have encountered a giant aneurysm situated exactly in the pineal region arising from a medial branch of the posterior cerebral artery which on CT mimicked a pineal tumor.

The biopsy path is selected so as to avoid contact with the major draining veins. A transparenchymal route through the frontal or parietal lobe has been used without difficulty. At the M.D. Anderson Hospital and Tumor Institute, the Todd-Wells base ring has been modified by the use of nylon pins and support posts. The base ring attaches to the GE 8800 scan table in exactly the manner that it is secured to the Todd-Wells stereotactic instrument (Fig. 12.3A). The position of the head, therefore, remains constant from the scanner to the frame and the numerical information contained on the individual CT slices can be directly assigned to the Todd-Wells frame millimeter for millimeter along the x, y, and z axes (Fig. 12.3B). When using the GE 8800, the base ring can be centered along the x and y axes of the scanner itself. Alternatively, the pair of localizing plates can be fixed to the base ring. The points visualized from the localizing plates can be used to calculate the stereotactic coordinates without regard to the type of CT scanner used as long as the base ring remains parallel with the CT images obtained (Fig. 12.4). The localizing plates correspond exactly to the x, y, and z scales of the Todd-Wells frame. The stereotactic coordinates can then be read from each CT scan containing the desired target(s). A transparent grid, scaled to the particular magnification of the CT image can be overlaid for the direct determination of stereotactic coordinates, or the same measurements can be made using the interactive cursor on the CT console.

The x coordinate on the Todd-Wells is defined from the midpoint of the base ring. The y coordinate defines the anterior to posterior movement and is obtained by determining the distance in millimeters from the top of the grid to the target level along the y axis. The z coordinate is also obtained from the two-dimensional CT image by measuring the distance from the diagonal mark to the posterior post. This is possible because the localizing plates were designed as equilateral triangles and therefore the horizontal distance equals the vertical distance or height. The z coordinate could also be measured by accurately determining the amount of table movement from the zero base line or from the reconstructed scout view. Figure 12.5 shows the actual CT image used to determine the stereotactic coordinates. The four nylon corner posts are seen but produce no artifact. A medium body scanning mode is used in order to incorporate all of the external markers within the scanned image. The localizing plates were visualized on either side of the head. The diagonals are drawn between the opposite corner posts in order to

determine the zero point of the x axis. On the Todd-Wells instrument this point also corresponds to the 60 mm distance along the y axis. Thus, by using a scaled ruler or the CT cursor, the x and y coordinates are readily determined. The z coordinate is read as stated above. Any number of target coordinates can be determined from the CT images available.

Following the CT, the patient is taken to the operating room where under fluoroscopic visualization the biopsy probe is inserted through a burr hole to the target site and tissue samples obtained. A number of biopsy instruments are available including an aspiration cannula, a cup forceps, and a spiral wire needle. The procedure is generally done under a local anesthesia, after which the patient is returned to his room for overnight observation.

RESULTS OF STEREOTACTIC BIOPSY

The Karolinska experience with 345 patients undergoing stereotactic biopsy in all regions of the brain has been reviewed by Edner in 1981 (13). An updated series of 48 patients seen at the Karolinska Hospital from 1969 to 1981 having a diagnosis of a pineal region mass has more recently been presented, of which 46 underwent stereotactic biopsy (24). Figure 12.6 gives the age and sex distribution of this group. Stereotactic radiosurgery was performed in 20 of these and the results will be discussed later. Stereotactic biopsy was recommended in all cases where high resolution CT did not suggest a resectable benign lesion. The histological findings are presented in Table 12.1. Only two germinomas were found, giving a 4% incidence. Six biopsies failed to yield sufficient tissue for definitive diagnosis (12%) and in two patients no biopsy was obtained. Thus, the incidence of germinoma in this predominantly Scandinavian population is much less than reported in other series. Even if all eight patients whose diagnosis could not be determined were to have germinomas, the incidence would only be 21%. Parapineal astrocytomas made up the largest number of tumors. These lesions may arise from the region of the posterior third ventricle, the quadrigeminal plate, and the pineal gland itself. On the basis of the clinical presentation and the CT radiological examination, it can be difficult to distinguish the site of origin. The two meningiomas were biopsied prior to the availability of CT scanning and the only significant complications in this series of biopsies developed in these

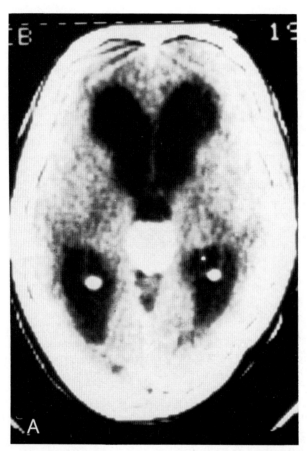

Figure 12.2. *A*, an enhancing pineal region tumor is clearly demonstrated on CT in this 64-yr-old male. Stereotactic biopsy revealed a malignant pineal tumor consistent with a pineocytoma/pineoblastoma. *B*, this 62-yr-old male without evidence of any systemic tumor underwent stereotactic biopsy and was found to have a malignant melanoma of the pineal region.

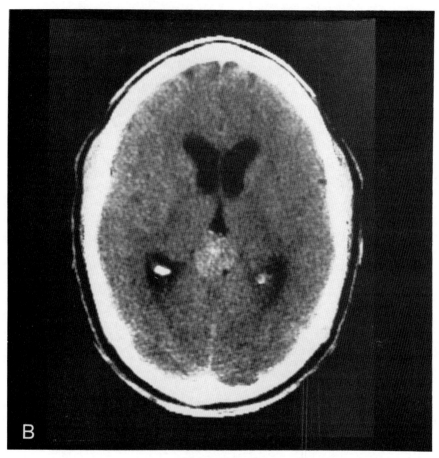

Figure 12.2. *B.*

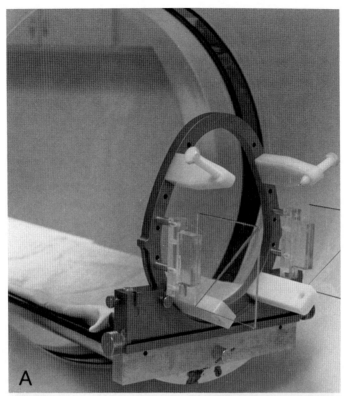

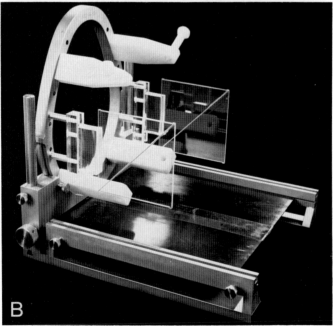

Figure 12.3. *A*, the modified Todd-Wells base ring is fixed to the GE 8800 CT table in exactly the same orientation as it is secured in the stereotactic frame. The nylon post and pins are CT compatible. The localizing plates are precisely attached to each side of the base ring. *B*, following the CT scan, the base ring along with the holder is returned to the stereotactic frame. The localizing plates are designed to correspond exactly (millimeter for millimeter) with the coordinate scales of the Todd-Wells frame. Thus, if the CT scan is obtained parallel with the base ring, the stereotactic coordinates can be measured directly from the CT images.

3D Stereotactic Representation

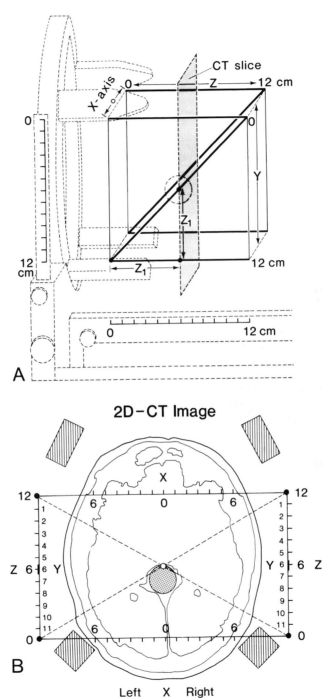

A

2D−CT Image

B

Left   X   Right

Figure 12.4. *A*, this schematic drawing illustrates how the three-dimensional stereotactic coordinates are obtained from the two-dimensional CT images. The only requirement is that the CT slice obtained be parallel with the stereotactic base ring. The localizing plates consist of two equilateral triangles and are secured to the base ring, precisely defining the *x*, *y*, and *z* axis of the Todd-Wells frame. *B*, the CT image contains all of the information to determine the stereotactic coordinates. The point of intersection of the diagonals defines zero along the *x* axis. The *y* coordinate is simply read from top to bottom along the *y* scale. The *z* coordinate is read from the bottom to the diagonal marker along the *z* scale.

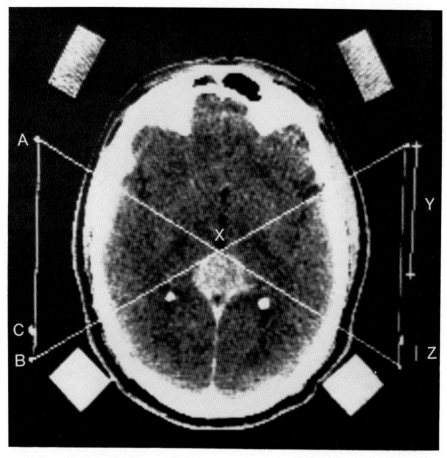

Figure 12.5.   The stereotactic coordinates are read directly from the CT scan. The *x* coordinate is zero given its midline position. The *y* coordinate is read from the top post to the level of the tumor. The *z* coordinate is read from the bottom post to the diagonal.

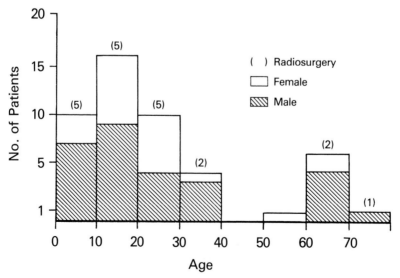

Figure 12.6.   The age and sex distribution of 48 patients seen with a diagnosis of a pineal region tumor. A male predominance and a modest bimodal distribution is noted.

cases. In the first patient the biopsy procedure resulted in a fatal intracranial hemorrhage, and in the second a transient hemiparesis occurred. With modern imaging technology, these meningiomas would have been better appreciated and most likely approached by a direct surgical exploration.

Several other surgical series have been reported employing either direct surgical exploration or stereotactic biopsy. Table 12.2 reviews seven series comprising 203 patients. Overall, the incidence of germinoma remains low. While Pecker et al (27) did report a 48% incidence in 12 of 25 stereotactic biopsies, the average incidence within the whole group was only 23%. The discrepancy between the Pecker study and the other series may reflect the tendency of the Paris group to exclude more of the parapineal lesions. The only reported complications in the Pecker series were those of transient meningismus in two patients thought to be secondary to subarachnoid hemorrhage and of a Parinauds' syndrome in one patient which regressed completely in 6 weeks. One death occurred during postoperative radiation which was attributed to the extent of disease rather than the biopsy procedure itself. No complications were reported in the Weigel et al (35) series from the University of Frieburg. The four other series review the pathology from open surgical procedures. Jooma and Kendall, 1983, (17) reported no operative mortality and minimal morbidity. Stein and Post (32) have had two operative deaths and Neuwelt et al (26) reported one operative death. Bruce (7), in his series of 26 operative cases, reported no mortality and one patient with severe neurologic impairment as the result of surgery.

On the basis of these studies, one can conclude that either open surgical exploration or stereotactic biopsy in the pineal region can be done with little mortality or permanent morbidity. The stereotactic approach will generally involve a much shorter hospitalization and reduce surgical discomfort. Whether or not the debulking of the malignant tumor improves the quality and length of survival following radiation and chemotherapy remains to be seen. This fact will have a significant bearing on future decisions

Table 12.1
Summary of Pineal Region Pathology 1969–1981 (48 Cases)

Type (WHO)	No.	Ages (Mean)
Germ cell		16
Teratoma	1	16
Germinoma	2	11–25 (18)
Pinealoma		
Pineoblastoma	5	1–64 (18)
Pineocytoma	5	12–68 (31)
Parapineal tumors		
Astrocytoma I–II	12	6–64 (19)
Astrocytoma III–IV	5	3–70 (24)
Ependymoma	3	7–64 (34)
Meningioma	2	57–65 (61)
Metastatic	1	68
Other		
Cyst	4	17–32 (25)
Nondiagnostic biopsy	6	7–68 (26)
No biopsy	2	2–7 (04)

Table 12.2
Incidence of Most Common Tumors in Pineal Region

Author	No. Biopsied	Astrocytoma (%)	Germinoma (%)	Pinealoma (%)
Bruce (7) (1982)	26	10 (38)	1 (4)	6 (23)
Jooma et al (17) (1983)	26	3 (11)	8 (31)	4 (15)
Moser et al (24) (1982)	40	17 (42)	2 (5)	10 (25)
Neuwelt et al (26) (1979)	23	5 (22)	3 (13)	3 (13)
Pecker et al (27) (1979)	25	5 (20)	12 (48)	2 (8)
Stein et al (31) (1982)	42	12 (29)	13 (31)	7 (17)
Weigel et al (34) (1979)	21	12 (57)	7 (30)	2 (9)
	203	64 (31)	46 (23)	34 (17)

regarding stereotactic biopsy vs open surgical resection.

The incidence of the various tumor types appears to depend on geographic location, racial population, and local referral patterns. The number of germinomas found in most surgical series is small compared to the incidence frequently quoted to justify blind radiation therapy. Bloom (4) in his review of the primary intracranial germ cell tumors stated an incidence of 45% for germinomas of the pineal region based on 12 published series in which the histology was available in a total of 278 out of 486 cases. This compares with the 23% incidence seen in the seven surgical series quoted in Table 12.2. In the latter group there were 203 of 211 definitive histological diagnosis made at the time of open surgical exploration or stereotactic biopsy. The physician confronted with a pineal region mass cannot assume that the majority of tumors will be radiosensitive germinomas. The discrepancy between these two literature reviews requires further examination. As illustrated by Abay et al (1), of the 27 cases reported, the only histological diagnosis was obtained at the time of autopsy in 9 of 11 patients. No germinomas were found in these nine patients. Since the period of case accumulation was from 1950 to 1978, the majority of radiologic diagnoses were probably without the benefit of CT.

One reason for the high number of germinomas reported in some series is the tendency to combine suprasellar germinomas, which frequently have been biopsied, with all of the pineal region tumors, most of which have not been biopsied. This would, therefore, bias the overall incidence toward that of germinoma in such series. Among the most frequently quoted articles is the report by the Children's Cancer Study (34), which included 118 cases having a histological diagnosis in 57, of which 36 were germinomas (63%). This included both pineal and suprasellar germinomas, but the number of the latter was not given separately. It would be reasonable to assume that since the study period covered the time from 1960 to 1975, the suprasellar lesions were more likely to be biopsied than the pineal region lesions. Thus, any quotation of this figure must include the understanding that the incidence of the pineal germinomas would be less than the 63% so frequently used. This is further exemplified in the series reported by Sung et al (33). Only 12 of 61 midline pineal tumors were verified histologically and only 4 were found to be germinomas,

whereas 11 of 16 suprasellar lesions were biopsied and found to be germinomas. Rao and associates (29) reported on their experience up to 1977 with 17 patients having pineal region masses. The histological diagnosis of a germinoma was made in only one patient. Yet the authors quoting Wara et al (34) and Sung et al (33) (all series having less than 50% histological verification) were able to conclude that germinomas make up over 60% of all pineal tumors. Another article frequently quoted as illustrating the high incidence of germinomas is by De-Girolami (12) in 1973. Thirty-five of 53 cases were histologically verified at the Massachusetts General Hospital. Only 10 of the 35 (28%) were considered to be pineal germinomas. Thus, based upon the review of the majority of surgical series and a critical evaluation of the radiation therapy literature, it is not possible to support the claim that the majority of pineal region tumors are radiosensitive germinomas.

FREE-HAND BIOPSY

The technique of obtaining needle biopsies in the CT scanner has been used by this author and others. With CT guidance it is possible to direct the needle to the target site of interest and obtain adequate samples for histological evaluation. Unfortunately, the free-hand technique may necessitate that several passes or needle adjustments be done in order to direct the biopsy probe to the target site. In addition, the biopsy needle is seldom fixed in its position with respect to the target site. Therefore, when the biopsies are being obtained, considerable movement of the needle can occur with untoward disruption of the brain substance leading to excessive trauma and potentially increased morbidity. The CT scan room, as a general rule, is not adequately equipped to deal with potential complications that might arise, and the risk of infection may be higher. The surgeon's control over the tissue sampling is also limited since one is generally restricted to an aspiration of the area in question. One cannot readily choose between aspiration, cup forceps, or spiral needle depending on the tissue consistency. Nonetheless, while the CT guided free-hand procedure cannot be encouraged, the definitive tissue diagnosis obtained under direct CT guidance is still preferable to no biopsy at all.

THE ROLE OF STEREOTACTIC BIOPSY

The Karolinska series had only three benign lesions (8%) which would have been best treated by direct surgical exploration. Also, it would appear that the radiosensitivity of the true germinomas and the excellent results apparently obtained with radiation therapy would preclude the need for debulking these tumors. Pineocytomas may at times be amenable to gross excision, but XRT would almost surely be administered postoperatively. A solitary metastatic lesion may be removed surgically if the radioresistance of the primary tumor and the patient's overall prognosis would warrant an aggressive intracranial approach. Good resolution CT and angiography should aid in selecting the relatively uncommon benign lesions. No reliable CT criteria exists to distinguish the malignant germ cell tumors from pinealomas, gliomas or metastatic disease. In addition, the irradiation technique and newer therapeutic approaches, including chemo- and immunotherapy, should be tailored to the specific tumor type. The chemotherapeutic agents showing the highest degree of activity against other similar systemic tumors should be used for the pineal region lesions. The primary intracranial germ cell tumors would be expected to respond best to those combinations of drugs used for the treatment of germ cell tumors in other locations (20). Metastatic tumors should be treated with the most effective systemic therapy for that particular tumor type (23). Given the relatively low incidence of germinomas, there is little merit in using the response to initial radiation therapy as indirect diagnostic technique. The concern about leptomeningeal spreading as a result of surgical manipulation remains though no definite correlation has been established (17). Therefore, lesions of uncertain histology can be stereotactically biposied and, if found to be benign, an open surgical procedure can be done without increased difficulty. The value of subtotal tumor resection in the majority of malignant pineal region tumors, especially in view of the potential morbidity associated with manipulation in this region, remains questionable. A careful preoperative evaluation is necessary in order to determine the best surgical approach to the diagnosis and subsequent management of pineal region tumors.

STEREOTACTIC RADIOSURGERY

A unique therapeutic approach to selected pineal region tumors using stereotactic techniques has been developed at Karolinska Hospital under the direction of Professor Leksell (22). The idea as first presented by Leksell in 1951 (21) is to utilize the precision of stereotactic localization to deliver very high doses of ionizing radiation to sharply defined volumes of tissue intracranially. In its first stage of development, Leksell used low-energy X-rays which had poor penetrance and collimation parameters. A proton beam was then used to cross fire at deep brain structures defined stereotactically. While the proton beam was an excellent source of precisely collimated, deeply penetrating ionizing radiation, technical and logistic problems made its routine clinical applicability exceedingly cumbersome. The gamma unit was therefore designed to serve as a clinically useful tool for the neurosurgeon. With this instrument it would be possible to destroy small volumes of precisely defined tissue deeply situated in the brain without the need for open surgical exposure. A schematic of the gamma unit is illustrated in Figure 12.7. One hundred seventy-nine individual narrow gamma beams, emanating from sources distributed over a hemispherical shell, cross fire exactly at the center of the collimator helmet contained within this shell. The center of the target volume defined by the stereotactic coordinates is positioned at the cross fire point or isocenter. The radiation received from any individual beam is quite small, but the single point of intersection receives the cumulative effect of all 179 beams. The exact geometry of the treatment volume depends on the distribution of the cobalt sources along the spherical sector and the beam collimation parameters used. The goal is to maintain a very steep isodose curve whereby the 90% isodose level is separated from the 50% isodose curve by only a few millimeters. Thus, a radionecrosing dose of ionization radiation can be delivered to the tumor while the surrounding brain receives a relatively small dose. The treatment is given at one time, requiring only a single stereotactic localization. The need to maintain the sharp isodose curves inherently limits the size of the volume that can be treated. As illustrated in the computer-generated isodose curves (Fig. 12.8), the lesions greater than 2 cm in diameter are not well contained within the 50% isodose curve for the largest 1.4 cm collimator helmet.

TREATMENT RESULTS

Between 1969 and 1981, 20 patients with pineal region tumors underwent stereotactic radiosurgery. Table 12.3 outlines the pathological lesions according to size. All but two had undergone stereotactic biopsy and those two were

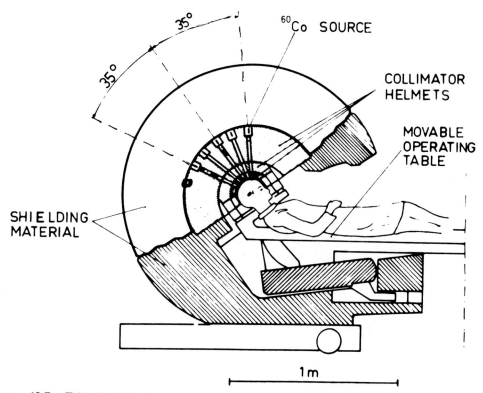

Figure 12.7. This schematic drawing illustrates the basic features of the Radiosurgical unit at the Karolinska Hospital. The center of the tumor is positioned at that point where all of the individual ^{60}Co photon beams intersect.

young children for whom permission could not be obtained. Germinoma patients were not considered for radiosurgery because of the feeling that conventional radiation therapy with larger fields would be more appropriate for this radio-sensitive lesion. Except in young children, only a local anesthesia was required. The procedure was well tolerated, with the patient generally being discharged on the following day. Lesions larger than 3.0 cm in diameter were not considered appropriate for this radiosurgery study and therefore were treated with open surgical resection and/or conventional radiation. The radio-surgical procedure is done completely under the direction of the neurosurgeon. Over the years various techniques have been developed for the transfer of the stereotactic coordinates to the gamma unit. The coordinates for the intracranial lesion are identified and this information is used to set the position of the head in the gamma unit using a special head holder. In the majority of patients a total radiation dose of 50 Gy is given at one time, directed from a remote control panel.

The follow-up study as of 1982 covered an average observation period of 5.4 yr. A definitive pathological diagnosis was made in only 15 of the 18 biopsies performed. The biopsy failures all occurred at the beginning of the study period prior to the use of CT. In these cases repeat contrast ventriculography was done prior to radiosurgery in order to confirm that the tumor lesion persisted after the biopsy attempt. The patients can be divided into two groups, those with tumors smaller than 2.1 cm and those between 2.1 to 3 cm in diameter. The survival for the smaller tumor group was quite favorable. Excluding the two patients with malignant astrocytomas, all of the other patients (11) are currently living. Nine of these 11 are alive and well, while 2 have residual neurologic deficits which were present prior to radiosurgery. Both patients with histological diagnosis of malignant astrocytoma died of their disease. The larger lesions have a much poorer prognosis. Obvious recurrences have developed in some of these patients and they have subsequently been treated with varying combinations of open sur-

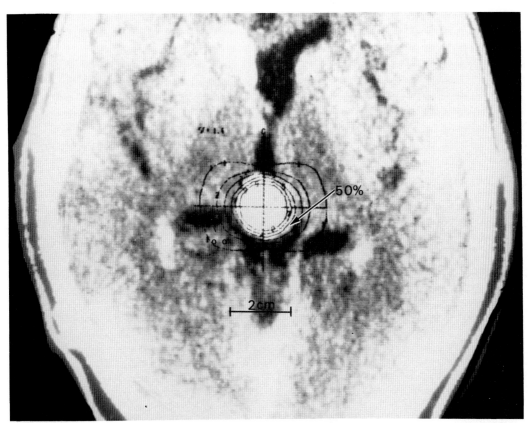

Figure 12.8. The idealized fitting of the computer-generated isodose curves for the radiosurgery unit is illustrated. As closely as possible the interface of the tumor with the surrounding brain should be positioned along the 50% isodose curve. The maximum diameter of a lesion that can be included in this isodose curve is slightly more than 2.0 cm.

Table 12.3
Initial Tumor Diameter (Number Alive)

Pathology	Under 2.1 cm	Over 2.1 cm
Pineocytoma	2 (2)	2 (0)
Pineoblastoma	0	2 (1)
Astrocytoma I–II	4 (4)	1 (1)
Astrocytoma III–IV	2 (0)	0
Ependymoma	0	2 (1)
Nondiagnostic	3 (3)	0
No biopsy	1 (1)	1 (1)

gery, conventional radiation therapy, and chemotherapy. In patients who have remained asymptomatic, the follow-up CTs generally showed decrease in the lesion size and in some increased calcification. Figure 12.9 shows a 64-yr-old patient with a malignant pineocytoma treated with a single radiosurgical lesion. Approximately 16 months later, the CT scan showed a substantial decrease in the tumor size. A similar response was seen in a young girl with a Grade II astrocytoma. It is not possible at this time to say whether the tumor has been completely devitalized or merely growth arrested. No mortality or morbidity has been associated with the radiosurgical procedure.

While the poor survival seen in the larger tumors may simply represent a more biologically aggressive neoplasm, we feel that the failures are in part due to the inability to adequately encompass the tumor margins completely within the high-dose irradiation field. The 2-cm diameter appears to represent the effective limit for a single radiosurgical lesion. Overlapping fields can be made but the geometry of the isodose curves becomes complex and the risks increased.

The development of newer radiosurgical techniques may offer improvement in both beam geometry and spatial distribution so that larger lesions up to 3 cm in diameter can be accurately

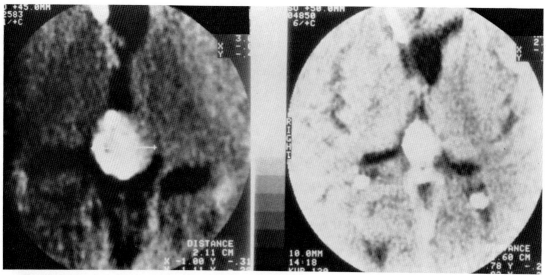

Figure 12.9. Follow-up CT scan on patient with a malignant pineocytoma. The tumor diameter has decreased from 2.11 to 1.60 cm.

ablated with a single well-defined irradiation volume. Advances in CT/three-dimensional reconstruction will aid in obtaining a more precise fit of the tumor within the effective volume of radionecrosis while excluding all but the thin margin of surrounding brain. Stereotactic radiosurgery has been used in other pathological conditions including arteriovenous malformations, pituitary adenomas, and acoustic neuromas (2). Its applicability is currently limited by the size of the lesion which can be treated and its effectiveness by the accuracy with which the tumor boundaries can be outlined radiographically. The new Gamma III unit will offer further refinement in these technical parameters. The advantages of radiosurgery include: a) the extremely low morbidity, and b) the reduced potential for CNS seeding as opposed to open surgical resection, the use of local anesthesia, a short hospital stay, a single treatment session, reduced hospital costs, its applicability to many tumor types, and the ability to still use other forms of therapy, including open surgical exploration, conventional radiation, chemotherapy and repeated radiosurgical lesions, depending on the tissue diagnosis and the presence of recurrence.

INTERSTITIAL THERAPY

Conway (9) in 1973 described the use of the cryoprobe, stereotactically inserted into the pineal tumors of two patients, in which definitive histological recurrence was documented on repeat biopsy. At the time of his report, both patients were doing well. Interstitial radiation, using both permanent implants and temporary isotopes for CNS tumors, has been used extensively in Europe over the last 30 yr. A renewed interest in this country for the use of interstitial isotopes has developed recently due to the attractive concept of being able to deliver a high dose of radiation to a limited volume of tissue and the fact that CT imaging has greatly contributed to our ability to define precisely the tumor borders and thus improve the fit of the isodose curves. Refinements in the isotopes themselves have also become available which allow for sharper isodose curve distributions. In addition, CT/three-dimensional reconstruction should continue to enhance the role of interstitial radiation in tumor management. One large series of patients using interstitial radiation for the management of pineal region tumors is from the University Clinic in Freiburg. In 1979, Weigel et al (35) reported in detail on their experience with interstitial radiation therapy for pineal region tumors. In particular, they presented their last 19 cases done since the introduction of computerized tomography. Their case material consisted of 7 germinomas, 10 low-grade astrocytomas, 1 anaplastic astrocytoma, 2 pinealomas, and 1 ependymoma. Iridium-192 was used in 17 cases and iodine-125 in the last 2. Of the six germinoma patients implanted, four died of progressive tumor extension in the base of the skull and into the ventricles. Nine of 10 patients implanted for low-grade tumors were alive at the time of this report. The patient with a malignant astrocytoma died, while the two pineocytomas and the ependymoma patient were still alive. One of the pineocytomas developed spinal metastasis resulting in quadraplegia.

Based on the limited experience available, it would appear that interstitial radiation probably is not justified in germ cell tumors and primary pineal tumors where extensive subarachnoid and intraventricular seeding may occur, or at least the interstitial radiation should be combined with a larger external radiation field. A definite role may develop for the use of low-dose rate interstitial radiation using iodine-125 in the management of low-grade gliomas (Fig. 12.10). As more experience is gained with the use of iodine-125 and other isotopes, a broader application of this technique may be in order.

SUMMARY

While considerable controversy may remain regarding the best means of obtaining the definitive tissue diagnosis, there is no question that a tissue diagnosis should be obtained whenever possible. Blind radiation therapy, based on the premise that the majority of pineal region tumors are highly radiosensitive germinomas can no longer be supported given the relatively low incidence reported in several biopsy series. Modern multimodality therapy, especially combination chemotherapy, must be tailored to the specific cell type in question. Further advances in the management of the patients will require that the medical oncologist have tissue available for histological exam, tissue culture, and chemosensitivity assay.

The use of microsurgical techniques and the increased experience of selected neurosurgeons, has resulted in marked decrease in mortality and morbidity of pineal region exploration. The transient neurological deficits that may occur, the intensive care, and the length of hospital stay must all be considered in deciding on the optimal approach in the management of a pineal region tumor. Certain tumors most clearly would be best managed by direct surgical resection. Most teratomas, meningiomas, and epidermoids in which CT and angiography may be quite suggestive, should be approached primarily by direct microsurgical exploration. Malignant germ cell tumors, pineoblastomas, and gliomas of all types probably do not benefit significantly from subtotal resection. Also, the risk of seeding and injury may increase with such surgical manipulation. Some surgeons have found that certain of these tumors, and especially the pineocytomas, may at times be sufficiently well delineated from the surrounding structures to suggest that a gross total removal can be accomplished. Whether the quality and the length of survival in this operated group justifies the risk involved

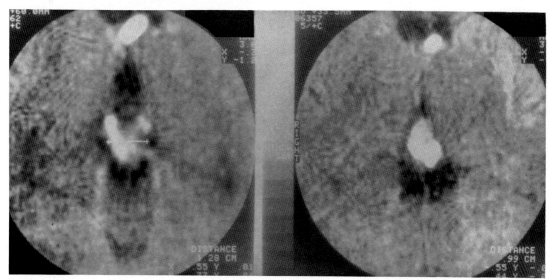

Figure 12.10. Pre- and post-CT scans following stereotactic radiosurgery CT scans for low-grade astrocytoma. A decrease in the size of the tumor is noted along with an increase in calcification.

remains to be seen. Given the outstanding results with radiation therapy in selected tumors, the morbidity of open surgery will have to remain extremely low. In addition, the reported series reflect the experience of a few selected experts and one must be fearful of the results obtained by the occasional practitioner of pineal region surgery. In no case do we see a role for blind irradiation, though in some situations CSF cytology and biochemical markers may preclude the need for a tissue biopsy.

If one exludes the obvious benign tumors demonstrated on CT and angiography, the vast majority of remaining lesions may be best managed by CT stereotactic biopsy, followed by the appropriate treatment. The mortality and morbidity is quite low. The hospital stay is brief, normally not more than 2 days. The hospital cost is significantly less and the benefit to the patient in terms of an accurate guide to further therapy is the same. Thus, the modern neurosurgical center should be prepared to offer either direct surgical exploration or stereotactic biopsy, depending on the particular appearance of the lesion and the needs of the patient. The stereotatic instrument should be used by the neurosurgeon as another specialized operative tool which, when applied appropriately, may represent the optimal approach in selected pineal region lesions. For all pineal region tumors it is essential that we tailor the therapeutic options to the specific pathological process at hand and thereby offer the best opportunity of obtaining a lasting remission with the least possible morbidity.

References

1. Abay EO, Laws ER, Grado GL, Bruckman JE, Forbes GS, Gomez MR, Scott M: Pineal tumors in children and adolescents. *J Neurosurg* 55:889–895, 1981.
2. Backlund EO: Stereotactic radiosurgery in intracranial tumor, and vascular malformation. In Krayenbuhl H (ed): *Advances and Technical Standards in Neurosurgery.* Vienna, Springer-Verlag, 1979, vol 6.
3. Birg W, Mundinger F: Direct target point determination for stereotactic brain operation from CT data and the calculation of setting parameters for polar coordinate stereotactic devices. Proceedings of the 8th Meeting World Society Stereotactic and Functional Neurosurgery, Part III, Zurich 1981. *Appl Neurophysiol* 45:387–395, 1982.
4. Bloom HJG: Primary intracranial germ cell tumors. *Clin Oncol* 2:233–257, 1983.
5. Boethius J, Bergstrom M, Greitz T: Stereotaxic computerized tomography with GE 8800 Scanner. *J Neurosurg* 52:794–800, 1980.
6. Brown RA: A computerized tomographic-computer graphics approach to stereotactic localization. *J Neurosurg* 50:715–720, 1979.
7. Bruce D: Pediatric brain tumor. *Surg Rounds* April 1982, p 22–31.
8. Chapman PH, Linggood RM: The management of pineal area tumors: A recent reappraisal. *Cancer* 46:1253–1257, 1980.
9. Conway LW: Stereotaxis diagnosis and treatment of intracranial tumours including an initial experience with cryosurgery for pinealomas. *J Neurosurg* 38:453–460, 1973.
10. Cushing H: Intracranial tumors: Notes upon a series of two thousand verified cases with surgical mortality pertaining thereto. Springfield, IL, Charles C Thomas, 1932.
11. DeGirolami U, Schmidek H: Clinicopathological study of 53 tumors of the pineal region. *J Neurosurg* 39:455–462, 1973.
12. DeGirolami U: Pathology of tumors of the pineal region. In Schmidek HH (ed): *Pineal Tumors.* New York, Masson Publishing USA, 1977, pp 1–19.
13. Edner G: Stereotactic biopsy of intracranial space occupying lesion. *Acta Neurochirurgica* 57:213–234, 1981.
14. Futrell NN, Osborn AG, Cheson BD: Pineal region tumors: Computed tomographic-pathologic spectrum. *Am J Radiol* 137:951–956, 1981.
15. Goerss S, Kelly P, Kall B, Alker G: A computed tomoraphic stereotactic adaptor system. *Neurosurgery* 10:30, 375–379, 1982.
16. Horsley V, Clark RH: The structure and function of the cerebellum examined by a new method. *Brain* 31:45–124, 1908.
17. Jooma R, Kendall BE: Diagnosis and management of pineal tumors. *J Neurosurg* 58:654–665, 1983.
18. Kelly PJ, Alker G, Goerss S: Computer-assisted stereotactic laser microsurgery for the treatment of intracranial neoplasms. *Neurosurgery* 10:324–331, 1982.
19. Kiessling M, Anagnostopoulos J, Lombeck G, Kleihues P: Diagnostic potential of stereotactic biopsy of brain tumors. In Voth D, Gutjahr P, Langnaid C (eds): *Tumors of the Central Nervous System in Infancy and Childhood.* Berlin, Springer-Verlag, 1981, pp 247–256.
20. Kirshner JJ, Ginsberg SJ, Fitzpatrick AV, Comis RL: Treatment of a primary intracranial germ cell tumor with systemic chemotherapy. *Med Ped Oncol* 9:361–365, 1981.
21. Leksell L: The stereotaxic method and radiosurgery of the brain. *Acta Chir Scand* 102:316–319, 1951.
22. Leksell L: Stereotaxis and radiosurgery. An operative system. Springfield, IL, Charles C Thomas, 1971.
23. Logothetis CJ, Samuels ML, Trindale A: The management of brain metastases in germ cell tumors. *Cancer* 49:12–18, 1982.
24. Moser RP, Backlund EO: Stereotactic radiosurgery in the management of pineal region tumors. *American Association of Neurological Surgeons Meeting,* Hawaii, 1982.
25. Mundinger F: CT-stereotactic biopsy of brain tumors. In Voth D, Gutjahr P, Langnaid C (eds):

Tumors of the Central Nervous System in Infancy and Childhood. Berlin, Springer-Verlag, 1981, pp 334–346.

26. Neuwelt EA, Glasberg M, Frenkel E, Clark WK: Malignant pineal region tumors. *J Neurosurg* 51:597–607, 1979.

27. Pecker J, Scarabin JM, Vallee B, Brucher JM: Treatment of tumours of the pineal region: Value of stereotaxic biopsy. *Surg Neurol* 12:341–348, 1979.

28. Perry JH, Rosenbaum AE, Lundsford LD, Swink CA, Zosul DS: Computed tomography-guided stereotactic surgery: Conception and development of a new stereotactic methodology. *Neurosurgery* 7:376–381, 1980.

29. Rao YTR, Medini E, Haselow RE, Jones TK, Levitt SH: Pineal and ectopic pineal tumors: The role of radiation therapy. *Cancer* 48:708–713, 1981.

30. Rougier A, DaSilva NN, Cohadon F: Tumoral volume assessment: Contributions of SEEG. In Szikla G (ed): *Stereotactic Cerebral Irradiation. Inserm Symposium No. 12*, 1979, pp 63–88.

31. Spiegel EA, Wycis HT, Marks M, Lee AJ: Stereotactic apparatus for operations on the human brain. *Science* 106:349–350, 1947.

32. Stein B, Post KO: Current management of pituitary and pineal tumor. *Curr Concepts Oncol* Winter 1982, pp 3–17.

33. Sung D, Harisiadis L, Chang CH: Midline pineal tumors and suprasellar germinomas: Highly curable by radiation. *Radiology* 128:745–751, 1978.

34. Wara WM, Jenkin RDT, Evans A, Ertel I, Hittle R, Ortega J, Wilson CB, Hammond D: Tumors of the pineal and suprasellar region: Childrens cancer study group treatment results 1960–1975. *Cancer* 43:698–701, 1979.

35. Weigel K, Ostertag CB, Mundinger F: Interstitial long-term irradiation of tumors in the pineal region. Stereotactic cerebral irradiation. *Inserm Symp No. 12*, 1979, pp 283–292.

36. Zimmerman RA, Bilaniuk LT, Wood JH, Bruce DA, Schut L: Computed tomography of pineal, parapineal, and histologically related tumors. *Radiology* 137:669–677, 1980.

CHAPTER 13

Surgical Therapy of Benign Pineal Tumors

BENNETT M. STEIN, M.D.

In categorizing my series of 65 pineal tumors, I have utilized a slight modification of Rubinstein's classification of pineal tumors (3). We have utilized four basic categories (Table 13.1). The *first category* of germ cell tumors includes: (1) the germinoma; (2) the teratoma of two or three embryonic layers which are mature and benign; and (3) the dermoid or epidermoid and a miscellaneous, mostly malignant group, including teratocarcinoma, choriocarcinoma and embryonal carcinoma. The *second category* of parenchymal cell tumors includes: the pineocytoma and the pineoblastoma. The *third category* includes tumors arising from supporting tissue in and around the pineal gland including astrocytomas, ependymomas, and meningiomas; the latter arising from the tela choroidea. The *fourth category* is a minor one comprising non-neoplastic arachnoid cysts. It is realized that in each category there are benign tumors. Although there is much to be learned from more elegant histological evaluation of these tumors including tissue culture and electron microscopy, this scheme appears to suffice especially when one hopes to distinguish benign tumors from malignant tumors. In the first category, benign tumors would include the mature teratomas, dermoids, and epidermoids. In the second category, some of the pineocytoma tumors are encapsulated and appear to be benign. In the third category some astrocytomas, especially the low-grade cystic variety, ependymomas and meningiomas, would be considered benign. The fourth category is only benign lesions. In my series of pineal tumors, approximately 30% of the tumors fall into the benign encapsulated category (Table 13.1) (5). The tumors of this group carry a high potential for surgical resection and cure.

Currently, there is no way that I know to satisfactorily distinguish the benign lesions from their malignant cousins without a shadow of doubt (1). This includes preoperative evaluation

Table 13.1
Classification of Pineal Tumors

A. Germ cell tumors
 1. Germinoma
 2. Teratoma
 3. Dermoid—epidermoid
 4. Teratocarcinoma, choriocarcinoma, embryonal carcinoma
B. Pineal parenchymal tumors
 1. Pineocytoma
 2. Pineoblastoma
C. Tumors of supporting or adjacent structures
 1. Astrocytoma
 2. Ependymoma
 3. Meningioma
 4. Sarcoma
D. Non-neoplastic masses
 1. Arachnoid cysts

of the clinical history, biological markers in serum and CSF, CT scans with and without contrast in various projections including the horizontal, coronal and sagittal cuts, and arteriography (Fig. 13.1). Because we have personally encountered difficulty in precisely diagnosing these tumors at routine light microscopy, especially when fragments are small, I have a personal aversion to the technique of diagnosis which enlists the use of a stereotactically placed biopsy needle. I have observed cases where even open surgical biopsy with resultant small fragments has led to a confusing diagnosis with different conclusions being reached by a variety of pathologists. Therefore, I feel that virtually all of the pineal tumors require surgical exposure and sufficient tissue removal to ensure an accurate histological diagnosis. With experience, I believe the surgeon can tell as he exposes the posterior and lateral aspects of these tumors whether or not they are encapsulated and therefore potentially resectable. We have come to rely more and more upon the gross features of the tumor and use the histological data from frozen section as a secondary indicator as to whether or not the tumor should be resected. Certainly some of the potentially malignant tumors, such as germinoma, even pineoblastoma may be cystic and partially encapsulated. However, the surgeon will be able to determine where the apparent encapsulation fades into the surrounding tissue as a malignant tumor reveals itself to be infiltrating in nature and thereby unresectable.

Table 13.2 summarizes the benign encapsulated tumors in my series. These included teratomas, epidermoids, pineocytomas, astrocytomas, meningiomas, and an arachnoid cyst. The most common benign tumors in my series were the astrocytomas arising in or around the pineal gland and the meningiomas. Many of these tumors were not recognized for their true nature prior to surgical intervention. While a shunt was placed to relieve hydrocephalus, a number were treated with maximum dose radiotherapy in the hope that this would cure the tumor. When the tumor did not disappear after sufficient radiation then surgical intervention was requested (Fig. 13.2).

All of the benign tumors were operated on via the supracerebellar infratentorial approach (6). The limiting factors in this operative exposure include the following: (1) tumors which extend superiorly toward the splenium of the corpus callosum, (2) tumors which extend laterally to either side toward or into the trigone of the lateral ventricle, (3) extension in a ventral direction compressing the tectum of the midbrain. Obviously the portion of a large tumor that is easiest to resect is that located in the center of the field in the direct trajectory of this posterior fossa exposure. Nevertheless, it is possible to reach to the sides to obscure locations in all regions. It may be necessary in some instances to cut the tentorial edge posteriorly from below in order to provide more lateral exposure. The superior extent of the operation depends upon the location of the deep venous system including the internal cerebral veins and the vein of Galen. We have found in almost all instances that these veins are either displaced along the dorsal surface of the capsule of the tumor or join collateral channels laterally and superiorly so that the normal anatomical relations of the internal cerebral veins and the vein of Galen are destroyed. The collateral veins usually reach the straight sinus either directly or via the veins of Rosenthal. This anatomical variation may be identified prior to operative intervention by an arteriogram especially with injection of large quantities of dye into the carotid system. However, the position of these veins is generally predictable in the presence of a benign tumor. I have not found patent and important veins in this system lying in the interior of the tumor, rather they are displaced to the margins of the capsule as previously noted, usually dorsal or dorsolateral. The arterial supply to these benign tumors generally comes from the posterior choroidal arteries. There may be small branches from the superior cerebellar arteries and other small branches besides the choroidal arteries from the posterior cerebral arteries. Rarely do the penetrating branches of the basilar, posterior communicating or posterior cerebral arteries participate in the blood supply to these tumors via midbrain or diencephalon.

With the advent of the CUSA (Cavitron Lasersonics, Cooper Medical Device Corporation, Stamford, CT), we have used this instrument with increased facility and benefit in the removal of benign relatively avascular tumors of the pineal region. This instrument is ideal in coring out the interior of the tumor while creating little displacement of the tumor capsule. When the CUSA is used, it is necessary to use a long focal-length objective for the operating microscope, and if possible, the long straight or the long curved tip of the CUSA. Some of the benign tumors, especially the meningiomas may be partially or heavily calcified and this instrument exhibits particular usefulness in these cases. Once the interior of the tumor has been removed and hemostasis secured, the capsule may be brought down and dissected free of the surrounding tissues by microsurgical dissection techniques. In the sitting position it is relatively easy to dissect the capsule away from the velum interpositum. Because of the effect of gravity, the tumor tends to fall away from these structures. Using a fine long tipped bipolar cautery with low current and intermittent irrigation it is possible to cauterize and divide with special long scissors the connections of the tumor capsule. The lateral margins of these benign tumors may be adherent to the lateral wall of the third ventricle or the ependymal surface overlying the medial thalamic nuclei. The adhesions in this area are modest to nonexistent. It is with the inferior or ventral portion of the tumor, especially large tumors that severely compress the midbrain, that the surgeon may have a problem

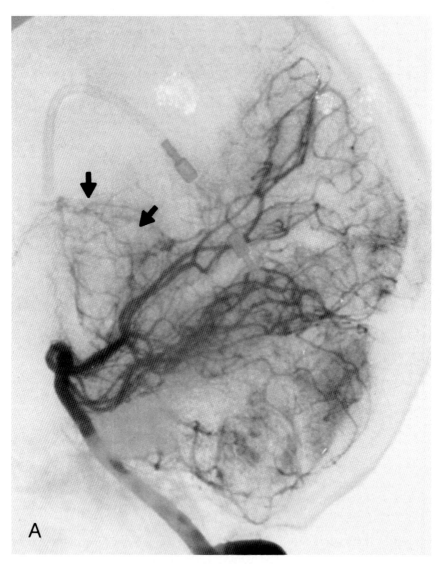

Figure 13.1. *A*, lateral vertebral arteriogram showing an area of increased vascularity (*arrows*), initially interpreted as representing a malignant tumor. At surgery this was a meningioma which could be totally resected.

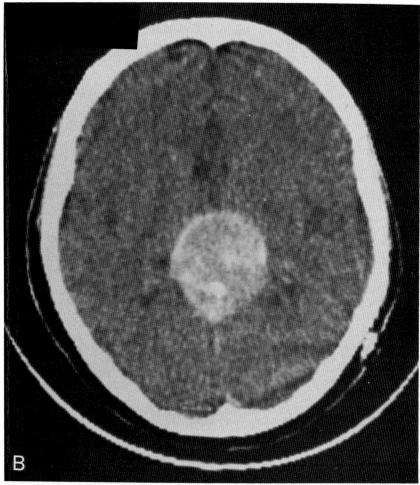

Figure 13.1. *B*, CT scan of the same patient indicating a large contrast enhancing tumor. The true diagnosis was not established until surgery.

Table 13.2
Relation to tumor type[a]

Germ cell	
Germinoma	0/20[b]
Teratoma	5/1
Dermoid	1/0
Pineal cell	
Pineocytoma	1/7
Pineoblastoma	0/2
Supporting cell	
Astrocytoma	4/14
Meningioma	6/0
Sarcoma	0/1
Colloid cyst	1/0
Choroid plexus tumor	1/0
Nontumor	
Cyst	1/0
	20/65

[a] Total cases operated = 65. Benign resectable tumors = 20.
[b] First number indicates resectable tumor, second number indicates nonresectable tumor.

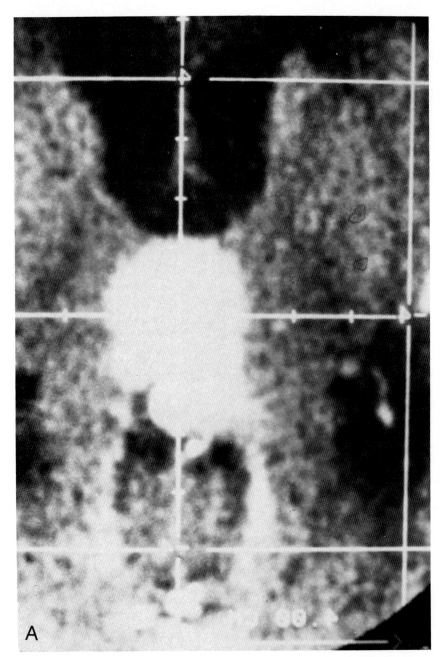

Figure 13.2. *A*, CT scan showing a large contrast enhancing tumor in the posterior third ventricle that was interpreted as a malignant tumor. The arteriogram was avascular. Nevertheless, the patient received 7000 rad of radiation.

with the posterior fossa operation. This presents a difficult technical exercise where the residual tumor capsule must be elevated with an instrument while dissection is carried out between tumor and the surface of the quadrigeminal region. The fourth cranial nerves also may be involved in the dissection and should be spared. Vascular adhesions in this area are minimal except for branches of the choroidal arteries which may be pushed anterior or anterolateral to the tumor. These may be cauterized and divided at the capsular surface of the tumor and

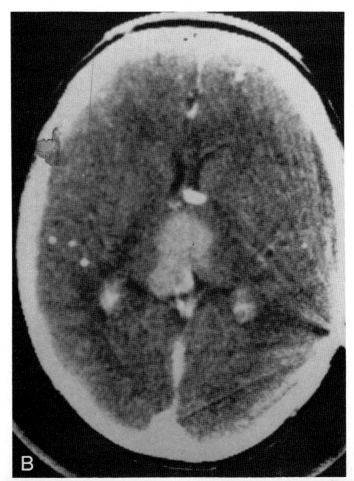

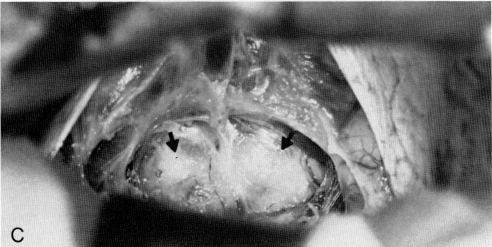

Figure 13.2. *B*, CT scan following radiation showing no appreciable change in the size of the tumor. At surgery this was a meningioma which was totally removed. The hydrocephalus has been controlled in this CT by a shunt established during radiotherapy. *C*, operative exposure of the meningioma (*arrows*) (14.2, *A* and *B*) in the pineal region without dural attachment.

hemostasis must be accurate, precise, and continuous. If hemostasis is not obtained during the removal of these benign tumors, then it is impossible to pack the wound afterwards to secure hemostasis. Once the tumor has been removed and the field dry even though it is in direct continuity with the third ventricle and the CSF, we have routinely lined the cavity with hemostatic substances. If necessary to ensure a total removal of these benign tumors, small largyngeal-type mirrors may be inserted into the wound to inspect obscure areas of the tumor bed. In every case, a postoperative scan ensures that a total removal was carried out (2, 4, 5).

Special consideration should be given to the various types of benign tumors that exist in this region, all being candidates for surgical resection.

TERATOMA

These tumors can generally be recognized from the preoperative CT scan in that they contain areas of calcification, fat, cholesterol and sometimes ossification or dentition (Fig. 13.3). These substances all add to the variegated appearance of these tumors. These tumors are encapsulated, may be lobulated with pseudopods that extend in various directions taking advantage of the varying density of the brain planes in this deep central region. The tumors often work their way in and around the velum interpositum and into the regions of the choroid fissure of the lateral ventricle and thereby the trigone of the lateral ventricle. Generally, the tumor capsule is shiny, smooth, relatively avascular, and not adherent to surrounding struc-

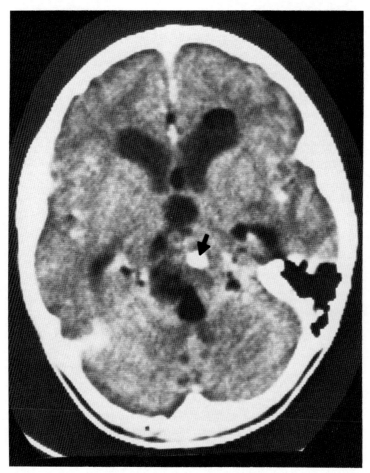

Figure 13.3.   CT scan with contrast enhancement showing a large irregular variegated tumor of the pineal representing a benign teratoma. A malformed tooth is indicated by the *arrow.*

tures provided that the area has not been radiated. I have not encountered a highly vascular teratoma in this region. In order to resect the tumor, a large opening must be made in the posterior capsule of the tumor and then some technique, preferably the CUSA, used to core out the interior of the tumor. Because of the extensive and circuitous nature of these tumors, operations on them to ensure a total removal are long and tedious (Fig. 13.4).

Postoperatively because of the potential spill of the tumor contents into CSF, there is a moderately high incidence of aseptic meningitis. There were five tumors in this category that were totally removed. Follow-up has ranged from 2 to 16 yr and there has been no evidence of recurrence.

DERMOID-EPIDERMOID

These tumors are generally a joy to encounter in the pineal region, but unfortunately are rare. In my series there was one dermoid tumor. As elsewhere in the central nervous system, these tumors contain a massive interior of sebaceous material often with hair which is easily removed with the aid of the CUSA (Fig. 13.5). The problem is related to the adherent capsule of these tumors. This often defies total removal because of its marked adherence to vital structures. However, experience indicates that portions of this capsule may be left and long-term follow-up has not shown recurrence of tumors after this type of surgical treatment either in the pineal region or elsewhere in the brain. Therefore, if difficulty is encountered, and it usually is, in removing every last scrap of the capsule, it is better to resist at this point and settle for a less than total removal of the capsule. Presumably the remaining capsular tissue, either stays static or grows at such a slow rate that it is not a threat to the patient. In the single dermoid tumor in this series, we now have a 16-yr follow-up with CT scan and no evidence of recurrence knowing that small scraps of the capsule were left in place (Fig. 13.6).

PINEOCYTOMA

This tumor varies tremendously in its potential for malignancy. Rarely the pineocytoma has been small and capsulated and apparently benign. In this case the potential for removal is recognized at surgery. It can be determined that a total removal is feasible and this should be

carried out. There was one case of a removable tumor with an 8-yr follow-up (Fig. 13.7).

ASTROCYTOMA

The benign astrocytoma includes the Grade I and possibly Grade II tumors of this region. In many instances this type of tumor, which may contain macrocysts, is encapsulated and benign and can be resected. It has a gross resemblance to the cystic astrocytoma of the cerebellum in children and generally occurs in childhood or adolescence. Its potential for resection can be recognized at surgery as the surgeon notes a consistent well-defined capsule around all margins of the tumor (Fig. 13.8). These tumors are modestly vascular and can be resected in toto. Postoperative scans have determined the completeness of resection in four cases and follow-up has been carried out for a period of 8½ yr without evidence of recurrence.

EPENDYMOMA

Strangely, I have not encountered an ependymoma in this series and therefore cannot speak from personal experience about this tumor. However, we do know that ependymomas which are located elsewhere in the ventricular system, i.e. anterior third ventricle and fourth ventricle are benign and when totally resected a cure may be obtained.

MENINGIOMAS

Meningiomas have occurred with an unusually high incidence in my series (2). I now have six meningiomas of the pineal region without dural attachment, i.e. without attachment to the tentorium. These meningiomas have been fully encapsulated and totally resectable. A number of them had been subjected to preoperative radiation on the mistaken assumption that they were malignant tumors even when they did not respond to radiation, it was felt that this was further indication of their malignancy (Fig. 13.9). However, the longevity of the patient belied this presumption. On CT scan they appear uniformly dense and contrast enhancing (Fig. 13.10). There have been no cystic meningiomas. Angiograms have shown a mixed pattern. In some the vascular pattern is striking and suggests a malignant tumor. In others, there is an avascular mass with only displacement of the vessels. In all cases the deep venous system has been displaced to the periphery of the tumor

(*Text continues on p. 269*)

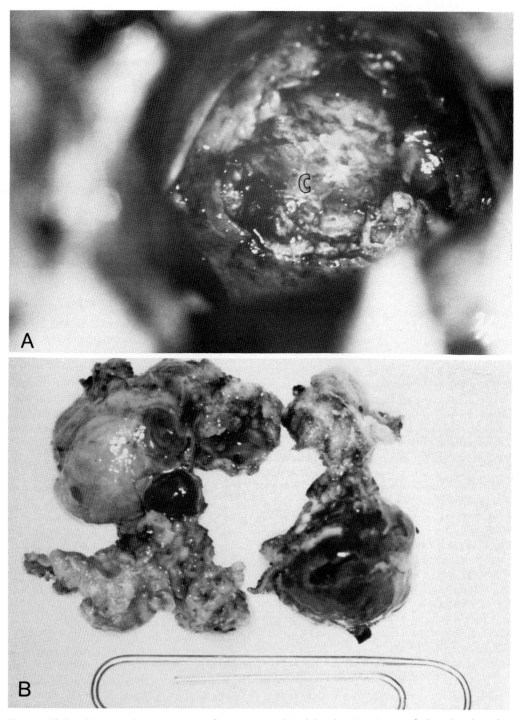

Figure 13.4. *A*, operative exposure of an encapsulated benign teratoma of the pineal region. Opening has been made into a large tumor cyst (*C*). *B*, portions of this tumor following removal show the encapsulated nature of the tumor and the large size compared to a paper clip at the bottom of the figure.

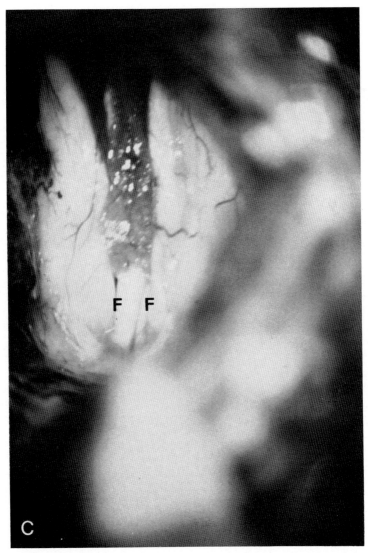

Figure 13.4. *C*, View through the opening left by tumor removal showing the roof of the third ventricle and the foramina of Monro (*F*).

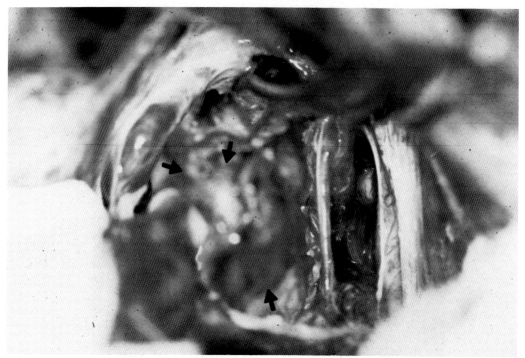

Figure 13.5.   Exposure of a pineal dermoid with a major portion of the interior contents removed (*arrows*).

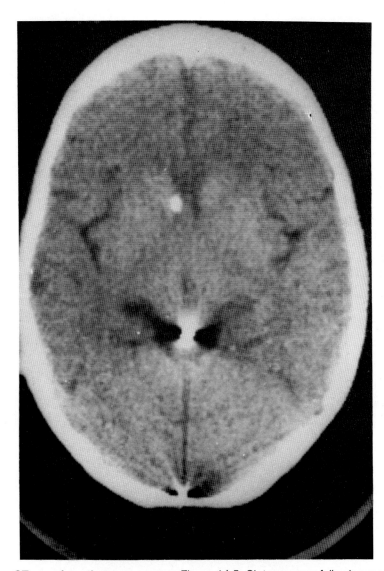

Figure 13.6.   CT scan from the same case as Figure 14.5. Sixteen years following resection of this tumor showing no evidence of residual tumor. The patient had been previously shunted.

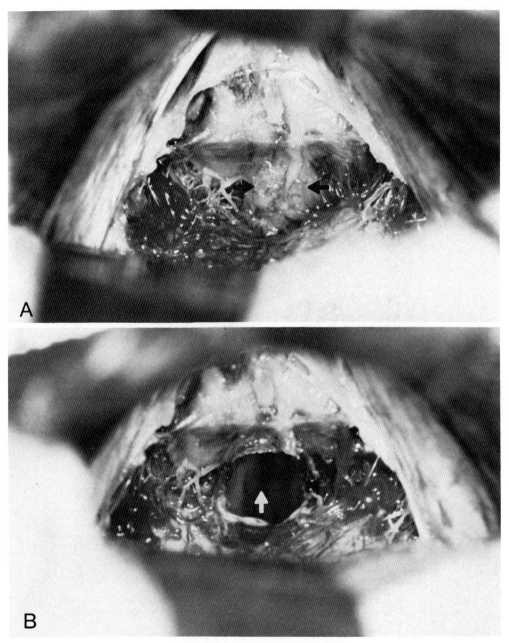

Figure 13.7. *A*, operative exposure of the pineal region showing a small discrete pineocytoma (*arrows*). *B*, operative exposure of the same patient following total removal of this tumor with the resultant opening into the posterior third ventricle (*arrow*).

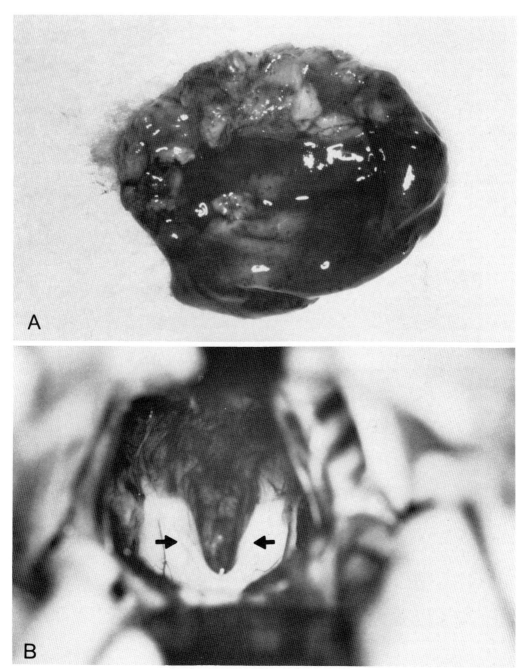

Figure 13.8. *A*, astrocytoma cystic and solid Grade I removed en toto from the pineal region. *B*, operative exposure showing view of the roof of the third ventricle (*arrows*) seen through the opening in the posterior third ventricle following total removal of the astrocytoma.

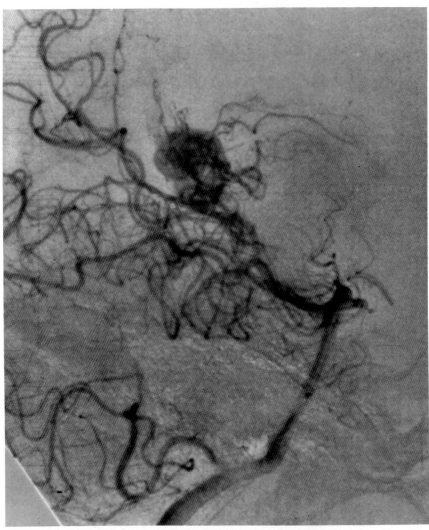

Figure 13.9. Lateral vertebral arteriogram showing a vascular pattern in the region of the tumor suggestive of a malignancy. This was a meningioma which was totally removed.

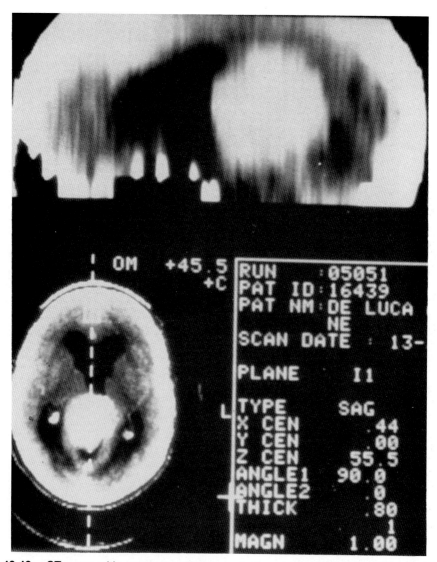

Figure 13.10. CT scan with contrast enhancement observed in horizontal plane and saggital reconstruction showing a large densely enhancing tumor mass which was a meningioma totally removed at surgery.

usually dorsal and dorsolateral. The gross appearance of the tumor at surgery varies. One case had an onset with hemorrhage and an intracapsular hemorrhage could be observed at the time of surgery (Fig. 13.11). This turned out to be an angioblastic meningioma or a hemangiopericytoma. Generally, these tumors have not been highly vascular, but do present a problem as some are extremely firm and fibrous and therefore difficult to remove piecemeal except with the use of a CUSA. Some have been lightly calcified. Other meningiomas are soft and can

be removed easily by suction and cautery (Fig. 13.12). Once the interior of the tumor has been debulked, then the capsule whether it be vascular or avascular is gradually withdrawn into the cavity left by the interior removal of tumor and dissected by microdissection techniques from the surrounding structures. The area of attachment is usually along the velum interpositum and here great care must be taken not to injure the internal cerebral veins or the great vein of Galen where the attachment may be quite firm. In all of these cases, postoperative CT scans

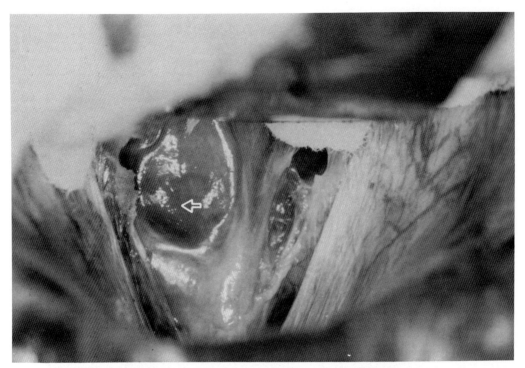

Figure 13.11.   Operative exposure showing hemorrhage (*arrow*) into the capsule of an angioblastic meningioma in a patient presenting with subarachnoid hemorrhage. This tumor was totally removed.

confirmed the total removal of the tumor and follow-up has ranged from 2 to 10 yr without evidence of recurrence.

CYSTS AND MISCELLANEOUS TUMORS

There is one arachnoid cyst in this series occurring in an infant. It was mistaken for a solid posterior third ventricle tumor. Its identity was only revealed at the time of surgery. It appeared to be a part of a greater process of cystic or inflammatory arachnoiditis which led to a communicating hydrocephalus after this cyst which blocked the aqueduct was removed. Such cysts have been previously described. Other single benign tumors included a choroid plexus tumor and a colloid cyst.

SUMMARY

The most interesting category of benign tumors that we have found is the meningioma group. These have been described as free-standing tumors by a number of authors and appear to arise from arachnoidal cluster cells which lie in or about the tela choroidea. They may attain massive size, especially when hydrocephalus has been corrected by a shunt. They appear to grow at a very slow rate, are universally benign and present with a slowly progressive syndrome of dementia rather than the usual characteristic syndrome of Parinaud's syndrome and symptoms of midbrain compression. Perhaps this unusual presentation is related to their very slow growth and intolerance for compression of the surrounding cerebral structures. One case as previously noted presented as an unlocalized subarachnoid hemorrhage. Because of its vascularity on arteriography, it was interpreted as a malignant tumor. Fortunately, no radiation was given and a total surgical resection could be carried out.

The prognosis for the group of benign lesions appears to be uniformly good. They comprise about 30% of the whole group. This is the major reason why I feel all pineal tumors should be confirmed histologically so as not to pass up a golden opportunity for the removal of a benign tumor without the threat of radiation to the normal brain. Unfortunately, in many of these benign tumors, radiation therapy had been given blindly with the adjuvant of a CSF shunt prior to referral of the patient to our center. My personal feeling is that radiation to the surrounding normal brain makes it less resilient to

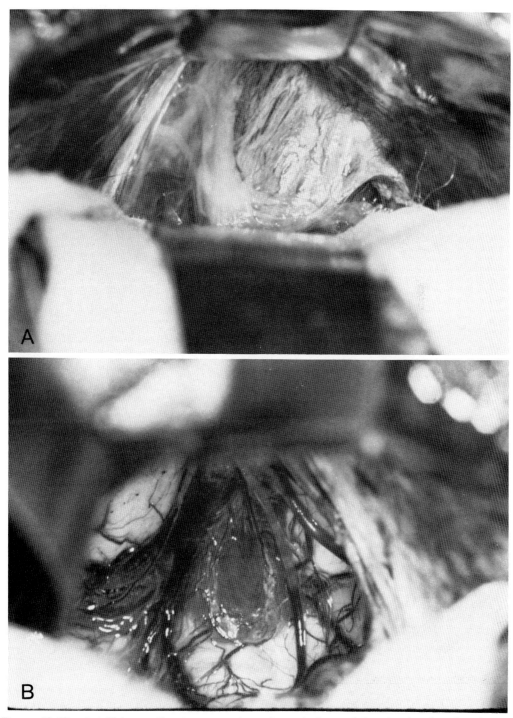

Figure 13.12. *A*, initial operative exposure of a soft meningioma of the pineal region. Attachment was to the area of the tela choroidea. *B*, operative photograph following total removal of this soft relatively avascular meningioma.

tolerate major surgical procedures in this area. Fortunately, there has been no morbidity of significance in any of these patients in the postoperative period whether they were radiated or not prior to surgery. Admittedly, the follow-up is short in some to confirm that these patients are cured. However, their recovery from surgery has been gratifying without mortality and without permanent morbidity.

References

1. Jooma R, Kendall BE: Diagnosis and management of pineal tumors. *J Neurosurg* 58:654–665, 1983.

2. Rozario R, Adelman L, Prager RJ, Stein BM: Meningiomas of the pineal region and third ventricle. *Neurosurgery* 5:489–495, 1979.

3. Rubinstein LJ: Cytogenesis and differentiation of pineal neoplasms. *Hum Pathol* 12:441–448, 1981.

4. Schmidek, HH: *Pineal Tumors.* Brady LW, De Vita VT (eds). New York, Masson Publishing USA, 1977, pp 1–138.

5. Stein BM: Surgical treatment of pineal tumors. *Clin Neurosurg* 26:490–510, 1979.

6. Stein BM: Supracerebellar approach for pineal region neoplasms. In Schmidek HH, Sweet WH (eds): *Operative Neurosurgical Techniques.* Grune & Stratton, 1982, vol 1.

CHAPTER 14

Surgical Treatment of Malignant Pineal Region Tumors

EDWARD A. NEUWELT, M.D.

INTRODUCTION

Krabbe proposed the term "pinealoma" for all tumors arising from the pineal gland and posterior third ventricle (18). This has led to much confusion in that a variety of different types of tumors have been called by that designation. A common malignant pineal tumor, the germinoma (atypical teratoma), has been commonly classified as a pinealoma. We prefer to reserve the term "pinealoma" for malignant tumors of the pineal parenchymal cells. Tumors of mature cells are "pineocytomas" and those of immature cells "pineoblastomas" (39).

It is the purpose of this communication to review the experience at the University of Texas Southwestern Medical School between 1972 and 1980 and the more recent experience of the author at the Oregon Health Sciences University with malignant pineal region tumors. More specifically, our purpose is: (*a*) to show that surgical exploration and biopsy of these lesions can be safe when the operating microscope is used; (*b*) to show that even malignant pineal tumors are surprisingly well encapsulated, permitting total gross excision; (*c*) to demonstrate the lack of criteria to make an accurate histological diagnosis on the basis of neuroradiological studies; (*d*) to point out the clinical importance of the tumor markers associated with these tumors, particularly the beta subunit of human chorionic gonadotropin (HCG) and alpha fetoprotein (AFP); (*e*) to relate ultrastructural and immunopathological studies of these tumors; and (*f*) to demonstrate the role that chemotherapy can play in the treatment of these tumors, particularly when a histological diagnosis is available. The initial eight patients in this series have been reported previously (26).

CLINICAL MATERIAL AND METHODS

Thirty-four patients with pineal region lesions have been treated in this series (Table 14.1).

Table 14.1
Pineal Region Lesions Seen at the University of Texas Southwestern Medical School from 1972–1981 and the Oregon Health Sciences University from 1981–1984

Lesions	No. of Cases
Benign, operative	
Meningiomas	2
Epidermoid cyst	1
Cystic astrocytoma—superior vermis	1
Thrombosed vein of Galen aneurysm	1
Vein of Galen aneurysm	1
Hematoma of splenium—cryptic arteriovenous malformation	1
Cysticerosis—quadrigeminal cistern	1
Dermoid cysts	3
Teratoma	1
Malignant, operative	
Thalamic gliomas	3
Metastatic adenocarcinoma	1
Ependymoma—posterior third ventricle	1†
Germinomas	2†
Germinoma + astrocytoma	1†
Pineocytomas	2†
Pineoblastoma	3†
Pineoblastoma + astrocytoma*	3†
Embryonal cell	1†
Malignant, nonoperative	
Germinoma	1†
Pineoblastoma	1†
Unknown	3
GRAND TOTAL	34

* Two cases were predominantly pineoblastoma with areas of well differentiated astrocytoma, the other case was vice-versa.

† Primary malignant pineal tumor, n = 15.

Twenty-nine of these patients have undergone direct surgical tumor exploration. Of these 34 patients, 15 had primary malignant pineal tumors (excluding thalamic gliomas), which were explored surgically. These 15 malignant pineal tumors are the basis of this report (Table 14.2). Patients with gliomas involving the pulvinar and 1 metastatic tumor have been excluded from this surgical series of primary malignant pineal tumors.

The occipital transtentorial approach was used in most of the patients who underwent direct surgical exploration. The details of this approach as used are described in Chapter 9.

Immunological studies were carried out on fresh aliquot specimens of three resected tumors. Identification of surface immunoglobulin (SIG), and erythrocyte rosetting was recognized by methods involving separated cells isolated from the tumor by gentle teasing (25).

CASE REPORTS

Case 1

(D.K.) This 16-yr-old boy presented with Parinaud's syndrome and mild right-sided weakness. A CT scan revealed a massive pineal region lesion which enhanced markedly with parenteral contrast administration. Angiography revealed that the tumor was essentially avascular. The patient underwent an occipital transtentorial exploration of this lesion. A subtotal decompression was performed and the histological diagnosis was a germinoma, as revealed by a diffuse proliferation of large cells against a background of small round cells with a lymphocytic appearance. Immunopathological studies performed on an aliquot revealed that the majority of the small cells could be classified as T-lymphocytes by virtue of their ability to form erythrocyte rosettes. A small proportion of the lymphocytes were found to have surface immunoglobulins indicative of B-lymphocytes (25). Serum and cerebrospinal fluid (CSF) levels of HCG and AFP were undetectable. The patient's parents refused postoperative radiotherapy and the patient received Laetrile, as prescribed by an outside physician, and he died while on this drug.

Case 2

(J.T.) This 16-yr-old boy had presented at another institution 3½ yr previously with headaches, a sixth-nerve palsy, and diabetes insipi-

dus. Metrizamide ventriculography and CT scans demonstrated two lesions involving the anterior and posterior third ventricles, respectively. A ventriculoperitoneal (VP) shunt was placed, and, on the presumptive diagnosis of germinoma, craniospinal irradiation was given (Table 14.3). The patient's symptoms resolved, although the diabetes insipidus persisted in a mild form, and he returned to school.

He noted a protuberant abdomen 2½ yr after his initial presentation. Chest film revealed elevation of the right hemidiaphragm and a large pleural effusion. Panmyelography was normal. The CSF cytology was normal. Cranial CT and metrizamide ventriculography were normal, except for a large pineal calcification. A CT scan of the abdomen demonstrated massive intraperitoneal and retroperitoneal tumor involvement as well as beaded tumor nodules along the thoracic portion of the thoracic shunt and on the superior surface of the diaphragm. Laboratory investigation revealed a serum HCG level of 67 ng/ml (normal is less than 3 ng/ml). Biopsy revealed a massive tumor filling the abdominal cavity which, on histological study, was found to be a germinoma.

The patient was started on multi-agent systemic chemotherapy with cis-platinum, bleomycin, and vinblastine (13). Excellent cytocellular reduction was achieved and, after four courses of chemotherapy, his serum HCG returned to normal and he had achieved a complete remission with no evident tumor by all measurable criteria. His stable condition has persisted for 5 yr. His VP shunt has been removed.

Case 3

(P.M.) This 17-yr-old boy presented with Parinaud's syndrome, headaches, and papilledema. A pneumoencephalogram and angiogram revealed a tumor in the pineal region, which was confirmed by CT scan (Fig. 14.1). His symptoms were transiently relieved by a VP shunt, but progressive headaches, increasing limitation of upward gaze, and lethargy precipitated a subtotal decompression via an occipital transtentorial approach. Pathological examination of the tumor revealed two types of cells, large cells and small cells with a lymphoid appearance, characteristic of pineal germinoma. Postoperative myelography was normal and he was treated with radiation therapy (Table 14.3). Serial CT

Table 14.2
Clinical Course in 15 Patients with Primary Malignant Pineal Tumors

Case No.	Patient's Initials	Histological Diagnosis	Shunt	Occipital Transtentorial Craniotomy	Radiation	Chemo-therapy	Outcome
1	DK	Germinoma	VP	Subtotal decompression	None	–	Died 1 yr postoperatively, received Laetrile only postoperatively
2	JT	Germinoma	VP		Craniospinal	+	Alive and well; tumor-free after 5 yr
3	PM	Germinoma	VP	Subtotal decompression	Craniospinal	–	Alive and well; tumor-free after 7 yr
4	RM	Embryonal cell pineocytoma	VP	Complete excision	Craniospinal	–	Died of spinal metastases
5	QA	Pineocytoma	VP	Complete excision	Craniospinal	–	Alive and well; tumor-free after 5 yr
6	RG	Pineocytoma	VP	Complete excision	Craniospinal	–	Alive and well; tumor-free after 6 yr
7	RM	Pineoblastoma	VP		Cranial only	–	Died of spinal metastases
8	SW	Pineoblastoma + astrocytoma	VP	Complete excision	Craniospinal	–	Alive and well; tumor-free after 5 yr
9	WK	Astrocytoma + pineoblastoma	VP	Complete excision	Cranial only	–	Alive and well; tumor-free after 2 yr
10	PH	Pineoblastoma	VP	Biopsy	Cranial	+	Died of metastatic renal carcinoma 1 yr following pineal surgery (i.e. of a 2nd primary)
11	TN	Pineoblastoma	VP	Complete excision	Craniospinal	–	Alive and well; tumor-free after 18 months
12	SS	Pineoblastoma + astrocytoma	VP	Complete excision	None	–	Alive and well; CT scan, recurrence at 8 months
13	EG	Pineoblastoma	VP	Biopsy	Craniospinal	+	Died 1 yr postoperatively
14	RJ	Malignant ependymoma	VP	Complete excision	Cranial only	–	Alive and well; tumor-free after 6 yr
15	GS	Germinoma + astrocytoma	VP	Complete excision	Cranial only	–	Alive and well; tumor-free after 4 months

Table 14.3
Details of Radiation Therapy of Patients with Primary Malignant Pineal Tumors

Case* No.	Patient's Initial	Cranial Irradiation		Spinal Dose (rad)
		Port	Dose (rad)	
2	JT	Whole head, boost to pineal	3800 1000	2500
3	PM	Whole head, boost to pineal	4000 1000	4000
4	RM	Whole head, boost to pineal	4000 1500	4000 (cervical only)
5	QA	Whole head, boost to pineal	4000 1000	4300
6	RG	Whole head, boost to tumor	4000 1500	2250†
7	RM	Whole head, boost to tumor	4000 1000	2700
8	SW	Whole head	5000	3400
9	WK	6 × 6 cm Tumor port	5000	None
10	PH	Cranial	5000	—
11	TN	Whole head, boost to tumor	4000 1500	4000
13	EG	Whole head, boost to tumor	4500 900	4000
14	RJ	7 × 7 cm Tumor port	5000	None
15	GS	Whole head, boost to tumor	4000 1500	None

* Cases no. 1 and 12 did not receive radiation therapy.

† Spinal irradiation given 1 yr after cranial irradiation when patient presented with quadriplegia. Patient died before planned dose of 4000 rad to spinal canal could be given.

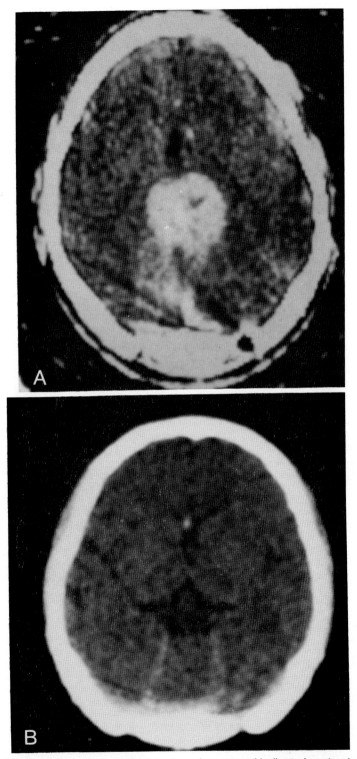

Figure 14.1.   CT scan following the administration of parenteral iodinated contrast agent showing a pineal germinoma (Case 3, P.M.): *A*, after occipital transtentorial craniotomy and biopsy; *B*, following the completion of cranial irradiation.

scans revealed progressive disappearance of the tumor, and 18 months after surgery he appears to be free of tumor (Fig. 14.1).

Case 5

(Q.A.) This 23-yr-old woman presented with severe progressive headaches. On physical examination she was lethargic, had anisocoria, decreased upward gaze, and bilateral ptosis. Her initial CT scan revealed moderate hydrocephalus and an enhancing mass in the pineal region. The levels of AFP and of the beta subunit of HCG in the serum and CSF were normal. The patient underwent a VP shunt with marked resolution of her headaches and lethargy. Two weeks later, she underwent an occipital transtentorial exploration of her pineal region. A well-encapsulated, well-demarcated tumor was totally excised microsurgically. Microscopic ex-

amination of the tumor revealed nests, sheets, and rosettes of neoplastic pineal cells. Mitoses and focal necrosis were also present. This neoplasm was believed to be a pineocytoma. The patient developed a posterior fossa epidural clot 48 hr postoperatively, which was evacuated. Her recovery was excellent, her shunt was removed, and she then received craniospinal radiotherapy. She is alive and well without evidence of recurrence 5 yr postoperatively (Table 14.3).

Case 6

(R.G.) This 58-yr-old man presented with Parinaud's syndrome and ataxia. A CT scan revealed a well-circumscribed spherical 3-cm mass in the pineal region (Fig. 14.2). Angiography confirmed a vascular pineal-region mass. A VP shunt was inserted which relieved him of his headaches. Two weeks later the lesion was en-

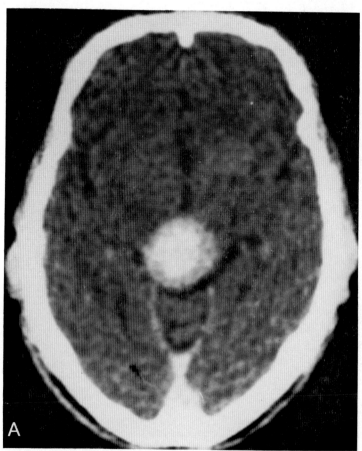

Figure 14.2. CT scans following administration of parenteral contrast, showing a pineocytoma (Case 6, R.G.): *A*, transverse cut; *B*, sagittal cut; *C*, coronal cut. The ventricular catheter can be seen as a small high-density just above the tumor mass; *D*, transverse scan done in the immediate postoperative period demonstrating absence of any evidence of residual tumor.

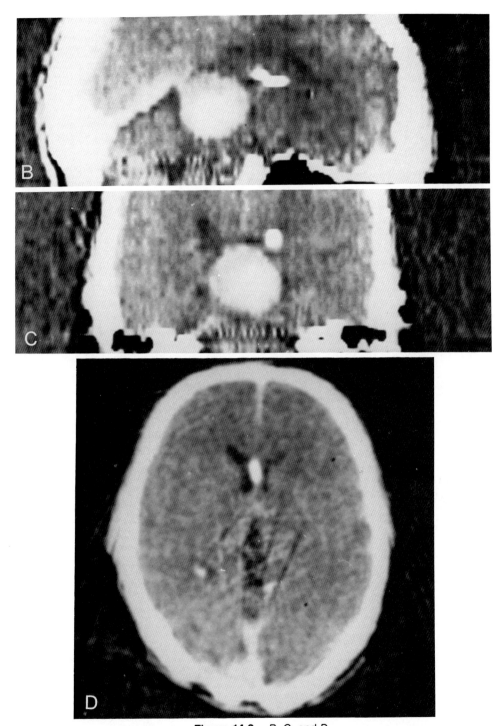

Figure 14.2. *B*, *C*, and *D*.

tirely removed via an occipital transtentorial craniotomy.

Microscopic examination of the tumor revealed a repetitious pattern of interlacing columns and rosettes of differentiating pineal cells. Occasional Homer-Wright pseudorosettes were present. The neoplasm was thought to have a degree of differentiation consistent with a pineocytoma.

Postoperatively, radiation was given (Table

14.3). All neurological abnormalities cleared. Repeat CT scan and metrizamide myelography 18 months postoperatively revealed no evidence of tumor recurrence (Fig. 14.2). The patient continues to do well 6 yr postoperatively.

Case 7

(R.M.) This 23-yr-old woman presented to another institution with limitation of upward gaze and papilledema. A CT scan revealed an enhancing tumor of the pineal region, pineal calcification, and hydrocephalus. A VP shunt was inserted with excellent resolution of her signs and symptoms. She then received cranial radiotherapy (Table 14.3).

Ten months after radiotherapy she developed back pain and progressive motor and sensory symptoms in all four extremities. The symptoms progressed over 2 months until she was essentially quadriplegic. She was transferred to our service. A myelogram done via C1-2 puncture revealed a complete block at the C2-3 level. Radiotherapy to her entire spinal axis was begun immediately. Cytological examination of the CSF revealed the presence of malignant CSF cells. The patient became septic and died 15 days following admission.

Postmortem examination revealed a 1-cm mass in the pineal region which on microscopic examination contained viable tumor despite a normal CT scan just prior to her death. The tumor filled the subarachnoid space from C-2 to C-7. Microscopic examination of the tumor showed sheets of small cells with round-to-oval nuclei and scanty cytoplasm. Homer-Wright rosettes were present. Electron microscopy showed membrane-bound vesicles within most processes that may represent secretory granules. A diagnosis of pineoblastoma was made.

Case 8

(S.W.) This 38-yr-old woman presented with papilledema, titubation of the head, and no other focal neurological abnormalities. A CT scan revealed a 3–4-cm spherical mass in the pineal region with multiple calcifications; enhancement was seen with parenteral iodinated contrast (Fig. 14.3). Marked hydrocephalus was also noted. Angiography confirmed a pineal neoplasm. A VP shunt was inserted which markedly decreased her head-bobbing. Search for tumor markers (HCG and AFP) in the serum and CSF was negative. An occipital transtentorial resec-

tion of her tumor was performed. The lesion was well circumscribed; a very definitive capsule permitted total surgical resection. Microscopic examination of the tumor revealed a small primitive neuroectodermal neoplasm with prominent pseudorosette formation and focal areas of glial differentiation. There was one prominent region of pilocytic astrocytoma with dense glial processes and Rosenthal's fibers. This tumor was diagnosed as a pineoblastoma with associated pilocytic astrocytoma. The postoperative course was uneventful, her shunt was removed and she was given prophylactic craniospinal irradiation (Fig. 14.3). She is alive and well 5 yr postoperatively with no evidence of recurrence (Table 14.3).

Case 14

(R.J.) This 12-yr-old girl presented with severe headaches and dystonic movements of her head and neck. Four-vessel cerebral angiography revealed marked hydrocephalus but no evidence of tumor. Ventriculography showed a large tumor arising from the right posterior third ventricle ependymal wall. A VP shunt was inserted and radiation therapy initiated to the tumor bed (Table 14.3). Three months after treatment, angiography and ventriculography revealed a progressive increase in tumor size. The pineal region was explored via an occipital transtentorial approach, and the tumor was located anterior to the vein of Galen and between the two basilar veins of Rosenthal. It had a well-defined capsule permitting total piecemeal tumor resection. Postoperatively, she had Parinaud's syndrome but no other deficits. Although shunt revision was needed, the patient has continued to be well 9 yr later. Histological examination of the tissue revealed a vascular glial stroma with perivascular pseudorosettes and papillomatous configurations; focal areas of necrosis were present. The histological diagnosis was anaplastic ependymoma.

SUMMARY OF CASES

Fourteen patients showed enhancing pineal region tumors on CT scan, and the diagnosis in the 15th patient was made by angiography and ventriculography. There was no accurate correlation of radiological appearance and tumor histology. Indeed, several of the cases clinically and radiologically (i.e. Case 6, R.G.; Case 8, S.W.) easily could have been a pineal region meningiomna (see Chapter 1, Case 6 and Chapter 13).

The initial therapeutic step in all 15 patients was insertion of a VP shunt. In 12 cases this was followed by direct surgical exploration (usually 7–10 days postoperatively), and postoperative irradiation (Tables 14.2 and 14.3). In 1 case, irradiation preceded surgery and in the other 2 cases, radiation therapy only was given. One patient (Case 12, S.S.) was not irradiated due to her age (6 months). The ports and doses of radiation are summarized in Table 14.3.

Complete gross microsurgical excision of well encapsulated tumors was possible in 9 of 13 patients who underwent definitive surgical exploration. Subtotal excision only was possible in two of the other patients. In the remaining two patients who had pineal germinomas, a less aggressive subtotal excision was done because of the known radiosensitivity of this tumor. Postoperative CT scans confirmed these results. The operative complications were: 3 patients developed a persistent homonymous hemianopsia (several patients had transient field defects), 1 patient had a mild transient hemiparesis, 1 an epidural hematoma of the posterior fossa, 1 an epidural hygroma, and several patients had a postoperative increase in their Parinaud's syndrome, which was almost always transient. Tissue obtained at surgery or autopsy revealed that 3 of these lesions were germinomas, 1 was an embryonal cell tumor, 4 were pineoblastomas, 4 were mixed tumors (pineoblastomas + astrocytoma; germinoma and astrocytoma), 2 were pineocytomas, and 1 was an anaplastic ependymoma.

The two patients treated with a shunt and radiation therapy but without craniotomy both developed metastases outside their radiation ports. One of the patients who developed metastases (Case 2, J.T.) had a germinoma which secreted HCG. His massive metastatic tumor burden totally disappeared with chemotherapy. Ten other patients were evaluated for tumor markers (HCG and AFP) in their serum and CSF, but none were found.

One patient (Case 7, R.M.), who developed spinal metastases from her pineoblastoma, was initially treated with a shunt and cranial radiation. Despite complete tumor regression by CT scan, she seeded her unirradiated spinal canal with tumor. Interestingly, at postmortem examination, she had 1 cm of residual viable tumor in the pineal region which was not apparent on her enhanced CT scan done 2 weeks earlier.

In summary, one has evidence of recurrence

by CT scan, 9 patients appear to be in complete remissions, and 5 patients died. One patient (Case 1, D.K.) with a germinoma received Laetrile only, postoperatively, against our advice, and died; Case 4 (R.M.) with embryonal cell cancer died with spinal metastases despite craniospinal irradiation. Case 7 (R.M.) died from spinal seeding of her pineoblastoma 10 months after VP shunt and cranial irradiation. Patient 10 (P.H.) died 1 year postoperatively of a second neoplasm (clear cell cancer of the kidney). Patient E.G. (Case 13) died of progressive disease 1 year postoperatively. His tumor progressed 3 months after radiation and he transiently responded to chemotherapy with methotrexate, cytoxan and procarbazine in association with osmotic blood-brain barrier opening (24, 27), before succumbing to his tumor.

DISCUSSION
The Role of Surgery

An important aspect of the present series is its deviation from some of the classic tenets of therapeutic intervention in pineal region tumors. In the past, radiotherapy has been the generally accepted primary treatment for pineal tumors. Schmidek's recent extensive review of therapy led him to conclude that "the mortality and morbidity associated with surgery of the pineal region would confirm the impression that primary excision of these lesions at the time they are diagnosed is not warranted" (39). He believes that a small fraction (10–15%) with classical neurodiagnostic criteria of benignity merited consideration for surgical resection, but that for most pineal region tumors, primary removal was associated with a 25–70% mortality (6–8, 14, 15, 20, 31–33, 46). Similarly, Donat et al (12) reviewed 53 years' experience at the Mayo Clinic and concluded that surgery should be reserved for tumors that are radioresistant or that progress after radiotherapy. Another basis for concern regarding operative attack on the tumor was expressed by Jenkins et al (17), who suggested that surgical intervention increased the risk of distant subarachnoid metastases. Two of their 10 patients whose pineal germinomas were biopsied and treated with only cranial irradiation developed meningeal seeding.

An alternative view was expressed by Jamieson (16), who advocated primary surgical exploration of all pineal region tumors. In his series of nine cases, successful complete excision of four germinomas and two pineocytomas was per-

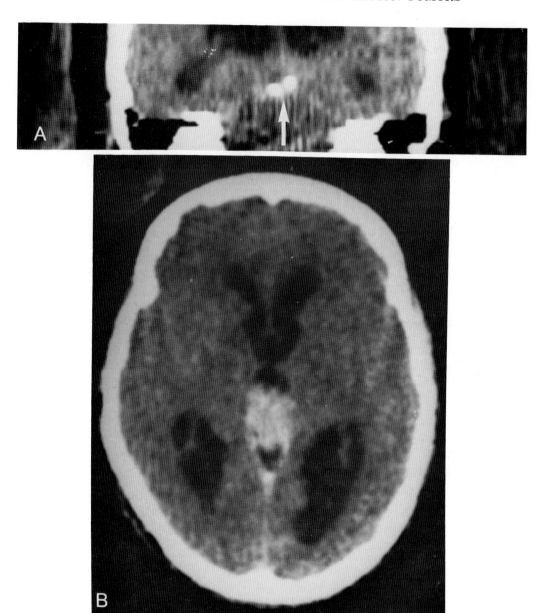

Figure 14.3. CT scans showing a pineoblastoma (Case 8, S.W.): *A,* coronal section (unenhanced) showing tumor calcification (*arrow*); *B,* enhanced transverse section; *C,* enhanced saggital section; *D,* normal enhanced CT scan (transverse section) 3 yr postoperatively and after radiotherapy.

formed with "minimal morbidity." One postoperative death occurred in a patient in whom biopsy only was attempted, and four patients with invasive or ectopic lesions were treated nonoperatively. Stein (44) has also advocated that surgery precede a decision regarding radiotherapy. However, in spite of these exceptions, the prevailing attitude has been the use of radiotherapy as the initial therapeutic modality for

all pineal region tumors except for those with clearly benign features on CT scan, that is, lesions with mixed fat and CSF density indicative of the presence of an epidermoid tumor, dermoid or teratoma.

Of the 34 patients (Table 14.1) with pineal region lesions seen over the past 11 yr, 28 have undergone microsurgical exploration and 1 patient had a needle biopsy. The occipital trans-

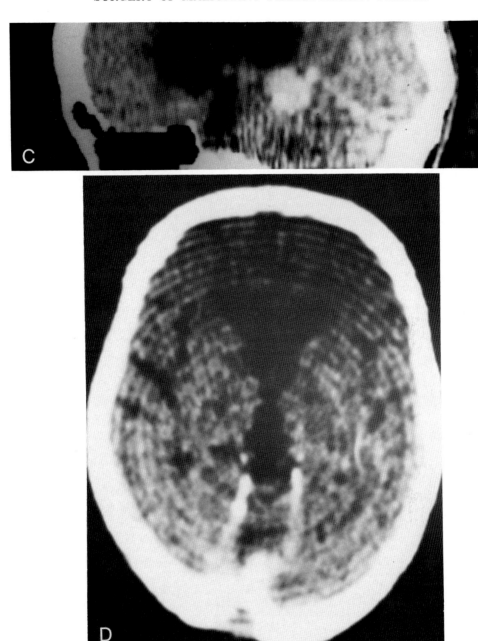

Figure 14.3. *C* and *D*.

tentorial approach was used in 24 cases and the infratentorial approach in 4 cases. These approaches have been described and compared previously (35). The operative microscope has provided the major therapeutic advance and with it, injury to the large venous structures in this region can be avoided. There has been only 1 operative death, and that in a patient with metastatic adenocarcinoma. Morbidity has been minimal in the overall series of 29 procedures. We have not had any persistent visual field deficits since 1978, probably because we have increased the size of the bone flap to give more room to retract the occipital lobe. Surgery has been safe and even malignant tumors have been completely excised!

This experience provides evidence that a wide variety of lesions in the pineal region can be microsurgically excised safely. In those circumstances where excision is not possible, the operative approach has provided important histological material that has been helpful in planning appropriate postoperative therapy. It is of further interest that in the patients with known histology, only 19 of 31 (61%) malignant lesions were encountered (in 3 of the 34 cases the histology is unknown). This is in marked contrast to Schmidek's calculation that only 10–15% of pineal region lesions are benign (39). These malignant lesions included 15 primary pineal region tumors, 3 thalamic gliomas, and 1 metastatic adenocarcinoma. Since benign lesions are more radioresistant, their relative frequency is of importance in the strategy of therapy. Empiric radiation in a benign lesion not only risks radiation damage to the CNS parenchyma, but also increases scarring of the thick arachnoid which encases the pineal and the deep venous system. The latter increases the difficulty and risks of subsequent surgery. It is also striking that only 1 of the 15 surgically treated malignant primary tumors of the pineal region have developed metastases, whereas the 2 nonoperative cases have.

These data from our clinical experience strongly support the importance of surgical exploration and biopsy or excision as the initial therapeutic modality in pineal region tumors. Indeed, these results, at least initially, are better than those achieved with radiotherapy alone and provide a more rational approach for the application of other therapeutic modalities, such as chemotherapy, which in the past has not been available nor tried. As discussed by Dr. Moser in Chapter 12, stereotactic biopsy is another alternative. The limited tissue sample and the risk of damage to the deep veins surrounding pineal lesions must be considered with stereotactic biopsy.

Neuroradiological Studies

Although it has been stated that a number of pineal region tumors can be identified neuroradiologically as either benign or malignant (39), this was not substantiated in the series of pineal tumors at our institution (Table 14.2) nor in another similar-sized series (43). In addition, no consistent neuroradiological criteria for the excisability of pineal tumors were detected. This topic is examined in more detail by Dr. Anderson in Chapter 3.

Pathological Studies

The pathological diagnosis of the 15 malignant primary pineal tumors is as follows: 3 germinomas, 2 pineocytomas, 4 pineoblastomas, 3 pineoblastoma + astrocytoma, 1 astrocytoma + germinoma, and 1 anaplastic ependymoma. The classification of pineal tumors has been described previously (39). Although most series consider the germinoma to be the most common pineal tumor (9, 39), there have been other series (5), including our own, in which tumors of the pineal parenchymal cells (pineoblastoma and pineocytoma) are more common.

The diagnosis of the three pure germinomas was straightforward, as these tumors are composed of two distinct cell populations: (a) large rounded germ cells with prominent, rounded, vesicular nuclei; and (b) clusters of cells of lymphoid appearance. The pathological evaluation of our one patient whose tumor was a mixture of germinoma and astrocytoma is reviewed in Chapter 1, case 7.

The microscopic picture of the well-differentiated pineocytoma is quite distinctive and resembles the normal pineal gland. Mitotic figures, necrosis, and hemorrhage are not usually present. The two pineocytomas in this series are less well differentiated and more closely resemble the lobular structure of the embryonal pineal gland. Cells within the lobules are more rounded and have less cytoplasm than in the better-differentiated pineocytomas. One of our cases also had a significant degree of mitotic activity and necrosis.

Our seven pineoblastomas are composed of dense cellular aggregates of small rounded or oval cells with scanty cytoplasm, and are indistinguishable from primitive neuroectodermal tumors in other locations. Three of the cases showed a prominent focus of differentiation toward an astrocytoma. In two of the cases, the tumor was primarily pineoblastoma with small areas of astrocytoma, whereas the third case was primarily a low-grade astrocytoma. Although previously reported in a medulloblastoma, these cases, to our knowledge, are unique.

Electron microscopy was performed in several of the cases of the pineal parenchymal cell tumors. Prior reports in the literature include one published case (30), and one abstract (23), reporting the ultrastructure of the pineocytoma. Our cases (26) showed similar findings, with numerous cell processes, often rich in microtubules, resembling neuronal processes, and an overall similarity in the normal adult pineal gland. The pineoblastomas in this series are the first, to our knowledge, to have their ultrastructure reported (26). They also had some features resembling normal pineal gland; however, overall there was even more of a resemblance to the undifferentiated cells of the medulloblastoma. One of the tumors contained membrane-bound vesicles that may represent secretory granules. A more detailed report of the ultrastructure of the pineocytoma and pineoblastoma is given by Dr. Herrick in Chapter 2.

Immunopathological evaluation of the tumor from Case 1 revealed that 81% of the "small cells" formed rosettes with sheep red blood cells as is characteristic of T-lymphocytes. The remainder of the "small cells" appear to be B-lymphocytes as evidenced by the presence of surface immunoglobulins. The details of our immunopathological study of this pineal germinoma have been reported (25). Similar studies on a pineocytoma (from Case 5) and a pineoblastoma (from Case 8) were negative for B- and T-cell markers. These immunological studies corroborate the morphological impression at the light and electron microscope level that the "small cells" are lymphocytes. The predominance of T-lymphocytes in this pineal germinoma is analogous to the predominance of T-lymphocytes in the perivascular spaces of malignant gliomas (42). The presence of lymphoid cells in tumors of the CNS may have pathogenic significance (25).

Tumor Markers

The most important marker of pineal germinomas appears to be the beta chain of HCG. Elevated HCG has been reported in a number of patients with this tumor (10, 19, 37, 40), and its plasma level correlates with tumor growth or regression. Unfortunately, it is not secreted by all germinomas and indeed is not necessarily associated with a malignant tumor (Dr. Mike Edwards, University of California, San Francisco, personal communication). Only one of our three patients with a germinoma in this series whose serum HCG was assayed had increased plasma levels (Case 2). As expected, when the tumor regressed following the administration of chemotherapy, the plasma level of HCG returned to normal. In highly invasive tumors, or in tumors that have already metastasized, the detection of increased levels of plasma or CSF

HCG may be sufficiently diagnostic to eliminate the need for a tissue diagnosis.

The carcinoembryonic antigen and the AFP have also been reported to be secreted by germ-cell tumors. Lee et al (21), reported increased levels of AFP in serum and CSF in a patient with an endodermal sinus tumor of the pineal region. At present, there are not any known markers of nongerminomatous pineal tumors, although melatonin (28) and luteinizing hormone-releasing hormone have been suggested as possible candidates (40, 48, 49). Preoperative evaluation of melatonin was carried out in two of our patients with pineal tumors (Cases 9 and 15, Table 14.2). One patient had a normal pattern of plasma melatonin levels, and the other patient had no evidence of any melatonin. Drs. Jennings, Gelman, and Hochberg discuss tumor markers in pineal germ cell tumors in Chapter 6.

Role of Radiotherapy

Except for a 6-month-old who was felt to be too young and another patient who refused all therapy except for Laetrile, all patients with malignant tumors were treated with postoperative radiotherapy regardless of whether a complete surgical excision was accomplished. The incidence of meningeal seeding can be as high as 57% with malignant pineal tumors (45). Pineal germinomas seem to have the greatest propensity for meningeal seeding (45). Brady (4) recommends a dose of 4000 rads to the entire craniospinal axis with a 1000- to 1500-rad boost to the tumor bed in subtotally resected tumors. A lesser dose is associated with an increased recurrence rate. For instance, Sung et al (45), reported intracranial relapses in 14 of 27 patients with midline pineal tumors treated with 3800–4500 rads, but only 2 of 30 midline pineal tumors recurred after 5000–5500 rads.

Not all radiotherapists advocate prophylactic spinal irradiation (41). Wara et al (47) reviewed the experience at the University of California at San Francisco over a 25-yr period. None of 19 patients developed spinal seeding. They advocated CSF cytology following cranial irradiation to screen for meningeal seeding. However, Sung et al (45), obtained a positive CSF cytology in only 3 of 12 patients with meningeal metastases. Periodic myelography with or without a CT scan plus periodic CSF cytology might be an alternative to prophylactic spinal radiation. Drs.

Danoff and Sheline discuss the radiotherapy of pineal tumors in detail in Chapter 16.

Metastases

Two of the three patients with metastases in this series did not undergo surgical exploration of the pineal region. They were initially treated elsewhere with VP shunts and irradiation. The shunted but not operated (Case 7, Table 14.2) patient with meningeal seeding and resultant quadriplegia was given only cranial irradiation, which resulted in a complete cranial remission as shown by CT scan. In retrospect, spinal irradiation may have averted or delayed the meningeal seeding.

The one patient who developed postoperative CSF seeding had an embryonal cell tumor. In this patient a well-encapsulated spherical embryonal cell carcinoma of the pineal 4 cm in diameter was grossly excised without complication. The serum and CSF were evaluated for the presence of AFP by radioimmunoassay and no increased levels were observed. Similarly, no increased levels of the beta chain of HCG were seen in serum. The absence of AFP in serum and CSF is contrary to the results of Allen et al (1). Postoperatively the patient received whole head (5800 rads) and cervical spine (4000 rads) irradiation. An attempt to initiate chemotherapy was made (cis-platinum, bleomycin, and vinblastine), but the patient did not tolerate the regimen due to intractable nausea and vomiting. The patient developed recurrent tumor, initially in the spine, and died. In retrospect, this recurrence may have been prevented or delayed if total craniospinal irradiation had been given.

Nineteen embryonal cell pineal tumors reported previously have recently been reviewed (2). As the authors point out, this malignancy is relatively radioresistant and most patients survive only a few months. Our case is important since it was possible to completely excise this radioresistant tumor. Having a histological diagnosis has also given us the opportunity to give postoperative chemotherapy. Embryonal carcinoma of the testes is highly sensitive to chemotherapy with cis-platinum, bleomycin, and vinblastine. These drugs may well have access to any microscopic foci of residual tumor since there is no blood-brain barrier in the pineal gland.

One patient (Case 2, J.T.) with a germinoma was treated with craniospinal irradiation which resulted in a complete CNS tumor remission, but he has developed massive peritoneal metastases probably secondary to his VP shunt. Extraneural metastasis is very rare with pineal tumors. Of the eight known cases reviewed by Sakata et al (38), all were either typical teratomas or germinomas, and all appeared to disseminate by a hematogenous route as evidenced by pulmonary metastases. Only one of these patients had a VP shunt, and his metastases were to the lung, urinary bladder, and pancreas. Therefore, our case appears to be relatively unique. Although the use of a filter in this boy's shunt may have prevented his peritoneal metastases, the increased incidence of shunt obstruction when filters are used probably outweighs their prophylactic value in patients with pineal tumors. However, as has been done in this series, the shunt should be removed after the tumor burden has been minimized.

Chemotherapy

Another therapeutic modality is now available that increases and expands the approach to pineal region tumors. Histologically the pineal germinoma is identical to the seminoma of the testes, a tumor which is highly responsive to chemotherapy. A complete remission rate with testicular seminomas of 82% in response to bleomycin, vinblastine, and cis-platinum has been reported (13). The response of the massive tumor burden of Case 2 to this regimen is, therefore, not surprising, although his cell burden was greater than most patients so treated.

There have been a few previous reports of the use of chemotherapy with pineal tumors. Sakata et al (38), used bleomycin without success to treat an embryonal cell pineal tumor that metastasized to the spinal canal and to extraneural organs. On the other hand, de Tribolet and Barrelet (11) treated a patient with a large pineal region tumor and malignant cells in the CSF with a combination of daunorubicin, vincristine, and bleomycin. There was a dramatic decrease in tumor size shown by CT scan over a 3-month period. The absence of a blood-brain barrier in the pineal gland may contribute to the sensitivity of this tumor to systemic chemotherapy (34). Borden et al (3), have also demonstrated objective tumor regression of a pulmonary metastasis from a pineal germinoma with a combination of chlorambucil, methotrexate, and dactinomycin. There is no evidence that pineal tumors of glial origin are sensitive to chemotherapy. In fact, glial tumors are well known to be very unresponsive to chemotherapy. Again, this interest in a new treatment modality adds another strong basis for a specific tissue diagnosis in planning therapy in patients with pineal tumors. The chemotherapy of pineal tumors is discussed further in Chapters 6 and 20.

Prognosis

The prognosis in pineal region tumors with shunting procedures and radiotherapy without a tissue diagnosis has been fairly well established. For instance, Camins and Schlesinger (5) reported a 64% survival in a series of 50 cases of pineal region tumors with a mean follow-up period for the survivors of more than 10 yr. However, the median survival of their 18 patients who died was only 2 months. The tumor type, heterogeneity, the ability to completely remove some tumors with microsurgery, and the exciting vistas of alternative therapeutic modalities (chemotherapy and immunotherapy) poses a new and strong bias in favor of an aggressive initial surgical approach to pineal region tumors.

Summary

Our current pineal region tumor series (n = 34) now spans 11 yr and currently includes 15 patients with primary malignant pineal tumors, only 3 of whom had pure germinomas. Complete gross microsurgical excision of well encapsulated tumors was possible in 9 of 13 patients who underwent definitive surgical exploration. Subtotal excision only was possible in two of the other patients. In the remaining two patients who had pineal germinomas, a less aggressive subtotal excision was done because of the known radiosensitivity of this tumor. Four of the operative patients had a tumor of mixed histology with benign and malignant components emphasizing the need for adequate tissue sampling (Table 14.2). Eleven of the 13 surgical patients received postoperative craniospinal radiation; a 6-month-old girl who had a gross total excision of a pineoblastoma was too young to be irradiated. Ten of the patients continued to do well up to 9 yr postoperatively. In view of the fact that only 3 of the 15 patients had pure germinomas, these results appear to be better than those reported with shunting and radiotherapy. Only one of our surgical patients developed postoperative metastases, an embryonal cell tumor that spread to the spinal canal. In the 34 total patients in this series with lesions of the pineal region, surgical exploration was associated with only one death (a patient with metastatic adenocarcinoma). As is common with the occipital transtentorial approach, a postoperative hemanopsia is common, but usually transient. We have also shown the importance of tumor markers and that germinomas are very sensitive to chemotherapy. Thus, microsurgery for pineal tumors provides a viable potential for complete tumor extirpation even with malignant lesions, and/or adequate tissue for diagnosis which is necessary in appropriate therapeutic planning for radiotherapy and/or chemotherapy. The traditional therapeutic approach of empiric radiotherapy without a tissue diagnosis for pineal lesions may no longer be acceptable.

Acknowledgments. We would like to express our gratitude to Dr. Joel Kirkpatrick and to the Armed Forces Institute of Pathology for their consultations on the cases described. Portions of the material in this chapter have been published previously (26) and are reprinted with permission.

References

1. Allen JC, Nisselbaum J, Epstein F, et al: Alphafetoprotein and human chorionic gonadotropin determination in cerebrospinal fluid. An aid to the diagnosis and management of intracranial germ cell tumors. *J Neurosurg* 51:368–374, 1979.
2. Arita N, Ushio N, Abekura M, et al: Embryonal carcinoma with teratomatous elements in the region of the pineal gland. *Surg Neurol* 9:198–202, 1978.
3. Borden IV S, Weber AL, Toch R, Wang CC: Pineal germinoma. *Am J Dis Child* 126:214–216, 1973.
4. Brady LW: The role of radiation therapy. In Schmidek HH (ed): *Pineal Tumors.* New York, Masson Publishing, 1977, pp 127–132.
5. Camins MB, Schlesinger EB: Treatment of tumours of the posterior part of the third ventricle and the pineal region: A long term follow-up. *Acta Neurochir* 40:131–143, 1978.
6. Cummins FM, Taveras JN, Schlesinger EB: Treatment of gliomas of the third ventricle and pinealomas. *Neurology* 10:1031–1036, 1960.
7. Dandy WE: *Benign Tumors in the Third Ventricle of the Brain. Diagnosis and Treatment.* Springfield, Illinois, Charles C Thomas, 1933, pp 171.
8. Davidoff LM: Some considerations in the therapy of pineal tumors. *Bull NY Acad Med* 43:537–561, 1967.
9. DeGirolami U, Schmidek H: Clinicopathological study of 53 tumors of the pineal region. *J Neurosurg* 39:455–462, 1973.
10. Demura R, Demura H, Shizume K, Kubo O, Kitamura K: A female case of the HCG-producing ectopic pinealoma associated with precocious puberty. *Endocrinol Jpn* 23:215–219, 1976.
11. deTribolet N, Barrelet L: Successful chemotherapy of pinealoma. *Lancet* 12:1228–1229, 1977.

12. Donat JF, Okazaki H, Gomez MR, Reagan TJ, Baker HL, Laws ER: Pineal tumors. *Arch Neurol* 35:736–740, 1978.

13. Einhorn LH: Combination chemotherapy of disseminated testicular carcinoma with cis-diamminedichloroplatinum, vinblastine, and bleomycin (PVB): An update. *Proc Amer Assoc Clin Oncolog*, Washington DC, April, 1978.

14. Horrax G: Treatment of tumors of the pineal body. Experience in a series of twenty-two cases. *Arch Neurol Psychiat* 64:227–242, 1950.

15. Horrax G, Daniels JT: The conservative treatment of pineal tumors. *Surg Clin North Am* 22:649–659, 1942.

16. Jamieson KG: Excision of pineal tumors. *J Neurosurg* 35:550–553, 1971.

17. Jenkins RDT, Simpson WJK, Keen CW: Pineal and suprasellar germinomas: Results of radiation treatment. *J Neurosurg* 48:99–107, 1978.

18. Krabbe KH: Histologische und Embryologische Untersuchungen uber die Zirbeldruse des Mechen. *Anat Hefte* 54:187–319, 1916.

19. Kubo O, Yamasaki N, Kamijo Y, Amano K, Kitamura K, Demura R: Human chorionic gonadotropin produced by ectopic pinealoma in a girl with precocious puberty. *J Neurosurg* 47:101–105, 1977.

20. Kunicki A: Operative experiences in 8 cases of pineal tumors. *J Neurosurg* 17:815–823, 1960.

21. Lee SH, Sundararesan N, Jereb B, et al: Endodermal sinus tumor of the pineal region: A case report. *Neurosurgery* 3:407–411, 1978.

22. Mincer F, Meltzer J, Botstein C: Pinealoma. A report of twelve irradiated cases. *Cancer* 37:2713–2718, 1976.

23. Nakazato Y, Ishida Y, Kawabuchi J: Ganglioneuroblastic differentiation in a pineocytoma. 8th Intl Congress Neuropathology, Abstract #255.

24. Neuwelt EA, Specht HD, Howieson J, Haines JE, Bennett MJ, Hill SA, Frenkel EP: Osmotic blood-brain barrier modification: Clinical documentation by enhanced CT scanning and/or radionuclide brain scanning. *Am J Neuroradiol* 4:907–913, 1983.

25. Neuwelt EA, Smith RG: Presence of lymphocyte membrane surface markers on "small cells" in a pineal germinoma. *Ann Neurol* 6:133–136, 1979.

26. Neuwelt EA, Glasberg M, Frenkel E, Clark WK: Malignant pineal region tumors: A clinico-pathological study. *J Neurosurg* 51:597–607, 1979.

27. Neuwelt EA, Balaban E, Diehl J, Hill S, Frenkel E: Successful treatment of primary central nervous system lymphomas with chemotherapy after osmotic blood-brain barrier opening. *Neurosurgery* 12:662–671, 1983.

28. Neuwelt EA, Lewy A: Disappearance of plasma melatonin after removal of a neoplastic pineal gland. *N Engl J Med* 308:1132–1135, 1983.

29. Neuwelt EA, Clark WK: *Clinical Aspects of Neuroimmunology.* Baltimore, Williams & Wilkins, 1978, pp 277.

30. Nielsen SL, Wilson CB: Ultrastructure of a "pineocytoma". *J Neuropathol Exp Neurol* 34:148–158, 1975.

31. Olivecrona H: Acoustic tumors. *J Neurosurg* 26:6–13, 1967.

32. Poppen JL, Marino R, Jr: Pinealomas and tumors of the posterior portion of the third ventricle. *J Neurosurg* 28:357–364, 1968.

33. Rand RW, Lemmen LJ: Tumors of the posterior portion of the third ventricle. *J Neurosurg* 10:1–18, 1953.

34. Rapoport SI: *Blood-Brain Barrier in Physiology and Medicine.* New York, Raven Press, 1976, pp 77–78.

35. Reid WS, Clark WK: Comparison of the infratentorial and transtentorial approaches to the pineal region. *Neurosurgery* 3:1–8, 1978.

36. Ringertz N, Nordenstam H, Flyger G: Tumors of the pineal region. *J Neuropathol Exp Neurol* 13:540–561, 1954.

37. Romshe CA, Sotos JF: Intracranial human chorionic gonadotropin-secreting tumor with precocious puberty. *J Pediatr* 86:250–252, 1975.

38. Sakata K, Yamada H, Sakai N, Hosono Y, Kawasako T, Sasaoka I: Extraneural metastasis of pineal tumor. *Surg Neurol* 3:49–54, 1975.

39. Schmidek HH: *Pineal Tumors.* Brady LW, De Vita VT (eds): Masson Publishing USA, Inc., NY. 1977, pp 1–138.

40. Scully RE, Galdabini JJ, McNeely BU: Case records of the Massachusetts General Hospital (Case 38-1975). *N Engl J Med* 293:653–660, 1975.

41. Smith NJ, El-Mahdi AM, Constable WC: Results of irradiation of tumors in the region of the pineal body. *Acta Radiologica Ther Phy Bio* 15:17–22, 1976.

42. Stavrou D, Anzil AP, Wiedenback W, et al: Immunofluorescence study of lymphocytic infiltration in gliomas. Identification of T-lymphocytes. *J Neurol Sci* 33:275–282, 1977.

43. Stein B: Personal communication, 1979.

44. Stein BM: The infratentorial supracerebellar approach to pineal lesions. *J Neurosurg* 35:197–202, 1971.

45. Sung D, Harisiadis L, Chang CH: Midline pineal tumors and suprasellar germinomas: Highly curable by radiation. *Radiology* 128:745–751, 1978.

46. Suzuki J, Iwabuchi T: Surgical removal of pineal tumors (pinealomas and teratomas). *J Neurosurg* 23:565–571, 1965.

47. Wara WM, Fellows CF, Sheline GE, Wilson CB, Townsend JJ: Radiation therapy for pineal tumors and suprasellar germinomas. *Radiology* 124:221–223, 1977.

48. Wurtman RJ, Moskowitz MA: The pineal organ (Part I). *N Engl J Med* 296:1329–1333, 1977.

49. Wurtman RJ, Moskowitz MA: The pineal organ (Part II). *N Engl J Med* 296:1383–1386, 1977.

CHAPTER 15

Surgical Therapy of Pineal Region Tumors

CLAUDE LAPRAS, M.D.

INTRODUCTION

Primary tumors of the pineal body can develop from any cell found in the gland during embryological or adult life: germ cells, pineal gland cells, glial, ependymal, arachnoid, or choroid plexus cells. The tumor destroys the gland, grows in the pineal region, extends anteriorly in the third ventricle or posteriorly in the ambient cistern, and always has a close relationship with the quadrigeminal plate and the thalamus. If the pineal gland tumor is small, diagnosis is easy, whereas, it may be impossible to determine the primary site of a large tumor infiltrating the pineal body and adjacent structures. As a result, all tumors in this area are called pineal region tumors.

At the beginning of our series, between 1964 and 1969, we used the transcallosal approach, according to Dandy, to approach eight cases of pineal region tumors. We found this approach difficult and dangerous. One patient died postoperatively; the seven other patients died within 10 yr. The deaths were not exclusively related to the pathology of the tumor, but also to the fact that all these initial cases had only a partial removal. After this short and unsuccessful experience we stopped performing the transcallosal approach. Since 1970, we have routinely used the occipital transtentorial approach according to Poppen (5) and to Jamieson (2). The 75 cases of tumors of the pineal region occurring between 1970 and 1982 and treated by the occipital transtentorial approach were reviewed for this study. Portions of these series have been reported previously (1, 3, 4, 6).

CLINICAL MATERIAL
Histology

The histology of the cases in this series is summarized in Table 15.1. We use the classification of Rubinstein, revised by deGirolami and

Table 15.1
Histology of 75 Cases of Pineal Tumors

Tumors	No. of Cases
Pineal cell tumors	
Pineocytomas	8
Pineoblastomas	13
TOTAL	21
Germ cell tumors	
Germinomas	8
Malignant teratomas	4
Benign teratomas	4
TOTAL	16
Epidermoid tumors	2
Benign cysts (arachnoid, glial)	7
Gliomas	
Astrocytomas	16
Ependymomas	4
Oligodendrogliomas	4
TOTAL	24
Meningiomas	2
Choroid plexus papilloma	1
Inflammatory process	2
GRAND TOTAL	75

Schmidek. Pineal parenchymal cell tumors were seen in 28% of our patients and 21% had germ cell tumors. The latter statistic is quite different from other reports. Parasellar germinomas were excluded from this series, which may in part explain the low proportion of germ cell tumors.

Age

The age of patients is given in Figure 15.1. The age range was 5 months to 63 yr. Forty-one patients were less than 15 yr of age, 34 older than 15 yr of age, 7 were infants under 2 yr, and 3 were infants under 1 yr.

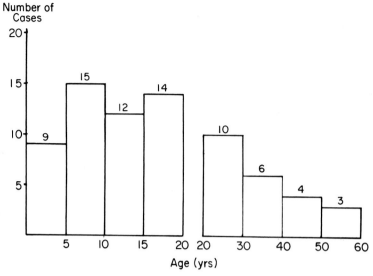

Figure 15.1.   Age range.

Sex

The overall male-female ratio was 40/35. As in previous series we noted the predominance for germ cell tumors in male patients (14 male/2 female), but we did not find the same predominance for pineal parenchymal cell tumors (10 male/11 female).

SYMPTOMS AND SIGNS

Intracranial Pressure

All except two patients had symptoms of increased intracranial pressure as evidenced by headache, nausea, vomiting, diplopia, and lethargy, and signs such as papilledema or abducens nerve palsy. In 20 cases these symptoms were not associated with localizing neurological signs. In 14 cases there were cerebellar or vestibular signs. Hydrocephalus was the presenting symptom in six patients. Other patients presented with papilledema (1 case), meiosis (1 case), and hypotonia or hypertonia (1 case each).

Parinaud's Syndrome

In 31 cases, we found a Parinaud's syndrome. In 18 cases there was a predominant upward gaze palsy with downward gaze more or less impaired. In six cases the Parinaud's syndrome was complete with Argyll Robertson pupils; in four cases the paralytic dilatation of the pupil was not associated with a gaze palsy; in three cases there was retraction nystagmus associated with upward gaze.

Infrequent Disorders

Infrequent neurologic and endocrine disorders are summarized in Tables 15.2 and 15.3. Out of five cases with diabetes insipidus before surgery, we found three germinomas, one choroid plexus papilloma, and one oligodendroglioma. The five patients had a well circumscribed tumor without any sign of extension to the hypothalamus. Only one patient, a boy 7-yr-old, had precocious puberty. He has been operated for a pineocytoma Grade II-III with a total removal. Before surgery, he had high plasma titers of human chorionic gonadotropin (HCG) as evidenced by a value of 209 ng/ml (normal under 1.50 ng/ml), and an elevated alpha-fetoprotein (AFP) at 1200 ng/ml (normal 0 to 20 ng/ml). After surgery the titers of HCG and AFP fell to normal levels. The titers rose again 9 months later without any sign of local recurrence in the pineal region, but with CSF tumor cell seeding. After craniospinal radiation, the titers of HCG and AFP fell again. Since then we have frequently assayed plasma levels of HCG, AFP, and melatonin, pre- and postoperatively. In our experience, these markers do not correlate well with the histologic diagnosis, but they are often helpful to follow the course of therapy.

SURGICAL TECHNIQUE

Anesthesia

All the patients are placed in the sitting position with positive-end expiratory pressure. Monitoring includes electrocardiogram, arterial

Table 15.2
Infrequent Neurologic Symptoms and Signs

Hemiparesis	5
Epileptic seizures	5
Facial palsy	4
Decreased vision	3
Hemianesthesia	2
Coma	2
Dyskinesia	1
Hemianopsia	1
Facial anesthesia	1
Paralysis of the soft palate	1
Swallowing paralysis	1
Dementia	1
Memory loss	1
Behavior changes	1

Table 15.3
Endocrine Dysfunction

Diabetes insipidus	5
Polyphagia—obesity	2
Anorexia—loss of weight	2
Anterior pituitary insufficiency	1
Impaired growth	1
Precocious puberty	1

blood pressure with a radial artery catheter, central venous pressure with a right atrial catheter, and expiratory pCO_2 with capnograph. We don't use Doppler ultrasound monitoring to detect air embolism, because of the ease and efficacy of the capnograph. The capnograph has less back-noise and the same efficacy. Monitoring also includes parameters like body temperature, urine output, and an esophageal stethoscope.

Position

In the sitting position, the patient's legs have special antigravity stockings and are elevated with the feet at the level of the heart. A large belt is fastened around the abdomen. The head is slightly turned to the right and anteriorly bent. The approach is usually performed on the right (nondominant) hemisphere, but the rotation of the head and the side of the approach is adjusted as a function of the lateral extension of the tumor on the CT scan.

The Occipital Transtentorial Approach

The scalp-flap is larger than necessary for the bone-flap to see precisely the landmarks of the midline on the sagittal suture. The free bone-flap is the shape of a trapezoid. The superolateral burr-hole is placed as far as possible from the midline, to give extra space during the retraction of the occipital lobe. The inferolateral burr-hole is less lateral to protect the inferior temporal veins. It is enlarged inferiorly by craniectomy to see the margin of the transverse sinus. The superomedial burr-hole is placed just at the margin of the sagittal sinus. The inferiomedial burr-hole is placed over the torcula. It is enlarged by craniectomy to see the margin between the torcular and the dura. The bone-flap is obliquely crossed in its middle by the lambdoid suture. In young children, special care is necessary when the bone-flap is elevated because the dura adherent to the suture can be torn. The dura is opened 1 cm from the transverse sinus and reflected toward the sagittal sinus. Usually a ventricular tap is not necessary. The parietal veins are immediately apparent upon opening the dura. They appear stretched between the parietal lobe and the sagittal sinus. They are wrapped with a piece of Surgicel: this coating reinforces their wall and prevents them from being torn. The same technique is used for the inferior temporal veins. Some rare arachnoid granulations between the medial surface of the occipital lobe and the falx are coagulated. Usually the occipital lobe is free of bridging veins and can be safely retracted; but sometimes we found one or two small veins bridging the inferior surface of the occipital lobe and the middle of the tentorium. These veins are carefully divided during the beginning of the retraction.

It is not necessary to vigorously retract the occipital lobe. The occipital lobe is retracted superiorly and laterally. It should only be elevated from the tentorium enough to visualize the tentorial notch. The tentorium is divided lateral and parallel to the straight sinus as far as possible posteriorly. Aberrant venous sinuses in the tentorium should be avoided. The tentorial notch is transected 1.5 cm from the vein of Galen. The lateral flap is retracted by generous coagulation. The medial flap of the tentorium is reflected by one or two sutures.

A self-retaining retractor and microscope are utilized at this stage. The quadrigeminal cistern is exposed. The culmen of the cerebellum and the superior cerebellar veins are apparent through the thick but usually translucent arachnoid. Sometimes very large tumors invade the cistern and are immediately visible. Usually, however, the tumor is not yet visible. The cistern is opened near the cerebellum as far as possible from the vein of Galen. The dissection of the arachnoid remains near the cerebellum and is extended laterally in both directions. Veins (two to three groups) cross the cistern through its middle, passing upward from the culmen and the quadrigeminal plate to the inferior surface of the vein of Galen. They can be transected without neurological complication. Using the sitting position allows the cerebellum to slip inferiorly in the posterior fossa and widely opens the operative field. The posterior part of the tumor appears outlined by a continuous venous arch formed laterally by the basilar veins of Rosenthal and medially by the vein of Galen. These veins are still protected by their arachnoid sheet. They must be preserved. The small internal occipital vein going from the medial surface of the occipital lobe to the basilar vein at the level of the tentorial notch must be preserved too. An unlucky coagulation on this vein can produce a postoperative hemianopsia. The splenium of the corpus callosum is far above the venous arch, it is unnecessary to split it. The quadrigeminal plate is below the tumor, sometimes it is distended by the development of the tumor in the lowest part of the third ventricle.

Surgical Management of the Tumor

The dissection of the tumor begins at the level of the quadrigeminal plate, where its extension is examined. The posterior commissure is not clearly visualized. Separation of the tumor from the quadrigeminal plate gives access to the floor of the third ventricle. If the tumor extends to the quadrigeminal plate, or the brain stem, the removal is stopped.

If the tumor is not invading, the arterial pedicles are dissected. The branches of the posterior choroidal arteries emerge laterally when they turn around the upper part of the brain stem. They go vertically upward from the lateral expansion of the ambient cistern in the groove between the tumor and the thalamo-pulvinar mass where they send branches to both sides. The arteries to the tumor are easily coagulated. This arterial control is the first step of the lateral dissection. The tumor is progressively separated from the lateral walls of the third ventricle. The dissection is bloodless in the inferior part of the third ventricle where the tumor has no important vascular pedicles. In the anterosuperior part of the lateral wall, an additional vascular pedicle is found with small arteries going from the membrana tectoria and small

veins going to the internal cerebral veins. With a right occipital approach, we can see the left lateral wall of the third ventricle more easily than the right one.

The tumor remains attached at the inferior part of the vein of Galen by its venous pedicle. Piecemeal resection is performed without pulling the tumor to avoid tearing the vein of Galen. It is easier to begin the removal of the tumor anteriorly. In some large tumors it is safer to dig a tunnel into the tumor mass to reach the anterior pole of the tumor. When the resection is almost complete, a little piece of tumor remains fixed at the vein of Galen by two or three short veins surrounded by thickened arachnoid. These veins are dissected and divided to achieve the removal. Sometimes, this last dissection appears too dangerous, in which case, the last piece of tumor is reduced by coagulation.

Surgical Removal

The removal of the tumor was felt to be complete in 48 of 75 (64%) cases. The correlations with histology are given in Table 15.4. The removal was subtotal or partial in 21 cases. A biopsy only was performed in six patients with invasive tumors.

Advantages

The occipital transtentorial approach has many advantages. At the beginning of the procedure it permits a wide view of the extent of the tumor and an assessment of whether the dissection is feasible. The tumor arterial supply

Table 15.4
The Correlation of Total Tumor Removal and Histology

Pineocytomas	8/8
Pineoblastomas	6/13
Germinomas	5/8
Malignant teratomas	1/4
Benign teratomas	4/4
Epidermoid tumors	2/2
Benign cysts	7/7
Gliomas	12/24
Astrocytomas	4/16
Ependymomas	4/4
Oligodendrogliomas	4/4
Meningiomas	1/2
Choroid plexus papilloma	1/1
Inflammatory process	1/2
Total	48/75

is visualized early and cut. This approach provides excellent exposure of the deep venous system (the vein of Galen in the middle, the internal cerebral veins in the roof of the third ventricle, and the basilar veins of Rosenthal laterally), the dissection of which can be delayed until the final stages of the procedure. Damage to these veins constitute the major cause of morbidity and mortality with this procedure. There are no blind corners, even for large tumors. Anterior extensions in the third ventricle are precisely removed; posterior expansions between the cerebellum and the brain stem or in the posterioinferior part of the third ventricle are resected under direct view.

SHUNT PROBLEMS
Shunt Before Surgery

Out of 75 cases, 57 had a shunt before direct surgery. The procedure is generally safe and efficient, but there can be problems. Initially, we used a ventriculoatrial shunt with a low pressure Holter valve. Extradural hematomas developed some hours after insertion of the shunt in two patients. Direct surgery on the pineal tumor had to be delayed. These two patients had a long clinical evolution and large ventricles on the CT scan. Even so, when direct surgery was performed some weeks later, the retraction of the occipital lobe was not as easy as it could have been with recently decompressed ventricles. Generally, long delays between shunt insertion and direct surgery should be avoided because the ventricles become smaller, making retraction more difficult. A medium pressure valve is adequate to treat the increased intracranial pressure and prevents excessive ventricular collapse. Clinical symptoms after shunt placement improved so dramatically that three patients declined direct surgery. They accepted surgery only some months later, when new symptoms appeared or when the tumor growth was obvious on repeated CT scan. In five cases the shunt, inserted in another hospital, was placed in the right parietooccipital region. This complicated the approach; we had to remove the proximal catheter at the beginning of the procedure and introduce it again at the conclusion of surgery in a collapsed lateral ventricle. Thus, we recommend shunt insertion either on the left side or in the right frontal horn with the distal catheter crossing to the left side of the neck.

During the evolution of malignant tumors, we did not observe seeding of tumor cells via the shunt. Meningitis was not observed in the patients receiving a shunt before direct surgery.

After tumor resection, eight patients are known to remain shunt-dependent. In seven of these cases the shunt had to be revised, and in one case, we tried to occlude the shunt and failed. Two patients are known to be shunt-independent because their shunt has been removed. Shunt dependency is unknown in all the other surviving patients since their shunts remain in place.

No Shunt Before Surgery

In 18 patients with a pineal tumor, tumor resection was carried out without a shunt. In six patients the shunt was unnecessary or dangerous because of the absence of ventriculomegaly. The no-shunt technique affords extra room for the cerebral retraction, but must be avoided when the ventricles are grossly enlarged because of the increased risk of a postoperative subdural hematoma.

In one case, after removal of the pineal tumor, we were able to insert a catheter between the third and the fourth ventricles. The catheter was introduced downward through the aqueduct. This patient had no shunt before or after surgery.

Only 7 patients out of 18 without a shunt before surgery needed a shunt after surgery. Thus, one-third of the patients never need a shunt after removal of a pineal tumor.

RADIATION THERAPY
Preoperative Radiation Therapy

Ventriculoperitoneal shunting and radiation therapy without a biopsy can be efficacious if the tumor is a germinoma. On the other hand, if the tumor enlarges, despite radiation, surgery is more difficult. Three patients had such "conservative treatment" in another hospital. The pathology was a meningioma, a benign teratoma, and a malignant teratoma. The "conservative treatment" delayed resection and the three tumors were then huge and difficult to manage surgically. We achieved a total removal only with the benign teratoma; this patient is still alive. Total removal was impossible for the other two patients because we found a thick, dense adherent arachnoid reaction and fibrotic tumor. Both patients subsequently died from tumor growth (the meningioma after 7 yr, the malignant teratoma after 3 months). It is better to avoid preoperative radiation therapy if a direct approach is possible.

Radiation therapy with shunt, without direct surgery, has to be integrated in a different therapy program. It requires an initial stereotaxic biopsy. Germinoma is the only lesion where "conservative treatment" is justified. Like Sano, we believe that "reduction of tumor bulk by direct surgery, even if that neoplasm is radiosensitive, is important to maximize the effectiveness of radiotherapy." In our experience germinomas and pineoblastomas, like medulloblastomas, do far better when the tumor burden is minimized prior to radiotherapy.

Postoperative Radiation Therapy

We treated 32 cases with postoperative radiation therapy. Cobalt therapy was routinely administered to highly radiosensitive tumors: germinoma (8/8), and pineoblastomas (11/13). Two pinealoblastoma patients were not irradiated because one died early after surgery and the other was in poor condition. The four malignant teratomas in the series were also irradiated (one preoperatively without benefit). Nine gliomas were irradiated and one patient with a pineocytoma (precocious puberty with a late recurrence diagnosed by elevated levels of HCG and AFP).

The modalities of radiation therapy and the volume of the irradiated central nervous system varied with the years. Four different protocols have been followed: focal irradiation (22 cases) or total craniospinal axis irradiation (10 cases), with or without chemotherapy.

The irradiation of the tumor bed was never less than 4500 rad. The normal dose was 5500 rad delivered during a period of 7 weeks. The spinal axis radiation ranged between 3000 and 3500 rad.

RESULTS

Postoperative Mortality

Within the first postoperative month, 2 out of 75 patients died giving a mortality rate of 2.6%. Both were adults. One had an invasive pineoblastoma. When attempting a gross total excision, the vein of Galen was entered. The patient remained comatose postoperatively and died 3 days later. The second patient, a 47-yr-old man, had a large epidermoid cyst. His initial postoperative course was uneventful, but on the 2nd day, he had an acute postoperative hematoma

and died. Two other patients died between 1 and 2 months after partial tumor removal giving an overall operative mortality of 5.3% (4/75). These latter postoperative deaths were the result of both postoperative central nervous system damage and rapid growth of a malignant tumor.

Postoperative Complications

One patient developed an intraoperative intracerebral hematoma. He was cured by a rapid surgical evacuation. During this evacuation we found a piece of tumor not seen during what was felt to be a complete surgical removal. This fact must be taken in account when the patients are classified as having had a complete resection.

Two patients developed postoperative meningitis which resolved with antibiotics. Two patients had two other infections requiring removal of the bone-flap. These two cases evolved during radiation therapy. Three patients had repeated seizures during the early postoperative period and needed intravenous anticonvulsant therapy. One of these patients had epilepsy prior to surgery. Four patients were lethargic during the initial postoperative period.

Five other patients became drowsy several hours to 1 day after surgery. A large bubble of air was found by CT scan in the frontal horn or the subdural space. One patient required a ventricular tap, but all the patients recovered. Another five patients had a subdural hematoma with symptoms appearing about 1 month after surgery. The symptoms were minimal and appeared during radiation therapy. Radiation may be the factor complicating asymptomatic, small, subdural hygromas since they are sometimes found on routine postoperative CT scan. These subdural effusions of fluid are related to the degree of hydrocephalus before surgery and are a consequence of the sitting position during surgery. One of these patients was treated medically by corticosteroid therapy; the other four required drainage (unilateral in three cases and bilateral in one case).

Overall Survival

Twenty-five of 75 patients died within the 13 yr of this study. Fifty patients are still alive (66%). Survival rates are illustrated in Figure 15.2. In Figure 15.3, there is no significant difference between the two age groups illustrated (under 15 yr and over 15 yr).

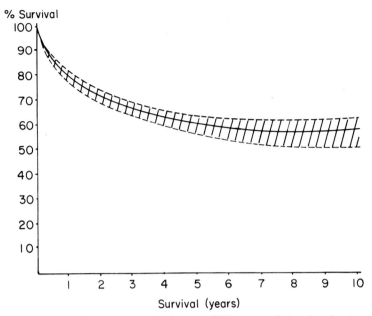

Figure 15.2. Observed survival rates of 75 cases of pineal region tumors.

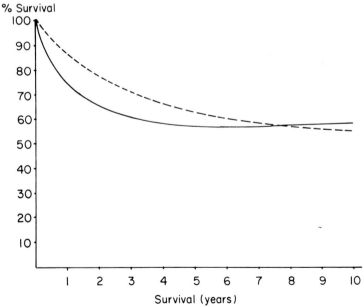

Figure 15.3. Observed survival rates of 75 cases of pineal region tumors aged less than 15 yr (*dotted line*) and 15 yr or over (*solid line*).

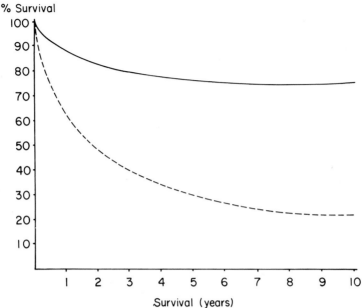

Figure 15.4. Observed survival rates of 75 cases of pineal region tumors according to the surgical removal (*dotted line*, partial removal; *continuous line*, total removal).

Late Deaths

In addition to the 4 early postoperative deaths, we had 21 late deaths, 6 after a total removal, and 15 after a partial removal or biopsy (Table 15.5). Fourteen deaths were related to a local recurrence of the tumor (1 germinoma, 1 meningioma, 2 malignant teratomas, 2 pineoblastomas, and 8 gliomas). Whereas, seven deaths (all pineoblastomas) were related to a diffuse tumor seeding of the subarachnoid space. Spinal seeding without local recurrence was seen in four cases.

Factors of Prognosis

Neither neurologic symptoms nor age clearly affect prognosis. The only clear prognostic factor is impaired consciousness not improved by shunt and/or a total Parinaud's syndrome associated with dilated pupils and convergence palsy.

In Table 15.6, we summarized the survival of each histologic tumor group. It shows a striking difference between pineoblastomas and germinomas. Pineoblastomas are the most difficult tumor to treat; surgery is not easy, total removal is often impossible, and total irradiation of the craniospinal axis is not sufficient to prevent seeding of the tumor. Tumor cells are frequently

Table 15.5
Late Deaths

Pathology	No. of Cases	Partial Removal or Biopsy	Total Removal
Pineoblastomas	9	5	4
Gliomas	8	6	2
Germinoma	1	1	0
Malignant teratomas	2	2	0
Meningiomas	1	1	0
Total	21	15	6

found in CSF even after radiotherapy. Perhaps, pineoblastomas will require a combination of radiotherapy and chemotherapy.

One of the most important prognostic factors is achieving a total removal, regardless whether the tumor is benign or malignant (Fig. 15.4). Out of 27 patients treated by a partial removal or biopsy, 10 are still alive (37%) in contrast to 40 of 48 (83%) patients treated by a total resection. At the beginning of our experience, during surgery for two benign tumors, a meningioma and a glioma, we performed a partial removal; later we had to operate again on these two patients but we were unable to achieve a complete resection. The result was several years of

Table 15.6
Survival Related to Histology

Histology	No. of Cases	Dead	Alive (%)
Pineocytomas	8	0	8 (100.0)
Pineoblastomas	13	11	2 (15.4)
Germinomas	8	1	7 (87.5)
Malignant teratomas	4	2	2 (50.0)
Benign teratomas	4	0	4 (100.0)
Epidermoid tumors	2	1	1 (50.0)
Benign cysts	7	0	7 (100.0)
Gliomas	24	9	15 (62.5)
Meningiomas	2	1	1 (50.0)
Papilloma	1	0	1 (100.0)
Inflammatory process	2	0	2 (100.0)
Total	75	25	50 (66.6)

survival in poor condition. Perhaps we should have taken more risk during the first operation to attain a total removal in these two cases.

The tumor size as estimated on the CT scan is not as important a factor as histology. By the occipital transtentorial approach, it is possible to completely remove large tumors as shown in Figure 15.5. Conversely some small tumors can invade the brain stem early and defy total resection.

Preoperative radiation therapy produces a fibrous reaction which greatly complicates surgery. It is a bad prognostic factor. The different protocols used for postoperative radiation therapy seem justified. Except for pineoblastomas, there is no clear difference in prognosis between local or total craniospinal radiation therapy. Out of 11 pineoblastomas, 5 patients received total cerebrospinal irradiation, and 2 of them are still alive; 6 had just a cranial irradiation, and they all died of spinal seeding or diffuse tumor invasion. In contrast, one out of eight irradiated germinomas has died. The death occurred in the group treated by total craniospinal irradiation (five cases). These results can be compared with the patients with suprasellar germinomas. Some of these patients are treated by focal radiation therapy and do not develop late spinal seeding. Thus, radiation of the spinal axis seems necessary for pineoblastomas, but it does not seem necessary for germinomas.

In our experience, radiation therapy did not significantly change the prognosis of gliomas: 3 out of 9 died with radiation (33.3%), 6 out of 15 died without radiation (44%). Radiation does have complications: it may increase the rate of infection or subdural hygromas, and in one case, cerebral radionecrosis was diagnosed after a dose of only 3500 rad. The child, 14-yr-old, remains alive but in a vegetative state. Thus, we don't recommend radiation therapy for glial tumors of the pineal region, especially after a gross total removal.

LATE RESULTS

Fifty patients who are still alive, are reviewed for this follow-up.

NEUROLOGIC SYMPTOMS AND SIGNS

During the early postoperative period, 34 of 50 patients had a Parinaud's syndrome (17 had the syndrome before surgery). For seven patients, the syndrome disappeared within 1 (three cases) to 12 (five cases) months. Three out of seven patients with a total resection had the syndrome preoperatively. Twenty-seven patients had a gaze palsy (54%), which improved in all except nine patients. Fifteen patients had a dissociated upward gaze palsy with recovery of the automatic upward gaze reflex (Bell's phenomenon). The voluntary upward gaze remains paralyzed or asymmetrical with diplopia. Three patients had only a downward gaze palsy. In ten patients, an oculo-motor paralysis and/or Parinaud's syndrome was observed. Two patients have impaired vision with optic atrophy, and five have hemianopsia. Three patients are deaf; in two the deafness is probably related to radiation therapy and in one, to antibiotic therapy. Two other patients had an auditive agnosia

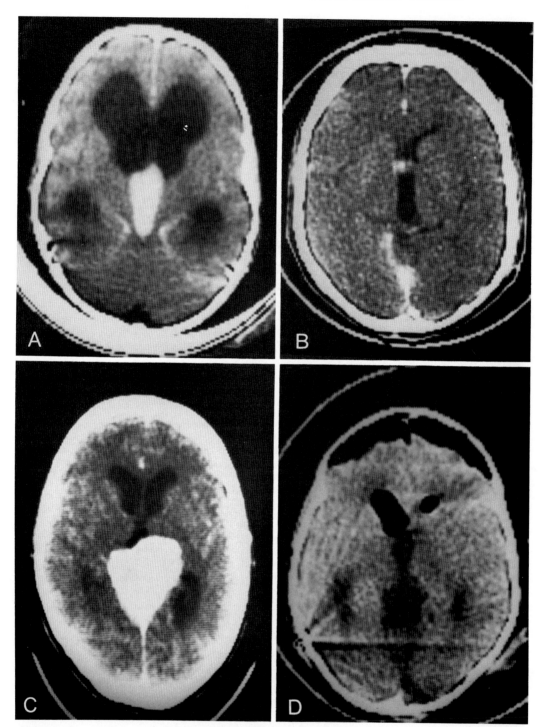

Figure 15.5. CT scan of two cases of pineal region tumors. *A*, enhanced CT scan of a pineocytoma. *B*, postoperative enhanced CT scan after total removal without preoperative shunt. *C*, preoperative enhanced CT scan of a meningioma of the pineal gland. *D*, early postoperative CT scan of the patient after total removal of the pineal tumor. A bubble of air is visible in the frontal subdural space and the frontal horns. The patient became drowsy 1 hr after awakening and needed a emergency frontal tap. Ultimately, the patient made a good recovery.

probably related to a lesion of the quadrigeminal plate.

Out of five patients with epileptic seizures prior to surgery, two died, two have had no more seizures on anticonvulsant therapy, and only one patient is still having seizures. Twelve patients without epilepsy before surgery developed postoperative seizures. Two patients had repeated seizures early during the postoperative period, but none later. Ten patients remain epileptic with rare (eight cases) or frequent (two cases) seizures.

ENDOCRINE DYSFUNCTION

The patient with precocious puberty required hormonal manipulation. Two patients had a postoperative growth defect probably related to radiation therapy, and needed growth hormone treatment. One patient developed pituitary insufficiency and amenorrhea related to radiation therapy and receives hormonal therapy.

No patient developed postoperative diabetes insipidus. Of the five patients with preoperative diabetes insipidus, two still require vasopressin, but with a smaller dose than before surgery. The other three no longer have diabetes insipidus.

QUALITY OF LIFE

Three patients are severely handicapped, 2 are in a vegetative state, and 15 patients are handicapped and unable to attend normal school or work, but are independent.

Thirty patients lead normal lives (60%). The adults are working full time, and the children are attending a normal school. Of these 30 patients, eight have two or more symptoms such as epilepsy, ataxia, impaired vision, or oculomotor paralysis associated with Parinaud's syndrome. Ten have only one symptom (nine a partial Parinaud's syndrome, and one a left hemianopsia). Only 12 of 30 patients (24% of all

living patients, 30% of cases with a normal life) are free of any symptom or sign.

SUMMARY

The prognosis of pineal region tumors depends on two main factors: the histology of the tumor and the extent of the tumor removal. The occipital transtentorial approach provides an easy and generous exposure of the pineal region. It permits the surgeon to know at the beginning of the removal if the tumor is infiltrative and if a total resection is possible. Total removal was possible for 64% of our patients. After a gross total resection, 83% of patients are still alive.

Some surgical problems such as the depth of the tumor and the proximity of the internal cerebral vein and the brain stem are the same for all the surgical approaches. However, the width of the transtentorial exposure is unmatched. Morbidity is not high, and 60% of our patients have a normal life after surgery by the occipital transtentorial approach. Even large tumors can be safely excised by this approach.

References

1. Izquierdo JM, Rougerie J, Lapras C, Sanz F: The so-called ectopic pinealomas—a cooperative study of 15 cases. *Childs Brain* 5:505–512, 1979.
2. Jamieson KG: Excision of pineal tumors. *J Neurosurg* 35:550–553, 1971.
3. Lapras C: Experience with direct surgical approach in 52 tumors of the pineal region. In Paoletti P, Walker MD, Butti G, Kuerich R (eds): *Multidisciplinary Aspects of Brain Tumor Therapy.* New York, Elsevier-North Holland, 1979, vol 1, pp 173–176.
4. Lapras C, Bret P, Nicolas A: Experience with the direct surgical approach in 52 tumors of the pineal region. *Childs Brain* 8:54–55, 1981.
5. Poppen JL, Marino Jr, R: Pinealomas and tumors of the posterior portion of the third ventricle. *J Neurosurg* 28:357–364, 1968.
6. Schafer M, Lapras C, Thomalske G, Grau H, Schobe R: Sarcoidosis of the pineal gland. Case reports. *J Neurosurg* 47:630–632, 1977.

CHAPTER 16

Radiotherapy of Pineal Tumors

BARBARA DANOFF, M.D. and **GLENN E. SHELINE, M.D.**

Radiotherapy has universally been used in the treatment of pineal tumors and suprasellar germinomas. Historically, radiation treatment usually was instituted following placement of a shunt for the relief of obstructive hydrocephalus without the benefit of a histologic diagnosis because of the high mortality and morbidity rates that were associated with the operative approach (3, 7, 9, 19, 22). Recently however, major technical advances related to the use of the operating microscope and development of microsurgical techniques have prompted a renewed interest in the direct surgical approach for biopsy and/or excision. This interest has resulted in a controversy regarding the role of surgery prior to radiotherapy. Because of the heterogeneity of tumors occurring in the pineal region (i.e., germ cell tumors, pineal parenchymal tumors, glial tumors, and cysts) and their differing biological behavior, controversy also surrounds aspects of radiotherapy such as: the optimal radiation dose, the volume to be irradiated, and indications for prophylactic spinal irradiation. A review of the available data is presented in an attempt to answer these questions.

ROLE OF SURGERY PRIOR TO RADIOTHERAPY

Advocates of the conservative surgical approach (i.e. ventricular shunting) (5, 7, 9, 11, 20, 22, 29, 33, 34) for pineal tumors have stressed the high mortality and morbidity rates historically associated with biopsy or resection (Table 16.1). With an operative mortality ranging from 0 to less than 8%, ventricular shunting for relief of obstructive hydrocephalus was considered the appropriate surgical procedure. An additional argument against the direct surgical approach was the observation that most pineal tumors could not be completely excised (9), and, therefore, would require routine postoperative radiotherapy irrespective of the attempted resection (23). As well, surgical series with histologic verification have demonstrated that the majority of pineal tumors are those expected to be highly radiosensitive, i.e. germinomas or pineoblastomas (Table 16.2). Furthermore, partial or subtotal resection of these radiosensitive tumors has not resulted in an improved survival (15). Certain authors (6, 15, 29, 33, 35) have suggested that surgical intervention is responsible for dis-

Table 16.2
Histologically Verified Tumors

Reference		% Radiosensitive[a]
Chapman and Linggood (6)	37	(3/8)[b]
DeGirolami and Schmidek (9)	54	(19/35)
Maier and Dejong (16)	83	(5/6)
Sung et al (29)	74	(17/23)
Obrador et al (19)	49	(128/262)

[a] Radiosensitive, i.e. germinoma, pineoblastoma.

[b] No. in parentheses is the number with germinoma or pineoblastoma compared to the total number of patients with pineal tumors.

Table 16.1
Operative Mortality Pineal Tumors

Reference	Mortality (%)		
	Shunt	Biopsy	Resection
DeGirolami and Schmidek (9)	< 8	33	60
Cummins et al (7)	5	34	
Poppen and Marino (22)		0	40
Bradfield and Perez (3)		0	67
Abay et al (1)	0		
Obrador et al (19)			38

semination of tumor cells within the cerebrospinal fluid resulting in an increased incidence of spinal seeding in patients with histologically verified tumors (Table 16.3). Others (18, 23), reporting small numbers of patients, have noted no such increase. A high incidence of spinal seeding, of course, would require irradiation of the entire spine, a procedure not without morbidity.

Currently available nonoperative predictors of histology include the initial CT appearance of the tumor (38), tumor markers (12), and the response of the tumor to radiotherapy as demonstrated by serial CT (11, 13, 20). Inoue et al (13) noted complete disappearance of the mass as seen on CT scans in nine cases of intracranial germinoma following 1600 to 3300 rad. With CT monitoring of tumor response, direct surgical intervention can be reserved for those tumors not responding to radiation (2, 5, 9, 15, 23, 26, 29, 33). A repeat CT scan is performed at 2000 to 3000 rad (2, 11, 13, 20, 26) and if there is complete tumor disappearance, radiotherapy is continued without surgical intervention. The presence of tumor markers (i.e., alpha-fetoprotein and human chorionic gonadotrophin) in the serum and CSF (12) may also establish the histologic diagnosis nonoperatively and aid in the evaluation of response to treatment as well as serving as a predictor of recurrence.

In terms of survival, there appears to be no significant difference between patients who have undergone direct surgery followed by radiotherapy and those undergoing radiotherapy with or without a shunt (Tables 16.4–16.6).

Advocates of the direct surgical approach (6, 18, 26, 27, 31) note the decreased mortality rates associated with the use of operating microscope and microsurgical techniques (Table 16.7). Histologic verification allows for individualization of treatment and perhaps identification of patients requiring craniospinal irradiation or chemotherapy (6, 18, 37). Surgical debulking, especially of the less radiosensitive tumors, may be beneficial (19, 26). Complete gross microsurgical excision of well encapsulated benign tumors may be possible (18) thereby obviating the need for radiotherapy. Postoperative radiotherapy is recommended for all malignant tumors regardless of the extent of surgical resection (18). Pecker et al (21) recommend stereotaxic biopsy prior to a direct surgical approach. The pathologic diagnosis of a radiosensitive tumor would then eliminate the need for further surgery.

Suprasellar germinomas are surgically more readily accessible. Operative mortality for tumors in this region has ranged from 0 (3, 9) to

Table 16.4
Survival Pineal Tumors and Suprasellar Germinomas

Reference	Survival %		Follow-up (yr)
	Histologically Verified	Unverified	
Wara et al (35)	58 (50)[a]	71 (59)	2–15
Onoyama et al (20)	82 (21)	69 (26)	5
Waga et al (33)	56 (23)	66 (39)	5

[a] Number in parentheses is the total number of patients.

Table 16.3
Incidence of Spinal Seeding as Related to Surgical Intervention

Reference	Spinal Seeding (%)			
	Unverified Tumor (No Surgery)		Histologically Verified Tumor (Surgery)	
Wara and Sheline (35)	1.7	(1/59)[a]	16	(8/50)
Jenkin et al (15)	6	(2/31)	19	(3/16)
Sung et al (29)	6	(3/50)	36	(8/22)
Rao et al (23)		(0/16)		(0/2)
Neuwelt et al (18)				(0/6)
Waga et al (33)		(0/39)	22	(5/23)
Chapman and Linggood (6)	8	(1/12)	25	(2/8)
Griffin et al (11)	11	(1/9)		
Total	4	(8/216)	21 (26/127)	

[a] Number in parentheses is the number of patients with spinal seeding compared to the total number of patients.

Table 16.5
Direct Surgical Approach (Biopsy and/or Resection) Pineal Tumors Followed by Irradiation

Reference	Survival %	Follow-up (yr)
Chapman and Linggood (6)	62 (5/8)[a]	2–4
Cummins et al (7)	75 (3/4)	>5
Poppen and Marino (22)	27 (3/11)	1.5–23
Maier and Dejong (16)	75 (3/4)	>5
Bradfield and Perez (3)	67 (2/3)	1.5–4.3
Camins and Schlesinger (4)	43 (6/14)	>5
Neuwelt et al (18)	100 (6/6)	1 mo–6 yr
Suzuki and Iwabuchi (31)	89 (8/9)	.5–5.5

[a] Number in parentheses is the number of survivors compared to the total number of patients.

Table 16.6
Survival Following Irradiation ± Shunt Pineal Tumors

Reference	Survival (%)		Follow-up (yr)
Chapman and Linggood (6)	75	(9/12)[a]	1–4.5
Griffin et al (11)	75	(6/8)	>5
Cummins et al (7)	33	(3/9)	>5
Poppen and Marino (22)	91	(21/23)	0.25–21
Maier and Dejong (16)	50	(2/4)	>5
Bradfield and Perez (3)	50	(3/6)	>5
Mincer et al (17)	62	(5/8)	>5
Smith et al (28)	50	(7/14)	>5
Onoyama et al (20)	69	(26)	>5
Salazar et al (25)	59	(10/17)	>5
Camins and Schlesinger (4)	66	(23/35)	>5
Rao et al (23)	87	(13/15)	>5
Abay et al (1)	70	(27)	>5

[a] Number in parentheses is the total number of patients or survivors compared to the total number of patients.

Table 16.7
Operative Mortality and Morbidity Pineal Tumors Microsurgical Technique

Reference	Morbidity (%)	Mortality (%)
Suzuki and Iwabuchi (31)	60	16
Chapman and Linggood (6)		0/8
Neuwelt et al (18)	50	0/6
Sano and Matsutani (26)		0/32
Jamieson (14)		0/6
Wood et al (37)		0/29

18% (27). There appears to be general agreement that suprasellar germinomas should be biopsied and/or resected prior to radiotherapy to allow for decompression of the optic nerves (26, 27, 29).

In summary, there appears to be no survival advantage for patients undergoing direct surgery prior to radiotherapy. There is a suggestion that surgical intervention may increase the incidence of spinal seeding. However, histologic verification allows for individualization and optimization of treatment. Surgical debulking may be of value in radioresistant tumors. The evaluation of the tumor response to radiotherapy on serial CT scans raises the possibility of reserving direct surgery for those patients who do not demonstrate tumor regression with relatively low dose radiotherapy.

Radiotherapy

Radiotherapy represents the primary treatment of pineal tumors and suprasellar germinomas. Controversy, however, has arisen regarding the optimal tumor dose, volume to be irradiated, and role of elective spinal irradiation.

Tumor Dose

For irradiation of the primary tumor mass, total doses of 4500 and 5500 rad with daily fractions of 180 to 200 rad have generally been employed in the treatment of pineal tumors and suprasellar germinomas (2, 10, 17, 20, 29, 32, 34, 36). Since the majority of these tumors are germinomas and exhibit a radiosensitivity similar to that of testicular seminomas, the ability of lower doses (i.e. 2500 to 3000 rad) to achieve equal results has been questioned (15). Table 16.8 demonstrates the incidence of intracranial relapse as related to the total tumor dose. Doses less than 5000 rad appear to be associated with an increased incidence of relapse. Table 16.9 relates survival to radiation tumor dose. There is a suggestion of a survival advantage for patients receiving 5000 rad or more. The need for higher doses than commonly used in the treatment of seminomas probably reflects the heterogeneity of pineal tumors and the inclusion of unverified radioresistant tumors.

Volume Irradiated

Historically, the volume irradiated for pineal tumors and suprasellar germinomas included the tumor plus an "adequate margin" (i.e., local field) (7, 16). The observation that these tumors frequently extend by direct contiguity or by seeding along the ventricular system (25) led to the recommendation for treatment to the entire ventricular system initially, usually followed by a boost to the area of gross tumor (3, 20, 25, 29, 34, 36). Certain authors (23, 24, 32) have extended the initial fields to include whole brain irradiation. Tables 16.10 and 16.11 compare the incidence of intracranial relapse and overall survival for patients treated with local fields as opposed to the entire ventricular system or whole brain. Chapman and Linggood (6), Jenkin et al (15) and Rao et al (23) noted a decreased incidence of intracranial relapse associated with the use of the larger treatment fields. Mincer et al (17), Sung et al (29) and Abay et al (1) did not confirm this finding. Wara et al (34), Bradfield and Perez (3), and Salazar et al (25) found a survival benefit for the use of larger fields, although in the latter series (25) this difference was evident only up to 5 yr. Rao et al (23) noted no significant difference.

The question of local vs extended fields remains somewhat unsettled, however, the average survival rates (Table 16.11) suggest that the larger volume irradiation is preferable. It should also be kept in mind that if intracranial recurrence follows less than total cranial irradiation, it is difficult, if not impossible, to adequately irradiate the volume at risk.

Indications for Craniospinal Irradiation

The overall incidence of spinal seeding from pineal tumors and suprasellar germinomas is

Table 16.8
Intracranial Relapse as Related to Radiation Tumor Dose Pineal Tumors and Suprasellar Germinomas

Reference	Intracranial relapse (%)	
	<5000 Rad	>5000 Rad
Sung et al (29)	47 (15/32)[a]	10 (4/40)
Jenkin et al (15)	0 (0/9)	9 (2/22)
Rao et al (23)	33 (1/3)	13 (2/15)
Abay et al (1)	37 (7/19)	12 (1/8)
Total	37 (23/63)	11 (9/85)

[a] Number in parentheses is the number of patients with relapse compared to the total number of patients.

Table 16.9
Survival as Related to Radiation Tumor Dose Pineal Tumors and Suprasellar Germinomas

Reference	Survival (%)		Follow-up (yr)
	<5000 Rad	>5000 Rad	
Wara et al (35)	63 (12/19)		2–15
Onoyama et al (20)	47	90	5
Salazar et al (25)	50	67	5
Bradfield and Perez (3)	57 (4/7)	75 (6/8)	3

[a] Number in parentheses is the number of survivors compared to the total number of patients.

Table 16.10
Intracranial Recurrence as Related to Field Size Pineal Tumors and Suprasellar Germinomas

| Reference | Intracranial Recurrence (%) | | Total |
	Local Field	Entire Ventricular System/Whole Brain	
Chapman and Linggood (6)	66 (2/3)	25 (1/4)	43 (3/7)
Mincer et al (17)	30 (3/10)	50 (1/2)	33 (4/12)
Sung et al (29)	17 (5/29)	32 (14/43)	26 (19/72)
Jenkin et al (15)	40 (2/5)	0 (0/26)	6 (2/31)
Rao et al (23)	33 (2/6)	8 (1/12)	17 (3/18)
Abay et al (1)	44 (8/18)	55 (5/9)	48 (13/27)
Total	31 (22/71)	23 (22/96)	26 (44/167)

Table 16.11
Survival as Related to Field Size Pineal Tumors and Suprasellar Germinomas

| Reference | Survival (%) | | Follow-up (yr) |
	Local field	Entire Ventricular System/Whole Brain	
Wara et al (34)	50 (3/6)	92 (12/13)	2–21
Bradfield and Perez (3)	43 (3/7)	67 (6/9)	3
Salazar et al (25)	20 (1/5)	75 (9/12)	5
Rao et al (23)	83 (5/6)	90 (9/10)	5
Total	50 (12/24)	82 (36/44)	

Table 16.12
Incidence Spinal Seeding Pineal Tumors and Suprasellar Germinomas

Author	Tumor	Suprasellar Germinoma
Chapman and Linggood (6)	3/22	
Cummins et al (7)	2/31	0/5
El-Mahdi et al (10)	1/4	0/2
Griffin et al (11)	1/9	1/4
Maier and Dejong (16)		
Personal Series	0/10	
AFIP	8/100	
Rubin and Kramer (24)		4/36
Bradfield and Perez (3)	3/16	1/2
Mincer et al (17)	1/10	0/2
Smith et al (28)	1/14	
Onoyama et al (20)	3/41	1/17
Sung et al (29)	5/57	4/15
Salazar et al (25)	2/19	0/3
Jenkin et al (15)	4/41	1/6
Rao et al (23)	0/17	0/1
Neuwelt et al (18)	1/8	
Sano and Matsutani (26)	2/32	0/20
Abay et al (1)	5/26	
Camins and Mount (5)		2/11
Total	42/457 (9%)	14/124 (11%)

Table 16.13
Incidence Spinal Seeding Pineal Tumors and
Suprasellar Germinomas

Reference	Spinal Seeding
Wara et al (35)	9/118
Dayan et al (8)	11/114
Wara et al (34)	0/19
Total	20/251 (8%)

approximately 10% (Tables 16.12 and 16.13). Therefore, routine craniospinal irradiation for all tumors as initially advocated by Jenkin et al (15) is not indicated. However, if possible, identification of any subset of patients who would benefit from craniospinal irradiation is important.

In the absence of a biopsy, positive cerebrospinal fluid cytology or myelogram are generally accepted as indications for craniospinal irradiation (6, 29). Unfortunately, CSF cytology may be unreliable in predicting the presence or subsequent development of spinal metastases (21). Sung et al (29) found it to be positive in only 25% of patients with spinal subarachnoid seeding. A positive myelogram is a definite indication for extending radiation to include the entire craniospinal axis.

Biopsy-proven germinomas and pineoblastomas may exhibit a greater propensity for spinal seeding. Sung et al (29) noted a 57% incidence of cerebral or spinal subarachnoid metastases in patients with biopsy proven germinomas. Wara et al (35) reported spinal metastases occurring in 14% of the patients with a diagnosis of germinoma while Sano and Matsutani (26) noted only a 3% incidence. The extent or nature of the surgical manipulation may be responsible for the variation in the reported incidence of seeding. A histologic diagnosis of germinoma or pineoblastoma, therefore, may be considered as an indication for craniospinal irradiation.

Some authors have recommended that histologically unverified tumors exhibiting CT evidence of regression following 2000 to 3000 rad should receive craniospinal irradiation (2, 11) as this finding provides indirect evidence for a diagnosis of germinoma or pineoblastoma. The coexistence of a suprasellar mass and a pineal region tumor also implies a diagnosis of germinoma, and, therefore, might be an indication for craniospinal irradiation. Sung et al (29) also recommend craniospinal irradiation for locally extensive or diffusely infiltrating tumors.

However, the subset of patients that merit full craniospinal irradiation remains small. As shown in Table 16.12, the incidence of seeding even after biopsy is approximately 10%. There appears to be no survival advantage to the use of craniospinal irradiation (Table 16.14), although patients receiving this form of treatment may represent a select group. The majority of patients with pineal tumors and suprasellar germinomas are young with a relatively long life expectancy. Adequate radiotherapy to the craniospinal axis carries little mortality, but a substantial morbidity, both early and late.

In summary, there is data to suggest that total tumor doses of 5000 to 5500 rad for the treatment of pineal tumors and suprasellar germinomas result in a decreased rate of intracranial relapse and an improved survival. The volume irradiated should initially include at least the entire ventricular system to 4500 rad. Routine craniospinal irradiation is not justified. Indications for craniospinal irradiation are discussed.

Survival Following Radiotherapy and Patterns of Relapse

Overall, 5-yr survival rates of 43 to 87% for pineal tumors (Table 16.15) and 33 to 100% for suprasellar germinomas (Table 16.16) have been achieved with radiotherapy. The majority of treatment failures are due to persistent or recurrent intracranial disease (Table 16.10) (20, 29), irrespective of whether or not spinal irradiation is given.

Response to Radiotherapy

Approximately 50% of patients experience improved visual function following radiotherapy (10, 20, 30). Smith et al (28), however, noted no improvement in Parinaud's syndrome. Pre-existing endocrine deficiencies have not improved with radiotherapy (10, 20). The incidence of a second intracranial malignancy has varied from 0 (30) to 2% (22).

Radiographic follow-up has demonstrated tumor regression or disappearance following treatment (6, 13, 30). Sung (30) noted no residual tumor in 10 of 12 patients with a suprasellar germinoma. Chapman and Linggood (6) reported significant tumor reduction in eight of nine patients with pineal tumors postradiotherapy. Inoue et al (13) noted complete disappearance of mass effect in nine patients with intracranial germinomas following 1600 to 3300 rad.

Table 16.14
Survival Midline Pineal Tumors and Suprasellar Germinomas Following Irradiation

Reference	Midline Pineal		Suprasellar Germinomas		Follow-up (months)
	CR[a]	CS[b]	CR	CS	
Salazar et al (25)	6/10[c]	2/2	1/3	1/1	18–60+
Smith et al (28)	7/14				60+
Mincer et al (17)	6/9		2/2		60+
Bradfield and Perez (3)	3/7		1/2		60+
Cummins et al (7)	6/13		2/3		60+
Griffin et al (11)	6/8		2/3	1/1	30–60+
Chapman and Linggood (6)	8/10	5/9			12–60
Rao et al (23)	13/15		1/1		60+
Takeuchi et al (32)			8/10	5/9	12–192
Jenkin et al (15)			2/5	0/1	60+
El-Mahdi et al (10)	2/3				60+
Maier and Dejong (16)	5/8				60+
Simson et al (27)			3/6		60+
Total	62/97 (64%)	7/11 (64%)	22/35 (63%)	7/12 (58%)	

[a] CR, cranial irradiation.
[b] CS, cranial plus prophylactic spinal irradiation.
[c] Number of survivors compared to the number of patients.

Table 16.15
Five-Yr Survival Midline Pineal Tumors Following Irradiation

Reference	5-Yr Survival %
Onoyama et al (20)	55 (41)[a]
Mincer et al (17)	67 (6/9)
Sung et al (29)	79 (61)
Maier and Dejong (16)	62 (5/8)
Bradfield and Perez (3)	43 (3/7)
Cummins et al (7)	46 (6/13)
Smith et al (28)	50 (7/14)
Salazar et al (25)	60 (6/10)
Griffin et al (11)	75 (6/8)
El-Mahdi et al (10)	67 (2/3)
Rao et al (23)	87 (13/15)
Abay et al (1)	70 (27)

[a] Number in parentheses is the total number of survivors compared to the total number of patients.

Table 16.16
Five-Yr Survival Suprasellar Germinomas Following Irradiation

Reference	5-Yr Survival %
Onoyama et al (20)	82 (17)
Mincer et al (17)	100 (2/2)
Sung et al (29)	77 (16)
Bradfield and Perez (3)	50 (1/2)
Rubin and Kramer (24)	50 (2/4)
Cummins et al (7)	67 (2/3)
Salazar et al (25)	33 (1/3)
Griffin et al (11)	67 (2/3)
Jenkin et al (15)	33 (2/6)
Takeuchi et al (32)	75 (6/8)
Rao et al (23)	100 (1/1)
Sano and Matsutani (26)	100 (32)
Simson et al (27)	50 (3/6)

Prognostic Factors

Patients with suprasellar germinomas appear to have a slightly higher survival rate than those with pineal tumors (Tables 16.15 and 16.16). This may reflect the varied nature (i.e., teratomas, gliomas, etc) of tumors occurring in the midline location or be related to the surgical procedure or radiation technique employed.

However, when comparing only histologically verified germinomas, those in the suprasellar location still appear to do better than those in the pineal region. Sano and Matsutani (26) reported a 65% 5-yr survival for pineal germinomas compared to 100% for suprasellar germinomas. The authors attributed this difference to the greater degree of surgical debulking possible in the suprasellar region. Onoyama et al (20) reported none of the patients with gliomas or teratomas alive at 5 yr. Sung et al (29) confirmed this finding for gliomas, however, all four patients with teratomas were alive at periods of 6 to 14 yr.

Age appears not to be a consistent prognostic factor. Onoyama et al (20) noted no difference in 5-yr survival when comparing patients less than or equal to 15 yr of age with those greater than 15 (59% vs 65%). Sano and Matsutani (26) reported an 87% 5-yr survival for patients less than 15 yr of age and a 65% 5-yr survival for those greater than 15 yr. Salazar et al (25) and Rao et al (23) found no effect of age on prognosis while Wara and Sheline (35) and Jenkin et al (15) noted an improved survival in younger patients.

References

1. Abay EO, Laws ER, Grado GL, Bruckman JE, Forbes GS, Gomez MR, Scott M: Pineal tumors in children and adolescents. *J Neurosurg* 55:889–895, 1981.
2. Bloom HJG: Intracranial tumors: Response and resistance to therapeutic endeavors, 1970–1980. *Int J Radiat Oncol Biol Phys* 8:1083–1113, 1982.
3. Bradfield JS, Perez CA: Pineal tumors and ectopic pinealomas. Analysis of treatment and failures. *Radiology* 103:399–406, 1972.
4. Camins MB, Schlesinger EB: Treatment of tumours of the posterior part of the third ventricle and the pineal region: A long-term follow-up. *Acta Neurochir* 40:131–143, 1978.
5. Camins MB, Mount LA: Primary suprasellar atypical teratoma. *Brain* 97:447–456, 1974.
6. Chapman PH, Linggood RM: The management of pineal area tumors: A recent reappraisal. *Cancer* 46:1253–1257, 1980.
7. Cummins FM, Taveras JN, Schlesinger EB: Treatment of gliomas of the third ventricle and pinealomas. *Neurology* 10:1031–1036, 1960.
8. Dayan AD, Marshall AHE, Miller AA, Pick FJ, Rankin NE: Atypical teratomas of the pineal and hypothalamus. *J Pathol Bacteriol* 92:1–28, 1966.
9. DeGirolami U, Schmidek H: Clinicopathological study of 53 tumors of the pineal region. *J Neurosurg* 39:455–462, 1973.
10. El-Mahdi AM, Philips E, Lott S: The role of radiation therapy in pinealoma. *Radiology* 103:407–412, 1972.
11. Griffin BR, Griffin TW, Tong DYK, Russell AH, Kurtz J, Laramore GE, Groudine M: Pineal region tumors: Results of radiation therapy and indications for elective spinal irradiation. *Int J Radiat Oncol Biol Phys* 7:605–608, 1981.
12. Haase J, Norgaard-Pedersen B: Alpha-feta-protein (AFP) and human chorionic gonadotrophin (HCG) as biochemical markers of intracranial germ cell tumors. *Acta Neurochir* 50:67–69, 1979.
13. Inoue Y, Takeuchi T, Tamaki M, Nin K, Hakuba A, Nishimura S: Sequential CT observations of irradiated intracranial germinomas. *Am J Roentgenol* 132:361–365, 1979.
14. Jamieson KG: Excision of pineal tumors. *J Neurosurg* 35:550–553, 1971.
15. Jenkin RDT, Simpson WJK, Keen CW: Pineal and suprasellar germinomas. *J Neurosurg* 48:99–107, 1978.
16. Maier JG, Dejong D: Pineal body tumors. *Am J Roentgenol* 99:826–832, 1967.
17. Mincer F, Meltzer J, Botstein C: Pinealoma. A report of twelve irradiated cases. *Cancer* 37:2713–2718, 1976.
18. Neuwelt EA, Glasberg M, Frenkel E, Clark WK: Malignant pineal region tumors. *J Neurosurg* 51:597–607, 1979.
19. Obrador S, Soto M, Gutierrez-Diaz JA: Surgical managment of tumours of the pineal region. *Acta Neurochir* 34:159–171, 1976.
20. Onoyama Y, Ono K, Nakajima T, Hiraoka M, Abe M: Radiation therapy of pineal tumors. *Radiology* 130:757–760, 1979.
21. Pecker J, Scarabin JM, Vallee B, Brucher JM: Treatment of tumours of the pineal region: Value of stereotaxic biopsy. *Surg Neurol* 12:341–348, 1979.
22. Poppen JL, Marino Jr, R: Pinealomas and tumors of the posterior portion of the third ventricle. *J Neurosurg* 28:357–364, 1968.
23. Rao YTR, Medini E, Haselow RE, Jones TK, Levitt SH: Pineal and ectopic pineal tumors: The role of radiation therapy. *Cancer* 48:708–713, 1981.
24. Rubin P, Kramer S: Ectopic pinealoma: A radiocurable neuroendocrinologic entity. *Radiology* 85:512–523, 1965.
25. Salazar OM, Castro-Vita H, Bakos RS, Feldstein ML, Keller B, Rubin P: Radiation therapy for tumors of the pineal region. *Int J Radiat Oncol Biol Phys* 5:491–499, 1979.
26. Sano K, Matsutani M: Pinealoma (germinoma) treated by direct surgery and postoperative irradiation. *Childs Brain* 8:81–97, 1981.
27. Simson LR, Lampe I, Abell MR: Suprasellar germinomas. *Cancer* 22:533–544, 1968.
28. Smith NJ, El-Mahdi AM, Constable WC: Results of irradiation of tumors in the region of the pineal body. *Acta Radiol Ther Phys Bio* 15:17–22, 1976.
29. Sung D, Harisiadis L, Chang CH: Midline pineal tumors and suprasellar germinomas: Highly curable by radiation. *Radiology* 128:745–751, 1978.
30. Sung DI: Suprasellar tumors in children. A review of the clinical manifestations and managments. *Cancer* 50:1420–1425, 1982.
31. Suzuki J, Iwabuchi T: Surgical removal of pineal tumors (pinealomas and teratomas). *J Neurosurg* 23:565–571, 1965.
32. Takeuchi J, Handa H, Nagata I: Suprasellar germinoma. *J Neurosurg* 49:41–48, 1978.
33. Waga S, Handa H, Yamashita J: Intracranial germinomas: Treatment and results. *Surg Neurol* 11:167–172, 1979.
34. Wara WM, Jenkin RDT, Evans A, Ertel I, Hittle R, Ortega J, Wilson CB, Hammond D: Tumors of the pineal and suprasellar region: Childrens cancer study group treatment results 1960–1975. *Cancer* 43:698–701, 1979.
35. Wara WM, Sheline GE: Radiation therapy of

malignant brain tumors. *Clin Neurosurg* 25:397–402, 1978.

36. Wara WM, Fellows CF, Sheline GE, Wilson CB, Townsend JJ: Radiation therapy for pineal tumors and suprasellar germinomas. *Radiology* 124:221–223, 1977.

37. Wood JH, Zimmerman RA, Bruce DA, Bilaniuk LT, Norris DG, Schut L: Assessment and management of pineal-region and related tumors. *Surg Neurol* 16:192–210, 1981.

38. Zimmerman RA, Bilaniuk LT, Wood JH, Bruce DA, Schut L: Computed tomography of pineal, parapineal, and histologically related tumors. *Radiology* 137:669–677, 1980.

CHAPTER 17

Nonsurgical Pineal Tumor Therapy—The Japanese Experience

KINTOMO TAKAKURA, M.D.

INTRODUCTION

The biological characteristics of intracranial germ cell tumors have gradually been clarified in recent years. Germ cell tumors are divided into three major histological types; radiation sensitive germinoma, radiation resistant mature teratoma, and malignant teratoma. Radiation, surgery, or chemotherapy as the principal therapeutic procedure for each type is selected based on the tumor's biological nature. Mature teratomas are surgically treated. Most germinomas can usually be treated by simple radiation even though a shunting procedure is sometimes required. Since malignant teratomas often produce HCG or AFP, these tumors can be diagnosed by the presence of such tumor markers in the serum without histological verification. Patients having functioning germ cell tumors can not be completely cured today by surgery alone and/or by simple radiation; they definitely require adjuvant chemotherapy or immunotherapy. In this paper, the statistical analysis of germ cell tumors in Japan and the results of treatment mainly by radiotherapy for germinoma and functioning germ cell tumors treated in our clinic will be summarized.

STATISTICAL ANALYSIS

It is well recognized that pineal tumors are more frequently found in the Japanese than in Caucasians (2, 3, 10, 17, 22), and intracranial germ cell tumors including germinoma, teratoma, and malignant teratoma constitute about 4% of all primary intracranial tumors in Japan (7). Three-quarters of these tumors are located in the pineal region and the rest in the suprasellar or other regions. Of 13,065 intracranial verified primary brain tumors registered between 1969 to 1977 by most of the neurosurgical clinics in Japan, there were 535 (4.1%) pineal and germ cell tumors. They consisted of 376 germinoma, 23 pineocytoma, 21 pineoblastoma, 72 teratoma, and 43 malignant teratoma (including choriocarcinoma) cases. In children 272 (12.7%) cases of germ cell tumors were found in 2,135 verified primary brain tumors.

In our 128 cases of tumors located in pineal region (Table 17.1), 74 (57.8%) were germino-

Table 17.1
Tumors in Pineal Region—(University of Tokyo)

Histological Type of Tumor	No. of Cases	Sex Ratio Male:Female	Age < 15 yr:> 15 yr
Germinoma	74	68:6	23:51
Teratoma	18	17:1	12:6
Malignant teratoma	11	11:0	9:2
Epidermoid	3	1:2	1:2
Ependymoma	8	4:4	3:5
Other gliomas	12	8:4	4:8
Meningioma	1	1:0	0:1
Metastatic tumor	1	1:0	0:1
Totals	128	111:17	52:76

mas, 18 (14.4%) were teratomas, and 11 (8.6%) were malignant teratomas. The occurrence of other tumors such as ependymoma, other gliomas, or epidermoid tumors in the pineal region was less frequent. Although the peak incidence of all germ cell tumors occurred between the ages of 10 and 15 (Fig. 17.1), germinoma was detected two and one-half times more frequently in patients over 15 yr, whereas teratoma and malignant teratoma were found two to four times more often in children.

The sex ratio of germ cell tumor incidence was quite significant. Especially in tumors of the pineal region, there were 11 times as many male germinoma patients (68 males out of a total 74 cases) and 17 times as many male teratoma patients. No malignant teratoma was found in any female patient. On the contrary, no significant sex difference was noted in suprasellar germ cell tumors.

The sex ratio of patients largely differs with age and the histological type of tumor (Fig. 17.2). As for germinoma, no sex difference of incidence was noted in children under the age of 10 yr. The number of male patients increased with age. There was a 1.5-fold male predominance in adolescents, a 5- to 6-fold increase at ages from 20 to 40 yr, and an eleven-fold increase in adults over 40 yr. In cases of benign teratoma, the sex ratio difference was not so great. Although there were six times as many 10- to 20-yr-old male patients, the occurrence in ages over 20 yr was almost the same in both sexes. The most significant sex difference was noted in cases of malignant teratoma. Male patients were seen 10 times more frequently between the ages of 10 to 20 yr, and no female patients from 20 to 40 yr have ever been found.

These statistical data strongly suggested hormonal control of germ cell tumors. Immature teratomas can produce tumor makers such as HCG or AFP. The tumor disseminates in the central nervous system and metastasizes to other organs. The prognosis is generally extremely poor and most patients die within a few years after the onset of the disease. Our data

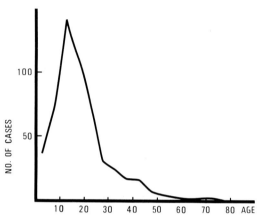

Figure 17.1. Age distribution of intracranial germ cell tumors including germinoma, teratoma, and malignant teratoma (7).

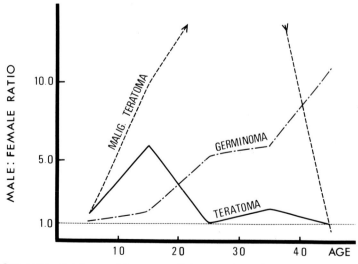

Figure 17.2. Sex ratio of intracranial germ cell tumors (germinoma, teratoma, and malignant teratoma) and age.

revealed that 14 out of 16 malignant teratomas, and 37 out of 96 germinomas were found in children. Although hormonal control of tumor growth is also evident in cases of germinoma, its growth rate is not as rapid as that of the malignant teratoma, therefore, more adult germinoma than malignant teratoma patients might be found.

PATIENTS AND METHOD OF TREATMENT

Twenty germ cell tumor patients were treated by radiotherapy without surgery. One of them showed recurrence and the tumor was surgically removed 7 yr after radiotherapy, and the tumor was verified to be a mature teratoma. Before 1978, radiotherapy was generally given after surgical removal and histological verification of the tumor. Sixty-one cases of germinoma (32 pineal region, 21 suprasellar region, and 8 cases with tumors of other sites) were treated by radiotherapy after surgical removal of the tumor. Seventeen cases of functioning malignant teratoma (HCG- and/or AFP-producing tumors, Table 17.2) were treated by surgery and radiotherapy. Postsurgical irradiation of all germ cell tumors except teratoma was given by supervoltage X-ray (^{60}Co or Linac). The total dose of local irradiation (6 x 6 to 8 x 8 cm field) was 50 to 60 gray.

Methotrexate (total dose 20 to 40 mg) and BUdR (bromouridine, total dose 2 to 4 gm) as a radiosensitizer were administered intraventricularly via an Ommaya reservoir concomitant with radiotherapy (19, 21) in eight cases of germ cell tumors. HCG- and AFP-producing tumors were treated by chemotherapy with actinomycin D, methotrexate, vinblastine, cisplatin, or VM-26 as a Phase II trial.

TREATMENT RESULTS
GERMINOMA
RADIOTHERAPY WITHOUT SURGERY

Since germinomas are quite radiosensitive, (Fig. 17.3) simple radiotherapy after ventriculoperitoneal shunt, if necessary, has been the standard initial treatment for this type of tumor. Radiotherapy without surgery was given to 20 germ cell tumors, of which five cases were treated before the introduction of CT. In these cases, diagnosis was established by ventriculography and cytological examination of the cerebrospinal fluid. The therapeutic result was quite satisfactory. Almost all cases showed complete tumor regression after 20 Gy of radiation over 2 to 3 weeks. Typical examples of tumor regression on CT are illustrated in Figures 17.4 and 17.5. None were functioning tumors producing HCG or AFP. The actuarial survival rate is 100% (14/14) at 3 yr after radiotherapy and 91% (10/11) after 5 yr.

The following case was a patient with mature teratoma. The tumor was surgically removed 7 yr after radiotherapy and the patient remains well 14 yr after the initial radiotherapy.

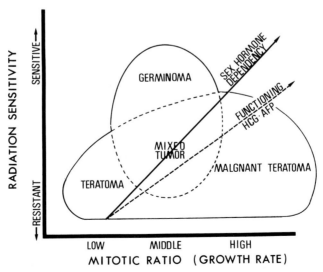

Figure 17.3. Relationship among intracranial germ cell tumors, sensitivity to radiation, mitotic ratio, sex difference, and tumor markers.

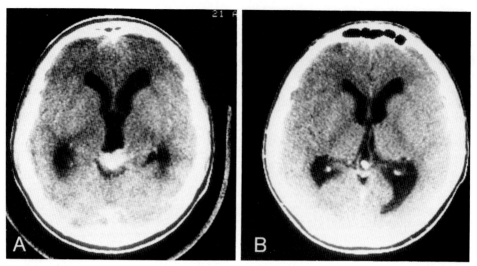

Figure 17.4.   Effect of radiotherapy on pineal germinoma (contrast enhancement). *A*, before radiation; *B*, after radiation (20 gray).

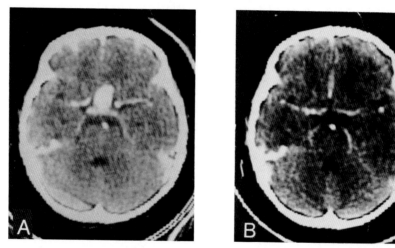

Figure 17.5.   Effect of radiotherapy on suprasellar germinoma (contrast enhancement). *A*, before radiation; *B*, after radiation (20 gray).

Case 1

A 19-yr-old male (No. TU 79047) had a teratoma in the pineal region. Headache, nausea, and vomiting appeared at age 5. Since hydrocephalus was detected, a ventriculoperitoneal shunt was inserted. Six months later headaches, polydipsia, and Parinaud's syndrome were noted. Ventriculography revealed a large nodular tumor in the pineal region. Local irradiation (57 gray by Linac) was given with intraventricular administration of methotrexate (25 mg) and bromouridine (2.5 gm as a radiosensitizer). The tumor size considerably decreased and the symptoms soon disappeared. The patient could return to school after this treatment regimen. After 7 yr, the headaches reappeared. CT revealed a large, irregular, and nodular mass filling the third ventricle. It was a low density mass with calcification. Extensive removal of the tumor using the interhemispheric, transcallosal approach was performed. Pathological diagnosis was mature teratoma. He has since been well controlled without desmopressin acetate administration. He is now 19-yr-old, and has survived 14 yr after detection of the disease. In this case, radiotherapy was beneficial for 7 yr. Since the initial treatment started before the CT age, the regression rate could not be confirmed. This case, however, strongly suggests that the radiosensitive cells in the teratoma tissue might have been destroyed at the initial radiotherapy.

Case 2

Another boy was treated by radiotherapy when he was 4-yr-old. CT later revealed an irregular calcified mass in the pineal region which was felt to be a mature teratoma. The size of the tumor by CT has remained unchanged during 8 yr of follow-up. He remains well (Karnofsky's performance status 100%) 8 yr after radiotherapy.

Case 3

One case of pineal germinoma (a 7-yr-old girl, No. NCC 69244) was initially treated with simple local irradiation (40 gray). Headache and nausea reappeared 1 yr later. Ventriculography revealed nodular masses in both lateral ventricles. Direct visualization with a ventricular fiberscope demonstrated dissemination of the tumor on the wall of the lateral ventricles in the form of several large nodules. Cytological examination of cerebrospinal fluid showed abundant epithelioid tumor cells. Methotrexate and BUdR were infused via an Ommaya reservoir concomitant with radiotherapy (40 gray) to her whole brain. The nodular tumor disappeared on ventriculography after the chemoradiotherapy. She has been well more than 10 yr since. This case suggests that chemotherapy of methotrexate and BUdR may potentiate the effect of radiation.

The other 18 cases were felt to be germinomas. Eight patients received intraventricular methotrexate (1 mg/day, total 20–40 mg) and BUdR (bromouridine, 100 mg/day, total 2 to 4 gm) via an Ommaya reservoir, concomitant with radiotherapy.

RADIOTHERAPY WITH SURGICAL REMOVAL OF THE TUMOR

Radiotherapy was given to 61 cases of germinoma after surgical removal and histological verification of the tumor. There was no surgical mortality. The survival rates of this tumor were 95.1% at 1 yr, 81.4% at 3 yr, 74.8% at 5 yr, and 69.3% at 10 yr after the surgery. Suprasellar

germinoma (21 cases) had a much better prognosis and the survival rates were 100% at 5 yr and 92.3% at 10 yr after surgery. The survival rates of pineal germinoma (32 cases) were, however, 93.5% at 1 yr, 72.7% at 3 yr, 64.7% at 5 yr, and 60.1% at 10 yr after the surgery. Germinoma in children showed a better prognosis than in adult patients. The survival rates of germinoma at 5 and 10 yr treated by surgery and radiation were both 86.9% in 33 children and 65.0% and 60.7% in 28 adult cases, respectively.

Functioning Germ Cell Tumor

Functioning germ cell tumors have generally shown a poor prognosis. Eleven patients demonstrated a high titer of serum HCG ranging from 81 to 700×10^3 IU/liter and 11 patients showed serum AFP ranging from 37 to 56,700 ng/ml, of which four cases showed elevation of both HCG and AFP (Table 17.2). The survival rates of these 17 functioning germ cell tumors were 88.2% at 1 yr, 68.8% at 2 yr, and 53.8% at 3 yr after the treatment. Histological examination revealed that all HCG-producing tumors contained a choriocarcinoma component and all AFP-producing tumor had an endodermal sinus tumor component.

High titers of serum HCG or AFP is a sign of a poor prognosis. Four out of five cases demonstrating serum HCG titer over 1,000 IU/liter and two cases demonstrating serum AFP over 10,000 ng/ml, have died within a few years. The longest survivor was a 19-yr-old male showing 32,000 ng/ml of AFP and 3,200 IU/liter of HCG, who died 3 yr and 7 months after the radiotherapy.

Either HCG- or AFP-producing tumors do not appear to be adequately treated by surgical treatment alone. They need adjuvant radiotherapy and chemotherapy. An extremely fulminant case of a functioning tumor is introduced as follows.

Case 4

A 14-yr-old male (No. TU 83040) with a malignant teratoma and choriocarcinoma (Figs. 17.6 and 17.7) began to complain of headaches in July 1981. The headaches gradually increased and nausea and vomiting appeared on January 7, 1982. A CT revealed hydrocephalus and a mass in the pineal region. A ventriculoperitoneal shunt was inserted and biopsy of the tumor was performed. The pathological diagnosis was an epidermoid tumor. The patient was transferred

Table 17.2
Functioning Germ Cell Tumors—(University of Tokyo)

No.	Age	Sex	Maximum Value of Markers		Survival Time		
			HCG IU/liter	AFP ng/ml		(yr)	(month)
1	14	M	93		Alive	3	
2	11	F	81		Alive	3	
3	22	M	691		Alive	4	
4	14	M	2,300		Died		10
5	15	M	7,380		Died	1	6
6	14	M	700×10^3		Died	1	2
7	8	M		40,000	Died	3	4
8	7	M		3,350	Alive	4	
9	4	M		139	Alive	2	
10	7	M		91	Died	1	4
11	12	M		749	Died		6
12	16	M		56,700	Died	2	7
13	6	M		37	Alive	2	
14	11	M	770	1,810	Alive	2	
15	19	M	3,200	32,000	Died	3	7
16	11	F	598	66	Alive	1	
17	14	M	2,570	528	Alive	3	

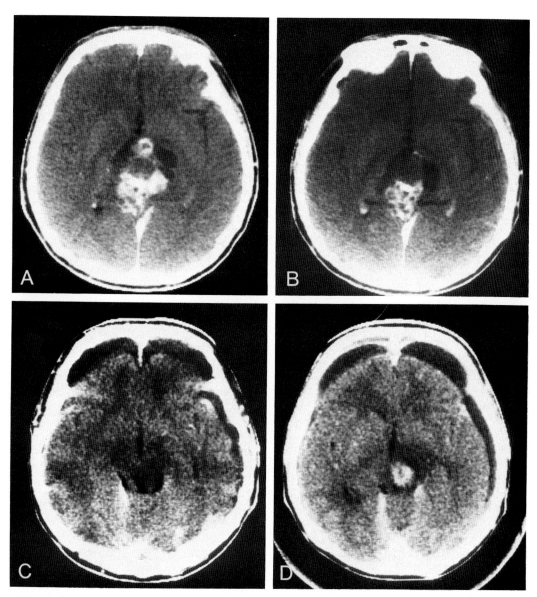

Figure 17.6. Malignant teratoma (Case 4, contrast enhancement), 14-yr-old boy. Serum HCG showed 700,000 IU/liter. A, before treatment; B, after radiotherapy (50 gray) with VM-26 and ACNU; C, after surgical removal of residual tumor; D, recurrent tumor 6 months after surgical removal.

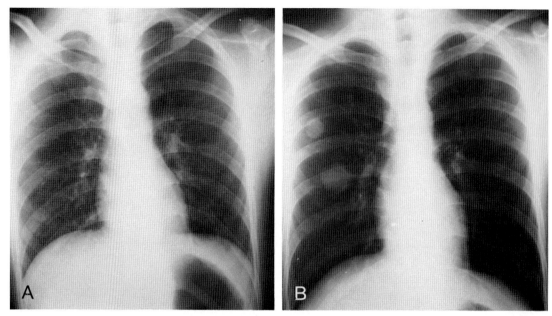

Figure 17.7. Same patient as shown in Figure 17.6 (Case 4). *A*, no metastasis was found at time of admission; *B*, two metastatic tumor nodules were found 5 months after removal of the tumor in the pineal region.

to our clinic on May 29, 1982 in a stuporous state. There was no light reflex and Parinaud's syndrome was noted. He could not stand or walk. The serum HCG was 6,050 IU/liter (Fig. 17.8). Local radiotherapy (50 gray) combined with chemotherapy using 100 mg of VM-26 (Epipodophyllo toxin) and 100 mg of ACNU (4 times every 2 weeks) was given. Serum HCG decreased to 80 IU/liter on August 9. Only slight regression of the tumor was noted, while his clinical signs and symptoms, however, markedly disappeared. He could talk, stand, and walk at that time. As the tumor remained on CT, total removal of the tumor by supratentorial transcallosal approach was performed. Pathological diagnosis was choriocarcinoma with teratomatous components. Although the serum HCG decreased after removal of the tumor, it increased again to 15,000 IU/liter on November 15. A chest X-ray revealed the presence of a round nodular metastasis in the right lower lobe. Radiotherapy to the lung was performed (40 gray) and also to the whole brain (20 gray). Serum HCG decreased again to 450 IU/liter on December 19. Radiotherapy was also given to whole spinal cord, but the serum HCG increased again to 9,300 IU/liter on January 21, 1983 and his chest X-ray showed a second metastatic coin lesion. Serum HCG increased without any beneficial effects by chemo-

therapy using actinomycin D, methotrexate, cisplatin, and vinblastine. Dissemination of the tumor to both lungs soon appeared and the serum HCG reached 700,000 IU/liter on March 25, and the patient died on April 12. Changes of the serum HCG over his clinical course is illustrated in Figure 17.8. This case demonstrates the typical course of a highly malignant teratoma of the pineal region.

Temporary remission only can be obtained by simple radiotherapy for tumors producing both HCG and AFP.

Case 5

An 11-yr-old girl (No. 820080) with a suprasellar malignant teratoma presented with polyuria and polydipsia which appeared at age 10. Poor appetite, general malaise, and sleepiness in the daytime followed. In January 1982 (at age 11), she began to loose the temporal visual field of her left eye. At the time of admission, she was vomiting and was in a pan-hypopituitary state with diabetes insipidus. CT revealed a suprasellar tumor mass. Serum HCG was 598 IU/liter and AFP was 66 ng/ml. Irradiation (local 30 gray and whole brain 20 gray) was given. The whole brain was irradiated because the tumor was a functioning tumor and suspected to be a

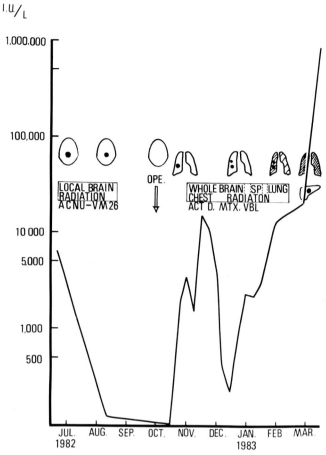

Figure 17.8. Change of serum HCG in the clinical course of malignant teratoma (Case 4, 14-yr-old boy). Pictures in the figure illustrate the size of tumor in brain, lung, and liver. OPE indicates the time of surgery.

malignant teratoma. Supplemental treatment was started with prednisolone, 10 mg per day, 30 mg of Thyradin S per day, and desmopressin acetate nasal administration. The tumor completely regressed on CT within a month. Serum AFP decreased to 5 ng/ml and 1.3 IU/liter of HCG 40 days after the start of radiotherapy. Her general condition recovered and she returned to school. One year later, tumor was not detected on CT and serum HCG and AFP was maintained within normal limits. Recent hormonal examination (April 1983), however, revealed the return of AFP to 50 ng/ml without evidence of recurrence on CT. This case demonstrates that HCG- or AFP-producing tumors probably cannot be completely cured by simple radiotherapy and suggests the necessity of combined chemotherapy.

Four cases of functioning tumors received combined chemotherapy with actinomycin D,

methotrexate, vinblastine, or cisplatin. It has not been concluded, however, that these chemotherapeutic agents have any significant suppressive effect even though they afforded temporary relief to patients and decreased the levels of tumor markers for a few weeks to several months.

DIFFERENTIAL DIAGNOSIS

Differential diagnosis is important for establishing the therapeutic schedule. CT, nuclear magnetic resonance (NMR), and angiographic findings, as well as tumor marker levels in serum are the basis for differential diagnosis. Irregular shape with calcification and various tumor densities in the third ventricle on CT (Fig. 17.9) suggest the possibility of teratoma. Small tumor masses in the pineal region are detected more clearly by the NMR sagittal view. Figure 17.10 demonstrates a large germinoma which disap-

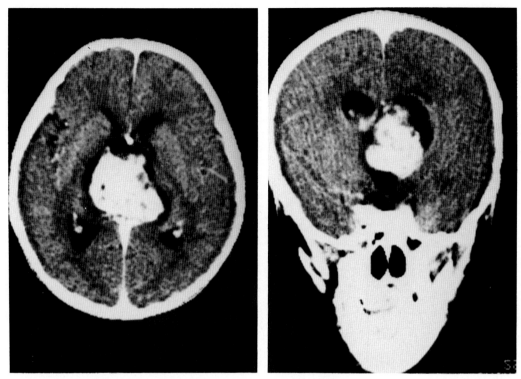

Figure 17.9. Teratoma (contrast enhancement) of a 4-yr-old boy. Irregular shape and variable density of the tumor are characteristic.

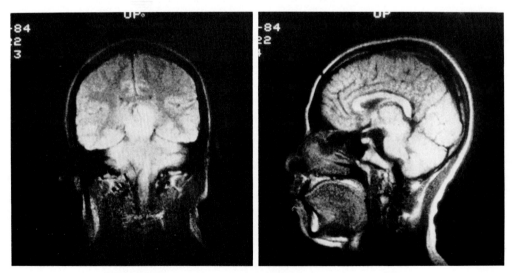

Figure 17.10. NMR images of germinoma in the pineal region.

peared after simple radiotherapy. Dissemination of tumor cells in the ventricular system is also well diagnosed by CT and cytological examination of cerebrospinal fluid.

Figure 17.11 demonstrates a 14-yr-old boy with tumor masses in both the pineal and suprasellar regions. The wall of both lateral ventricles showed a high density coating with tumor cells.

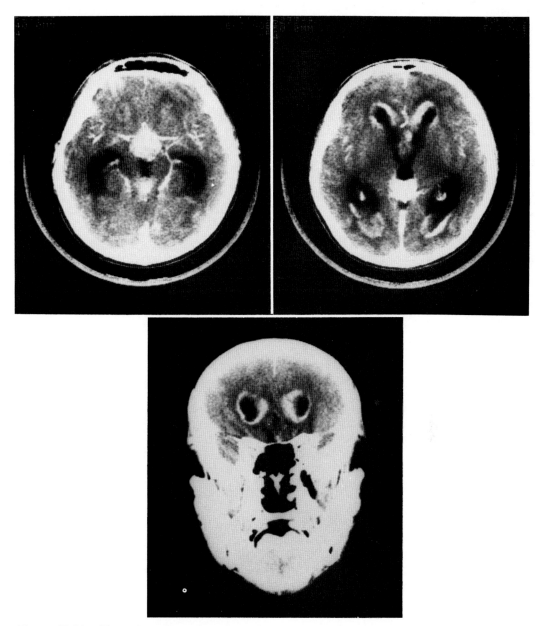

Figure 17.11. Disseminated germinoma (contrast enhancement). Tumors are located in the pineal and suprasellar regions, and on the wall of lateral ventricles.

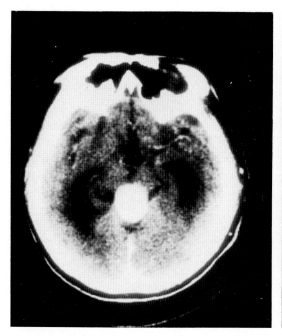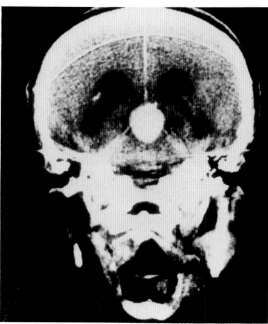

Figure 17.12.   Falcotentorial meningioma (contrast enhancement). Smooth surface and homogenous density of the tumor are noted.

Tumor dissemination to the subarachnoid space was also clearly demonstrated. Cell culture of cerebrospinal fluid showed growth of abundant epithelioid cells and lymphoid cells. This patient had not shown elevation of serum HCG or AFP but was diagnosed as germinoma. The tumor was quite sensitive to radiation and symptoms of headache, nausea, and loss of visual field disappeared with 20 gray of radiation. Most of the high density mass in the ventricles also disappeared.

Several non-germ cell tumors or vascular anomalies are often found in the pineal region. Falcotentorial meningioma is sometimes erroneously diagnosed as germ cell tumor. Figure 17.12 demonstrates a 50-yr-old man with falcotentorial meningioma which was treated by radiotherapy at another hospital without favorable response. Angiography revealed a homogeneous round tumor stain in the capillary phase and demonstrated a feeding tentorial artery. The tumor was totally removed and he returned to his job without any neurological deficit. Most vascular anomalies can be easily diagnosed by angiography. Examination of serum tumor marker levels is especially important for diagnosing malignant immature teratoma as increases of serum HCG or AFP have definite

significance in the diagnosis of malignant functioning germ cell tumor.

DISCUSSION

Since the nomenclature of pineal tumors is still controversial, three terms for the major histological types are used here, namely germinoma, teratoma, and malignant teratoma. Germinoma is the most frequent type of tumor and is composed of large spherical epithelioid cells and lymphoid cells (possibly a mixture of lymphocytes and plasmacytes) which has often been called the "two cell pattern pinealoma." The cell population ratio of epithelioid and lymphoid cells differs case by case and proliferation of lymphoid cells is regarded as an expression of immunological response to the tumor cells. The histological resemblance of germinoma to seminoma and dysgerminoma of the ovary has been pointed out (9). Teratoma is used for mature, slow growing tumors composed of various tissues from the three germinal layers of origin, excluding simple epidermoid tumors. The term malignant teratoma is applied to immature teratomatous tumor including all tumors such as endodermal sinus tumor, yolk sac tumor, choriocarcinoma, teratocarcinoma, and embryonal carcinoma. The tumors in this category often produce HCG, AFP, and possibly other tumor markers, and so are called functioning germ cell tumor.

It is quite important to note that these three histological types of pineal tumors are often found in the same tumor tissue. Mixed histological findings such as germinoma and teratoma, teratoma and choriocarcinoma, HCG- and AFP-producing tumors, or HCG-producing tumor with germinoma component, are not rarely encountered. It seems, therefore, to be reasonable to integrate these tumors under the single nomenclature of intracranial germ cell tumor and to classify them into subtypes. The terms of pineocytoma and pineoblastoma are more complicated. According to the Japanese Brain Tumor Registry, 23 (5.5%) pineocytoma, 21 (5.0%) pineoblastoma, and 376 (89.5%) pinealoma (germinoma) patients have been registered. The term pineocytoma is used for tumors composed of a homogeneous mass of small epithelioid cells without lymphoid cell infiltration. Russell and Rubinstein (15) regarded this type of tumor as of true pineal parenchymal origin and divided it into pineocytoma and malignant pineoblastoma. It has not yet been confirmed that the registered pineocytoma and pineoblastoma exactly fit this criteria. Future consensus will be needed to use these terminologies for the intracranial germ cell tumor subtypes.

Germ cell tumors can be further classified by two biological characteristics; namely, mitotic ratio (growth rate) and sensitivity to radiation (Fig. 17.4). Mature teratoma is a slow growing benign tumor and resistant to radiation. Germinoma has a moderate mitotic ratio and is very sensitive to radiation (1, 4–6, 8, 11–14, 16, 18, 20, 23). Immature teratoma grows rapidly and disseminates intrathecally and to other organs. Its mitotic ratio is high and its radiosensitivity is variable, but it is not as sensitive as germinoma.

Hormonal steroids might significantly influence the genesis and growth of the tumor. The secretion of HCG, AFP, or of other nondetected marker proteins depends on the presence of functional cells. The therapeutic schedule for intracranial germ cell tumor should be established based on these biological characteristics. Benign teratomas should be removed surgically. Germinoma can be treated by radiotherapy alone. Malignant teratomas appear to require multimodal treatment using surgery, radiation and chemoimmunotherapy. It is important to stress here the existence of mixed tumors. Such tumors should be treated by combined therapy. There is no doubt that chemotherapy and hormonal control will soon take major roles in the treatment of malignant teratoma.

Acknowledgments. This work was supported by a Cancer Research Grant from the Ministry of Health and Welfare and a Scientific Research Grant from the Ministry of Education, Science, and Culture. The author wishes to thank Emeritus Professor Keiji Sano, Drs. Masao Matsutani, Tatsuya Kondo, Akira Teramoto, and Associate Professor Shinya Manaka for preparing this study.

References

1. Abay EO, Laws ER, Grado GL, Bruckman JE, Forbes GS, Gomez MR, Scott M: Pineal tumors in children and adolescents. *J Neurosurg* 55:889–895, 1981.
2. Albrechtsen R, Klee JG, Møller JE: Primary intracranial germ cell tumors including five cases of endodermal sinus tumor. *Acta Pathol Microbiol Scand* [A]80:(Suppl)233:32–38, 1972.
3. Araki C, Matsumoto S: Statistical reevaluation of pinealoma and related tumors in Japan. *J Neurosurg* 30:146–149, 1969.
4. Bradfield JS, Perez CA: Pineal tumors and ectopic pinealomas. Analysis of treatment and failures. *Radiology* 103:399–406, 1972.
5. Brady LW: The role of radiation therapy. In Schmidek HH (ed): *Pineal Tumors.* New York, Masson Publishing, 1977, pp 127–132.
6. Camins MB, Schlesinger EB: Treatment of tumours of the posterior part of the third ventricle and the pineal region: A long-term follow-up. *Acta Neurochir* 40:131–143, 1978.
7. Committee of Japanese Brain Tumor Registry: *All Japan Brain Tumor Registry*, vol 4, 1982.
8. DeGirolami U, Schmidek H: Clinicopathological study of 53 tumors of the pineal region. *J Neurosurg* 39:455–462, 1973.
9. Friedman NB: Germinoma of the pineal. Its identity with germinoma ("seminoma") of the testis. *Cancer Res* 7:363–368, 1947.
10. Jellinger K: Primary intracranial germ cell tumours. *Acta Neuropathol* 25:291–306, 1973.
11. Jenkin RDT, Simpson WJK, Keen CW: Pineal and suprasellar germinomas. *J Neurosurg* 48:99–107, 1978.
12. Mincer F, Meltzer J, Botstein C: Pinealoma. A report of twelve irradiated cases. *Cancer* 37:2713–2718, 1976.
13. Onoyama Y, Ono K, Nakajima T, Hiraoka M, Abe M: Radiation therapy of pineal tumors. *Radiology* 130:757–760, 1979.
14. Rao YTR, Medini E, Haselow RE, Jones TK, Levitt SH: Pineal and ectopic pineal tumors: The role of radiation therapy. *Cancer* 48:708–713, 1981.
15. Russell DS, Rubinstein LJ: *Pathology of Tumors of the Nervous System*, ed 4. Baltimore, Williams & Wilkins, 1977, pp 287–290.
16. Sang II D, Harisiadis L, Chang CH: Midline pineal

tumors and suprasellar germinomas: Highly curable by irradiation. *Radiology* 128:745–751, 1978.

17. Sano K: Diagnosis and treatment of tumors in the pineal region. *Acta Neurochir* 34:153–157, 1976.

18. Sano K, Matsutani M: Pinealoma (germinoma) treated by direct surgery and postoperative irradiation. *Childs Brain* 8:81–97, 1981.

19. Sano K, Hoshino T, Nagai M: Radiosensitization of brain tumor cells with a thymidine analogue (Bromouridine). *J Neurosurg* 28:530–538, 1968.

20. Smith NJ, El-Mahdi AM, Constable WC: Results of irradiation of tumors in the region of the pineal body. *Acta Radiol Oncol Radiat Phys Biol* 15:17–22, 1976.

21. Takakura K, Matsutani M, Koyama K, Sing OK: Intrathecal BAR therapy for malignant brain tumors. *Brain Nerve* (Tokyo) 24:585–593, 1972.

22. Ueki K, Tanaka R: Treatments and prognoses of pineal tumors—experience of 110 cases. *Neurol Med Chir* 20:1–26, 1980.

23. Wara WM, Fellows CF, Sheline GE, Wilson CB, Townsend JJ: Radiation therapy for pineal tumors and suprasellar germinomas. *Radiology* 124:221–223, 1977.

CHAPTER 18

Conservative Management of Pineal Tumors—Mayo Clinic Experience

EDWARD R. LAWS, Jr., M.D., EUSTACIO O. ABAY III, M.D.,
GLENN S. FORBES, M.D., GORDON L. GRADO, M.D.,
JAMES E. BRUCKMAN, M.D., and MARK SCOTT, Ph.D.

Although pineal tumors are rare, comprising about 2% of primary brain tumors in most series, they remain a subject of interest and some controversy (12, 19, 31). With the advent of CT scanning, the diagnosis of these tumors and the hydrocephalus which so commonly accompanies them has been greatly facilitated, allowing for earlier detection and greater precision in delineating the lesions. The ability to follow accurately the size of the tumor and the extent of hydrocephalus by serial CT scanning has altered both the concepts and the practice of management.

Our current concepts of the management of presumed primary pineal neoplasms are based on our review of 54 cases with autopsy or histopathologic analysis, evaluated at the Mayo Clinic between 1923 and 1976, and on a review of the literature, especially those cases treated primarily by shunting and radiation therapy (1, 4, 8, 15, 23, 24, 28, 39, 45, 46, 49, 52, 55, 56, 61, 66, 70, 71–73, 76, 80, 82–84).

Primary tumors affecting the pineal region may be of glial, pineal cell, or germ cell origin (18, 20, 22, 34, 58, 62, 64, 88). Although gliomas of the pineal region or quadrigeminal plate may mimic true pineal tumors, their natural history and response to therapy are no different from other supratentorial gliomas and they will not be discussed further in this chapter. The differential diagnosis of tumors of the pineal region is presented in Table 18.1. In most cases, excellent radiologic studies can differentiate among primary pineal tumors, cysts, epidermoids, aneurysms, and other nonpineal lesions in the area.

Of the true pineal tumors, approximately two-thirds are of germ cell origin. Of these, about

Table 18.1
Tumors of the Pineal Region: Differential Diagnosis

A. Pineal cell tumors
   1. Pinealocytoma
   2. Pinealoblastoma
B. Germ cell tumors
   1. Germinoma
   2. Benign teratoma
   3. Malignant teratoma
   4. Embryonal carcinoma
   5. Choriocarcinoma
C. Gliomas
   1. Astrocytoma, glioblastoma, spongioblastoma, astroblastoma, oligodendroglioma
   2. Ganglioma, ganglioneuroma
   3. Ependymoma
   4. Medulloblastoma, neuroblastoma
   5. Choroid plexus papilloma
D. Others
   1. Meningioma, angioblastoma, hemangiopericytoma
   2. Dermoid, epidermoid
   3. Colloid cyst
   4. Metastatic carcinoma
E. Nontumors
   1. Aneurysm, vein of Galen
   2. Arachnoid cyst
   3. Tuberculoma

half are germinomas (seminomas) and half are teratomas (50% benign, 50% malignant) (7, 30, 63, 65). Pineal cell tumors comprise approximately one-third of the true pineal tumors, and are pinealocytomas and pinealoblastomas (22, 33, 40). Long-term survival has followed successful management of germinoma, benign teratoma, and pineal cell tumors. The more malignant lesions have a uniformly poor prognosis.

The age and sex distribution of primary pineal tumors are quite distinctive (9). The mean age at diagnosis is 17 yr and there is a marked male preponderance (8:1). They are more common in Orientals than in people of other races (3). These data can be used, in conjunction with the CT scan, as predictors of pathology in those patients treated presumptively without histopathologic confirmation.

The most frequent presenting symptoms are those of generalized increased intracranial pressure, namely headache, vomiting, and drowsiness (11, 18). Visual symptoms are nearly as common, and include blurring of vision and decrease in acuity. Symptoms of hypothalamic dysfunction such as precocious puberty, diabetes insipidus, or emaciation are less common, occurring in only about 15% of patients (6, 27).

The most prominent pathologic signs of pineal tumors are neuro-ophthalmologic, with some abnormality present in virtually every case. Papilledema, diminished pupillary reflexes, and paresis of upward gaze (Parinaud's syndrome) are the most common findings. Other signs related either to hydrocephalus or local extension of the tumor may occur, namely ataxia, corticospinal tract dysfunction with spasticity, visual field defect, or hemi-sensory loss.

Radiologic findings on plain skull x-rays consist of abnormal calcifications in the pineal region in about 25%, and of signs of increased intracranial pressure (separation of sutures, erosion of the dorsum sellae) in a significant proportion of cases (13). The CT scan has all but replaced pneumoencephalography and ventriculography as the definitive neuroradiologic procedure for pineal tumors. The CT scan shows virtually 100% of the lesions, usually as high-density abnormalities, with contrast enhancement a common occurrence (37, 43, 74, 79, 87). The CT scan shows the degree of hydrocephalus when present, and a contrast CT scan may also demonstrate ependymal seeding, which may occur with pinealoblastoma, germinoma, or malignant teratoma. Angiography is occasionally helpful; a highly vascular tumor pattern may be seen with malignant germ cell tumors such as embryonal carcinoma. A giant aneurysm simulating pineal tumor can be ruled out. Most importantly, especially if surgery is planned, angiography will show the venous drainage of the pineal area and its relationship to the bulk of the tumor.

Other laboratory tests may be helpful. Although no specific endocrine abnormalities are present in pinealoma, baseline hypothalamic-pituitary evaluation should be done. Melatonin assays in blood and CSF are currently of limited usefulness. Lumbar puncture should be avoided in the presence of obstructive hydrocephalus. However, if lumbar or ventricular samples of CSF are obtained, cytologic evaluation should be performed both for help in the diagnosis of the primary lesion and for documentation of seeding when it occurs. Human chorionic gonadotropin (HCG) and alpha fetoprotein (AFP) may be detected in the CSF of patients with germ cell tumors, and may be useful in planning therapy (2).

The neurosurgical management of pineal tumors has gone through several phases, and still is in a state of flux (10, 14, 32, 35, 36, 38, 41, 47, 48, 50, 53, 54, 57, 67, 69, 77, 85, 86). Walter Dandy (16, 17) reported his early experience with a right occipito-parietal transcallosal approach, but was discouraged by a very high operative mortality. Later, Poppen (53) recommended a right occipital transtentorial approach, and reported some success with this mode of direct attack. Van Wagenen (81) utilized a right transcortical, transventricular approach. Kempe (42) embellished and beautifully illustrated the approach through the splenium of the corpus callosum in his atlas. With the advent of the operating microscope and micro-neurosurgical techniques, direct attack has become more readily recommended and much less dangerous (26). Using these methods, Stein has popularized a posterior fossa infratentorial supracerebellar approach (75), and others have utilized one or another of the transcallosal or transtentorial approaches.

Some of the earliest shunting procedures were performed for hydrocephalus resulting from pineal tumors. Dandy had one patient with a red rubber tube passed through the aqueduct. Some of Torkildsen's (78) first patients treated with ventriculo-cisternal shunts likewise had pineal lesions. Shunting became more widely and effectively applied in the 1950's after ventriculo-atrial and ventriculo-peritoneal shunts were developed. A functioning unit will effectively eliminate those symptoms and signs related to hydrocephalus.

The beneficial effects of radiation therapy on many pineal tumors have been recognized for some time. The CT scan has given dramatic evidence of the disappearance of some lesions following radiotherapy. Germinomas, like semi-nomas, and pineal cell tumors (pineoblastoma and pineocytoma), like medulloblastomas, are highly sensitive to radiation therapy. Whole brain and spinal axis radiation is usually recommended in those tumors where seeding has been documented or is likely to occur (29). Radiation therapy, either as primary therapy or when given following surgery, can be given accurately and safely, and virtually every known long-term surviving patient with a pineal tumor has been treated with radiation therapy.

Stereotactic surgery has been utilized for the biopsy of pineal tumors (51). This has been accomplished both by endoscopic guidance through an enlarged lateral ventricle (25), and by more traditional means using a stereotactic device. CT coupled stereotactic devices are under development and should make such a procedure relatively simple.

The various recent reports advocating direct surgical approach emphasize the following points:

(a) Tissue diagnosis is desirable for planning adjunctive therapy, especially chemotherapy for germinomas (21).

(b) "Total" removal of benign lesions can be accomplished.

(c) Successful removal of a pineal tumor may eliminate obstructive hydrocephalus and the need for a shunt.

(d) Unnecessary radiation therapy may be avoided.

The significant improvements which have occurred in direct surgical mortality and morbidity make these arguments more persuasive (44). On the other hand, improvements in neuroradiologic diagnosis have made the diagnosis and follow-up of presumed pineal tumors much more secure.

THE MAYO CLINIC EXPERIENCE

This study includes 44 patients seen at the Mayo Clinic between November 1950 and April 1978 diagnosed to have a pineal tumor and treated by radiotherapy and CSF shunting when hydrocephalus was a problem. Of the 44, 32 had both CSF shunting and radiotherapy at the Mayo Clinic, 1 had a shunt elsewhere but radiotherapy was done at the Mayo Clinic, and 7 had radiotherapy at the Mayo Clinic and required no CSF shunting procedure.

Fifteen other patients who had both CSF shunting and radiotherapy in other institutions were evaluated at the Mayo Clinic during the period but were excluded from the study because most of them were seen at the Mayo Clinic 2–10 yr after initial therapy, and more than 60% of the deaths from disease in our study occurred within 2½ yr of diagnosis. Patients who had the same diagnosis but were seen prior to 1950, and those that had had direct surgical management as initial therapy have also been excluded.

Age and Sex Distribution

Tumors of the pineal gland area were more common in males (3:1), with the highest incidence in the second decade. The ages of the patients ranged from 1–50 yr (Table 18.2).

Basis of Diagnosis

Twenty-five of the 44 patients of this series had CT examinations; 40 had skull radiographs, 17 underwent arteriography; 32 underwent pneumoencephalography or ventriculography.

The pineal gland was identified in all 25 patients who had a CT examination. Pineal calcification was observed in 21 of 25 (84%). The calcification measured over 10 mm in 20 of 25 (80%). Homogeneous dense calcifications were seen in 12 of 25 patients while an irregular amorphous pattern was observed in 13 of 25. Nine of the 12 patients (75%) with the dense pattern were alive at the time of follow-up, while 5 of 13 with the amorphous pattern were alive. Seventeen of 25 demonstrated some degree of ventricular obstruction, and 21 of the 25 CT examinations were considered abnormal with either abnormal size of the pineal, abnormal calcification, or ventricular obstruction. Intravenous contrast was administered in 15 of 25 exams, and 9 of 15 tumors demonstrated contrast enhancement. Four of 9 patients with enhancing tumors died during the course of the study.

Significant regression of tumor size was demonstrated in 5 patients who had serial CT ex-

Table 18.2
Age/Sex Distribution of Patients with Pineal Tumors

	Yr					
	1–10	11–20	21–30	31–40	41–50	Total
Male	4	17	5	3	4	33
Female	2	4	2	1	2	11
Total	6	21	7	4	6	44

amination following radiation treatment. Several tumors showed a denser, more even pattern of calcification after radiation treatment. In general, tumors with larger size, more amorphous calcification and contrast enhancement were more likely to show regressive changes with radiation treatment.

Surgery-CSF Shunting

Thirty-seven patients underwent CSF shunting prior to radiotherapy; all had hydrocephalus. Eighteen had ventriculocisternal shunts (Torkildsen, 78), 12 had ventriculoperitoneal shunts, and 7 had ventriculo-atrial shunts. The average hospitalization of these patients was 7 days.

Immediate improvement in symptomatology was the usual result of the shunt. Two patients with mental confusion and one with altered consciousness became worse after shunting; these patients were moribund with severe hydrocephalus and disseminated disease upon admission.

There was no operative mortality. None of the patients developed subdural hematoma, intracranial hemorrhage, or seizures. One patient developed a shunt infection (*Staphylococcus epidermidis*) 7 months postoperatively, and subsequently died at another institution.

Malfunction and Revisions

Ten patients required shunt revision because of malfunction and 2 required a second revision. Of the 4 Torkildsen shunts which required revision, 1 had a ventriculoperitoneal shunt 1 day after the former procedure. Two others, 14 days and 3 months later, respectively, had a ventriculo-atrial shunt. The last patient had all shunts eventually removed.

The ventriculo-atrial shunt which required revision 1 day after surgery was obstructed by tumor cells.

Five ventriculoperitoneal shunts required revision 3 months to 33 months after the procedure, 2 of which required second revisions 1 month and 19 months, respectively, after the first.

Radiation Therapy

Patients with pinealomas presenting for radiation therapy at the Mayo Clinic Division of Therapeutic Radiology were evaluated and treated by many different radiotherapists and no one uniform treatment policy was incorporated in the planning of the treatment program. Generally, however, radiation therapy was delivered to the pineal region in a dose thought to be adequate for control of this tumor, usually 3500–5000 rads in 3.5–5 weeks of treatment.

Generally, radiation therapy was delivered to the pineal region and field sizes ranged from 56–300 cm^2, with the majority being treated with 8 × 8 cm to 10 × 10 cm sized fields. As with field sizes, doses ranged from 1850–6000 rads (one patient received 651 rads and was unable to complete treatment because of his rapidly deteriorating condition).

RESULTS

Survival and Follow-up

The mean survival in this study is 24.0 yr. One yr survival is 80%; 5 yr, 70%; 10 yr, 64%; and 15 yr, 58%. Twenty patients (45%) are alive and well, and 7 (15.5%) are alive with mild residual neurologic deficits (Fig. 18.1).

Of the 17 dead, 14 died from the disease—3 in less than 1 yr, 8 within 1–4 yr, and 1 each after 5, 10, and 20 yr. Three died of other causes, 1 from a shunt infection 7 months postoperatively, another committed suicide 4 yr later, and the third died from accidental asphyxiation 17 yr later.

A dose-response relationship to radiation therapy was demonstrated (Table 18.3).

Recurrence

Nineteen of the 44 (43%) patients developed recurrences: 4 at the primary site; 4 at other sites in the brain; 2 in the spinal cord; 6 in both the primary site and other sites in the brain; 2 in other sites in the brain and spinal cord; and 1 in the primary and other sites in the brain and spinal cord. A total of 5 patients developed spinal axis metastasis out of a total of 42 patients who were at risk (2 patients received prophylactic spinal axis irradiation) for an incidence of 11.9%. Fifteen (34%) of the patients failed at extrapineal sites within the CNS.

Of the 19 that recurred, 1 had subsequent craniotomy at another institution, 6 had a second course of radiotherapy, and 3 had chemotherapy.

Histology and Survival

Fourteen had histologic diagnoses from later surgery (2) or autopsy (12). Most of the deaths occurred within the first 2 years. It is noteworthy

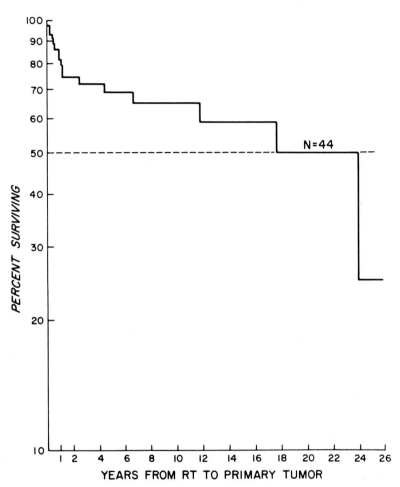

Figure 18.1. Survival after radiation ± ventricular shunting in patients with pineal tumors at the Mayo Clinic.

Table 18.3
Pineal Tumors: Local Control Related to Dose and Treatment Field

Dose in Rads	Recurrence Site	No. of Patients	% Local Failure	% Local Control
≤2999	Inside field	2	(2/5) 40.0	
	Outside field	0		(3/5) 60.0
	None	3		
	Total	5		
3000–3999	Inside field	3	(3/8) 37.5	
	Outside field	4		(5/8) 62.5
	None	1		
	Total	8		
4000–4999	Inside field	3	(3/15) 20.0	
	Outside field	4		(12/15) 80.0
	None	8		
	Total	15		
≧5000	Inside field	2	(2/16) 12.5	
	Outside field	1		(14/16) 87.5
	None	13		
	Total	16		

Table 18.4
Survival of 14 Patients with Histology from Autopsy or Later Surgery*

No. of Patients	Histology	Survival Time	Status
3	Pineocytoma	6 yr	Dead
		4.5 yr	Alive and well
		6 months	Dead
2	Pineocytoma/blastoma	3 yr	Dead
		3 months	Dead
2	Pineoblastoma	11 yr	Dead
		1 yr	Dead
1	Malignant teratoma	2 yr	Dead
1	Benign teratoma	2 months	Dead
1	Embryonal carcinoma	1 month	Dead
1	Neuroblastoma	1 yr	Dead
1	Embryonal rhabdomyosarcoma	1 yr	Dead
1	Grade IV astrocytoma	1 yr	Dead
1	Ependymoma had craniotomy + RoRx 1 yr later at another institution	4 yr	Alive with deficit VI CN
1	Meningioma	24 yr	Dead

* NB: 5 others who had died, 2 from disease and 3 from other causes, expired at other institutions and histology could not be obtained.

that only 1 of the 12 autopsied patients had a truly benign pineal tumor (benign teratoma). None of these patients with proven histologic diagnosis had a germinoma; one had a meningioma (59, 60) (Table 18.4).

DISCUSSION

If the incidence and natural history of the various pineal tumors are considered, several facts are evident:

(a) 85% of pineal tumors are either very sensitive to radiation therapy or highly malignant.

(b) All long-term survivors have been treated with radiation therapy.

(c) The effects of radiation therapy, shunting, or direct surgery may be followed closely by serial CT scans.

Because of these considerations, it is our general policy to recommend shunting and radiation therapy as primary treatment for nearly all pineal tumors. If symptoms related to mass effect do not resolve and if the lesion on CT scan does not respond to radiation therapy, then direct surgery is recommended. The route chosen, either infratentorial supracerebellar, or supratentorial through the splenium of the corpus callosum, depends on the angiographic demonstration of the venous anatomy in each case. If tissue confirmation is thought to be essential prior to recommending radiation therapy or chemotherapy, direct or stereotactic surgery is recommended.

In summary, the typical pineal tumor occurs in an adolescent boy with subacute increased intracranial pressure and Parinaud's syndrome. Diagnosis is confirmed by CT scanning, and long-term survival usually following shunting and radiation therapy. Direct surgical methods for successful treatment of suitable pineal tumors have evolved and may be utilized with relatively low risk in appropriate cases.

References

1. Abay EO, Laws ER, Grado GL, Bruckman JE, Forbes GS, Gomez MR, Scott M: Pineal tumors in children and adolescents. *J Neurosurg* 55:889–895, 1981.
2. Allan JC, Nisselbaum J, Epstein F, Rosen G, Schwartz MK: Alphafetoprotein and human chorionic gonadotropin determination in cerebrospinal fluid. *J Neurosurg* 51:368–374, 1979.
3. Araki C, Matsumoto S: Statistical reevaluation of pinealoma and related tumors in Japan. *J Neurosurg* 30:146–149, 1969.
4. Backlund ED, Rahn T, Sarby S: Treatment of pinealomas by stereotaxic radiation surgery. *Acta Radiol Ther* 13:368–376, 1974.
5. Baggenstoss AH, Love JG: Pinealomas. *Arch Neurol Psychiat* 41:1187–1206, 1939.
6. Balagura S, Shulman K, Sobel EH: Precocious puberty of cerebral origin. *Surg Neurol* 11:315–326, 1979.
7. Bochner SJ, Scarff JE: Teratoma of the pineal body. Classification of embryonal tumors of the pineal body: Report of a case of teratoma of the pineal body presenting formed teeth. *Arch Surg* 36:303–309, 1979.
8. Bradfield JS, Perez CA: Pineal tumors and ectopic

9. Brodeur GM, Howarth CB, Pratt CB, Caces J, Hustu HO: Malignant germ cell tumors in 57 children and adolescents. *Cancer* 48:1890–1898, 1981.
10. Camins MB, Schlesinger EB: Treatment of tumours of the posterior part of the third ventricle and the pineal region: A long term follow-up. *Acta Neurochir* 40:131–143, 1978.
11. Castleman B, McNeely BU: Case records of the Massachusetts General Hospital. *N Engl J Med* 284:1427–1434, 1971.
12. Chapman PH, Linggood RM: The management of pineal area tumors: A recent reappraisal. *Cancer* 46:1253–1257, 1980.
13. Cole H: Tumours in the region of the pineal. *Clin Radiol* 22:110–117, 1971.
14. Conway LW: Stereotaxis diagnosis and treatment of intracranial tumours including an initial experience with cryosurgery for pinealomas. *J Neurosurg* 38:453–460, 1973.
15. Cummins FM, Taveras JN, Schlesinger EB: Treatment of gliomas of the third ventricle and pinealomas. *Neurology* 10:1031–1036, 1960.
16. Dandy WE: Operative experiences in cases of pineal tumor. *Arch Surg* 51:1–14, 1945.
17. Dandy WE: An operation for the removal of pineal tumors. *Surg Gyn Obst* 33:113–119, 1921.
18. David M, Vernard-Weik E, Dilenge D: Les tumeurs de la glande pineale. *Ann Endocrinol* (Paris) 24:286–330, 1963.
19. Davidoff LM: Some considerations in the therapy of pineal tumors. *Bull NY Acad Med* 43:537–561, 1967.
20. DeGirolami U, Schmidek H: Clinicopathological study of 53 tumors of the pineal region. *J Neurosurg* 49:455–462, 1973.
21. deTribolet N, Barrelet L: Successful chemotherapy of pinealoma. *Lancet* 12:1228–1229, 1977.
22. Donat JF, Okazaki H, Gomez MR, Reagan TJ, Baker HL, Laws ER: Pineal tumors. *Arch Neurol* 35:736–740, 1978.
23. El-Mahdi AM, Philips E, Lott S: The role of radiation therapy in pinealoma. *Radiology* 103:407–412, 1972.
24. Fowler FD, Alexander E Jr, Davis CH Jr: Pinealoma with metastases in the central nervous system—a rationale of treatment. *J Neurosurg* 13:271–288, 1956.
25. Fukushima T. Endoscopic biopsy of intraventricular tumors with the use of a ventriculoscope. *Neurosurg* 2:110–113, 1978.
26. Glasauer FE: An operative approach to pineal tumors. *Acta Neurochir* 22:177–180, 1970.
27. Globus JH: Pinealoma. *Arch Path* 31:533–568, 1941.
28. Griffin BR, Griffin TW, Tong DYK, Russell AH, Kurtz J, Laramore GE, Groudine M: Pineal region tumors: Results of radiation therapy and indications for elective spinal irradiation. *Int J Rad Oncol Biol Phys* 7:605–608, 1981.
29. Haimovic IC, Sharer L, Hyman RA, Beresford R: Metastasis of intracranial germinoma through a ventriculoperitoneal shunt. *Cancer* 48:1033–1036, 1981.

pinealomas. Analysis of treatment and failures. *Radiology* 103:399–406, 1972.

30. Haldeman KO: Tumors of the pineal gland. *Arch Neurol Psychiat* 18:724, 1927.
31. Handa H, Yamashita J: Summary: Current treatment of pineal tumors. *Neurologia Medico-chirurgica* 21:147–148, 1981.
32. Harris W, Cairns H: Diagnosis and treatment of pineal tumors. *Lancet* 1:3–9, 1932.
33. Herrick MK, Rubinstein LJ: The cytological differentiating potential of pineal parenchymal neoplasms (true pinealomas). *Brain* 102:289–320, 1979.
34. Horrax G, Bailey P: Tumors of the pineal body. *Arch Neurol Psychiat* 13:423–470, 1925.
35. Horrax G: Treatment of tumors of the pineal body. Experience in a series of twenty-two cases. *Arch Neurol Psychiat* 64:227–242, 1950.
36. Horsley V: Discussion of paper by CMH Howell on tumors of the pineal body. *Proc R Soc Med* 3:77–78, 1910.
37. Hyman RA, Loring MF, Liebeskind AL, Naidich JB, Stein HL: Computed tomographic evaluation of therapeutically induced changes in primary and secondary brain tumors. *Neuroradiology* 14:213–218, 1978.
38. Jamieson KG: Excision of pineal tumors. *J Neurosurg* 35:550–553, 1971.
39. Jenkin RDT, Simpson WJK, Keen CW: Pineal and suprasellar germinomas. *J Neurosurg* 48:99–107, 1978.
40. Juif JG, Maitrot D, Pierson M, Heldt N, Buchheit F, Luckel JC: Les tumeurs cerebrales primitives d'origine germinale. *Arch Franc Ped* 34:335–346, 1977.
41. Kahn EA: Surgical treatment of pineal tumors. *Arch Neurol Psychiat* 38:833–842, 1937.
42. Kempe LG: *Operative Neurosurgery.* Berlin, Heidelberg, New York, Springer Verlag, 1968.
43. Kretzschmar K, Aulich A, Schindler E, Lange S, Grumme T, Meese W: The diagnostic value of CT for radiotherapy of cerebral tumors. *Neuroradiology* 14:245–250, 1978.
44. Lazar ML, Clark K: Direct surgical management of masses in the region of the vein of Galen. *Surg Neurol* 2:17–22, 1974.
45. Maier JG, Dejong D: Pineal body tumors. *Am J Roentgenol* 99:826–832, 1967.
46. Minger F, Meltzer J, Botstein C: Pinealoma. A report of twelve irradiated cases. *Cancer* 37:2713–2718, 1976.
47. Neuwelt EA, Glasberg M, Frenkel E, Clark WK: Malignant pineal region tumors. *J Neurosurg* 51:597–607, 1979.
48. Obrador S, Soto M, Gutierrez-Diaz JA: Surgical management of tumors of the pineal region. *Acta Neurochir* 34:159–171, 1976.
49. Onoyama Y, Ono K, Nakajima T, Hiraoka M, Abe M: Radiation therapy of pineal tumors. *Radiology* 130:757–760, 1979.
50. Page LK: The infratentorial-supracerebellar exposure of tumors in the pineal area. *Neurosurgery* 1:36–40, 1977.
51. Pecker J, Scarbarin JM, Vallee B, Brucher JM: Treatment of tumours of the pineal region: Value of stereotaxic biopsy. *Surg Neurol* 12:341–348, 1979.
52. Pertuiset B, Visot A, Metzger J: Diagnosis of pinealoblastomas by positive response to cobalttherapy. *Acta Neurochir* (Wien) 34:151–152, 1976.
53. Poppen JL, Marino Jr R: Pinealomas and tumors of the posterior portion of the third ventricle. *J Neurosurg* 28:357–364, 1968.
54. Rand RW, Lemmen LJ: Tumors of the posterior portion of the third ventricle. *J Neurosurg* 10:1–18, 1953.
55. Rao YTR, Medini E, Haselow RE, Jones TK, Levitt SH: Pineal and ectopic pineal tumors: The role of radiation therapy. *Cancer* 48:708–713, 1981.
56. Ray P, Olson MH, Sarivar M, Wright AE, Wu J, Allam AA: Pinealoma: Analysis of treatment and failure. Proceedings of the American Society of Therapeutic Radiologists. *Int J Radiat Oncol Biol Phys* (Suppl)1:144, 1976.
57. Reid WS, Clark WK: Comparison of the infratentorial and transtentorial approaches to the pineal region. *Neurosurgery* 3:1–8, 1978.
58. Ringertz N, Nordenstam H, Flyger G: Tumors of the pineal region. *J Neuropathol Exp Neurol* 13:540–561, 1954.
59. Roda JM, Perez-Higueras A, Oliver B, Alvarez MP, Blazquez MG: Pineal region meningiomas without dural attachment. *Surg Neurol* 17:147–151, 1982.
60. Rozario R, Adelman L, Prager RJ, Stein BM: Meningiomas of the pineal region and third ventricle. *Neurosurgery* 5:489–495, 1979.
61. Rubin P, Kramer S: Ectopic pinealoma: A radiocurable neuroendocrinologic entity. *Radiology* 85:512–523, 1965.
62. Rubinstein LJ: *Tumors of the Central Nervous System. Atlas of Tumor Pathology,* 2nd series, Fascicle 6. Washington, Armed Forces Inst of Pathology, 1972.
63. Rubinstein LJ: Cytogenesis and differentiation of pineal neoplasms. *Hum Pathol* 12:441–448, 1981.
64. Russel DS, Sachs E: Pinealoma. A clinicopathologic study of 7 cases with a review of literature. *Arch Path* 35:869–888, 1943.
65. Russell DS: The pinealoma: Its relationship to teratoma. *J Path Bact* 56:145–150, 1944.
66. Salazar OM, Castro-Vita H, Bakos RS, Feldstein ML, Keller B, Rubin P: Radiation therapy for tumors of the pineal region. *Int J Rad Oncol Biol Phys* 5:491–499, 1979.
67. Sano K: Diagnosis and treatment of tumors in the pineal region. *Acta Neurochir* 34:153–157, 1976.
68. Sano K: Pinealomas in children. *Childs Brain* 2:62–72, 1976.
69. Sano K, Matsutani M: Pinealoma (germinoma) treated by direct surgery and postoperative irradiation. *Childs Brain* 8:81–97, 1981.
70. Sharan VM: Management of pineal tumors by radiation therapy and CT scanning. (Meeting Abstract) *Int J Radiat Oncol Biol Phys* 2(2):154, 1978.
71. Sheline GE: Radiation therapy of tumors of the central nervous system in childhood. *Cancer* 35:957–964, 1975.
72. Smith NJ, El-Mahdi AM, Constable WC: Results of irradiation of tumors in the region of the pineal body. *Acta Radiologica Ther Phy Bio* 15:17–22, 1976.

73. So SC: Pineal tumours: A clinical study of 23 cases. *Aust NZ J Surg* 46:75–79, 1976.
74. Spiegel AM, Di Chiro G, Gorden P, Ommaya AK, Kolins J, Pomeroy TC: Diagnosis of radiosensitive hypothalamic tumors without craniotomy *Ann Int Med* 85:290–293, 1976.
75. Stein BM: Supracerebellar-infratentorial approach to pineal tumors. *Surg Neurol* 11(5):331–337, 1979.
76. Sung D, Harisiadis L, Chang CH: Midline pineal tumors and suprasellar germinomas: Highly curable by radiation. *Radiology* 128:745–751, 1978.
77. Suzuki J, Iwabuchi T: Surgical removal of pineal tumors (pinealomas and teratomas). *J Neurosurg* 23:565–571, 1965.
78. Torkildsen A: A new palliative operation in cases of inoperable occlusion of the Sylvian aqueduct. *Acta Chir Scand* 82:117–124, 1939.
79. Tucker WG, Leong ASY, McCulloch GAJ: Tumours of the pineal region—neuroradiological aspects. *Australas Radiol* 21:313–324, 1977.
80. Ueki K, Tanaka K: Study on treatment and prognosis of pineal neoplasms. *Seara Med Neurochir* 7(2):279–315, 1978.
81. Van Wagenen WP: A surgical approach for the removal of certain pineal tumors. *Surg Gyn Obst* 53:216–220, 1931.
82. Waga S, Handa H, Yamashita J: Intracranial germinomas: Treatment and results. *Surg Neurol* 11:167–172, 1979.
83. Wara WM, Jenkin RDT, Evans A, Ertel I, Hittle R, Ortega J, Wilson CB, Hammond D: Tumors of the pineal and suprasellar region: Childrens cancer study group treatment results 1960–1975. *Cancer* 43:698–701, 1979.
84. Wara WM, Fellows CF, Sheline GE, Wilson CB, Townsend JJ: Radiation therapy for pineal tumors and suprasellar germinomas. *Radiology* 124:221–223, 1977.
85. Wilson CB: Diagnosis and surgical treatment of childhood brain tumors. *Cancer* 35:950–956, 1975.
86. Wood JH, Zimmerman RA, Bruce DA, Bilaniuk LT, Norris DG, Schut L: Assessment and management of pineal-region and related tumors. *Surg Neurol* 16:192–210, 1981.
87. Zimmerman RA, Bilaniuk LT, Wood JH, Bruce DA, Schut L: Computed tomography of pineal, parapineal, and histologically related tumors. *Radiology* 137:669–677, 1980.
88. Zulch KJ: *Brain tumors: Their Biology and Pathology* (ed 2). New York, Springer Publishing Co., 1965, p 326.

CHAPTER 19

Germinomas and Other Pineal Tumors: Chemotherapeutic Responses

EDWARD A. NEUWELT, M.D. and EUGENE P. FRENKEL, M.D.

INTRODUCTION

There have been only a few reports of the successful use of chemotherapy in treatment of pineal region tumors. deTribolet and Barrelet (9) reported a patient with a large pineal region tumor and meningeal carcinomatosis who was treated with daunorubicin, vincristine, and bleomycin, and had a dramatic decrease in tumor size over a 3-month period as evaluated by CT scan. A report by Borden et al (4) documented regression of a pulmonary metastasis from a pineal germinoma following therapy with chlorambucil, methotrexate, and actinomycin D.

The known 82% complete response rate of testicular tumors treated with a combination of bleomycin, vinblastine, and cis-platinum and the histological similarity between seminomas of the testes and intracranial germinomas, led us to propose such a *cis*-platinum-based multidrug combination as the therapy of choice for recurrent suprasellar and pineal germinomas in 1978. Indeed, because of the complications inherent in craniospinal irradiation, particularly in young patients (38), we felt this chemotherapeutic regimen might in the future prove to be the initial treatment choice.

Our initial reports (29, 32) demonstrated that pineal region tumors are highly sensitive to the multi-agent chemotherapeutic regimen developed by Einhorn and Donohue (12) for testicular tumors, which includes *cis*-platinum, bleomycin, and vinblastine. Furthermore, therapeutic responsiveness could be monitored both by computed tomography and by the serial determination of serum and cerebrospinal fluid (CSF) for the β-subunit of human chorionic gonadotropin (β-HCG), a tumor marker that is sometimes secreted by this neoplasm. Despite an excellent tumor response in three of three patients, two of our three patients subsequently developed bleomycin-induced pulmonary fibrosis. This known potential complication of bleomycin therapy occurred at a dose considerably lower than that seen with the use of bleomycin in other tumors (2).

The present communication reviews our detailed experience with these three patients with intracranial germinomas who we began treating with the Einhorn regimen in 1978. An additional two patients who responded to two other chemotherapeutic drug regimens will also be discussed. Finally, the limited available experience of pineal tumor chemotherapy will be reviewed.

METHODS

The levels of β-HCG were determined using a radioimmunoassay kit (Nuclear Medical Systems, Newport Beach, CA). Alpha-fetoprotein (AFP) levels were measured in serum and CSF (Smith, Kline Clinical Laboratory, St. Louis, MO).

Cis-Platinum levels were determined by X-ray fluorescence spectroscopy on a Van de Graaff proton accelerator (through the auspices of Cecil Thompson, Ph.D., Professor of Physics, University of Texas at Arlington, Arlington, TX). The limit of assay sensitivity in plasma is 0.1 μg/ml; the limit of assay sensitivity in tissue is 0.5 μg/g of tissue.

CASE REPORTS

Case 1

H.K., a 22-yr old man, was seen in another institution in 1968 with headaches and evidence of diabetes insipidus. A mass in the anterior third ventricle was seen on a pneumoencephalogram and angiogram. At craniotomy a suprachiasmatic mass was visualized and a presumptive diagnosis of astrocytoma was made without biopsy. The patient was treated with 4500 rad of megavoltage cranial radiation via 5- × 5-cm fields over 6 weeks. His subsequent course was uneventful except for some difficulty in managing his diabetes insipidus and retarded growth.

He moved to Dallas and late in 1979 his diabetes insipidus became more difficult to control. He was found to have a recurrent 5- to 6-cm tumor that extended from the third ventricle into the temporal lobe (Fig. 19.1A). The tumor showed progressive enlargement on CT scans, and a new lesion developed in the roof of the fourth ventricle (Fig. 19.1B). In March 1980 the patient underwent a right anterior temporal lobectomy, and histologic examination of the tumor revealed that the lesion was a germinoma.

The cellular composition of the fresh, unfixed tumor obtained at operation was evaluated by the immunological techinques described (32). The commonly recognized histologic and cytologic pattern of the germinoma was seen. That is, two major cell types were evident, "large cells" and "small cells." Using the classical sheep red blood cell (SRBC) agglutination technique for the identification of T-lymphocytes, 80–90% of only the small cells were seen to form typical T-cell rosettes. The fluorescence-activated cell sorter was used to examine cell surface immunoglobulins characteristic of B-lymphocytes; the staining was nonspecific showing only Fc receptors on the cell surface. Therefore, on the basis of morphology and the presence of the SRBC receptor, 80–90% of the small cells in this suprasellar germinoma appeared to be T-lymphocytes. None of the large cells demonstrated lymphoid phenotype characteristics.

Based on the histological diagnosis, the patient was studied for the presence of a testicular tumor. He had no evidence of a testicular tumor or extraneural tumor by extensive clinical and radiographic evaluation. The patient's postoperative β-HCG levels were 52.8 mIU/ml in the serum (normal, less than 3.5 mIU/ml) and 179 mIU/ml in the CSF (normal, undetectable). AFP values were undetectable.

From these data, we interpreted the original lesion seen 12 yr earlier as a germinoma and that it has recurred in spite of the previous radiotherapy. Because of the considered risk of radiation necrosis with any additional radiotherapy, the patient was treated with chemotherapy consisting of cis-platinum, bleomycin, and vinblastine using the standard therapy protocol for testicular tumors (12). The cis-platinum total dose (100 mg/m^2) was given in divided

aliquots on each of 5 successive days, i.v. in an 8-hr infusion. Serum and CSF aliquots were obtained for the measurement of cis-platinum concentration during the last hr of the 8-hr infusion on two occasions. The cis-platinum levels (± SD) in the serum at these times were 1.2 ± 0.35 and 0.8 ± 0.44 μg/ml; no cis-platinum was detected in the CSF on either occasion.

Within 2 weeks of the initial course of chemotherapy, the serum β-HCG level had fallen markedly (to 4.4 mIU/ml), and the CSF β-HCG value was 28 mIU/ml. After the second course of chemotherapy the β-HCG values were no longer detectable in the serum or CSF (Fig. 19.2). A CT scan at this time demonstrated a dramatic decrease in the amount of (enhancing) tumor to but 10% of its postoperative size in each of the two lesions.

During chemotherapy the management of the diabetes insipidus was difficult. He had significant hyponatremia. In addition, he had a grand mal seizure and developed marked sensorineural hearing loss. No new neurological or other clinical events occurred. Routine laboratory studies were otherwise stable and his creatine clearance was unchanged from its initial value of 60 ml/min.

After a third course of chemotherapy, the supratentorial and infratentorial tumors were no longer apparent by CT scan (Fig. 19.1). By all criteria the patient was in a complete response; that is, he had no clinical, neuroradiological, or tumor-marker (i.e. serum and CSF β-HCG levels) evidence of tumor. He subsequently developed acute respiratory failure, which proved histologically to be due to pulmonary fibrosis. The presumptive cause of the pulmonary fibrosis was bleomycin. He died in spite of intensive supportive therapy; permission for postmortem examination was denied.

Case 2

J.T., a 16-yr old boy, was first seen at another institution 4½ yr previously with headaches, a 6th nerve palsy, and diabetes insipidus. Metrizamide ventriculography and CT scans demonstrated two lesions involving the anterior and posterior third ventricle, respectively. A ventriculoperitoneal (VP) shunt was placed. A presumptive diagnosis of a germinoma was made and craniospinal radiation was administered. The patient's symptoms resolved, although mild diabetes insipidus persisted, and he returned to school.

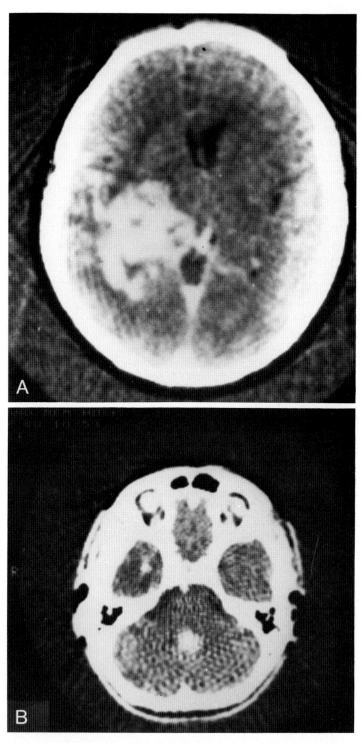

Figure 19.1. Case 1. *A*, enhanced cranial CT scan obtained after H.K.'s second craniotomy shows a large enhancing tumor extending from the third ventricle into the right temporal lobe. *B*, same CT scan as in *A*, but at the level of the fourth ventricle, shows a second enhancing mass in the roof of the fourth ventricle. *C*, enhanced CT scan at the level of the lateral and third ventricles after three courses of chemotherapy showing no evidence of residual tumor, compare with *A*. *D*, enhanced CT scan at the level of the fourth ventricle, 2 weeks after a single course of chemotherapy, shows marked regression of the tumor in the roof of the fourth ventricle (see *B*). With permission from *Neurosurgery*, 7:352–358, 1980, (Ref. 32).

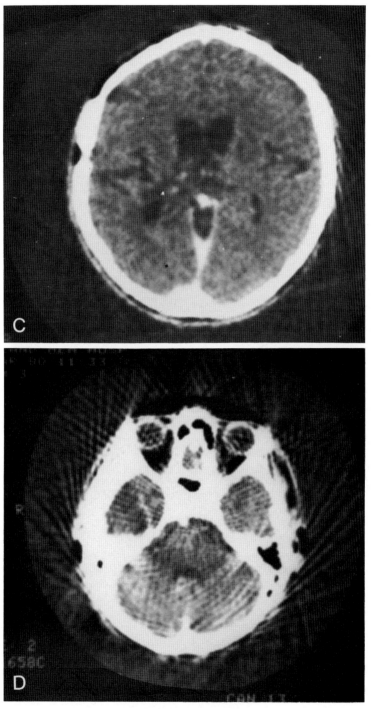

Figure 19.1. *C* and *D.*

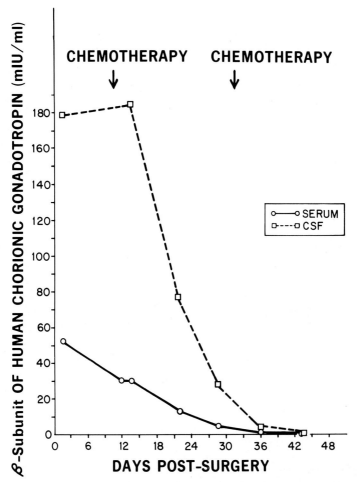

Figure 19.2. Case 1. Serum and cerebrospinal fluid levels of the β-HCG before and serially after the institution of systemic chemotherapy. An anterior temporal lobectomy and small biopsy were done on day 0. With permission from *Neurosurgery* 7:352–358, 1980, (Ref. 32).

The patient noted a protuberant abdomen 2½ years after his initial presentation. A chest film revealed elevation of the right hemidiaphragm and a large pleural effusion. A panmyelogram was normal, as was cytological examination of his CSF. A cranial CT scan and metrizamide ventriculogram were normal, except for a large pineal calcification. A CT scan of the abdomen (Fig. 19.3) demonstrated massive intraperitoneal and retroperitoneal tumor involvement, as well as beaded tumor nodules along the thoracic portion of the thoracic shunt and on the superior surface of the diaphragm. Laboratory investigation revealed a serum HCG level of 201 mIU/ml. AFP values were below the level of detection.

Biopsy revealed a massive tumor filling the abdominal cavity which, on histological study, was shown to be a germinoma.

The patient was started on multiagent systemic chemotherapy with *cis*-platinum, bleomycin, and vinblastine (as described above). Remarkable lysis of the tumor was achieved and, after four courses of chemotherapy, his serum HCG returned to normal and he had achieved a complete clinical remission with no evidence of tumor by any measurable criteria. The patient received two courses of chemotherapy beyond the point of a complete remission by all clinical criteria and a nondetectable β-HCG level. He has remained in complete remission and off of

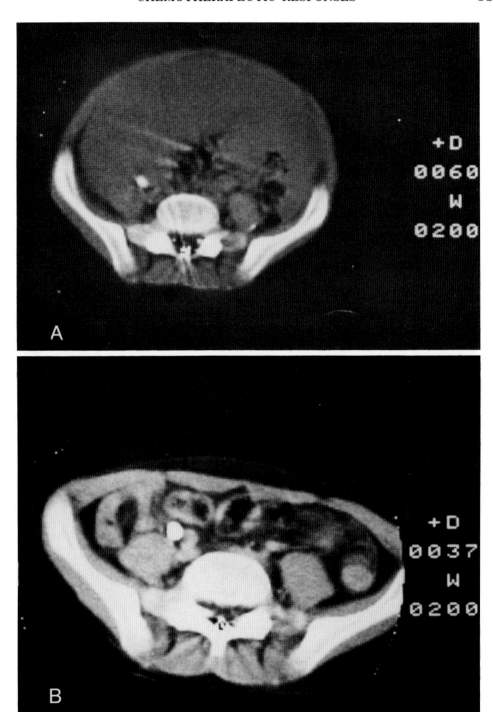

Figure 19.3. Case 2. Transverse cut body CT scan at the level of the superior iliac crest. *A*, a scan before the institution of chemotherapy shows essentially confluent tumor filling the distended abdominal cavity. *B*, a scan 6 months later, after four courses of chemotherapy, shows no residual evidence of tumor, just the normal abdominal contents. With permission from *Neurosurgery* 7:352–358, 1980, (Ref. 32).

all therapy for 6 yr. His VP shunt has been removed. He is currently a University student with normal functional capacity.

Case 3

J.G. presented in August of 1978 with multiple enhancing lesions on enhanced CT scan in the corpus callosum and hypothalamus. A transcallosal biopsy revealed tissue which appeared to consist of inflammatory cells and granulomas, and a diagnosis of sarcoidosis was made. The patient had had a clinical response to antibiotics and these plus adrenocortical steroids resulted in some improvement in his clinical status. The patient's neurologic status deteriorated in January, 1980, and a repeat biopsy was performed and again was consistent with a granulomatous process. Over the next 2 yr the patient required multiple revisions of his ventricular shunt, but was clinically stable until he again manifested new neurologic findings in January, 1982 (Fig. 19.4). A right frontal lobectomy was performed and tissue examined from this procedure showed the lesion to be a germinoma. By this time the patient's mental status was markedly impaired, in part probably the result of multiple surgical procedures. Our treatment plan was based on the precarious mental and neurologic status of the patient and our previous responses to multiagent chemotherapy. Considering the rapidity of our previous responses and the maintenance of the patient's neurologic and functional status, we planned initial therapy with chemotherapy. Any evident lack of tumor response would immediately lead us to radiation therapy with the risks of neurologic loss. The patient received two courses of *cis*-platinum, vinblastine, and bleomycin. After the second course of chemotherapy, the patient had no evidence of residual tumor by CT scan (Fig. 19.4). The patient was electively admitted for his third course of chemotherapy. An evident decrease in pulmonary function was noted and the patient developed progressive pulmonary symptoms. His total dose of bleomycin to this point was 180 units. His symptoms progressed and the patient died of pulmonary insufficiency. At autopsy, no evidence of residual germinoma was found in the brain. In the pineal region a mature teratoma was present which in retrospect upon review of the CT scan was also present on his previous CT scans. Pathologic examination of the lungs revealed diffuse pulmonary interstitial fibrosis.

DISCUSSION

In 1947, Friedman (16) made the classical observation that many pineal and suprasellar tumors were histologically identical to certain testicular and ovarian germ cell tumors. He proposed the term germinoma to denote these lesions. Since that time these tumors have been shown to be highly radiosensitive, with tumor-free intervals of at least 5 yr in 55–90% of cases treated with cranial radiation (7). These results were achieved with cranial radiation (5000–5500 rads) accompanied by radiation to the spinal axis because of the potential for these tumors to seed the subarachnoid space. The tumors that recur after such radiation present a major therapeutic dilemma because the incidence of radiation necrosis rises dramatically with additional radiotherapy (25).

The patients described in this report demonstrate that primary intracranial germinomas either totally within the CNS or having metastasized outside the CNS are highly responsive to the same chemotherapeutic regimen used in the histologically identical tumor of the testis, the seminoma (13). It is often difficult to evaluate the efficacy of therapy of tumors in the CNS. Clinical findings may not resolve significantly, particularly in patients who have had previous extensive surgery and radiation therapy. Computed tomography has provided a new and important dimension in the serial evaluation of therapeutic trials in such tumors. An additional powerful parameter is accessible in these germinomas in the form of tumor markers (β-HCG or AFP) which may be released to the CSF or blood. These markers provide a simple accessible and inexpensive parameter of tumor responsiveness during treatment trials. Using the CT scan and the tumor markers we were able to show rapid and dramatic tumor response to chemotherapy in the cases reported herein. Tottori et al (44), as well as others (1), have pointed out that, when the tumor secreting the β-HCG is located solely within the CNS, the serum-CSF ratio is lower than if the tumor is extraneural. Indeed, in Patient 1, the CSF β-HCG level was much higher in the CSF than in the serum.

The long-term sequelae of radiation therapy in the management of pineal region tumors has already been mentioned (see Chapter 16). However, chemotherapy also is not free of side effects. In most reports, the primary toxicity of

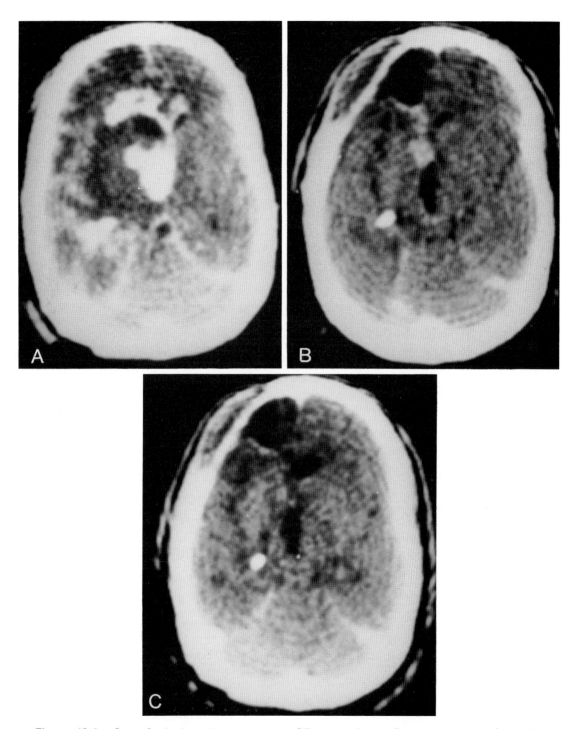

Figure 19.4. Case 3. *A*, An enhanced cranial CT scan prior to frontal lobectomy, 2 yr after presentation showing hypothalamic and right frontal germinoma. *B*, enhanced CT scan following right frontal lobectomy with residual enhancing tumor. *C*, after chemotherapy, the enhancing tumor is essentially gone.

the *cis*-platinum-vinblastine-bleomycin combination relates to the *cis*-platinum. The major toxicity related to the *cis*-platinum is renal, but this can be avoided by vigorous hydration and diuresis. Uncommon side effects include peripheral neuropathy and toxic injury of the VIII cranial nerve. The major toxicity related to the vinblastine is that of marrow injury with resultant pancytopenia. This is almost always transient and reversible. The present small series describe an uncommon incidence of a potential toxicity of bleomycin, that of pulmonary fibrosis. In general this is dose-related, leading to the usual discontinuation of bleomycin when 300 units has been administered and can be, in part, predicated by a falling pulmonary diffusing capacity. The rapidity of onset and progression of the pulmonary fibrosis, the failure to respond to steroids, and the fatal outcome in this small series of this subset of tumors, raises unanswered questions concerning the nature of the interrelationship of the bleomycin and this tumor form.

Following our initial report of the use of the *cis*-platinum-vinblastine-bleomycin regimen in the treatment of intracranial germ cell tumors in 1979 (29, 32) two other cases have been reported. Kirshner et al (21) described a partial remission using this program, and Siegal et al (42) treated a patient with recurrent CNS germinoma with subependymal and spinal metastases and achieved a complete response. The tumor subsequently recurred, but again responded to the same program. In the case reported by Kirshner et al in which a partial response was seen, the bleomycin was stopped after a total dose of 360 units because early pulmonary toxicity was present.

The problems of pulmonary toxicity to bleomycin in this tumor subset is troublesome. The uncommon incidence of the tumor precludes any meaningful dissection of the drug-tumor interrelationships. Since an alternative (to *cis*-platinum-vinblastine-bleomycin) treatment program exists, capable of the salvaging treatment failures as well as achieving excellent primary complete remission rate, it seems reasonable to utilize that program as the initial approach in recurrent tumors. The combination of *cis*-platinum and VP-16 can therefore provide the same potential treatment response rate as *cis*-platinum-vinblastine-bleomycin without the risk of the pulmonary toxicity (46). Since it is possible to serially evaluate the tumor prior to each course of chemotherapy, a failure to document

progressive decline in tumor markers and reduction in tumor size should then be used to turn to the more "conventional" *cis*-platinum-vinblastine-bleomycin regimen. Although radiation has a defined toxicity, particularly in younger patients, it remains a highly effective and durable standard treatment regimen (see Chapter 16).

The clinical response of the case reported by de Tribolet and Barrelet (9), as well as the response in two of our patients in whom the tumors were totally within the CNS, raises important questions relative to the role of the blood-brain barrier as a factor in the delivery of chemotherapeutic agents to tumors in the CNS.

Controversy exists as to whether the poor response of most tumors in the CNS to chemotherapy is due to inherent resistance of the tumor or poor drug delivery. Certainly the responses in these cases might suggest that the germinoma is simply a tumor highly responsive to chemotherapy. This view that drug delivery is irrelevant is fostered by the observation that the enhanced CT scan defines extravastion of contrast material and thereby identifies a defective blood-brain barrier. This conceptual view is weakened by the failure of chemotherapeutic response in other tumors (breast, small cell of the lung, etc) metastatic to the CNS, particularly where the systemic lesions in these same patients did respond. This suggests that the responsiveness of germinomas to chemotherapy may be related to a circumstance different from that existent in most other tumors in the CNS.

Inasmuch as the anterior pituitary and the pineal gland are two of the locations within the CNS that normally lack a blood-brain barrier (40), it may be that the suprasellar germinoma derives its vasculature from vessels similar to those that are present in the normal anterior pituitary and that pineal neoplasms derive their vasculature from the vessels supplying the normal pineal. Therefore, drug delivery may not represent the same problem in these lesions as it does in most other primary or metastatic CNS malignancies. Alternatively, these tumors may be exquisitely sensitive to chemotherapy despite reduced drug exposure due to a partially intact blood-brain barrier.

With regard to other germ cell tumors, our experience is limited to one patient. We have consulted on a 14-yr-old boy who in 1981 had a clinical diagnosis of a pineal region tumor and was treated with craniospinal radiation. There was a 75% decrease in the tumor size. One yr later the tumor rapidly increased in size and a subtotal resection of the tumor was performed. Pathologic examination revealed it to be an endodermal sinus tumor. Following the craniotomy the patients serum AFP level was 19,324 mIU/ml. The patient was treated with sequential multi-agent chemotherapy (vincristine, methylprednisolone, procarbazine, hydroxyurea, cis-platinum, cytosine arabinoside, and DTIC), with a decrease in the tumor size by CT scan. The serum AFP levels decreased to 74 mIU/ml. Six months later and after three courses of therapy the patient's tumor again increased in size and the serum AFP rose to 1,980 mIU/ml. At this point, the family refused further therapy.

There is very little evidence aside from the above-mentioned studies which indicate any kind of response of nongerm cell pineal tumors to chemotherapy. We have had one patient with a primitive neuro-ectodermal tumor, probably a pineoblastoma, in the pineal region, who had a transient but definite response to combination chemotherapy (methotrexate, cytoxan, and procarbazine) in association with osmotic blood-brain barrier disruption (26, 33). Thus, in large part, a successful chemotherapeutic regimen for nongerm cell tumors of the pineal remains to be determined.

SUMMARY

The results and potential future role of chemotherapy in the treatment of pineal region tumors are reviewed in this chapter. To date only a small number of patients with pineal region tumors have been treated with chemotherapy and this has commonly been done in association with radiation therapy. Very few patients have had a chemotherapy-induced tumor response that can clearly be attributed to only that therapy. In this chapter we review 5 patients from our series in whom a therapeutic response was observed that was clearly attributable to drug administration and not surgery, radiotherapy, or adrenal corticosteroids. Four of these patients had tumors of germ cell origin. These observations added to a limited number of other case reports suggest a promising therapeutic role for chemotherapeutic agents in the management of pineal region tumors. In particular, germ cell tumors of the pineal region appear to be especially responsive to chemotherapeutic agents. In spite of the limited observations to date, the pattern and responses of the pineal region tumors suggest that an important factor in therapeutic effectiveness is the absence of the blood-brain barrier in this area, thereby permitting appropriate drug delivery.

An exciting prospect is that the Japanese are currently conducting a national cooperative study on the use of chemotherapy in the treatment of pineal tumors. Because of the high incidence of these tumors in Japan, these studies will undoubtedly be of great value. Finally, Dr. Jeff Allen and associates at the 1984 meeting of the American Society for Clinical Oncology reported a number of chemotherapeutic regimens he had tried on seven patients with recurrent CNS germ cell tumors. Measurable responses were seen with cyclophosphamide alone (80 mg/kg), cis-platinum alone (120 mg/m^2) and using a combination of vinblastine, bleomycin, cyclophosphamide, actinomycin D, and cis-platinum.

Acknowledgments. This work was supported by the Ira Kassanoff Research Fund, the Southwestern Medical Foundation, the Mary Taxis Foundation, the Veterans Administration, and Grants CA23115, CA18132, and CA 27191 from the National Cancer Institute, U.S. Public Health Service.

The authors express their appreciation to Suellen Hill, R.N., for her help and assistance. Cecil Thompson, Ph.D., kindly performed the serum and CSF assays for evaluating the cis-platinum concentrations.

This chapter is an updated and expanded version of a previous communication (32).

References

1. Allen JC, Nisselbaum J, Epstein F, Rosen G, Schwartz MK: Alphafetoprotein and human chorionic gonadotropin determination in cerebrospinal fluid. *J Neurosurg* 51:368–374, 1979.
2. Bauer KA, Skarin AT, Balikian JP, Garnick MB, Rosenthal DS, Canellos GP: Pulmonary complications associated with combination chemotherapy programs containing bleomycin. *Am J Med* 74:557, 1983.
3. Benjamin RS, Wiernik PH, Bachur NR: Adriamycin chemotherapy—efficacy, safety, and pharmacologic basis of an intermittent single high-dosage schedule. *Cancer* 33:19–27, 1974.
4. Borden IV S, Weber AL, Toch R, Wang CC: Pineal germinoma. *Am J Dis Child* 126:214–216, 1973.
5. Brooks WH, Markesbery WR, Gupta GD, Roszman TL: Relationship of lymphocyte invasion and survival of brain tumor patients. *Ann Neurol* 4:219–224, 1978.
6. Burger PC, Mahaley MS, Jr, Dudka L, Vogel FS: The morphologic effect of radiation administered therapeutically for intracranial gliomas: A postmortem study of 25 cases. *Cancer* 44:1256–1272, 1979.

7. Camins MB, Schlesinger EB: Treatment of tumours of the posterior part of the third ventricle and the pineal region: A long term follow-up. *Acta Neurochir* 40:131–143, 1978.

8. Cline MJ, Haskell CM. *Cancer Chemotherapy*, (ed 3). Philadelphia, W. B. Saunders Co., 1980, p. 79.

9. de Tribolet N, Barrelet L: Successful chemotherapy of pinealoma. *Lancet* 2:1228–1229, 1977.

10. DiStefano A, Yap HY, Hortobagyi GN, Blumenschein GR: The natural history of breast cancer patients with brain metastases. *Cancer* 44:1913–1918, 1979.

11. Edelson RL, Hearing VJ, Dellon AJ, et al: Differentiation between B cells, T cells, and histiocytes in melanocytic lesions: Primary and metastatic melanoma and halo and giant pigmented nevi. *Clin Immunol Immunopathol* 4:557–568, 1975.

12. Einhorn LH, Donohue JP: Improved chemotherapy in disseminated testicular cancer. *J Urol* 117:65–69, 1977.

13. Einhorn LH: Combination chemotherapy of disseminated testicular carcinoma with *cis*-diammine-dichloroplatinum, vinblastine, and bleomycin (PVB): An update. *Proc Am Assoc Clin Oncol* 19:308, 1978.

14. Finkelman FD, Lipsky PE: Immunoglobulin secretion by human splenic lymphocytes in vitro: The effects of antibodies to IgM and IgD. *J Immunol* 120:1465–1472, 1978.

15. Frenkel EP, Smith RG, Ligler FS, Hernandez J, Himes JR, Sheehan R, Vitetta ES, Kettman JR, Uhr JW: Analysis and detection of B cell neoplasms. *Blood cells*, in press.

16. Friedman NB: Germinoma of the pineal. Its identity with germinoma ("seminoma") of the testis. *Cancer Res* 7:363–368, 1947.

17. Fröland SS, Natvig JB: Class, subclass and allelic exclusion of membrane-bound Ig of human B lymphocytes. *J Exp Med* 136:409–414, 1972.

18. Ginsberg S, Kirshner J, Reich S, Panasci L, Finkelstein T, Fandrich S, Fitzpatrick A, Shechtman L, Comis R: Systemic chemotherapy for a primary germ cell tumor of the brain: A pharmacokinetic study. *Cancer Treat Rep* 65(5–6):477, 1981.

19. Hamlin IME: Possible host resistance in carcinoma of the breast, a histological study. *Br J Cancer* 22:383–401, 1968.

20. Kaplan ME, Clark C: An improved rosetting assay for detection of human T lymphocytes. *J Immunol Methods* 5:131–135, 1974.

21. Kirshner JJ, Ginsberg SJ, Fitzpatrick AV, Comis RL: Treatment of a primary intracranial germ cell tumor with systemic chemotherapy. *Med Ped Oncol* 9:361–365, 1981.

22. Levy R, Warnke R, Dorfman RF, Haimovich J: The monoclonality of human B-cell lymphomas. *J Exp Med* 145:1014–1028, 1977.

23. Ligler FS, Smith RG, Kettman JR, Hernandex J, Himes JB, Vitetta ES, Uhr JW, Frenkel EP: Detection of tumor cells in the peripheral blood of nonleukemic patients with B cell lymphoma: Analysis of "clonal excess." *Blood*, in press.

24. Ligler FS, Vitetta ES, Smith RG, Himes JB, Uhr JW, Frenkel EP, Kettman JR: An immunologic approach for the detection of tumor cells in the peripheral blood of patients with malignant lymphoma: Implications for the diagnosis of minimal disease. *J Immunol* 123:1123–1126, 1979.

25. Martins AN, Johnston JS, Henry JM, Stoffel TJ, Chiro GD: Delayed radiation necrosis of the brain. *J Neurosurg* 47:336–345, 1977.

26. Neuwelt EA, Specht HD, Howieson J, Haines JE, Bennett MJ, Hill SA, Frenkel EP: Osmotic blood-brain barrier modification: Clinical documentation by enhanced CT scanning and/or radionuclide brain scanning. *Am J Neuroradiol* 4:907–913, 1983.

27. Neuwelt EA, Frenkel E: Is there a therapeutic role for blood brain barrier disruption? *Ann Intern Med* 93:135–137, 1980.

28. Neuwelt EA, Smith RG: Presence of lymphocyte membrane surface markers on "small cells" in a pineal germinoma. *Ann Neurol* 6:133–136, 1979.

29. Neuwelt EA, Glasberg M, Frenkel E, Clark WK: Malignant pineal region tumors: A clinico-pathological study. *J Neurosurg* 51:597–607, 1979.

30. Neuwelt EA, Clark WK: Unique aspects of central nervous system immunology. *Neurosurgery* 3:419–430, 1978.

31. Neuwelt EA, Maravilla KR, Frenkel EP, Barnett P, Hill S, Morse RJ: Use of enhanced computerized tomography to evaluate osmotic blood-brain barrier disruption. *Neurosurgery* 6:49–56, 1980.

32. Neuwelt EA, Frenkel EP, Smith RG: Supra-sellar germinomas (ectopic pinealomas): Aspects of immunologic characterization and successful chemotherapeutic responses in recurrent disease. *Neurosurgery* 7:352–358, 1980.

33. Neuwelt EA, Balaban E, Diehl J, Hill S, Frenkel E: Successful treatment of primary central nervous system lymphomas with chemotherapy after osmotic blood-brain barrier opening. *Neurosurgery* 12:662–671, 1983.

34. Neuwelt EA: Treatment of central nervous system neoplasms. In Rosenberg RN (ed): *The Treatment of Neurological Diseases*. New York, Spectrum Publications, 1979, pp 205–229.

35. Neuwelt EA, Clark WK: *Clinical Aspects of Neuroimmunology*. Baltimore, Williams & Wilkins, 1978, pp 93–94.

36. Nisonoff A, Wissler FC, Lipman LN, Woernley DL: Separation of univalent fragments from bivalent rabbit antibody molecule by reduction of disulfide bonds. *Arch Biochem Biophys* 89:230–244, 1960.

37. Nugent JL, Bunn PA, Jr, Matthews MJ, Ihde DC, Cohen MH, Gazdar A, Minna JD: CNS metastases in small cell bronchogenic carcinoma: Increasing frequency and changing pattern with lengthening survival. *Cancer* 44:1885–1893, 1979.

38. Onoyama Y, Abe M, Takahashi M, Yabumoto E, Sakamoto T: Radiation therapy of brain tumors in children. *Radiology* 115:687–693, 1975.

39. Palma L, DiLorenzo N, Guidetti B: Lymphocytic infiltrates in primary glioblastomas and recidivous gliomas: Incidence, fate, and relevance to prognosis in 228 operated cases. *J Neurosurg* 49:854–861, 1978.

40. Rapoport SI: *Blood-Brain Barrier in Physiology and Medicine*. New York, Raven Press, 1976, pp 77–78.

41. Rozencweig M, von Hoff DD, Slavik M, Muggia

FM: *Cis*-diamminedichloroplatinum (II): A new anticancer drug. *Ann Intern Med* 86:803–812, 1977.

42. Siegal T, Pfeffer MR, Catane R, Sulkes A, Gomori MJ, Fuks Z: Successful chemotherapy of recurrent intracranial germinoma with spinal metastases. *Neurology* 33:631–633, 1983.

43. Stavrou D, Anzil AP, Wiedenback W, et al: Immunofluorescence study of lymphocytic infiltration in gliomas. Identification of T-lymphocytes. *J Neurol Sci* 33:275–282, 1977.

44. Tottori K, Takahasi T, Hanaoka J, Sato Y, Takeuchi S: Approach to the early diagnosis of brain metastasis by the serum/CSF HCG and B-HCG ratio in patients with choriocarcinoma. In *Proceedings of the 38th Annual Meeting of the Japanese Cancer Association*, Tokyo, Japan, Sept. 1979, p 321, Tokyo, Japanese Cancer Association, 1979 (abstract).

45. Williams SD, Einhorn LH: Brain metastases in disseminated germinal neoplasms. *Cancer* 44:1514–1516, 1979.

46. Williams SD, Turner S, Loehrer PJ, Einhorn LH: Testicular cancer: Results of re-induction therapy. *Proc Am Soc Clin Oncol* 2:137, 1983.

CHAPTER 20

Suprasellar Germinomas

RICHARD P. MOSER, M.D.

INTRODUCTION

Primary intracranial germinomas may arise in the pineal gland, the suprasellar region, the basal ganglia, and the cerebral hemispheres (11, 16). The most common site is the pineal region, where direct extension into the suprasellar space can, on occasion, be documented radiographically. The incidence of isolated suprasellar germinomas varies in different series from 14 to 30% of intracranial germ cell tumors (2, 10, 15, 18, 20). No definite sex predominance has been noted and the tumors are generally diagnosed within the first three decades of life. Outside of the oriental population, these tumors occur with even greater rarity.

PATHOLOGY

Germinomas presenting in the suprasellar region are identical to the other primary intracranial germinomas. They share the same histological features as the pineal germinoma, gonadal seminoma, and ovarian dysgerminoma (5). The conflicting terminology for this neoplasm has created considerable confusion. The descriptive term of ectopic pinealoma, which has been used in reference to suprasellar germinomas, should be abandoned. Intracranial germ cell tumors should not be placed in the pineal category, but rather described in terms of the location in which they are found.

The suprasellar germinoma typically arises in the floor of the third ventricle and the pituitary stalk. They locally invade the hypothalamus, optic chiasm, and adjacent structures. We have seen one suprasellar germinoma initially present as an intrasellar mass, and only later was the suprasellar extension noted. They are macroscopically poorly defined and diffusely infiltrating. The microscopic histology is that of the testicular seminoma. Two distinct cell types are found, without evidence for an intermediate transitional form. Large polygonal cells with clear cytoplasm and frequent mitosis are seen surrounded by a stroma containing small cells with deeply basophilic nuclei, scant cytoplasm, and immunologic surface markers characteristic of lymphocytes.

Bloom (1) in his review of pineal and suprasellar tumors found only 69 of 576 cases (10%) where CSF seeding was documented. If only germinomas are reviewed, the reported incidence of CSF spread varies from 18 (21) to 85% (20). Sung and associates (18) showed a 10% incidence of seeding of pineal germinomas and a 33% incidence with suprasellar germinomas. It is reasonable to conclude that leptomeningeal involvement can be expected with greater frequency in suprasellar germinomas.

CLINICAL PRESENTATION

Schmidek (17) in his earlier monograph reviewed a classification system which categorized the clinical presentation on the basis of tumor origin and extension of growth within the suprasellar region. The most common initial symptom is that of diabetes insipidus which occurred first in 50% of the cases reported by Takeuchi and associates (19). Eventually, 83% of the patients went on to develop diabetes insipidus at some point in their disease. Visual disturbances occurred in only 17% initially, although as a later manifestation it was present in 78%. The diabetes insipidus itself may predate the onset of other signs and symptoms by several years. Obstruction of the third ventricle will result in hydrocephalus. Signs of increased intracranial pressure were present in only 11%, although 50% of the patients would at some time complain of headaches. Frank growth retardation and hypogonadism were noted in only a minority, although many patients would exhibit endocrine dysfunction with some degree of hormonal deficiency.

DIAGNOSTIC PROCEDURES

Computerized tomography has been the most helpful of diagnostic radiological procedures. The tumors generally appear as a homogenous isodense or slightly hyperdense lesion on non-contrast studies. With contrast infusion the tumor will enhance uniformly, although there is nothing pathognomonic in its apperance. Skull X-rays may show clinoid erosion, but they are frequently normal in the absence of hydrocephalus or involvement of the sella turcica directly. Calcification is not characteristic of the suprasellar germinoma, although its presence does not exclude the diagnosis. Carotid angiography may reveal tumor vascularity or a suprasellar mass with elevation of the A_1 segment of the anterior cerebral arteries. Contrast ventriculography will frequently show an anterior third ventricular-filling defect. In conclusion, while the radiological studies may be suggestive of a suprasellar germinoma, the definitive diagnosis is not possible.

Where feasible, CSF cytology should be obtained. Subarachnoid seeding occurs more commonly with the suprasellar lesions (3, 18). A positive cytology would obviate the need for diagnostic surgical intervention. Biochemical tumor markers, including alpha-fetoprotein and human chorionic gonadotropin are not generally characteristic of germinomas. Thus, in the absence of a positive cytology, a surgical procedure for a tissue diagnosis is indicated.

SURGICAL MANAGEMENT

The neurosurgeon's role in the management of suprasellar germinomas is to provide: (1) a definitive tissue diagnosis, (2) decompression of compromised neural structures, and (3) CSF shunting should symptomatic hydrocephalus be present. The numerous pathological lesions in the suprasellar region including craniopharyngiomas, gliomas, histiocytosis X, pituitary adenomas, meningiomas, and hamartomas demand either direct surgical exploration or stereotactic biopsy followed by exploration should an operable lesion be found.

Direct surgical exploration may be the procedure of choice for those suprasellar lesions where decompression of the tumor mass is indicated to relieve pressure causing impairment of vital neural functions. Tumors presenting in the suprasellar cistern, extrinsic to the hypothalamus, can be approached subfrontally or via the pterion depending on the particular features of the tumor and the preference of the surgeon. Intraventricular lesions, especially those associated with hydrocephalus, can be approached through a transcortical-transventricular route or via a

transcallosal section. A tumor mass extending into the sella may be exposed by a transsphenoidal procedure. Whenever possible, it is important to obtain a biopsy of the suspected tumor rather than to merely confirm the presence of a swollen optic chiasm or distorted hypothalamic surface.

In those patients where the tumor appears to be intra-axial and locally invasive in the hypothalamus, CT/stereotactic biopsy can be used with a a high degree of accuracy and little morbidity. Where a germinoma or glioma is suspected, sterotactic biopsy would appear to be the procedure of choice. The technical aspects of CT stereotaxis have been discussed elsewhere in this volume (see Chapter 12). The stereotactic procedure can be done using a local anesthesia and generally requires no more than a 48-hr hospital stay. Figure 20.1 illustrates the CT appearance of a suprasellar germinoma. The sterotactic device is secured to the head during the CT scan in order for the tumor coordinates to be determined. This particular patient had undergone a previous subfrontal craniotomy which on visual inspection of the suprasellar region failed to reveal any obvious pathology. A definitive tissue diagnosis was obtained as a result of the stereotactic biopsy, and subsequent radiation therapy resulted in the complete disappearance of the enhancing mass. There were no complications associated with the biopsy and the patient was discharged on the following day.

The demonstrable radiosensitivity of the suprasellar germinomas should compel the neurosurgeon at the time of open surgical exploration to limit the surgical resection to easily removable tumor. Decompression of the optic apparatus should be done if compromised by the tumor mass, and the tumor debulking may obviate the need for shunting in cases where obstructive hydrocephalus is present. Aggressive tumor resection of locally infiltrated hypothalamic tissue must be avoided. Irradiation will be more effective and of much less risk for the vast majority of suprasellar germinomas.

CSF shunting may be necessary in a few cases where ventricular obstruction dominates the clinical presentation. Tumor seeding through the shunt has been well documented, and therefore a filter should be included in the shunt device (7). Since the tumor will shrink rapidly in the radiosensitive cases, the shunt will not be needed on a long-term basis. Shunting may be the only surgical procedure necessary if CSF cytology is definitive.

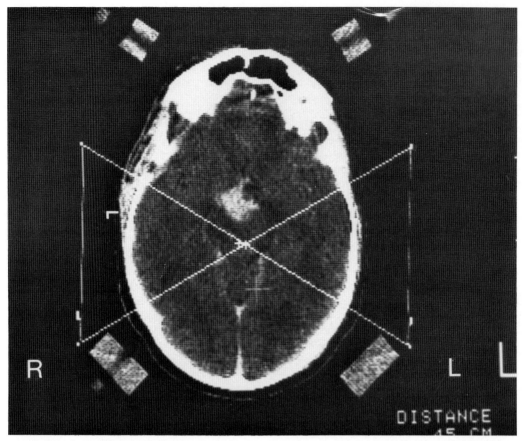

Figure 20.1. CT/stereotactic scan for biopsy of a suprasellar germinoma in a 29-yr-old male who had previously undergone a negative subfrontal exploration.

RADIATION THERAPY

Suprasellar germinomas, along with the other midline intracranial germinomas, are in general very radiosensitive and therefore irradiation should be considered the treatment of choice (1, 18). The major controversy in the use of radiation therapy centers on the extent of the radiation field to be used. Some authors have advocated craniospinal irradiation because of the incidence of leptomeningeal seeding, especially associated with suprasellar germinomas (1, 18). Others have suggested that spinal irradiation should be given only if cytological or radiological evidence of tumor seeding is present (15, 22). The role of surgery in promoting dissemination has not been established (9, 13, 23).

CHEMOTHERAPY

While whole cranial irradiation probably represents the treatment of choice (15, 20), germ cell tumors elsewhere in the body have been found to be quite sensitive to combination chemotherapy (12). Complete remission and possible cures have been documented in the literature for systemic germ cell tumors. Drug penetration into the intracranial germ cell tumors has been demonstrated (4, 6). Concern about the blood-brain barrier should not significantly influence the drug selection. The combination chemotherapy found most effective for the testicular seminoma or ovarian dysgerminoma should be considered for recurrent intracranial germinomas following initial radiation therapy (14). The biopsy material can be submitted for tissue culture and *in vitro* chemosensitivity assay in order to further select the most favorable drug regimen. Young children who are more adversely affected by the use or irradiation might be considered for chemotherapy as the primary treatment. One can assume, given the encouraging results seen with the treatment of systemic germ cell tumors, that chemotherapy for similar intracranial disease will be more aggressively applied in the future (14). The chemotherapy of CNS germ cell tumors is also discussd in the Chapters 6, 19, and 21.

CLINICAL COURSE

The prognosis for patients with suprasellar germinoma appears to differ widely between various authors. Hoffman (8) reported a dismal 25% survival in his series of five patients and as a result is quite pessimistic about the survival in these patients. Sano (16), however, showed an 82% survival in 11 patients, and Takeuchi et al (19), in 18 patients had a 66% survival. In all of these studies, a definitive diagnosis was made on the basis of a biopsy or CSF cytology.

The dramatically better survival statistics are seen with the Japanese series where the incidence is higher and the biologicl sensitivity of the tumor may make it more amenable to radiation therapy. To the extent that it was possible to compare, no substantial differences could be appreciated among these four series in terms of the tumor histology, patient's age, surgical procedures, or the irradiation techniques.

SUMMARY

Suprasellar germinomas are rare in the nonoriental population. The variety of possible pathological lesions, both neoplastic and nonneoplastic, benign and malignant, necessitate a definitive tissue diagnosis whenever possible. Lesions appearing to be predominately extraaxial, compressing the optic apparatus or compromising ventricular outflow are best explored and resected grossly. Lesions appearing to be intra-axial and locally invasive in the diencephalon are best biopsied using a CT/stereotactic technique. Most suprasellar germinomas would fall into the latter group. A positive CSF cytology would obviate the need for surgical intervention unless decompression were indicated to salvage neurological function.

Germinomas can be expected to respond to irradiation with doses up to 50 gray (5000 rad). Some experts have recommended prophylactic craniospinal irradiation because of the frequency of CSF seeding. Others would reserve this for patients with documented spread. Adjuvant chemotherapy has not been subjected to clinical trial due to the rarity of this tumor. Salvage chemotherapy based on the responsiveness of this tumor type systemically has been used with some encouraging initial results (14).

Further progress with combination chemotherapy and *in vitro* drug selection can be expected as more experience is gained with these modalities.

References

1. Bloom HJG: Primary intracranial germ cell tumors. *Clin Oncol* 2:233–257, 1983.
2. Chang CG, Kageyama N, Kobayashi T, Yoshida J, Negoro M: Pineal tumors: Clinical diagnosis, with special emphasis on the significance of pineal calcification. *Neurosurgery* 8:656–668, 1981.
3. Dayan AD, Marshall AHE, Miller AA, Pick FJ, Rankin NE: Atypical teratomas of the pineal and hypothalamus. *J Pathol* 92:1–28, 1966.
4. Feun LG, Samson MK, Stephens RL: Vinblastine, bleomycin, cis-diammine-dichloroplatinum in disseminated extragonadal germ cell tumors. *Cancer* 45:2543–2549, 1980.
5. Friedman NB: Cerminoma of the pineal. Its identity with germinoma ("seminoma") of the testis. *Cancer Res* 7:363–368, 1947.
6. Gensberg S, Kirshner J, Reich S, Panasci L, Finkelstein T, Fandrich S, Fitzpatrick A, Shechtman L, Comis R: Systemic chemotherapy for a primary germ cell tumor of the brain : A pharmacokinetic study. *Cancer Treat Rep* 65:477–483, 1981.
7. Haimovic IC, Sharer L, Hyman RA, Beresford R: Metastasis of intracranial germinoma through a ventriculoperitoneal shunt. *Cancer* 48:1033–1036, 1981.
8. Hoffman HJ: Suprasellar Germinomas. In *Pediatric Neurosurgery: Surgery of the Developing Nervous System.* New York, Grune and Stratton, 1982, pp 487–491.
9. Jenkin RDT, Simpson WJK, Keen CW: Pineal and suprasellar germinomas. *J Neurosurg* 48:99–107, 1978.
10. Kageyama N, Belsky R: Ectopic pinealoma in the chiasmal region. *Neurology* 11:318–327, 1961.
11. Kobayashi T, Kageyama N, Kida, Yoshida J, Shibuya N, Okamura K: Unilateral germinomas involving the basal ganglia and thalamus. *J Neurosurg* 55:55–62, 1981.
12. Logothetis CJ, Samuels ML, Trindade A: The management of brain metastases in germ cell tumors. *Cancer* 49:12–18, 1982.
13. Neuwelt EA, Galsberg M, Frenkel E, Clark WK: Malignant pineal region tumors. *J Neurosurg* 51:597–607, 1979.
14. Neuwelt EA, Frenkel EP, Smith RG: Suprasellar germinomas (ectopic pinealomas): Aspects of immunologic characterization and successful chemotherapeutic responses in recurrent disease. *Neurosurgery* 7:352–358, 1980.
15. Salazar OM, Castro-Vita H, Bakos RS, Feldstein ML, Keller B, Rubin P: Radiation therapy for tumors of the pineal region. *Int J Radiat Oncol Biol Phys* 5:491–499, 1979.
16. Sano K: Diagnosis and treatment of tumors in the pineal region. *Acta Neurochir* 34:153–157, 1976.
17. Schmidek HH: Suprasellar germinomas (ectopic pinealomas). In Schmidek H (ed): *Pineal Tumors.* New York, Masson (USA), 1977, pp 115–126.
18. Sung D, Harisiadis L, Chang CH: Midline pineal tumors and suprasellar germinomas: Highly cur-

able by radiation. *Radiology* 128:745–751, 1978.

19. Takeuchi J, Handa H, Nagata I: Suprasellar germinoma. *J Neurosurg* 49:41–48, 1978.

20. Ueki K, Tanaka R: Treatments and prognoses of pineal tumors—experience of 110 cases. *Neurol Med Chir* 20:1–26, 1980.

21. Waga S, Handa H, Yamashita J: Intracranial germinomas: Treatment and results. *Surg Neurol* 11:167–172, 1979.

22. Wara WM, Jenkin RDT, Evans A, Ertel I, Hittle R, Ortega J, Wilson CB, Hammond D: Tumors of the pineal and suprasellar region: Childrens cancer study group treatment results 1960–1975. *Cancer* 43:698–701, 1979.

23. Wood JH, Zimmerman RA, Bruce DA, Bilaniuk LT, Norris DG, Schut L: Assessment and management of pineal-region and related tumors. *Surg Neurol* 16:192–210, 1981.

CHAPTER 21

Brain Metastases with Extraneural Germ Cell Tumors: Incidence, Characteristics, and Treatment

BENTON M. WHEELER, M.D., STEPHEN D. WILLIAMS, M.D., and
LAWRENCE H. EINHORN, M.D.

INTRODUCTION

Brain metastases are an important problem for clinicians treating disseminated germ cell tumors. Solid parenchymal lesions are the most common neurological complication found. Although they occur infrequently, they are associated with a poor prognosis in the majority of patients in whom they occur. Long-term survivors have been rare enough. Because most patients with germ cell tumors are young with their lives and working potential ahead, the treatment of disseminated germ cell tumors is of great importance and the management of their complications deserves attention.

Extraneural germ cell tumors originate in the testis, ovary, and extragonadal sites. These tumors share common histological subtypes and, to some extent, a common clinical course and response to treatment. Germ cell neoplasms represent a very aggressive malignancy which spread rapidly by both lymphatic and hematogenous routes. Clearly a propensity for CNS metastases exists. The incidence of CNS metastases from extraneural germ cell tumors varies with the site of origin. In testis cancer, the incidence ranges from 6 to 40% (7, 21, 27, 34, 43, 47). Male extragonadal germ cell tumors may develop CNS disease more frequently than their testicular counterparts, as high as 40% in one series (26, 27). Female ovarian and extragonadal germ cell tumors are uncommon malignancies and CNS spread is unusual.

Testicular cancer makes up the bulk of extraneural germ cell tumors. Although testis cancer is uncommon, accounting for less than 1% of all cancers estimated for 1984, it is one of the most common solid tumors among men in the 15 to 35 yr age group with 5600 new cases predicted (36). Testis cancer usually presents with a scrotal mass, although patients may present with signs and symptoms of systemic disease. Fifteen to twenty percent of patients have disseminated disease at initial diagnosis. The diagnosis is usually made by high inguinal orchiectomy. Serial serum tumor markers, namely AFP and β-subunit of human chorionic gonadotropin (HCG), accurately reflect the clinical course and response to treatment. At least one tumor marker is elevated in 75 to 94% of patients with germ cell tumors (8, 21, 30). Histologically, testicular cancer can be classified as seminoma, embryonal carcinoma, teratoma, teratocarcinoma, choriocarcinoma, mixed germ cell tumor, or endodermal sinus tumor. For the clinician, the classification can be simplified into either pure seminoma or nonseminoma. This distinction is critical because the management of seminomatous and nonseminomatous tumors differs greatly. Seminoma is exquisitely radiosensitive and early-stage disease can be cured with radiotherapy alone in 90 to 95% of patients. Patients with "pure seminoma" diagnosed by orchiectomy who have an elevated serum AFP level have nonseminomatous elements present elsewhere and should be treated as their nonseminomatous counterparts. Early-stage nonseminomatous disease is often curable by surgery. Disseminated disease of any histologic type is treated with chemotherapy. Sixty-five to 75% of patients with disseminated disease can expect to be cured with modern cisplatin-based combination chemotherapy (8–10, 48).

Ovarian germ cell tumor (OGCT) occurs predominantly in young women in the second and third decade of life. These tumors are rare, accounting for only 5% of the 18,300 estimated new cases of ovarian cancer for 1984 (36). They typically present with abdominal pain or distention, abnormal vaginal bleeding, or an asymptomatic abdominal mass. At initial diagnosis, most are found confined to the ovary and only 3 to 10% are bilateral. Histologically, OGCT is classified as dysgerminoma, endodermal sinus tumor, embryonal carcinoma, immature teratoma, and mixed germ cell tumor. Dysgerminoma, like its testicular analogue, the seminoma, is highly radiosensitive with a 90 to 95% cure rate in early-stage disease using radiotherapy following surgery. OGCT other than pure dysgerminoma displays a more aggressive nature. Surgery alone or with radiotherapy offers little hope of long-term survival (6, 14, 24, 25, 31). Combination chemotherapy used adjuvantly or following maximal debulking surgery greatly improves results. In three studies using vincristine, actinomycin D, and cyclophosphamide (VAC), 43 of 64 (67%) patients remained disease free with median follow-up well over 2 yr (6, 14, 38). At Memorial, 17 patients, 14 with advanced disease, were treated with combination chemotherapy including vinblastine, actinomycin D, bleomycin, and cisplatin (VAB II-IV), 8 (47%) of whom are disease free with median follow-up of 17 months (4). CNS metastases have been noted in only one patient, who died with widely disseminated disease (4).

Gestational trophoblastic disease (GTD) is a rare tumor of the placenta that follows 1 in 50,000 term pregnancies and 1 in 30 hydatidiform moles. These tumors are known for their rapid growth and wide hematogenous dissemination as well as their remarkable response to chemotherapy. Serum HCG levels have been well documented to correlate accurately with the clinical course. The histologic subtype is choriocarcinoma although it differs from ovarian choriocarcinoma in both clinical course and response to treatment. Poor prognostic factors in GTD include CNS or liver metastases, initial serum HCG > 42,000 or urinary HCG > 100,000, duration of symptoms for greater than 4 months, inadequate response to prior chemotherapy and metastatic disease following term pregnancy (17, 29). Complete remissions with chemotherapy are lower in patients with poor risk factors compared to patients without those factors (66% vs 100%) (18).

The overall incidence of brain metastases in GTD varies from 3 to 28% but probably is between 5 and 10% in patients receiving modern chemotherapy. Three large studies have recently been reported (2, 19, 45) showing that roughly one-half of the patients presented with CNS disease at initial diagnosis (early CNS disease) and half developed brain metastases while on chemotherapy or at subsequent relapse (late CNS disease). The development of CNS disease and overall prognosis was related to extent of systemic disease and to responsiveness to initial chemotherapy. All patients with CNS disease had widely metastatic disease and virtually all had multiple pulmonary nodules. Patients with late CNS disease had refractory systemic disease which ultimately determined survival. Weed et al (45) found 23 patients with CNS metastases in over 400 patients with malignant GTD. Treatment consisted of systemic chemotherapy (usually a triple drug regimen) and whole brain irradiation (WBI); only one patient received primary intrathecal chemotherapy. Overall, 10 of 23 (43%) were long-term survivors with follow-up of 27 to 144 months, 7 out of 11 (64%) in the early CNS disease group and 3 out of 12 (25%) who developed late CNS relapse. Sixty-nine cases of brain metastases were found among 782 patients (8.8%) treated at Charing Cross Hospital (2). CSF to serum HCG ratios were measured in 46 patients before initial treatment. The ratio was abnormal (>1.7%) in 38 (83%) and normal in 8 (17%). Fourteen patients were found to have an abnormal ratio before any other clinical parameter of CNS disease became evident. All patients received systemic and intrathecal chemotherapy (3). Systemic treatment generally included intermediate to high dose methotrexate. Only 14 patients (20%) received WBI which was usually employed only when there was evidence of drug resistance. Since 1974, 80% of patients with early CNS disease and 25% with late CNS disease remain alive. Thus, cranial irradiation and intrathecal chemotherapy seem to be equally efficacious. The role of neurosurgery in these two series was small and was generally limited to surgical decompression, primarily because of the increased risk of hemorrhage associated with choriocarcinoma.

Extragonadal germ cell tumor (EGCT) arises most commonly in the anterior mediastinum, retroperitoneum, and pineal gland, with rare occurrences in other area (20, 28, 33, 37, 41). Although the overall incidence of EGCT is not known, the incidence among males with germ cell tumors ranges from 2.9 to 13% (10, 21, 27, 30). It is possible that many patients are labeled as malignancy of unknown primary and are not recognized as having a germ cell tumor. Female EGCT is thought to be very rare (28). The pathogenesis of EGCT can be explained in two ways. Primordial germ cells originating in the yolk sac migrate along the urogenital ridge (which extends from the sixth cervical to the second sacral vertebrae during embryonic development) to the primitive gonadal ridge (49, 50). Germ cells which fail to migrate into the gonadal ridge or to undergo physiologic dissolution in displaced locations, thus creating germ cell remnants, account for the midline occurrence in the vast majority of EGCT. Another theory is that totipotential cells, the precursors of germ cells, become dislodged or migrate during embryogenesis, explaining the rare occurrence in non-midline sites (33). Malignant transformation may occur with increased frequency in these extragonadal sites similar to that observed in the cryptorchid testis (5, 40).

The most frequent symptoms of primary mediastinal germ cell tumor are cough, chest pain, and dyspnea. Primary retroperitoneal germ cell tumor often presents with abdominal low back pain or palpable abdominal mass. These tumors can attain a very large size before initial detection and most patients present with advanced disease at initial diagnosis (11, 12, 15, 16, 28). Histologically, these tumors are identical to those arising in the testis and ovary. However, the pathologic specimen may be interpreted as "poorly differentiated adenocarcinoma" or "malignant neoplasm—primary unknown." The diagnosis of EGCT should be considered, especially in patients in the 20 to 50 yr age group with tumor originating in midline structures because of the potential curability by either radiotherapy or chemotherapy (32). Elevated serum AFP or HCG or positive tissue immunoperoxidase stains for AFP or HCG help confirm the diagnosis and should be performed in all patients.

Staging and treatment of EGCT should parallel that of their testicular counterpart. Orchiectomy or blind testis biopsy is not indicated in patients with normal testes on palpation (12, 16, 28, 41). Mediastinal and retroperitoneal seminoma can be treated with radiotherapy with excellent results (11). Nonseminomatous tumors or disseminated seminoma is treated with combination chemotherapy. Initial studies in EGCT were not encouraging. The poor results compared to disseminated testis cancer were felt to be secondary to the greater tumor bulk found in patients with EGCT at initial diagnosis rather than an inherent biologic difference in virulence or response to treatment (11). Recent studies using intensive cisplatin containing combination chemotherapy and surgical resection of residual disease are more promising. Garnick et al (15) reported a 67% complete remission (CR) among 15 patients with EGCT but only 4 (27%) remained disease free with median follow-up of 40 months. Funes et al (13) treated 14 patients with mediastinal germ cell tumor, 6 (43%) achieving CR with no relapses at a median follow up of 16 months. Hainsworth et al (16) found 21 of 31 patients (68%) achieved CR, 19 (58%) of whom are disease free with median follow-up of 30 months. In the latter study, dosage reductions were allowed only for severe and prolonged myelosuppression or documented bacterial sepsis. Newlands et al (30) using a sequential combination regimen, achieved CR in seven of nine patients (78%), but median follow-up was only 16.5 months. These results are comparable to those reported in germ cell tumors of testicular origin that have a similar initial tumor burden. Mediastinal endodermal sinus tumor represents a particularly aggressive subgroup with only rare long-term survivors (26).

Because brain metastases develop most often in male germ cell tumors and are generally associated with a poor prognosis, we found it useful to review our data in men with disseminated germ cell tumors concerning the incidence of brain metastases, the characteristics of patients who develop CNS spread, their presentation, clinical course, and response to treatment.

MATERIALS AND METHODS

Between October 1974 and August 1983, 408 men with germ cell tumors began cisplatin-based combination chemotherapy at Indiana University. Patients referred to our hospital for relapse after receiving prior chemotherapy elsewhere were excluded. Nineteen patients were excluded because of incomplete records; enough information was available in the majority of these patients to exclude CNS disease. Therefore, 389 patients were available for analysis.

Patients were treated with cisplatin, vinblastine, and bleomycin (PVB), with or without adriamycin (PVBA), or cisplatin, VP-16, and bleomycin (BEP). No differences between these regimens in systemic response rates have been noted. The details of these regimens are available in other publications (8–10). In brief, patients were generally treated with four courses of chemotherapy. Patients who failed to achieve complete remission (CR) underwent surgical resection of residual disease if possible. More recently, if the surgical specimen revealed residual carcinoma, patients also received adjuvant chemotherapy postoperatively. Patients who had unresectable disease were placed on maintenance chemotherapy (most often single agent vinblastine) and subsequently underwent salvage chemotherapy (usually cisplatin and VP-16) when progression was noted. A variety of salvage regimens were used, however. Patients who relapsed following initial CR or who had no evidence of disease after surgery (surgical NED) and subsequently relapsed were treated with similar salvage regimens.

Histologic material from initial specimens was available in almost all patients. Rare patients were treated with compatible history, exam, and marker data only. Histologic material of brain metastases was not routinely available.

Patients with signs or symptoms of CNS involvement underwent radioisotope brain scans, computerized tomography, or both. These were not employed routinely in asymptomatic patients. Specific treatment of brain metastases consisted of radiotherapy or surgery followed by radiotherapy. Patients also regularly received steroids, most often dexamethasone, (16 mg/day) at the time of diagnosis or onset of symp-toms. Dexamethasone was continued throughout radiation therapy and was then tapered as tolerated. Anticonvulsants, primarily phenytoin, were also given for seizure prophylaxis. Three patients received adjuvant systemic chemotherapy after CNS tumor removal while in systemic CR. Systemic therapy was continued in other patients when indicated.

RESULTS

The records of these 389 patients with disseminated germ cell tumor undergoing chemotherapy (PVB, PVBA, or BEP) were reviewed. Overall, 24 patients (6.2%) developed brain metastases. If patients with less than 2 yr follow-up after starting chemotherapy are excluded (108 patients), 21 of 281 patients (7.5%) developed CNS disease. Table 21.1 defines the patient population according to study protocol, chemotherapy, dates of initial treatment, survival, and incidence of CNS metastases.

The sites of disease at initiation of chemotherapy and at diagnosis of CNS spread are listed in Table 21.2. All patients who developed brain metastases had advanced disease at onset of chemotherapy. All 24 patients had pulmonary involvement at diagnosis. Twenty also had retroperitoneal disease including six patients with concomitant liver metastases.

Brain metastases generally occurred in the setting of disseminated disease. Eighteen of 24 (75%) patients had extensive disease at the time

Table 21.1
Patient Population

Protocol & Study Dates[a]	No. Patients	Followup (Months)	Alive, NED (%)	Alive With Disease (%)	Dead (%)	Brain Metastases (%)
PVB 10/74-9/76	46	83–106	24 (52)	2 (4)	20 (44)	5 (10.9)
PVB (0.3) vs PVB (0.4) vs PVBA[b] 11/76-5/78	71	63–81	51 (72)	0 (0)	20 (28)	3 (4.2)
PVB vs PVBA 6/78-1/82	179	19–62 (Median = 41)	137 (77)	8 (4)	34 (19)	14 (7.8)
PVB (off protocol) 4/81-1/83	26	7–29 (Median = 18)	21 (81)	1 (4)	4 (15)	0 (0)
PVB vs BEP[c] 5/83-8/83	67	0–15 (Median = 9)	39 (74)	8 (15)	6 (11)	2 (3.8)
Total[c]	389		272 (73)	19 (5)	84 (22)	24 (6.2)

[a] See text for abbreviations.
[b] See Reference 9.
[c] Fourteen patients have not finished initial chemotherapy and are not included in percent figures.

Table 21.2
Extent of Disease in 24 Patients with Brain Metastases

Sites of Disease Outside CNS	At Onset of Chemotherapy No. Patients	At CNS Diagnosis No. Patients
Pulmonary	24	18
Advanced[a]	22	17
Abdominal[b]	20	11
Advanced[a]	13	8
Liver	6	6
Elevated markers only	0	1
None		5

[a] Advanced criteria are by Samuels' classification, see Reference 8.
[b] All patients with abdominal disease had concomitant pulmonary involvement.

Table 21.3
Response to Initial Chemotherapy

Response	CNS Disease at Diagnosis No. Patients (No. Alive)	Subsequent CNS Relapse No. Patients (No. Alive)
Complete remission	2 (2)	5 (2)
Partial remission	3 (3)	13 (2)
No response	1	0
Total	6 (5)	18 (4)

of presentation of CNS metastases, all of whom had pulmonary involvement. Eleven had pulmonary and retroperitoneal disease and six had additional liver disease. One patient developed CNS metastases within 1 month of undergoing surgical excision of residual carcinoma (surgically NED), but relapsed systemically 1 month after CNS disease was found. Only five patients were in complete remission at the time of diagnosis of CNS disease.

The response to initial chemotherapy is given in Table 21.3. Development of CNS metastases correlated with the absence of a complete response to initial chemotherapy. Of 18 patients who had CNS relapse subsequent to initial diagnosis, only five had achieved initial CR. Of these five patients, two received adjuvant systemic chemotherapy when CNS relapse occurred while still in systemic CR and both are alive

without disease; one remained in systemic CR and died of CNS disease; one patient relapsed systemically and achieved second CR with salvage chemotherapy but later died of CNS disease; and one patient relapsed and died of progressive systemic disease. Thirteen patients achieved only PR with initial treatment and 11 eventually died of progressive disease. Only two patients were salvaged with further chemotherapy and surgery, one of whom remains alive and disease free and one who later died of CNS disease alone.

Six patients (25%) presented with CNS disease at the time of diagnosis of disseminated disease. One patient had no response to therapy and died of progressive disease. Three patients had PR only, two of whom later died of progressive disease and one who was salvaged with further chemotherapy and surgery and remains disease free 17 months off all treatment. Two patients achieved CR. One remains alive without disease, off treatment at 26 months. The other patient relapsed systemically after 3 yr off treatment and remains alive on salvage chemotherapy.

The median interval from diagnosis of testicular cancer to diagnosis of CNS metastases was 8 months (range 0–9½ yr). Twenty (83%) occurred within 18 months. The median time to development of CNS disease after starting cisplatin chemotherapy was 4.5 months (range 0–22 months).

The presenting signs and symptoms of brain metastases and their frequency are listed in Table 21.4. Complaints were those commonly associated with an intracranial mass. Headache, seizures, and focal weakness were the most com-

Table 21.4
Signs and Symptoms of Brain Metastases in 24 Patients

Signs and Symptoms	No. Patients	%
Seizure	11	46
Headache	10	42
Focal weakness	8	33
Altered mental status	7	29
Paresthesia	5	21
Visual changes	4	17
Nausea or vomiting	4	17
Other[a]	11	
None	1	4

[a] Papilledema, 3; aphasia, 2; vertigo, 2; cranial nerve palsy, 1; and unknown, 1.

mon features but altered mental status was also frequent. Symptoms tended to occur subacutely and generally within a few days of diagnosis of CNS disease, although one patient developed symptoms 6 months before a brain scan showed a right frontoparietal lesion. All patients except one had symptoms referrable to the central nervous system at the time of diagnosis of brain metastases. This patient was asymptomatic when a head CT showed two right parietal metastases.

Four patients (17%) who developed brain metastases had extragonadal germ cell tumors, three of retroperitoneal origin and one from the anterior mediastinum. Although the incidence for the entire series is not known, there were 29 cases of EGCT among the most recent 343 consecutive patients (8.4%).

Histologic diagnosis was available in 376 of the 389 patients overall and in 21 of the 24 patients with brain metastases. Table 21.5 relates the histology of the initial specimens to the incidence of CNS disease. Only choriocarcinoma is associated with an increased risk of development of brain metastases. Additionally, of the three patients with CNS disease without histologic diagnosis, all had advanced disease and HCG above 100,000 and may have had choriocarcinoma. Thus, these results may not indicate the true incidence of brain metastases in choriocarcinoma. Histologic information on the CNS lesion was available in four patients. In three cases, this correlated with the primary tumor (all three embryonal), while the fourth case could be described only as poorly differentiated carcinoma (the original orchiectomy specimen revealed embryonal carcinoma). Only one patient developed documented leptomeningeal disease.

The diagnosis of brain metastases was usually easily confirmed by computerized tomography (Figs. 21.1 and 21.2) or radionuclide brain scanning or both. CT scans were positive in 18 of 19 patients (95%) with CNS disease. The single false negative became positive 4 days later on repeat scan done for progressive symptoms. Brain scans never provided additional information when combined with CT scans and occasionally gave false results.

Ten patients who developed subsequent CNS relapse had prior scans in the absence of CNS symptoms 2 to 26 months (median, 5 months) before documentation of brain metastases; all were negative. One patient had an equivocal CT scan performed in March 1977 for choreoathetoid movements, which revealed a poorly visualized right parietal lucency without enhancement that was not thought to be clinically significant. A brain scan done in July 1977 for seizures was normal. He received no treatment except anticonvulsants. Severe headaches were noted in January 1978 when a brain scan showed a large right frontoparietal lesion. Thus, CNS disease may have been present for several months before radiologic confirmation.

Table 21.6 shows the treatment given and survival data according to treatment modality. Three patients received only steroids. They were critically ill at diagnosis and as expected, had a short survival.

Seventeen patients received radiation therapy as the only specific treatment for brain metastases. Seven patients were treated with 5000 rad in 25 fractions over 5 weeks and six patients received 3000 to 3300 rad in 300-rad fractions. There were no apparent differences in number of CNS lesions or status of systemic disease between patients selected for either 5000- or 3000-rad WBI. Four patients received other dosage schedules.

Among the seven patients treated with 5000-rad WBI (Fig. 21.2), three remain alive and without evidence of disease at 27+, 49+, 69+ months later. The median survival was 13 months after diagnosis of CNS disease. Of six patients treated with 3000 to 3300 rad, five patients died with a median survival of 4.5 months and one patient remains alive with systemic disease at 46 months. This patient relapsed systemically 41 months after initial diagnosis and remains alive on salvage chemotherapy without evidence of recurrent CNS dis-

Table 21.5
Incidence of Brain Metastases Related to Cell Type

Histology	No. Patients All Studies	No. Patients Brain Metastases (%)
Embryonal	201	13 (6.5)
Teratocarcinoma	76	2 (2.6)
Teratoma	23	1 (4.3)
Choriocarcinoma	23	4 (17.4)
Yolk Sac	7	0
Seminoma	46	1 (2.2)
Not available	13	3
Total	389	24

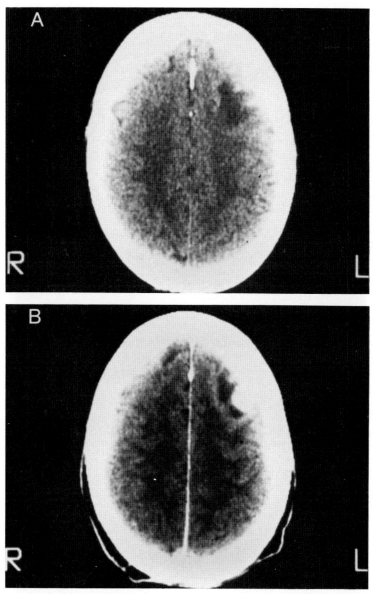

Figure 21.1. Solitary left frontoparietal metastases from testicular cancer. *A*, without contrast; *B*, with contrast.

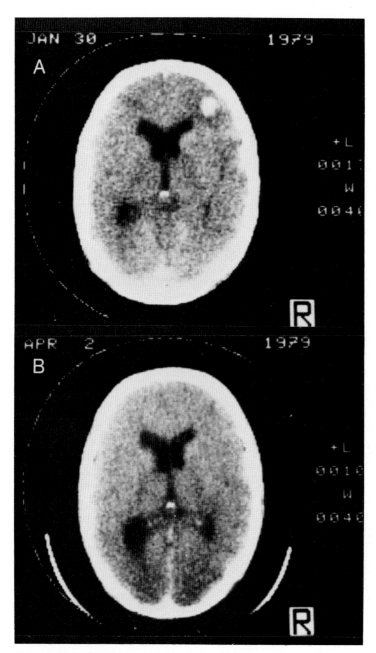

Figure 21.2. Solitary right frontal metastasis from testicular cancer. *A*, at diagnosis; *B*, after treatment with 5000-rad WBI. Note almost complete response.

Table 21.6
Treatment of Brain Metastases

Treatment	No. Patients	No. Brain Metastases[a]	Status of Systemic Disease[b]	Alive	Dead	Survival in Months Median (Range)
None	3	3S	1 CR, 1 DX, 1 PD	0	3	0, 0, 2
WBI, total	17	7S, 9M, 1?	1 CR, 5 DX, 11 PD	5	12	5 (0–69+)
5000 rad	7	2S, 5M	1 CR, 3DX, 3PD	3	4	13 (2–69+)
3000–3300 rad	6	2S, 4M	2 DX, 4 PD	1[c]	5	4.5 (1–46+)
Other	4	3S, 1?	4 PD	1[c]	3	0, 1, 1+, 2
Surgery + WBI	4	3S, 1M	3 CR, 1 PR	2	2[d]	16 (5–45+)
3000–5000 rad					Overall	5.0 (0–69+)

[a] S, solitary; M, multiple; ?, clinical only.
[b] CR, complete remission; PR, partial remission; PD, progressive disease; DX, CNS disease at initial diagnosis.
[c] Alive with systemic disease.
[d] Both died of CNS disease alone.

ease. Four additional patients received other irradiation schedules, all with progressive systemic disease. Three died within 2 months and one is alive with recurrent CNS symptoms 1 month after receiving 2000 rad in 10 treatments.

Four patients underwent CNS tumor removal followed by 3000- to 5000-rad WBI. Three patients had a solitary brain lesion and were in complete systemic remission at the time of surgery. One developed carcinomatous meningitis and died 5 months after surgery. Two remain alive and free of disease 12 and 45 months later. The fourth patient was in excellent partial remission and underwent craniotomy for a presumed solitary metastasis. Retrospective review of the CT scan revealed multiple lesions. He died of progressive CNS disease 20 months later.

Five of 17 patients treated with radiation therapy alone and two of four patients treated with surgery followed by radiation therapy are alive, although two patients in the radiation group have systemic relapse and will probably die of disseminated disease. The median survival in the radiotherapy group is 5 months while the surgical group had a median survival of 16 months. Comparison of survival and relapse rate between the surgery and radiotherapy groups are not meaningful because of the small numbers and obvious favorable selection factors in patients undergoing surgical excision.

Overall, symptomatic improvement was noted in the majority of patients who received treatment for brain metastases. Three patients who were not treated died within 2 months. Three patients with inadequate records died within 1 month with progressive systemic disease. Eleven patients had permanent control of CNS symptoms while seven patients had radiographic and/or symptomatic relapse. Eleven of these 18 patients have died, nine with systemic disease and two from CNS metastases. Three of these patients survived longer than 12 months. The overall median survival was five months (range 0–69+ months).

Five patients remain alive and free of disease at 12+, 27+, 45+, 49+, and 69+ months following diagnosis of brain metastases. These five patients have been off all therapy for 8 to 54 months and lead normal lives. The last four are probably cured of their disease, although rare late relapses do occur. The characteristics of these patients are listed in Table 21.7. Two patients remain alive with evidence of disease.

Analysis of the cause of death reveals that progressive systemic disease was present in 14 of the 17 patients who died. Only three patients were thought to have died of CNS disease alone. One patient presented with headache, nausea, emesis, and changing mental status, and was found to have a right frontoparietal lesion on CT scan. He aspirated and died from cardiopulmonary arrest the following day. Autopsy revealed a 4-cm brain metastasis but no evidence of systemic tumor was found. Another patient presented with seizures while in complete remission 2 months after completing salvage chemotherapy. He underwent CNS tumor removal and WBI. Unfortunately, he returned 2 months later with severe myalgias and nuchal rigidity. CSF cytology was consistent with carcinomatous

Table 21.7
Characteristics of Disease-free Survivors

Source (Ref. No.)	Histology	No. of Brain Metastases	Status of Systemic Disease	Treatment after Diagnosis of CNS Metastases	Survival after Diagnosis of CNS Metastases (Months)
Kaye et al (22)	Choriocarcinoma	Multiple	Presentation	CT (IT, systemic),[a] surgery, WBI 3930 rad	33+
Stolinsky (39)	Choriocarcinoma	Solitary	CR	CT (IT, systemic), surgery	196+
Logothetis et al (27)	Embryonal	Solitary	Controlled	CT (systemic), WBI 3000 rads	35+
Logothetis et al (27)	Teratocarcinoma	Solitary	Controlled	CT (systemic), WBI 3000 rad	14+
Present study	Embryonal	Multiple	CR	CT (systemic), WBI 5000 rad	69+
Present study	Embryonal	Solitary	CR	CT (systemic), surgery, WBI 5000 rad	45+
Present study	Embryonal	Solitary	Presentation	CT (systemic), WBI 5000 rad	49+
Present study	Choriocarcinoma (?)	Multiple	Presentation	CT (systemic), WBI 5000 rad	27+
Present study	Embryonal	Solitary	Surgical NED	CT (systemic), surgery, WBI 4000 rad	12+

[a] CT, chemotherapy; IT, intrathecal; surgery, solitary CNS metastatectomy; WBI, whole brain irradiation.

meningitis. He responded initially to cranio-spinal irradiation but later developed recurrent seizures and deteriorated, dying of CNS disease 2 months later. He received no further chemotherapy and remained in systemic CR during this time. The final patient presented with confusion while in partial remission on maintenance therapy. CT scan was initially thought to show a solitary left parietal lesion and he underwent craniotomy at an outside hospital. Review of the CT scan revealed three initial areas of disease. He was treated with 3600-rad WBI and salvage chemotherapy achieving a systemic CR. He later developed further CNS metastases which initially responded to further cranial irradiation and intracarotid artery cisplatin before subsequent neurologic deterioration. He died 20 months after initial CNS symptoms of progressive brain metastases while still in systemic remission.

DISCUSSION

Brain metastases are an important complication of disseminated germ cell neoplasms. Because female germ cell tumors other than GTD rarely spread to the CNS, the discussion that follows will focus on male extraneural germ cell tumors. Specific reference to female germ cell neoplasms will be made when appropriate.

CNS disease should be suspected in any patient presenting with the signs or symptoms listed in Table 21.4. The diagnosis is usually easily confirmed by computerized tomography. In our experience, CNS symptoms did not occur without previous or concomitant evidence of systemic disease. Thus, the diagnosis was never in doubt. As CNS disease tends to develop from widespread disseminated disease, it is unlikely that a patient will present solely with a brain metastasis from an obscure extraneural germ cell tumor primary. If after biopsy the histology of the CNS lesion is in doubt, in the appropriate clinical setting immunoperoxidase stains for AFP and HCG should be performed (1, 32). If a germ cell malignancy is confirmed, careful physical examination, serum and CSF tumor markers, chest X-ray, and abdominal CT scan will invariably reveal the site of an extraneural primary when present.

The ratio of cerebrospinal fluid (CSF) to serum HCG in male germ cell tumors has been correlated with the presence of brain metastases, although false negatives occur (21, 35, 44). Kaye et al (21) found that ratios >2.5% were restricted to patients with CNS disease but the false neg-

ative rate was 33% (3 of 9). Schold et al (35) simultaneously measured CSF and serum HCG levels in 15 patients with disseminated testicular cancer. In 10 patients without CNS disease, the ratio was <1% compared to >5% in five patients with documented brain metastases. Successful treatment was followed by normalization of CSF HCG. Partial response or relapse showed elevated levels. Although there is some evidence to suggest that an abnormal CSF/serum HCG ratio may predate clinically apparent CNS disease, its usefulness remains to be determined. CSF AFP levels have not been shown to be reliable in disseminated testicular cancer. The CSF/serum HCG ratio was measured in only one patient in our series with a false negative result. However, CSF HCG levels may occasionally aid in the diagnosis of CNS metastases.

Examination of the CSF for malignant cells in extraneural germ cell tumors has not been shown to be of benefit. The results of routine CSF cytology in patients with brain metastases have not been reported. Only three patients, one at Indiana University and two at M.D. Anderson, have been documented to have positive CSF cytology, all of whom had signs of leptomeningeal disease (27). No case of leptomeningeal disease was seen among 51 patients with CNS metastases at Memorial (34). In contrast, patients with primary CNS germ cell tumors often have positive CSF cytology (1).

The overall incidence of brain metastases in the current study was 6.2%. This incidence is lower than other studies for several reasons. Routine autopsies on all patients were not obtained in our series, although autopsy data was used when available. Autopsy series where most patients die of widespread systemic disease, yield higher rates of brain metastases as shown by the Memorial series (34) and also by Earle (7) and the Armed Forces Institute of Pathology (27), with a 30 and 40% incidence of brain metastases, respectively. Patients with refractory systemic disease have a higher incidence of CNS disease as evidenced by our earlier series (47) and by the higher incidence found among patients referred for salvage chemotherapy. Of 30 patients with refractory disease treated with ifosfamide, a Phase II agent, six (20%) had CNS metastases (45). It is the ability of modern chemotherapy to control a systemic tumor that reduces the overall rate of CNS spread. Control of systemic disease is probably the primary factor in determining the incidence of brain metastases.

Twenty-nine cases of EGCT were found among the most recent 343 consecutive patients (8.4%). Since four of these patients with EGCT developed CNS disease, the rate of brain metastases in EGCT was 13.8%. The higher incidence of CNS spread in patients with EGCT is probably explained by the increased tumor volume at initial diagnosis with subsequent poorer overall response to treatment compared to tumors of testicular origin. The incidence of brain metastases in EGCT at M.D. Anderson was also higher (33%, 2 of 6), but was not statistically different from those originating in the testis (27).

Patients who develop CNS spread present with more advanced disease and have a worse response to initial chemotherapy. The incidence of brain metastases at initial presentation is very low, occurring in only six patients (1.5%). Brain metastases are generally a late occurrence in the natural history of extraneural germ cell tumors, primarily occurring in patients with advanced refractory systemic tumor. Only three patients were thought to have died of CNS disease alone. Thus, control of systemic disease is the most important factor determining overall survival in patients who develop brain metastases. Although no study has shown the value of prophylactic WBI or intrathecal chemotherapy in preventing CNS relapse in male germ cell tumors, in only three of our 389 (0.8%) could such therapy have possibly been beneficial.

The development of brain metastases in five patients who were free of systemic tumor lends support to the concept that the central nervous system acts as a sanctuary for neoplastic growth. This finding is in contrast to that at Memorial where all patients had pulmonary involvement when the diagnosis of brain metastases was made (34). Although there may be some penetration of the blood-brain barrier by systemic antineoplastic agents, as discussed below, this effect is incomplete and does not entirely prevent or control CNS spread in all patients.

The prognosis for patients with CNS disease is generally poor. Overall, among the 24 patients in this study, median survival after diagnosis of CNS disease was 5 months. Five patients (21%) remain alive and disease free.

Only rare long-term survivors in patients with parenchymal brain lesions are reported (22, 27, 30, 34, 39). Overall 14 patients in the literature and our series remain alive and free of disease. Schold et al (34) reported four of 41 patients

still living, although none longer than 12 months and only one free of disease. Newlands et al (30) reported three of four patients who presented with CNS disease at initial diagnosis achieved CR using an alternating combination chemotherapy including cisplatin and intermediate dose methotrexate (1 gm/m^2/course) as well as intrathecal methotrexate but exact duration of follow-up was not given. These cases are not included in the subsequent analysis. Adequate information was available in nine cases and their characteristics are presented in Table 21.7. Six patients were in CR or had systemic disease controlled when CNS spread occurred and three patients presented with CNS disease at initial diagnosis.

All nine patients who remain alive and disease free received systemic chemotherapy following diagnosis of CNS disease. Cisplatin with other agents was given to all surviving patients in this study. The importance of systemic chemotherapy is not known. It may act by preventing peripheral relapse analogous to acute lymphoblastic leukemia, by enhancing the radiotherapy effect, or by a direct cytotoxic effect on the CNS tumor itself. The absence of a blood-brain barrier in fully developed CNS metastases, demonstrated by Vick and Bigner (42) may allow systemic chemotherapy to penetrate CNS lesions. Of interest, Khan et al (23) used intravenous cisplatin alone in two patients with recurrent brain metastases from germ cell neoplasms. Both patients responded (one CR) with responses lasting 5 and 10 months. One patient in our series received intra-arterial cisplatin with initial response before ultimately dying of progressive CNS disease. Thus, systemic cisplatin appears to have a direct effect on brain metastases and there is some suggestion that it may be important in management of CNS disease.

Current therapy of brain metastases remains inadequate. Most patients die of systemic disease within months. Mainstays of therapy are WBI or surgical resection followed by WBI with no clear evidence favoring one over another. The value of higher doses of WBI is also unclear with some suggestion that higher doses may give greater CNS control. Finally, systemic chemotherapy following diagnosis of CNS spread seems to have benefit.

Our current treatment recommendations for patients with male germ cell tumors who develop brain metastases are as follows. Patients who have refractory systemic disease or who are moribund are given 3000 rad in 10 fractions as palliative therapy or receive steroids alone. Most of these patients will ultimately die of systemic tumor. Patients who present with CNS disease at initial diagnosis and patients who have adequate control of systemic disease are treated with 5000 rad in 25 fractions with curative intent. Surgical resection is reserved for patients with good control of systemic disease who have a solitary brain metastasis. This is followed by 4000- to 5000-rad WBI. Systemic chemotherapy should be given to all patients treated for cure. The best therapy for OGCT and female EGCT metastatic to the CNS is not known because of the rarity of these diseases but should probably be similar to that used in male germ cell tumors.

The clinical course of GTD has several interesting parallels to male germ cell tumors in that CNS disease tends to develop in patients with widespread systemic disease which invariably includes multiple pulmonary metastases, late CNS relapse tends to occur in patients with refractory systemic disease, and control of systemic disease is the most important predictor of long-term survival. However, relatively more patients with GTD present with brain metastases at initial diagnosis and their overall prognosis is better. These patients should receive systemic combination chemotherapy and either WBI or intrathecal chemotherapy.

SUMMARY

The incidence of brain metastases in patients with extraneural germ cell tumors treated with modern combination chemotherapy is low. We attribute this to greater control of systemic disease than achieved with earlier regimens. CNS lesions occur more frequently in patients with advanced disease, in patients with EGCT, and in patients with choriocarcinoma. The most important factor in survival after diagnosis of CNS disease is control of systemic disease. Current treatment methods are inadequate but the addition of systemic chemotherapy may be beneficial in male germ cell tumors. Aggressive treatment in patients who develop brain metastases will produce 20% disease-free survivors in male germ cell tumors and 40 to 50% in patients with gestational trophoblastic disease. Other patients can expect significant improvement in symptoms and survival.

References

1. Allen JC, Nisselbaum J, Epstein F, Rosen G, Schwartz MK: Alpha-fetoprotein and human chorionic gonadotropin determination in cerebrospinal fluid: An aid to the diagnosis and management of intracranial germ cell tumors. *J Neurosurg* 51: 368–374, 1979.

2. Athanassiou A, Begent RHJ, Newlands ES, Parker D, Rustin GJS, Bagshawe KD: Central nervous system metastases of choriocarcinoma: 23 years' experience at Charing Cross Hospital. *Cancer* 52:1728–1735, 1983.

3. Begent RJH, Bagshawe KD: The management of high risk choriocarcinoma. *Semin Oncol* 9:198–203, 1982.

4. Bradof JE, Hakes TB, Ochoa M, Golbey R: Germ cell malignancies of the ovary: Treatment with vinblastine, actinomycin D, bleomycin, and cisplatin containing chemotherapy combinations. *Cancer* 50:1070–1075, 1982.

5. Campbell HE: The incidence of malignant growth of the undescended testis: A reply and re-evaluation. *J Urol* 81:663–668, 1959.

6. Curry SL, Smith JP, Gallagher HS: Malignant teratoma of the ovary: Prognostic factors and treatment. *Am J Obstet Gynecol* 131:845–849, 1978.

7. Earle KM: Metastatic and primary intracranial tumors of the adult male. *J Neuropathol Exp Neurol* 13:448–454, 1954.

8. Einhorn LH, Donohue JP: Cis-diamminedichloroplatinum, vinblastine, and bleomycin combination chemotherapy in disseminated testicular cancer. *Ann Int Med* 87:293–298, 1977.

9. Einhorn LH: Combination chemotherapy with cis-dichlorodiammineplatinum (II) in disseminated testicular cancer. *Cancer Treat Rep* 63:1659–1662, 1979.

10. Einhorn LH, Williams SD: Chemotherapy of disseminated testicular cancer: A random prospective trial. *Cancer* 46:1339–1344, 1980.

11. Einhorn LH: Extragonadal germ cell tumors. In Einhorn LH (ed): *Testicular Tumors: Management and Treatment.* New York, Masson Publishing, 1980, p 185–204.

12. Feun LG, Samson MK, Stephens RL: Vinblastine, bleomycin, cis-diamminedichloroplatinum in disseminated extragonadal germ cell tumors: A Southwest Oncology Group Study. *Cancer* 45:2543–2549, 1980.

13. Funes HC, Mendez M, Alonzo E, Oviben R, Manas A, Mediola C: Mediastinal germ cell tumors treated with displatin, bleomycin, and vinblastine (abstract). *Proc Am Ass Cancer Res* 22:474, 1981.

14. Gallion H, Van Nagell JR, Powell DF, Donaldson ES, Hanson M: Therapy of endodermal sinus tumor of the ovary. *Am J Obstet Gynecol* 135:447–451, 1979.

15. Garnick MB, Canellos GP, Richie JP: Treatment and surgical staging of testicular and primary extragonadal germ cell cancer. *JAMA* 250: 1733–1741, 1983.

16. Hainsworth JD, Einhorn LH, Williams SD, Steward M, Greco FA: Advanced extragonadal germ cell tumors: Successful treatment with combination chemotherapy. *Ann Int Med* 97:7–11, 1982.

17. Hammond CB, Borchet LG, Tyrey L, Creasman WT, Parker RT: Treatment of metastatic tropho-

blastic disease. Good and poor prognosis. *Am J Obstet Gynecol* 115:451–457, 1973.

18. Hammond CB, Currie JL, Weed JC: The role of operation in the current therapy of gestational trophoblastic disease. *Am J Obstet Gynecol* 136:844–858, 1980.

19. Ishizuka T, Tomoda Y, Kaseki S, Goto S, Hara T, Kobayashi T: Intracranial metastasis of choriocarcinoma: A clinicopathologic study. *Cancer* 52:1896–1903, 1983.

20. Johnson DE, Laneir JP, Mountain CF, Luna M: Extragonadal germ cell tumors. *Surgery* 73:85–90, 1973.

21. Kaye SB, Bagshawe KD, McElwain TJ, Peckham MJ: Brain metastases in malignant teratoma: A review of four years' experience and an assessment of the role of tumor marker. *Br J Cancer* 39:217–223, 1979.

22. Kaye SB, Regnet R, Newland B, Bagshawe KD: Successful treatment of malignant testicular teratoma and brain metastases. *Br Med J* 1(6158):233–234, 1979.

23. Khan AB, D'Souza BJ, Wharam MD, Champion L, Sinks L, Woo S, McCullough D, Leventhal B: Cisplatin therapy in recurrent childhood brain tumors. *Cancer Treat Rep* 66:2013–2020, 1982.

24. Kurman RJ, Norris HJ: Endodermal sinus tumor of the ovary: A clinical and pathologic analysis of 71 cases. *Cancer* 38:2404–2419, 1976.

25. Kurman RJ, Norris HJ: Embryonal carcinoma of the ovary: A clinicopathological entity distinct from endodermal sinus tumor resembling embryonal carcinoma of the adult testis. *Cancer* 38:2420–2433, 1976.

26. Kuzur ME, Cobleigh MA, Greco FA, Einhorn LH, Oldham RK: Endodermal sinus tumor of the mediastinum. *Cancer* 50:766–774, 1982.

27. Logothetis CJ, Samuels ML, Trindade A: The management of brain metastases in germ cell tumors. *Cancer* 49:12–18, 1982.

28. Luna MA: Extragonadal germ cell tumors. In Johnson DE (ed): *Testicular Tumors*, ed 2. New York, Medical Examination Publishing Co, 1976, p 261–265.

29. Miller JM, Surwit EA, Hammond CB: Choriocarcinoma following term pregnancy. *Obstet Gynecol* 53:207–212, 1979.

30. Newlands ES, Begent RHJ, Rustin GJS, Parker D, Bagshawe KD: Further advances in the management of malignant teratomas of the testis and other sites. *Lancet* 1:948–951, 1983.

31. Norris HJ, Zirkin HJ, Benson WL: Immature (malignant) teratoma of the ovary: A clinical and pathologic study of 58 cases. *Cancer* 37:2359–2372, 1976.

32. Richardson RL, Schoumacher RA, Fer MF, Hande KR, Forbess JT, Oldham RK, Greco FA: The unrecognized extragonadal germ cell cancer syndrome. *Ann Int Med* 94:181–186, 1981.

33. Schlumberger HG: Teratoma of the anterior mediastinum in the group of miliary age. *Arch Pathol* 41:398–444, 1946.

34. Schold CS, Vugrin D, Golbey RB, Posner JB: Central nervous system metastases from germ cell carcinoma of testis. *Semin Oncol* 6:102–108, 1979.

35. Schold SC, Fleisher M, Schwartz M, Posner JB: Cerebrospinal fluid biochemical markers of central nervous system metastases. *Trans Am Neurol Assoc* 103:179–181, 1978.

36. Silverberg E: Cancer statistics, 1984. *Ca-A Cancer J* 34:7–15, 1984.

37. Simson LR, Lampe I, Abell MR: Suprasellar germinomas. *Cancer* 22:533–544, 1968.

38. Slayton RE, Hreshchyshyn MM, Silverberg SG, Shingleton HM, Park RC, DiSaia PJ, Blessing JA: Treatment of malignant ovarian germ cell tumors: Response to vincristine, dactinomycin, and cyclophosphamide. *Cancer* 42:390–398, 1978.

39. Stolingsky DC: Prolonged survival after cerebral metastasis of testicular carcinoma. *Cancer* 47:978–981, 1981.

40. Thurzo R, Pinter J: Cryptorchism and malignancy in men and animals. *Urol Int* 11:216–231, 1961.

41. Utz DC, Buscemi M: Extragonadal testicular tumors. *J Urol* 105:271–274, 1971.

42. Vick N, Bigner D: Microvascular abnormalities in virally induced canine brain tumors: Structural basis from altered blood brain barrier function. *J Neurol Sci* 17:29–39, 1972.

43. Vugrin D, Vitkovic E, Posner JB, Golbey RB: Biology of brain metastases of testicular germ cell carcinomas. *Proc Am Soc Clin Oncol* (Abstr) 19:197, 1978.

44. Vugrin D, Nisselbaum J, Schold CS, Posner JB, Cvitkovic E, Schwartz M, Goldbey RB: Blood and cerebrospinal fluid tumor markers in the diagnosis of brain metastases from testicular cancer. *Proc Am Soc Clin Oncol* 20:115, 1979.

45. Weed JC, Woodward KT, Hammond CB: Choriocarcinoma metastatic to the brain: Therapy and prognosis. *Semin Oncol* 9:208–212, 1982.

46. Wheeler BM, Einhorn LH, Loehrer PJ, Williams SD: Ifosfamide, an active agent in refractory germ cell tumors. *Proc Am Soc Clin Oncol*, 1984, in press.

47. Williams SD, Einhorn LH: Brain metastases in disseminated germinal neoplasms: Incidence and clinical course. *Cancer* 44:1514–1516, 1979.

48. Williams SD, Turner S, Loehrer PJ, Einhorn LH: Testicular cancer: Results of reinduction therapy. *Proc Am Soc Clin Oncol* 2:137, 1983.

49. Willis RA: *Borderland of Embryology and Pathology*, ed 2. Washington, DC, Butterworth & Co, 1962, p 47–62.

50. Witschi E: Migration of the germ cells of human embryos from the yolk sac to the primitive gonadal folds. *Contrib Embryol* 209:67–80, 1948.

References

Abay EO, Laws ER, Grado GL, Bruckman JE, Forbes GS, Gomez MR, Scott M: Pineal tumors in children and adolescents. *J Neurosurg* 55:889–895, 1981.

Abell MR, Fayos JV, Lampe I: Pathology-Radiation Therapy Conference-Parapituitary germinoma. *Univ Mich Med Ctr J* 32:250–251, 1966.

Abreo K, Steele TH: Pineal cyst associated with polycystic kidney disease: Case report. *Am J Kidney Dis* 1:106–109, 1981.

Ahagon A, Yoshida Y, Kusano K, et al: Suprasellar germinoma in association with Klinefelter's syndrome. *J Neurosurg* 58:136–138, 1983.

Albrechtsen R, Klee JG, Møller JE: Primary intracranial germ cell tumors including five cases of endodermal sinus tumor. *Acta Pathol Microbiol Scand* [A] [80 Suppl] 233:32–38, 1972.

Alexander Jr, E: Benign subtentorial supracollicular cyst as a cause of obstructive hydrocephalus. *J Neurosurg* 10:317–323, 1953.

Allen JC, Nisselbaum J, Epstein F, Rosen G, Schwartz MK: Alpha fetoprotein and human chorionic gonadotropin determination in cerebrospinal fluid. *J Neurosurg* 51:368–374, 1979.

Allen SS, Lovell HW: Tumors of the third ventricle. *Arch Neurol Psychiatry* 28:990–1006, 1932.

Altman RP, Randolph JG, Lilly JR: Sacrococcygeal teratoma: American Academy of Pediatrics Surgical Section Survey-1973. *J Pediatr Surg* 9:389–398, 1974.

Anderson T, Waldmann TA, Javadpour N, Glatstein E: Testicular germ-cell neoplasms: Recent advances in diagnosis and therapy. *Ann Int Med* 90:373–385, 1979.

Aoyama I, Makita Y, Nabeshima S, Motomichi M: Intracranial double teratomas. *Surg Neurol* 17:383–387, 1982.

Appuzzo MLJ, Mitchell MS: Immunologic aspects of intrinsic glial tumors. *J Neurosurg* 55:1–18, 1981.

Apuzzo MLJ, Davey LM, Manuelidis EE: Pineal apoplexy associated with anticoagulant therapy. *J Neurosurg* 45:223–226, 1976.

Araki C: Meningeoma in the pineal region. A report of two cases removed by operation. *Arch Jpn Chir* 14:1181–1192, 1937.

Araki C, Matsumoto S: Statistical reevaluation of pinealoma and related tumors in Japan. *J Neurosurg* 30:146–149, 1969.

Arendt J, Forbes JM, Brown WB, Marston A: Effect of pinealectomy on immunoassayable melatonin in the sheep. *J Endocrinol* 85:1P–2P, 1980.

Arendt J, Wirz-Justice A, Bradtke J: Annual rhythm of serum melatonin in man. *Neurosci Lett* 7:327–330, 1977.

Arendt J: Current status of assay methods of melatonin. In Birau N, Schloot W (eds): *Melatonin—Current Status and Perspectives* (Advances in the Biosciences). New York, Pergamon Press, 1981, vol 29, 1981.

Arendt J: Radioimmunoassayable melatonin: Circulating patterns in man and sheep. *Prog Brain Res* 52:249–257, 1979.

Arita N, Bitoh S, Ushio Y, Hayakawa T, Hasegawa H, Fujiwara M, Ozaki K, Par-khen L, Mori T: Primary pineal endodermal sinus tumor with elevated serum and CSF alpha fetoprotein levels. *J Neurosurg* 53:244–248, 1980.

Arita N, Ushio Y, Hayakawa T, Uozumi T, Watanabe M, Mori T, Mogami H: Serum levels of alpha-fetoprotein, human chorionic gonadotropin and carcinoembryonic antigen in patients with primary intracranial germ cell tumors. *Oncodev Biol Med* 1:235–240, 1980.

Arita N, Ushio Y, Abekura M, Koshino K, Hayakawa T: Embryonal carcinoma with teratomatous elements in the region of the pineal gland. *Surg Neurol* 9:198–203, 1978.

Arlant PA, Grunnett ML, Heilbrun MP: Primary malignant melanoma of the pineal region. *Surg Neurol* 7:121–123, 1977.

Armstrong S, Ng KT, Coleman GJ: Influence of the pineal gland on brain-behavior relationship. In Reiter RJ (ed): *The Pineal Gland, Extra-Reproductive Effects.* Boca Raton, CRC Press, 1982, vol 3, pp 81–106.

Arnold H, Usbeck W: Tumoren des hirnstammes und 3. ventrikel im kindes- und entwicklungsalter. *Psychiat Neurol Med Psychol* 23:518–523, 1971.

Arseni C, Danaila L, Nicola L, et al: Intracranial teratomas. *Acta Neurochirurg* (Wien) 20:37–51, 1969.

Askanazy M: Die teratome nach ihrem ban, ihrem verlauf, ihrer genese und im vergleich zum experimentellen teratoid. *Verhandl d. Deutsch path Gesellesch* 11:39–82, 1907.

Auerbach SH, DePiero TJ, Romanul F: Sylvian aqueduct syndrome caused by a unilateral midbrain lesion. *Ann Neurol* 11:91–94, 1981.

Axelrod J, Weissbach H: Purification and properties of hydroxyindole-O-methyltransferase. *J Biol Chem* 236:211–213, 1961.

Axelrod J: The pineal gland: A neurochemical transducer. *Science* 184:1341–1348, 1974.

Backlund ED, Rahn T, Sarby S: Treatment of pinealomas by sterotaxic radiation surgery. *Acta Radiol Ther* 13:368–376, 1974.

Backlund EO: Stereotactic radiosurgery in intracranial tumor, and vascular malformation. In Krayenbuhl H (ed): *Advances and Technical Standards in Neurosurgery.* Vienna, Springer-Verlag, 1979, vol 6.

Bader JL, Meadows AT, Zimmerman LE, Rorke LB, Voute PA, Champion LAA, Miller RW: Bilateral retinoblastoma with ectopic intracranial retinoblastoma: Trilateral retinoblastoma. *Cancer Genet Cytogenet* 5:302–313, 1982.

Baggenstoss AH, Love JG: Pinealomas. *Arch Neurol Psychiat* 41:1187–1206, 1939.

Baghai P, Vries JK, Bechtel PC: Retromastoid approach for biopsy of brain stem tumors. *Neurosurgery* 10:574–579, 1982.

Bailey P, Jelliffe SE: Tumors of the pineal body. *Arch Int Med* 8:851–880, 1911.

Bailey P, Buchanan DN, Bucy PC: Intracranial tumors of infancy and childhood. The University of Chicago Press, Chicago-London, 1964.

Baker GS, Rucher CW: Metastatic pinealoma involving the optic chiasm. *J Neurosurg* 7:377–378, 1950.

Baker Jr, HL: The venous angiogram: A frequently overlooked phase of carotid angiography. *Clin Neurosurg* 10:130–150, 1964.

Balado M, Tiscornia A: Tumor de la hoz del cerebro pediculado a desarrollo subtentorial. *Arch Argent Neurol* 1:297–310, 1927.

Balagura S, Shulman K, Sobel EH: Precocious puberty of cerebral origin. *Surg Neurol* 11:315–326, 1979.

Banerjee AK, Kak VJ: Pineoblastoma with spontaneous intra and extracranial metastasis. *J Pathol* 114:9–12, 1973.

Barber SG, Smith JA, Hughes RC: Melatonin as a tumour marker in a patient with pineal tumour. *Br Med J* 2:328, 1978.

Barber SG, Smith JA, Cove DH, Smith SCH, London DR: Marker for pineal tumours? *Lancet* 2:372–373, 1978.

Bartke A: Role of prolactin in reproduction in male mammals. *Fed Proc* 39:2577–2581, 1980.

Bartlemez GW, Dekaban AS: The early development of the human brain. *Contrib Embryol* 37:13–32, 1962.

Bebin J: Seminar in neuropathology: Part III germinoma (atypical pineal teratoma, ectopic pinealoma). *Miss State Med Assoc* 15:329–330, 1974.

Becker DH, Silverberg GD: Successful evacuation of an acute pontine hematoma. *Surg Neurol* 10:263–265, 1978.

Beeley JM, Daly JT, Timperley WR, et al: Ectopic pinealoma an unusual clinical presentation and a histochemical comparison with seminoma of the testis. *J Neurol Neurosurg Psychiatr* 36:864–873, 1973.

Bender MB: Brain control of conjugate horizontal and vertical eye movements: A survey of the structural and functional correlates. *Brain* 103:23–69, 1980.

Benjamin RS, Wiernik PH, Bachur NR: Adriamycin chemotherapy—efficacy, safety, and pharmacologic basis of an intermittent single high-dosage schedule. *Cancer* 33:19–27, 1974.

Benson B, Ebels I: Other pineal peptides and related substances—Physiological implications for reproductive biology. In Reiter RJ (ed): *The Pineal Gland Vol 2, Reproductive Effects.* Boca Raton, CRC Press, 1981, pp 165–188.

Benson B, Ebels I: Pineal peptides. *J Neural Transm* [Suppl] 13:157–173, 1978.

Benson B: Current status of pineal peptides. *Neuroendocrinology* 24:241–258, 1977.

Berg JW, Baylor SM: The epidemiologic pathology of ovarian cancer. *Human Pathol* 4:537–547, 1973.

Berndtson WE, Desjardins C: Circulating LH and FSH levels and testicular function in hamsters during light deprivation and subsequent photoperiodic stimulation. *Endocrinology* 95:195–205, 1974.

Best PV: A medulloblastoma-like tumour with melanin formation. *J Pathol* 110:109–111, 1973.

Bestle J: Extragonadal endodermal sinus tumor originating in the region of the pineal gland. *Acta Pathol Microbiol Scand* 74:214–222, 1968.

Betz H: Das pneumotomogramm der cisterna laminae quadrigeminae. *Radiologe* 8:366–368, 1968.

Birau N: Melatonin in human serum: Progress in screening investigation and clinic. In Birau N, Schloot W (eds): *Melatonin—Current Status and Perspectives.* New York, Pergamon, 1981, pp 297–326.

Birg W, Mundinger F: Direct target point determination for stereotactic brain operation from CT data and the calculation of setting parameters for polar coordinate stereotactic devices. Proceedings of the 8th Meeting World Society Stereotactic and Functional Neurosurgery, Part III, Zurich 1981. *Appl Neurophysiol* 45:387–395, 1982.

Blackwood W, Borit A: Tumours of the pineal region. 8th International Congress of Neuropathology, Abstract #33.

Bloom HJG: Primary intracranial germ cell tumors. *Clin Oncol* 2:233–257, 1983.

Bloom HJG: Primary intracranial germ cell tumors. *Clin Oncol* 2:1, 233–257, 1983.

Bloom HJG: Intracranial tumors: Response and resistance to therapeutic endeavors, 1970–1980. *Int J Radiat Oncol Biol Phys* 8:1083–1113, 1982.

Bochner SJ, Scarff JE: Teratoma of the pineal body. Classification of embryonal tumors of the pineal body: Report of a case of teratoma of the pineal body presenting formed teeth. *Arch Surg* 36:303–309, 1979.

Bodenheimer S, Winter JSD, Faiman C: Diurnal rhythms of serum gonadotropins, testosterone, estradiol and cortisol in blind men. *J Clin Endocrinol Metab* 37:472–475, 1973.

Boethius J, Bergstrom M, Greitz T: Stereotaxic computerized tomography with G.E. 8800 Scanner. *J Neurosurg* 52:794–800, 1980.

Borden IV S, Weber AL, Toch R, Wang CC: Pineal germinoma. *Am J Dis Child* 126:214–216, 1973.

Borit A: History of tumors of the pineal region. *Am J Surg Pathol* 5:613–619, 1981.

Borit A, Blackwood W, Mair WGP: The separation of pineocytoma from pineoblastoma. *Cancer* 45:1408–1418, 1980.

Borit A, Blackwood W: Pineocytoma with astrocytomatous differentiation. *J Neuropathol Exp Neurol* 38:253–248, 1979.

Borit A: Embryonal carcinoma of the pineal region. *J Pathol* 97:165–168, 1969.

Bosl GJ, Lange PH, Fraley EE, et al: Vinblastine, bleomycin and cis-diamminedichloroplatinum in the treatment of advanced testicular carcinoma. Possible importance of longer induction and shorter maintenance schedules. *Am J Med* 68:492–496, 1980.

Bosman FT, Giard RWM, Nieuwenhuijen AC, et al: Human chorionic gonadotropin and alpha-fetoprotein in testicular germ cell tumors: A retrospective immunohistochemical study. *Histopathology* 4:673–684, 1980.

Bouchard J: Radiation therapy of tumors and diseases of the nervous system. Philadelphia, Lea & Febiger, 1966.

Bradac GB, Holdorff B, Simon RS: Aspects of the

venous drainage of the pns and the mesencephalon. *Neuroradiology* 3:102–108, 1971.

Bradfield JS, Perez CA: Pineal tumors and ectopic pinealomas. Analysis of treatment and failures. *Radiology* 103:399–406, 1972.

Brady LW: The role of radiation therapy. In Schmidek HH (ed): *Pineal Tumors.* New York, Masson Publishing, 1977, pp 127–132.

Brainard GC, Richardson BA, Peterborg LJ, Reiter RJ: The effect of different light intensities on pineal melatonin content. *Brain Res* 233:75–81, 1982.

Brainard GC, Richardson BA, King TS, Matthews SA, Reiter RJ: The suppression of pineal melatonin content and *N*-acetyltransferase activity by different light irradiances in the Syrian hamster: A dose-response relationship. *Endocrinology*, in press.

Brainard GC, Petterborg LJ, Richardson BA, Reiter RJ: Pineal melatonin in Syrian hamsters: Circadian and seasonal rhythms in animals maintained under laboratory and natural conditions. *Neuroendocrinology* 35:342–348, 1982.

Brammer M, Binkley S: Pineal glands of immature rats: Rise and fall in *N*-acetyltransferase activity *in vitro. J Neurobiol* 12:167–173, 1981.

Braun JP, Wackenheim A: Phlébographie mésencéphalique dans les tumeurs du tronc cérébral. *Acta Radiol* 13:45–53, 1972.

Bravo G, Vaquero J, Martinez R, Cabezudo J: Conservative management of a mesencephalic tuberculoma. *J Neurosurg* 55:287–288, 1981.

Breen JL, Maxson WS: Ovarian tumors in children and adolescents. *Clin Obstet Gynec* 20:607–623, 1977.

Bridges RS, Goldman BD: Diurnal rhythms in gonadotrophins and progesterone in lactating and photoperiod induced acyclic hamster. *Biol Reprod* 13:613–622, 1975.

Brodal A: Neurologic Anatomy, ed. 3, New York: Oxford University Press, 1981, p 747.

Brodeur GM, Howarth CB, Pratt CB, Caces J, Hustu HO: Malignant germ cell tumors in 57 children and adolescents. *Cancer* 48:1890–1898, 1981.

Brooks WH, Markesbery WR, Gupta GD, Roszman TL: Relationship of lymphocyte invasion and survival of brain tumor patients. *Ann Neurol* 4:219–224, 1978.

Brosman S, Gondos B: Testicular teratomas in children. In JH Johnston, WE Goodwin (eds): *Reviews in Pediatric Urology.* Amsterdam. *Excerpta Medica,* 1974, Ch 7, p 131.

Browder J, Kaplan H, Krieger AJ: Anatomical features of the straight sinus and its tribuatries. Clinical correlations. *J Neurosurg* 44:55–61, 1976.

Brown NJ: Yolk-sac tumor ('orchioblastoma') and other testicular tumors of childhood. In Hugh RCB (ed): *Pathology of the Testis.* Oxford, Blackwell Scientific Publications, 1976, pp 364–365.

Brown RA: A computerized tomographic-computer graphics approach to stereotactic localization. *J Neurosurg* 50:715–720, 1979.

Bruce D: Pediatric brain tumor. *Surg Rounds* April 1982, pp 22–31.

Brunner C, Rorschach: Uber einen fall von tumor der glandula pinealis cerebri. *Cor Blatt Schweiz Arzte* 642–643, 1911.

Bruton OC, Martz DC, Gerard ES: Precocious puberty due to secreting chorionepithelioma (teratoma) of the brain. *J Pediatr* 59:719–725, 1961.

Budka H: Intracranial lipomatous hamartomas (intracranial "lipomas"). *Acta Neuropathol* 28:205–222, 1974.

Budka H: Intrakranielle teratome. In Jellinger K, Gross H (eds): *Aktuelle Probleme der Neuropathologie, Band 4.* Wien, Facultas-Verlag, 1978, pp 88–93.

Burger PC, Mahaley Jr, MS, Dudka L, Vogel FS: The morphologic effect of radiation administered therapeutically for intracranial gliomas: A postmortem study of 25 cases. *Cancer* 44:1256–1272, 1979.

Burger PC, Vogel SF: Neoplasms in the pineal region. In *Surgical Pathology of the Nervous System and its Coverings,* ed 1. New York, Wiley, 1976, pp 398–407.

Burres KP, Hamilton RD: Pineal Apoplexy. *Neurosurgery* 4:264–268, 1979.

Büttner-Ennever JA, Buttner U, Cohen B, Baumgartner G: Vertical gaze paralysis and the rostral interstitial nucleus of the medial longitudinal fasciculus. *Brain* 105:125–149, 1982.

Butzow R: Luteinizing hormone-releasing factor increases release of human chorionic gonadotropin in isolated cell columns of normal and malignant trophoblasts. *Int J Cancer* 29:9–11, 1982.

Camins MB, Schlesinger EB: Treatment of tumours of the posterior part of the third ventricle and the pineal region: A long-term follow-up. *Acta Neurochir* 40:131–143, 1978.

Camins MB, Mount LA: Primary suprasellar atypical teratoma. *Brain* 97:447–456, 1974.

Camins MB, Takeuchi J: Normotopic plus heterotopic atypical teratomas. *Childs Brain* 4:157–160, 1978.

Capron JP, Debrun G, Sichez JP, Comoy J, Lacour P: Ligature des veines cerebrales internes et survie. A propos de deux pinealomectomies. *Neurochirurgie* 20:90–91, 1974.

Cardinali DC: Melatonin. A mammalian pineal hormone. *Endocrinol Rev* 2:327–346, 1981.

Cardinali DC, Vacas MI: Feedback control of pineal function by reproductive hormones—A neuroendocrine paradigm. *J Neurol Transm,* [Suppl] 13:175–204, 1978.

Cardinali DC: Molecular biology of melatonin: Assessment of the "microtubule hypothesis of melatonin action." In Birau N, Schloot W (eds): *Melatonin—Current Status and Perspectives.* New York, Pergamon, 1981, pp 247–256.

Carletti B, Kehyayan E, Fraschini F: Remarkable seasonal variations of urinary gonadotropin excretion in young girls. *Experientia* 20:383, 1964.

Caron JP, Nick J, Contamin F, Singer B, Comoy J, Keravel Y: Tolerance de la ligature et de la thrombose aseptique des veines cerebrales profondes chez l'homme. *Ann Med Interne* 128:899–906, 1977.

Carr JL: Cystic hydrops of the pineal gland. *J New Dis* 99:552–560, 1944.

Carrillo R, Ricoy JR, del Pozo JM, Garcia-Uria J, Herrero J: Dissemination with malignant changes from a pineal tumor through the corpus callosum after total removal. *Childs Brain* 3:230–237, 1977.

Castleman B, McNeely BU: Case records of the Massachusetts General Hospital. *N Engl J Med* 284:1427–1434, 1971.

Chandler WF, Farhar SM, Pauli FJ: Intrathalamic epidermoid tumor. Case report. *J Neurosurg* 43:614–617, 1975.

Chang CG, Kageyama N, Kobayashi T, Yoshida J, Negoro M: Pineal tumors: Clinical diagnosis, with special emphasis on the significance of pineal calcification. *Neurosurgery* 8:656–668, 1981.

Chang CG, Kageyama N, Kobayashi T, Yoshida J, Negoro M: Pineal tumors: Clinical diagnosis, with special emphasis on the significance of pineal calcification. *Neurosurgery* 8:656–668, 1981.

Chapman PH, Linggood RM: The management of pineal area tumors: A recent reappraisal. *Cancer* 46:1253–1257, 1980.

Charlton HM, Grocock CA, Ostberg A: The effects of pinealectomy and superior cervical ganglionectomy on the testis of the vole, *Microtus agrestis. J Reprod Fertil* 48:377–379, 1976.

Chen HJ, Reiter RJ: The combination of twice daily luteinizing hormone-releasing factor administration and renal pituitary homografts restores normal reproductive organ size in male hamsters with pineal-mediated gonadal atrophy. *Endocrinology* 106:1382–1385, 1980.

Chen HP: Intracranial teratoma of a newborn. *J Neuropathol Exp Neurol* 17:599–603, 1958.

Chretien PB, Milam JD, Foote FW, et al: Embryonal adenocarcinoma sacrococcygeal region. *Cancer* 26:522–535, 1970.

Christie SBM, Ross EJ: Ectopic pinealoma with adipsia and hypernatremia. *Br Med J* 2:669–670, 1968.

Christoff N: A clinicopathologic study of vertical eye movements. *Arch Neurol* 31:1–8, 1974.

Christoff N, Anderson PJ, Bender MB: Convergence and retractory nystagmus. *Trans Am Neurol Assoc* 85:29–32, 1960.

Clabough JW: Cytological aspects of pineal development in rats and hamsters. *Am J Anat* 137:215–230, 1973.

Clar HE, Reinhardt V, Gerhard L, Hensell V: Clinical and morphological studies of pineal tumours. *Acta Neurochir* 46:59–76, 1979.

Clar HE, Bock WJ, Grote W, Lohr E: Atlas der enzephalotomographie. Stuttgart, Thieme Verlag, 1976.

Cline MJ, Haskell CM: Cancer Chemotherapy, ed 3. Philadelphia, WB Saunders, 1980, p 79.

Clinicopathologic Conference: Pineal germinoma with endocrine manifestations. *Calif Medic* 106:196–202, 1967.

Clinicopathologic Conference: Case report of the Massachusetts General Hospital #25-1971. *N Engl J Med* 284:1427–1434, 1971.

Clinicopathologic Conference: Case report of the Massachusetts General Hospital #41-1974. *N Engl J Med* 291:837–843, 1974.

Clinicopathologic Conference: Case report of the Massachusetts General Hospital #38-1975. *N Engl J Med* 293:653–660, 1975.

Clinicopathologic Conference: Panhypopituitarism due to ectopic pinealoma. *Stanford Med Bull* 13:56–61, 1955.

Cogan DG: Convergence nystagmus. *Arch Ophthalmol* 62:295–298, 1959.

Cohen DN, Steinberg M, Buchwald R: Suprasellar germinomas: Diagnostic confusion with optic gliomas. *J Neurosurg* 41:490–493, 1974.

Cohen HN, Hoy ID, Annesley TM, Beastall GH, Wallace AM, Spooner R, Thomson JA, Eastwald P,

Klee GG: Serum immunoreactive melatonin in boys with delayed puberty. *Clin Endocrinol* 17:517–521, 1982.

Cole H: Tumours in the region of the pineal. *Clin Radiol* 22:110–117, 1971.

Collier J: Nuclear ophthalmoplegia with special reference to retraction of lids and ptosis and to lesions of the posterior commissure. *Brain* 50:488–498, 1927.

Collin JP: Differentiation and regression of the cells of the sensory line in the epiphysis cerebri. In Wolstenholme GEW, Knight J (ed): *The Pineal Gland.* Edinburgh-London, Churchill Livingstone, 1971, pp 127–146.

Committee of Japanese Brain Tumor Registry. *All Japan Brain Tumor Registry,* vol 4, 1982.

Conway LW: Stereotaxis diagnosis and treatment of intracranial tumours including an initial experience with cryosurgery for pinealomas. *J Neurosurg* 38:453–460, 1973.

Cooper ERA: The development of the thalamus. *Acta Anat* 9:201–225, 1950.

Copty M, Bedard F, Turcotte JF: Successful removal of an entirely calcified aneurysm of the vein of Galen. *Surg Neurol* 14:396–400, 1980.

Corbett JJ, Savino PJ, Thompson HS, Kansu T, Schatz NJ, Orr LS, Hopson D: Visual loss in pseudotumor cerebri: Followup of 57 patients from 5 to 41 years and a profile of 14 patients with permanent severe visual loss. *Arch Neurol* 39:461–474, 1982.

Cox DR: Regression models and life tables. *J R Stat Soc* (Series B) 34:187–202, 1972.

Cox JD: Primary malignant germinal tumors of the mediastinum. *Cancer* 36:1162–1168, 1975.

Cox JN: Hypothalamic syndrome caused by "pinealoma" occupying the 3rd ventricle. *Arch Dis Childhood* 49:75–76, 1974.

Cravioto H, Dart D: The ultrastructure of "pinealoma." *J Neuropathol Exp Neurol* 32:552–565, 1973.

Cummins FM, Taveras JN, Schlesinger EB: Treatment of gliomas of the third ventricle and pinealomas. *Neurology* 10:1031–1036, 1960.

Cushing H: Intracranial tumors: Notes upon a series of two thousand verified cases with surgical mortality pertaining thereto. Springfield, IL, Charles C Thomas, 1932.

Cushing H: *Intrakranielle Tumoren.* Berlin, Springer Verlag, 1935.

Cushing H: The establishment of cerebral hernia as a decompressive measure for inaccessible brain tumors. *Surg Gyn Obst* 1:297–314, 1905.

Czyba JC, Girod G, Durand N: Sur l'antagonisme epiphysohypophysaire et les variations saisonmiere de la spermatogenese chez le hamster dore (*Mesocricetus auratus*). *C R Soc Biol* 158:742–745, 1964.

Dakhil S, Ensminger W, Kindt G, Niederhuber J, Wheeler R: Outpatient intraventricular infusion of methotrexate in brain malignancies. *Clin Res* 27:637A, 1979.

Dandy WE: Operative experiences in cases of pineal tumors. *Arch Surg* 33:19–46, 1936.

Dandy WE: Operative experiences in cases of pineal tumor. *Arch Surg* 51:1–14, 1945.

Dandy WE: Benign Tumors in the Third Ventricle of the Brain. Diagnosis and Treatment. Springfield, IL, Charles C Thomas, 1933, p 171.

Dandy WE: Extirpation of the pineal body. *J Exp Med* 22:237–247, 1915.

Dandy WE: An operation for the removal of pineal tumors. *Surg Gyn Obst* 33:113–119, 1921.

Dandy WE: Surgery of the brain. In *Lewis' Practice of Surgery.* Hagerstown, MD, WF Prior, 1945, vol 12.

Daroff RB, Hoyt WF: Supranuclear disorders of ocular control systems in man: Clinical, anatomical and physiological correlations. In Bach-Y-Rita P, Collins CC (eds): *The Control of Eye Movements.* New York, Academic Press, 1971, pp 175–235.

David M, Vernard-Weik E, Dilenge D: Les tumeurs de la glande pineale. *Ann Endocrinol* (Paris) 24:286–330, 1963.

Davidoff LM: Some considerations in the therapy of pineal tumors. *Bull NY Acad Med* 43:537–561, 1967.

Davis L: The principles of neurological surgery. Philadelphia, Lea & Febiger, 1946.

Davis RL: Personal communication in Smith III, RA, Eastridge MN. Pineal tumors. In Vinken PJ, Bruyn GW (eds): *Handbook of Clinical Neurology.* Amsterdam, North-Holland Publishing Co., 1974, vol 17, pp 648–665.

Dayan AD, Marshall AHE, Miller AA, Pick FJ, Rankin NE: Atypical teratomas of the pineal and hypothalamus. *J Pathol Bacteriol* 92:1–28, 1966.

de Tribolet N, Barrelet L: Successful chemotherapy of pinealoma. *Lancet* 2:1228–1229, 1977.

DeGirolami U, Armbrustmacher VW: Juvenile pilocytic astrocytoma of the pineal region: Report of a case. *Cancer* 50:1185–1188, 1982.

DeGirolami U, Schmidek H: Clinicopathological study of 53 tumors of the pineal region. *J Neurosurg* 39:455–462, 1973.

DeGirolami U: Pathology of tumors of the pineal region. In Schmidek HH (ed): *Pineal Tumors.* New York, Masson Publishing, 1977, pp 1–19.

DeGirolami U: Pathology of tumors of the pineal region. In Schmidek HH (ed): *Pineal Tumors.* New York, Masson Publishing, 1977, pp 1–19.

DeGirolami U, Zvaigzne O: Modification of the Achúcarro-Hortega pineal stain for paraffin-embedded formalin-fixed tissue. *Stain Technol* 48:48–50, 1973.

Deguchi T: Sympathetic regulation of circadian rhythm of serotonin N-acetyltransferase activity in pineal gland of infant rat. *J Neurochem* 38:797–801, 1982.

Deguchi T, Axelrod J: Superinduction of serotonin N-acetyltransferase and supersensitivity of adenyl cyclase to catecholamines in denervated pineal gland. *Mol Pharmacol* 9:184–190, 1973a.

Deguchi T, Axelrod J: Induction and superinduction of serotonin N-acetyltransferase by adrenergic drugs and denervation in the rat pineal organ. *Proc Natl Acad Sci USA* 69:2208–2211, 1972.

Deguchi T, Axelrod J: Supersensitivity and subsensitivity of the β-adrenergic receptor in pineal gland regulated by catecholamine neurotransmitter. *Proc Natl Acad Sci USA* 70:2411–2414, 1973b.

Demakas JJ, Sonntag VKH, Kaplan AM, Kelley JJ, Waggener JD: Surgical management of pineal area tumors in early childhood. *Surg Neurol* 17:435–440, 1981.

Demura R, Demura H, Shizume K, Kubo O, Kitamura K: A female case of the HCG-producing ectopic pinealoma associated with precocious puberty. *Endocrinol Jpn* 23:215–219, 1976.

deTribolet N, Barrelet L: Successful chemotherapy of pinealoma. *Lancet* 12:1228–1229, 1977.

Deutsch M: Radiotherapy of primary brain tumors in very young children. *Cancer* 50:2785–2789, 1982.

DiStefano A, Yap HY, Hortobagyi GN, Blumenschein GR: The natural history of breast cancer patients with brain metastases. *Cancer* 44:1913–1918, 1979.

Donat JF, Okazaki H, Gomez MR, Reagan TJ, Baker HL, Laws ER: Pineal tumors. *Arch Neurol* 35:736–740, 1978.

Dooling EC, Chi Je G, Gilles FH: Melanotic neuroectodermal tumor of infancy. Its histological similarities to fetal pineal gland. *Cancer* 39:1535–1541.

Dupont MG, Gerard JM, Flamant-Durand J, et al: Pathognomonic aspects of germinoma on CT scan. *Neuroradiology* 14:209–211, 1977.

Duvernoy HM: Human brainstem vessels. Berlin, Springer Verlag 1978.

Ebadi M, Chan A, Hammad H, Govitrapong P, Swanson S: Serotonin N-acetyltransferase and its regulation by pineal substances. In Reiter RJ (ed): *The Pineal and Its Hormones.* New York, Alan R. Liss, 1982, pp 21–33.

Ebels I, Benson B: A survey of the evidence that unidentified pineal substances affect the reproductive system in mammals. *Prog Reprod Biol* 4:51–57, 1978.

Eberts TH, Ransburg RC: Primary intracranial endodermal sinus tumor. *J Neurosurg* 50:246–252, 1979.

Edelson RL, Hearing VJ, Dellon AJ, et al: Differentiation between B cells, T cells, and histiocytes in melanocytic lesions: Primary and metastatic melanoma and halo and giant pigmented nevi. *Clin Immunol Immunopathol* 4:557–568, 1975.

Edner G: Stereotactic biopsy of intracranial space occupying lesion. *Acta Neurochir* 57:213–234, 1981.

Einhorn LH: Testicular cancer as a model for a curable neoplasm. The Richard and Hilda Rosenthal Foundation Award Lecture. *Cancer Res* 41:3275–3280, 1981.

Einhorn LH, Donohue JP: Improved chemotherapy in disseminated testicular cancer. *J Urol* 117:65–69, 1977.

Einhorn LH: Combination chemotherapy of disseminated testicular carcinoma with *cis*-diamminedichloroplatinum, vinblastine, and bleomycin (PVB): An update. *Proc Am Assoc Clin Oncol* Washington, DC, April 1978.

Einhorn LH: Combination chemotherapy of disseminated testicular carcinoma with *cis*-diamminedichloroplatinum, vinblastine, and bleomycin (PVB): An Update. *Proc Am Assoc Clin Oncol* 19:308, 1978.

Einhorn LH: Combination chemotherapy of disseminated testicular carcinoma with *cis*-diamminedichloroplatinum, vinblastine, and bleomycin (PVB): An update. *Proc Am Assoc Clin Oncol* Washington, DC, April, 1978.

Eiser C: Psychological sequelae of brain tumors in childhood: A retrospective study. *Br J Clin Psychol* 20:35–38, 1981.

El-Mahdi AM, Philips E, Lott S: The role of radiation therapy in pinealoma. *Radiology* 103:407–412, 1972.

Elden CA: Sterility of blind women. *Jpn J Fertil Steril* 16:48–50, 1971.

Elliott J: Circadian rhythms and photoperiodic time measurement in mammals. *Fed Proc* 35:2339–2346, 1976.

Elschnig A: Nystagmus retractorius, ein cerebrales Herdsymptom. *Med Klin* 9:8–11, 1913.

Engel E: Pinealoma metastasizing within the central nervous system. *J Oslo City Hosp* 19:62–67, 1969.

Engel RM, Elkins RC, Fletcher BD: Retroperitoneal teratoma. *Cancer* 22:1068–1073, 1968.

Esslen E, Papst W: Die bedeutung der elektromyographie fur die analyse von motilitatsstorungen der augen. *Bibl Ophthalmol* 57:1–168, 1961.

Fedeleff H, Aparicio NJ, Guitelman A, Aebeluk L, Mancini A, Cramer C: Effect of melatonin on the basal and stimulated gonadotrophin levels in normal men and postmenopausal women. *J Clin Endocrinol Metab* 42:1014–1017, 1976.

Ferrier D, Turner WA: Experimental lesions of the corpora quadrigemina in monkeys. *Brain* 24:27–46, 1901.

Fatranska M, Repcekova-Jezova D, Jurcovicova J, Vigas M: LH and testosterone response to LH-RH in blind men. *Horm Metab Res* 10:82–83, 1978.

Feun LG, Samson MK, Stephens RL: Vinblastine, bleomycin, *cis*-diamminedichloroplatinum in disseminated extragonadal germ cell tumors. *Cancer* 45:2543–2549, 1980.

Fine BS, Yanoff M: Ocular Histology. A Text and Atlas, ed 2. Hagerstown, Harper and Row, 1979, p. 74.

Finkelman FD, Lipsky PE: Immunoglobulin secretion by human splenic lymphocytes *in vitro*: The effects of antibodies to IgM and IgD. *J Immunol* 120:1465–1472, 1978.

Fitzharris BM, Kaye SB, Saverymuttu S, Newlands ES, Barrett A, Peckham MJ, McElwain TJ: VP16-213 as a single agent in advanced testicular tumors. *Eur J Cancer* 16:1193–1197, 1980.

Foerster O: Ein Fall von Vierhügeltumor, durch Operation entfernt. *Arch Psychiatr* 84:515–516, 1928.

Foerster O: Das operative Vorgehen bei Tumoren der Vierhügelgegend. *Wien Klin Wochenschr* 41:986–990, 1928.

Foerster O: Uber das operative Vorgehen bei Operationen der Vierhigelgegend. *Zentralbl Ges Neurol Psychiat* 61:457–459, 1932.

Fossa SD, Klepp O, Barth E, et al: Endocrinological studies in patients with metastatic malignant testicular germ cell tumors. *Int J Androl* 3:487–501, 1980.

Fowler FD, Alexander Jr, E, David Jr, CH: Pinealoma with metastases in the CNS: A rationale for treatment. *J Neurol* 13:271–288, 1974.

Fowler FD, Alexander Jr, E, Davis Jr, CH: Pinealoma with metastases in the central nervous system—a rationale of treatment. *J Neurosurg* 13:271–288, 1956.

Fraley EE, Lange PH, Kennedy BJ: Germ cell testicular cancer in adults. *N Engl J Med* 301:1370–1377, 1420–1426, 1979.

Frankl-Hochwart L: Uber Diagnose der Zirbeldrüsentumoren. *Dtsch Z Nervenh* 37:455–465, 1909.

Frenkel EP, Smith RG, Ligler FS, Hernandez J, Himes JR, Sheehan R, Vitetta ES, Kettman JR, Uhr JW: Analysis and detection of B cell neoplasms. Blood cells. In press.

Friedman NB: Cerminoma of the pineal. Its identity with germinoma ("seminoma") of the testis. *Cancer*

Res 7:363–368, 1947.

Friedman NB: Comparative morphogenesis of extragenital and gonadal teratoid tumors. *Cancer* 4:256–276, 1951.

Fröland SS, Natvig JB: Class, subclass, and allelic exclusion of membrane-bound Ig of human B lymphocytes. *J Exp Med* 136:409–414, 1972.

Fujii T, Itakura T, Hayashi S, Komai N, Nakamine H, Saito K: Primary pineal choriocarcinoma with hemorrhage monitored by computerized tomography. Case report. *J Neurosurg* 55:484–487, 1981.

Fukushima T: Endoscopic biopsy of intraventricular tumors with the use of a ventriloscope. *Neurosurgery* 2:110–113, 1978.

Futrell NN, Osborn AG, Cheson BD: Pineal region tumors: Computed tomographic-pathologic spectrum. *AJR* 137:951–956, 1981.

Gachelin G: The cell surface antigens of mouse embryonal carcinoma cells. *Biochim Biophys Acta* 516:27–60, 1978.

Gale G: Malignant mediastinal germ cell tumors. *Med Ped Oncol* 9:375–380, 1981.

Garnica AD, Netzloff ML, Rosenbloom AL: Clinical manifestations of hypothalamic tumors. *Ann Clin Lab Sci* 10:474–485, 1980.

Gay AJ, Brodkey J, Miller JE: Convergence retraction nystagmus. *Arch Ophthalmol* 70:456–461, 1963.

Gefford MR, Puizillout JJ, Delaage MA: A single radioimmunological assay for serotonin, *N*-acetylserotonin, 5-methoxytryptamine, and melatonin. *J Neurochem* 39:1271–1277, 1982.

Germa-Lluch JR, Begent RH, Bagshawe KD: Tumour-marker levels and prognosis in malignant teratoma of the testis. *Br J Cancer* 42:850–855, 1980.

Gern WA, Ralph CL: Melatonin synthesis by the retina. *Science* 204:183–184, 1979.

Ghatak NR, Hirano A, Zimmerman HM: Intrasellar germinomas: A form of ectopic pinealoma. *J Neurosurg* 31:670–675, 1969.

Ghoshhajra K, Baghai-Naiini P, Hahn HS, et al: Spontaneous rupture of pineal teratoma. *Neuroradiology* 17:215–217, 1979.

Giarman NJ, Day M: Presence of biogenic amines in the bovine pineal body. *Biochem Pharmacol* 1:235–237, 1959.

Gindhart TD, Tsukahara YC: Cytologic diagnosis of cerebrospinal fluid and sputum. *Acta Cytol* 23:341–346, 1979.

Ginsberg S, Kirshner J, Reich S, Panasci L, Finkelstein T, Fandrich S, Fitzpatrick A, Shechtman L, Comis R: Systemic chemotherapy for a primary germ cell tumor of the brain: A pharmacokinetic study. *Cancer Treat Rep* 65:477–483, 1981.

Glasauer FE: An operative approach to pineal tumors. *Acta Neurochir* 22:177–180, 1970.

Glasberg MR, Kirkpatrick JB, Neuwelt EA: Pineal parenchymal cell tumors. A light microscopic and ultrastructural study. *J Neuropathol Exp Neurol* 38:314, 1979.

Glass JD, Lynch GR: Evidence for a brain site of melatonin action in the white-footed mouse, *peromyscus leucopus*. *Neuroendocrinology* 34:1–6, 1982.

Glass RL, Culbertson CG: Teratoma of the pineal gland with choriocarcinoma and rhabdomyosarcoma. *Arch Pathol* 41:552–555, 1946.

Globus JH: Pinealoma. *Arch Pathol* 31:533–568, 1941.

Goerss S, Kelly P, Kall B, Alker G: A computed

tomographic stereotactic adaptor system. *Neurosurgery* 10:30, 375–379, 1982.

Goldhahn WE, Goldhahn G: Hirntumore. Leipzig, JA Barth Verlag, 1978.

Goldman B, Hall V, Hollister C, Reppert S, Roychoudhury P, Yellon S, Tamarkin L: Diurnal changes in pineal melatonin content in four rodent species: Relationship to photoperiodism. *Biol Reprod* 24:778–783, 1981.

Goldman B, Hall V, Hollister C, Roychoudhury P, Tamarkin L, Westrom W: Effects of melatonin on the productive system in intact and pinealectomized male hamsters maintained under various photoperiods. *Endocrinology* 104:82–88, 1979.

Goldman BD, Carter DS, Hall VD, Roychoudry P, Yellin SM: Physiology of pineal melatonin in three hamster species. In Klein DC (ed): *Melatonin Rhythm Generating System.* Basel, Karger, 1982, pp 210–231.

Goldzieher M: Uber eine Ziebeldrusengeschwulst. *Virchows Arch [Pathol Anat]* 213:353–365, 1913.

Gonzales-Cruzzi F: Extragonadal Teratomas. *Atlas of Tumor Pathology,* 2nd series, Fascicle 18. Washington DC, Armed Forces Institute of Pathology, 1982.

Gonzalez-Crussi F, Winkler RF, Mirkin DC: Sacrococcygeal teratomas in infants and children. *Arch Pathol Lab Med* 102:420–425, 1978.

Graham S, Gibson R, West D, et al: Epidemiology of cancer of the testis in upstate New York. *J Natl Cancer Inst* 58:1255–1261, 1977.

Greenwald GS: Histologic transformation of the ovary of the lactating hamster. *Endocrinology* 77:641–649, 1965.

Greiner AC, Chan AC: Melatonin content of the human pineal gland. *Science* 199:83–84, 1978.

Greitz T: Tumours of the quadrigeminal plate and adjacent structures. *Acta Radiol* 12:513–538, 1972.

Griffin BR, Griffin TW, Tong DYK, Russell AH, Kurtz J, Laramore GE, Groudine M: Pineal region tumors: Results of radiation therapy and indications for elective spinal irradiation. *Int J Radiat Oncol Biol Phys* 7:605–608, 1981.

Grote E, Lorenz R, Vuia O: Clinical and endocrinological findings in ectopic pinealoma and spongioblastoma of the hypothalamus. *Acta Neurochir* 53:87–98, 1980.

Growdon JH, Winkler GF, Wray SH: Midbrain ptosis—a case with clinicopathologic correlation. *Arch Neurol* 30:179–181, 1974.

Guiffre R, DiLorenzo N: Evolution of a primary intrasellar germinomatous teratoma into a choriocarcinoma. *J Neurosurg* 42:602–604, 1975.

Gutzeit R: Ein Teratom der Zirbeldrüse. Thesis, E. Erlatis, Königsberg, 1896.

Haase J, Norgaard-Pedersen B: Alpha-feta-protein (AFP) and human chorionic gonadotropin (HCG) as biochemical markers of intracranial germ cell tumors. *Acta Neurochir* 50:67–69, 1979.

Haase J, Neilsen K: Value of tumor markers in the treatment of endodermal sinus tumors and choriocarcinomas in the pineal region. *Neurosurgery* 5:485–488, 1979.

Hahn FJY, Rim K, Schapiro RL: The normal range and position of the pineal gland on computed tomography. *Radiology* 119:599–600, 1976.

Haimovic IC, Sharer L, Hyman RA, Beresford R: Metastasis of intracranial germinoma through a ventriculoperitoneal shunt. *Cancer* 48:1033–1036, 1981.

Hainsworth JD, Einhorn LH, Williams SD, Stewart M, Greco A: Advanced extragonadal germ-cell tumors. *Ann Int Med* 97:7–11, 1982.

Hajdu SI, Porro RS, Lieberman PH, Foote Jr, FW: Degeneration of the pineal gland of patients with cancer. *Cancer* 29:706–709, 1972.

Hajdu SI: Pathology of germ cell tumors of the testis. *Semin Oncol* 6:14–25, 1979.

Haldeman KO: Tumors of the pineal gland. *Arch Neurol Psychiatr* 18:724, 1927.

Halsall AK, Fairweather DS, Bradwell AR, Blackburn JC, Dykes PW, Howell A, Reeder A, Hine KR: Localization of malignant germ-cell tumours by external scanning after injection of radiolabeled antialpha-fetoprotein. *Br Med J* 283:942–944, 1981.

Hamburger C: Gonadotropins, androgens and oestrogens in cases of malignant tumours of the testis. In Wolstenholme GEW, O'Connor M (eds): *Hormone Production in Endocrine Tumours.* Boston, Little, Brown and Co., 1958, p 200.

Hamlin IME: Possible host resistance in carcinoma of the breast, a histological study. *Br J Cancer* 22:383–401, 1968.

Hammock MK, Milhorat TH, Earle K, DiChiro G: Vein of Galen ligation in the primate. *J Neurosurg* 34:77–83, 1971.

Handa H, Yamashita J: Summary: Current treatment of pineal tumors. *Neurol Med Chir* 21:147–148, 1981.

Handa H, Yamashita J: Summary: Current treatment of pineal tumors. *Surg Neurol* 16:279–1981.

Hanks GE, Herring DF, Kramer S: Patterns of care outcome studies: Results of the national practice in seminoma of the testis. *Int J Radiat Oncol Biol Phys* 7:1413–1417, 1981.

Hansen T, Heyden T, Sundberg T, Wetterberg L: Effect of propranolol on serum melatonin. *Lancet* 2:309–310, 1977.

Harris W, Cairns H: Diagnosis and treatment of pineal tumors. *Lancet* 1:3–9, 1932.

Hasegawa H, Ushio Y, Hori M, et al: Primary intracranial choriocarcinoma in the pineal regions: a case report. *Med J Osaka Univ* 25:63–71, 1974.

Haase J, Nielsen K: Value of tumor markers in the treatment of endodermal sinus tumors and choriocarcinomas in the pineal region. *Neurosurgery* 5:485–488, 1979.

Hassoun J, Gambarelli D, Pellissier JF, Henin D, Toga M: Germinomas of the brain. Light and electron microscopic study. A report of seven cases. *Acta Neuropathol* 7:105–108, 1981.

Hassoun J, Gambarelli D, Choux M, Toga M: Macrophagic activity in intracerebral germinoma: Ultrastructural study of a case. *Hum Pathol* 2:207–210, 1980.

Hayashi S, Nishii T, Osaki A, et al: Akinetic mutism associated with pineal teratoma. *Brain Nerve* (Tokyo) 24:119–125, 1972.

Haymaker W, Liss L, Vogel FS, Johnson Jr, JE, Adams RD, Scharenberg K: The pineal gland. In Haymaker W, Adams RD (eds): *Histology and Histopathology of the Nervous System.* Springfield, Charles C Thomas, vol II, 1982, pp 1801–2023.

Hedges III, TR, Hoyt WF: Ocular tilt reaction due to an upper brainstem lesion: Paroxysmal skew deviation, torsion and oscillation of the eyes with head tilt. *Ann Neurol* 11:537–540, 1982.

Heppner F: Uber Meningeome des 3. Ventrikels. *Acta Neurochir* 4:55–67, 1956.

Heppner F: Zur Operationstechnik bei Pinealomen. *Zentralbl Neurochir* 19:219–224, 1959.

Herrick MK, Rubinstein LJ: The cytological differentiating potential of pineal parenchymal neoplasms (true pinealomas). *Brain* 102:289–320, 1979.

Higashi K, Katayama S, Orita T: Pineal apoplexy. *J Neurol Neurosurg Psychiatry* 42:1050–1053, 1979.

Hipkin LJ: Effect of 5-methoxytryptophol and melatonin on uterine weight responses to human chorionic gonadotrophin. *J Endocrinol* 48:287–288, 1970.

Hirano A, Llena JF, Chung HD: Some new observations on intracranial germinoma. *Acta Neuropathol* 32:103–113, 1975.

Hirsch LF, Rorke LB, Schmidek HH: Unusual cause of relapsin hydrocephalus. Congenital intracranial teratoma. *Arch Neurol* 34:505–507, 1977.

Ho K-L, Rassekh ZS: Endodermal sinus tumor of the pineal region. Case report and review of the literature. *Cancer* 44:1081–1086, 1979.

Hoffman HJ: Suprasellar Germinomas. In *Pediatric Neurosurgery: Surgery of the Developing Nervous System.* New York, Grune and Stratton, 1982, pp 487–491.

Hoffman HJ, Becker L, Craven MA: A clinically and pathologically distinct group of benign brainstem gliomas. *Neurosurgery* 7:243–284, 1980.

Hoffman HJ, Yoshida M, Becker LE, Hendrick EB, Humphreys PR: Pineal region tumors in childhood. *Concepts Pediatr Neursurg* 4:360–386, 1983.

Hoffman RA, Reiter RJ: Response of some endocrine organs of female hamsters to pinealectomy and light. *Life Sci* 5:1147–1151, 1966.

Hoffman RA, Reiter RJ: Pineal gland: Influence on gonads of male hamsters. *Science* 142:1609–1611, 1965.

Hoffmann K: Pineal involvement in the photoperiodic control of reproduction and other functions in the Djungarian hamster, *Phodopus sungorus.* In Reiter RJ (ed): *The Pineal Gland Vol. 2, Reproductive Effects.* Boca Raton, CRC Press, 1982, pp 45–82.

Hoffmann K: Photoperiod, pineal, melatonin and reproduction in hamsters. *Prog Brain Res* 52:397–415, 1979.

Hollwich F, Dieckhues B: Endokrines System und Erblindung. *Deut Med Wschr* 96:363–368, 1971.

Hollwich F, Neirmann H, Dieckhues B: Einfluss des Augenlichtes auf die Sexualsteuerung bei Mensch and Tier. *J Neurovisc Rel [Suppl] 10]* 247–255, 1971.

Hollwich F: *The Influence of Ocular Light Perception on Metabolism in Man and in Animal.* Springer, New York, 1979.

Hooper RJC, Silman RE, Leone RM, Young IM: The development of a plasma assay for 5-methoxytryptamine using gas chromatography-mass spectrometry. In Matthews CD, Seamark RF (eds): *Pineal Function.* Elsevier/North Holland, 1981, pp 1–6.

Horrax G, Bailey P: Tumors of the pineal body. *Arch Neurol Psychiat* 13:423–470, 1925.

Horrax G: Extirpation of a large pinealoma from a patient with pubertas praecox: a new operation approach. *Arch Neurol Psychiat* 37:385–397, 1937.

Horrax G: Treatment of tumors of the pineal body.

Experience in a series of twenty-two cases. *Arch Neurol Psychiat* 64:227–242, 1950.

Horrax G: The diagnosis and treatment of pineal tumors. *Radiology* 52:186–192, 1959.

Horrax G, Daniels JT: The conservative treatment of pineal tumors. *Surg Clin North Am* 22:649–659, 1942.

Horsley V, Clark RH: The structure and function of the cerebellum examined by a new method. *Brain* 31:45–124, 1908.

Horsley V: Discussion of paper by CMH Howell on tumors of the pineal body. *Proc R Soc Med* 3:77–78, 1910.

Hosoi K: Teratoma and teratoid tumors of the brain. *Arch Pathol* 9:1207–1219, 1930.

Houser R, Izant Jr, RJ, Persky L: Testicular germ cell tumors in children. *Am J Surg* 110:876–892, 1965.

Howell CMH: Tumours of the pineal gland. *Proc R Soc Med* 3:64–77, 1910.

Huang YP, Wolf BS: The veins of the posterior fossa—superior or Galenic draining group. *Am J Roentgenol* 95:808–821, 1965.

Hübner G: Intracerebral metastatic malignant teratoma in the region of the optic chiasm. *Beitr Pathol* 157:189–199, 1976.

Huckman MS, Robeson GM, Norton T: Radiology of suprasellar ectopic pinealoma. *Acta Radiol [Suppl]* 347:515–527, 1975.

Hurlbut EC, King TS, Richardson BA, Reiter RJ: The effects of the light:dark cycle and sympathetically-active drugs on pineal *N*-acetyltransferase activity and melatonin content in the Richardson's ground squirrel, *Spermophilus richardsonnii.* In Reiter RJ (ed): *The Pineal and Its Hormones.* New York, Alan R. Liss, 1982, pp 45–56.

Hutchinson JSM, Brooks RV, Barratt TM, Newman CGH, Prunty FTG: Sexual precocity due to an intracranial tumour causing unusual testicular secretion of testosterone. *Arch Dis Child* 44:732–737, 1969.

Hyman RA, Loring MF, Liebeskind AL, Naidich JB, Stein HL: Computed tomographic evaluation of therapeutically induced changes in primary and secondary brain tumors. *Neuroradiology* 14:213–218, 1978.

Iguchi H, Kato, Iboyashi H: Age-dependent reduction in serum melatonin concentration in healthy human subjects. *J Clin Endocrinol Metab* 55:27–29, 1982.

Illmensee K, Mintz B: Totipotentiality and normal differentiation of single teratocarcinoma cells cloned by injection into blastocysts. *Proc Natl Acad Sci USA* 73:549–553, 1976.

Illnerova H, Skopkova S: Regulation of the diurnal rhythm in rat pineal serotonin *N*-acetyltransferase activity and serotonin content during ontogenesis. *J Neurochem* 26:1051–1054, 1976.

Inoue Y, Takeuchi T, Tamaki M, Nin K, Hakuba A, Nishimura S: Sequential CT observations of irradiated intracranial germinomas. *Am J Roentgenol* 132:361–365, 1979.

Iraci G: Ectopic pinealoma. Report of a case and remarks on the treatment. *Acta Neurochir* 38:293–303, 1977.

Isamat F: Tumours of the posterior part of the third ventricle: Neurosurgical criteria. In *Advances and Technical Standards in Neurosurgery.* Wien-New

York, Springer-Verlag, 1979, vol 6, pp 171–184.

Isayama Y, Takahashi T, Inoue M: Ocular findings of suprasellar germinoma: Long-term followup after radiotherapy. *Neurol Ophthalmol* 1:53–61, 1980.

Izquierdo JM, Rougerie J, Lapras C, Sanz F: The so-called ectopic pinealomas. *Childs Brain* 5:505–512, 1979.

Jacob F: The Leeuwenhoek Lecture 1977: Mouse teratocarcinoma and mouse embryo. *Proc R Soc Lond [Biol]* 201:249–270, 1978.

Jahner D, Stuhlmann H, Stewart CI, et al: De novo methylation of retroviral genomes during mouse embryogenesis. *Nature* 298:623–628, 1982.

Jakobiec FA, Tso MO, Zimmerman LE, Danis P: Retinoblastoma and intracranial malignancy. *Cancer* 39:2048–2058, 1977.

James W, Dudley HR: Teratoma in the region of the pineal body. Report of a case. *J Neurosurg* 14:235–241, 1957.

Jamieson KG: Excision of pineal tumors. *J Neurosurg* 35:550–553, 1971.

Javadpour N, Bergman S: Recent advances in testicular cancer. *Curr Probl Surg* XV:5–53, 1978.

Javadpour N: The role of multiple tumor markers in the diagnosis and management of seminoma. In Anderson CK, Jones WG, Ward AM (eds): *Germ Cell Tumors.* New York, Alan R Liss Inc, 1981, pp 297–311.

Javadpour N: The value of biologic markers in diagnosis and treatment of testicular cancer. *Semin Oncol* 6:37–47, 1979.

Jellinger K: Primary intracranial germ cell tumours. *Acta Neuropathol* 25:291–306, 1973.

Jenkin RDT, Simpson WJK, Keen CW: Pineal and suprasellar germinomas. *J Neurosurg* 48:99–107, 1978.

Jimerson DC, Lynch HJ, Post RM, Wurtman RJ, Bunney WE: Urinary melatonin rhythms during sleep deprivation in depressed patients and normals. *Life Sci* 20:1501–1507, 1977.

Jirasek J: Development of the genital system and male pseudohermaphrotism. Baltimore: *Johns Hopkins Press* 1971, pp 3–10.

Johnson LY: The pineal gland as a modulator of the adrenal and thyroid axes. In Reiter RJ (ed): *The Pineal Gland Vol. 3 Extra-Reproductive Effects.* Boca Raton, CRC Press, 1982, pp 107–152.

Johnson LY, Vaughan, Reiter RJ: The pineal and its effects on mammalian reproduction. In Reiter RJ (ed): *The Pineal and Reproduction.* Basel, Karger, 1978, pp 116–156.

Johnson LY, Vaughan MK, Richardson BA, Petterborg LJ, Reiter RJ: Variation in pineal melatonin content during the estrous cycle of the rat. *Proc Soc Exp Biol Med* 169:416–419, 1982.

Johnson LY, Asch RH, Reiter RJ: Failure of pinealectomy to affect acute changes in plasma levels of luteinizing hormone and prolactin in ovariectomized rats following delta 9-tetrahydrocannabinol administration. *Subst Alcohol Actions Misuse* 1:355–359, 1980.

Jooma R, Kendall BE: Diagnosis and management of pineal tumors. *J Neurosurg* 58:654–665, 1983.

Jordan RM, Kendall JW, McClung M, et al: Concentration of human chorionic gonadotropin in the cerebrospinal fluid of patients with germinal cell

hypothalamic tumors. *Pediatrics* 65:121–124, 1980.

Judisch GF, Shivanand RP: Concurrent heritable retinoblastoma, pinealoma, and trisomy X. *Arch Ophthalmol* 99:1767–1769, 1981.

Juif JG, Maitrot D, Pierson M, Heldt N, Buchheit F, Luckel JC: Les tumeurs cerebrales primitives d'origine germinale. *Arch Fr Pediatr* 34:335–346, 1977.

Kabashima K, Harada M, Morabayashi T. A case of ectopic pinealoma: study on course and autopsy. *Brain Nerve* 29:453–458, 1977.

Kageyama N: Ectopic pinealoma in the region of the optic chiasm. Report of five cases. *J Neurosurg* 35:755–759, 1971.

Kageyama N, Belsky R: Ectopic pinealoma in the chiasmal region. *Neurology* 11:318–327, 1961.

Kahn EA: Surgical treatment of pineal tumors. *Arch Neurol Psychiatry* 38:833–842, 1937.

Kalumpaheti R, Thumnoon K, Thanaphum V: The pineal tumour in Thailand. 8th International Congress Neuropathology, Abstract #176.

Kalyanaraman UP: Primary glioblastoma of the pineal gland. *Arch Neurol* 36:717–718, 1979.

Kaplan EL, Meier P: Nonparametric estimation from incomplete observations. *J Am Stat Assoc* 53:457–481, 1958.

Kaplan ME, Clark C: An improved rosetting assay for detection of human T lymphocytes. *J Immunol Methods* 5:131–135, 1974.

Kappers JA: The development, topographical relations and innervation of the epiphysis cerebri in the albino rat. *Z Zellforsch* 52:163–215, 1960.

Katsura S, Suzuki J, Wada I: A statistical study of brain tumors in the neurosurgical clinics in Japan. *J Neurosurg* 16:570–580, 1959.

Kawakami Y, Yamada O, Tabuchi K, Ohmoto T, Nishimoto A: Primary intracranial choriocarcinoma. *J Neurosurg* 53:369–374, 1980.

Kazner E, Stochdorph O, Wende S, Grumme T: Intracranial lipoma: Diagnostic and therapeutic considerations. *J Neurosurg* 52:234–245, 1980.

Keane JR: Ocular skew deviation. Analysis of 100 cases. *Arch Neurol* 32:185–190, 1975.

Kebabian JW, Zatz M, Romero JA, Axelrod J: Rapid changes in rat pineal β-adrenergic receptor. Alterations in 1-(^{3}H) alprenolol binding and adenylate cyclase. *Proc Natl Acad Sci USA* 72:3735–3739, 1975.

Kelly PJ, Alker G, Goerss S: Computer-assisted stereotactic laser microsurgery for the treatment of intracranial neoplasms. *Neurosurgery* 10:3, 324–331, 1982.

Kempe LG: Operative Neurosurgery. Berlin, Springer-Verlag, 1968.

Kennaway DJ, McCulloch G, Matthews CD, Seamark RF: Plasma melatonin, luteinizing hormone, follicle-stimulating hormone, prolactin, and corticoids in two patients with pinealoma. *J Clin Endocrinol Metab* 49:144–145, 1979.

Kennaway DJ, Frith RG, Phillipou G, Matthews CD, Seamark RF: A specific radioimmunoassay for melatonin in biological tissue and fluid and its validation by gas chromatography-mass spectrometry. *Endocrinology* 101:119–127, 1977.

Kennaway DJ, Gilmore TA, Seamark RF: Effect of melatonin feeding on serum prolactin and gonadotrophin levels and the onset of seasonal estrous cyclicity in sheep. *Endocrinology* 110:1766–1772, 1982.

Kenning JA: Intrasellar-suprasellar mixed germ cell tumor.

Kiessling M, Anagnostopoulos J, Lombeck G, Kleihues: Diagnostic potential of stereotactic biopsy of brain tumors. In Voth D, Gutjahr, Langnaid C (eds): *Tumors of the Central Nervous System in Infancy and Childhood.* Berlin, Springer-Verlag, 1981, pp 247–256.

King TS, Richardson BA, Reiter RJ: Age-associated changes in pineal serotonin N-acetyltransferase activity and melatonin content in the male gerbil. *Endocr Res Commun* 8:253–262, 1981.

Kirshner JJ, Ginsberg SJ, Fitzpatrick AV, Comis RL: Treatment of a primary intracranial germ cell tumor with systemic chemotherapy. *Med Ped Oncol* 9:361–365, 1981.

Klein DC, Auerback DA, Namboodiri MAA, Wheler GHT: Indole metabolism in the mammalian pineal gland. In Reiter RJ (ed): *The Pineal Gland Vol. 1 Anatomy and Physiology.* Boca Raton, CRC Press, 1981, pp 199–227.

Klein DC, Weller JL: Adrenergic-adenosine 3′,5′-monophosphate regulation of serotonin N-acetyltransferase activity and the temporal relationship of serotonin N-acetyltransferase activity to synthesis of ³H-N-acetylserotonin and ³H-melatonin in the cultured rat pineal gland. *J Pharmacol Exp Ther* 186:516–527, 1973.

Klein DC, Weller J: Indole metabolism in the pineal gland: A circadian rhythm in N-acetyltransferase. *Science* 169:1093–1095, 1970.

Kline KT, Damjanov I, Katz SM, Schmidek H: Pineoblastoma: An electron microscopic study. *Cancer* 44:1692–1699, 1979.

Klintworth GK: The ontogeny and growth of the human tentorium cerebelli. *Anat Rec* 158:433–441, 1967.

Klintworth GK: The comparative anatomy and phylogeny of the tentorium cerebelli. *Anat Rec* 160:635–641, 1968.

Kneisley LW, Moskowitz MH, Lynch HJ: Cervical spinal cord lesions disrupt the rhythm in human melatonin excretion. *J Neural Transm* [Suppl] 13:311–323, 1978.

Kobayashi S, Sugita K, Tanaka Y, Kyoshima K: Infratentorial approach to the pineal region in the prone position: concorde position. *J Neurosurg* 58:141–143, 1983.

Kobayashi T, Kageyama N, Kida Y, Yoshida J, Shibuya N, Okamura K: Unilateral germinomas involving the basal ganglia and thalamus. *J Neurosurg* 55:55–62, 1981.

Koerber HL: Ueber drei falls von retraktronskewegung des bulbus. *Opthalmol Klin* 7:65–67, 1903.

Koide O, Watanabe Y, Sato K: A pathological survey of intracranial germinoma and pinealoma in Japan. *Cancer* 45:2119–2130, 1980.

Komatsu K, Hiratsuka H, Inaba Y: Pathologic study of four cases with tumors in the region of the pineal body. *Brain Nerve* 23:917–926, 1971.

Komrower GM: Precocious puberty in association with pineal seminoma. *Arch Dis Childhood* 49:822, 1974.

Koos WTH, Miller MH: Intracranial tumors of infants and children. Stuttgart, Thieme Verlag, 1971.

Krabbe KH: Histologische und Embryologische Untersuchungen uber die Zirbeldruse des Mechen. *Anat Hefte* 54:187–319, 1916.

Krabbe KH: The pineal gland, especially in relation to the problem of its supposed significance in sexual development. *Endocrinology* 7:379–414, 1923.

Krause F: Chirurgie des Gehirns und Rückenmarks. Vol. 1. Berlin, Urban und Schwarzenberg, 1911.

Krause F: Operative Freilegung der Vierhügel, nebst Beobachtungen über Hirndruck und Dekompression. *Zentralbl Chir* 53:2812–2819, 1926.

Kretzschmar K, Aulich A, Schindler E, Lange S, Grumme T, Meese W: The diagnostic value of CT for radiotherapy of cerebral tumors. *Neuroradiology* 14:245–250, 1978.

Kubo O, Yamasaki N, Kamijo Y, Amano K, Kitamura K, Demura R: Human chorionic gonadotropin produced by ectopic pinealoma in a girl with precocious puberty. *J Neurosurg* 47:101–105, 1977.

Kun LE, Tang TT, Sty JR, Camitta BM: Primary cerebral germinoma and ventriculoperitoneal shunt metastasis. *Cancer* 48:213–216, 1981.

Kundert JG: Pinealom und Tumoren des III. Ventrikels. Katamnestische Untersuchungen von 20 neurochirurgisch behandelten Patienten. Schweiz. *Arch Neurol Psychiat* 92:296–333, 1963.

Kunicki A: Operative experiences in eight cases of pineal tumors. *J Neurosurg* 17:815–823, 1960.

Kuramoto H, Hamano M, Suzuki M, et al: Study of so called "cellular effect" methotrexate on choriocarcinoma and its mode of manifestation. *Nippon Sanka Fujinka Gakkai Zasshi* 34:187–195, 1982.

Kurisaka M, Moriyasu N, Kitajima K: Immunohistochemical studies of brain tumors associated with precocious puberty, preliminary report of correlation between tumor secreting hormone and leydig cells in precocious puberty. *Neurol Med Chir* 19:675–682, 1979.

Kurman RT, Norris HJ: Endodermal sinus tumor of the ovary: A clinical and pathologic analysis of 71 cases. *Cancer* 38:2404–2419, 1976.

Kurumado K, Mori W: Virus like particles in human pinealoma. *Acta Neuropathol* 35:273–276, 1976.

Kurumado K, Mori W: Synaptic ribbon in the human pinealocyte. *Acta Pathol Jpn* 26:381–384, 1976.

Kurumado K, Mori W: A morphological study on the pineal gland of human embryo. *Acta Pathol Jpn* 27:527–531, 1977.

Lang J: Die äuBeren Liquorräume des Gehirna. *Acta Anat* 86:267–299, 1973.

Lapin V, Ebels I: The role of the pineal gland in neuroendocrine control mechanisms of neoplastic growth. *J Neural Transm* 50:275–282, 1981.

Larmande P, Henin D, Jan M, Elie A, Gouaze A: Abnormal vertical eye movements in the locked-in syndrome. *Ann Neurol* 11:100–102, 1982.

Lazar ML, Clark K: Direct surgical management of masses in the region of the vein of Galen. *Surg Neurol* 2:17–22, 1974.

Lee SH, Sundararesan N, Jereb B, et al: Endodermal sinus tumor of the pineal region: A case report. *Neurosurgery* 3:407–411, 1978.

Legait H, Legait E: Contribution a l'etude de la glande pineale humaine; etude faite a l'aide de 747 glandes. *Bull Assoc Anat* 61:107–121, 1977.

Lehman RAW, Torres-Reyes E: Cystic intracranial teratoma in an infant: Case report. *J Neurosurg*

33:334–338, 1970.

Lehrer S: Fertility and menopause in blind women. *Fertil Steril* 36:396–397, 1981.

Lehrer S: Fertility of blind women. *Fertil Steril* 38:751–753, 1982.

Leksell L: The stereotaxic method and radiosurgery of the brain. *Acta Chir Scand* 102:316–319, 1951.

Leksell L: Stereotaxis and radiosurgery. An operative system. Springfield, IL, Charles C Thomas, 1971.

Lenko HL, Lang U, Aubert ML, Paunier L, Sizonenko PC: Melatonin in plasma and urine before and during puberty. *Pediatr Res* 15:74–79, 1981.

Lerner AB, Nordlund JJ: Melatonin: Clinical pharmacology. *J Neural Transmis*, [Suppl] 13:339–347, 1978.

Levy R, Warnke R, Dorfman RF, Haimovich J: The monoclonality of human B-cell lymphomas. *J Exp Med* 145:1014–1028, 1977.

Lewis I, Baxter DW, Stratford JG: Atypical teratomas of the pineal. *Can Med Assoc J* 89:103–110, 1963.

Lewy AJ, Kern HA, Rosenthal NE, Wehr TA: Bright artificial light treatment of a manic-depressive patient with a seasonal mood cycle. *Am J Psychiat* 139:1496–1498, 1982.

Lewy AJ: Biochemistry and regulation of mammalian melatonin production. In Relkin R (ed): *The Pineal Gland*. New York, Elsevier, 1983, pp 77–128.

Lewy AJ, Newsome DA: Different types of melatonin circadian secretory rhythms in some blind subjects. *J Clin Endocrinol Metab* (in press).

Lewy AJ, Tetsu M, Markey SP, Goodwin FK, Kopin IJ: Pinealectomy abolishes plasma melatonin in the rat. *J Clin Endocrinol Metab* 50:204–205, 1980.

Lewy AJ, Markey SP: Analysis of melatonin in human plasma by gas chromatography negative chemical ionization mass spectrometry. *Science* 201:741–743, 1978.

Lewy AJ, Wehr TA, Goodwin FK, Newsome DA, Markey SP: Light suppresses melatonin secretion in humans. *Science* 210:1267–1269, 1980.

Ligler FS, Smith RG, Kettman JR, Hernandex J, Himes JB, Vitetta ES, Uhr JW, Frenkel EP: Detection of tumor cells in the peripheral blood of nonleukemic patients with B cell lymphoma: Analysis of "clonal excess." *Blood*, in press.

Ligler FS, Vitetta ES, Smith RG, Himes JB, Uhr JW, Frenkel EP, Kettman JR: An immunologic approach for the detection of tumor cells in the peripheral blood of patients with malignant lymphoma: Implications for the diagnosis of minimal disease. *J Immunol* 123:1123–1126, 1979.

Liliequist B: The subarachnoid cisterns. An anatomic and roentgenologic study. *Acta Radiol* (Suppl) 183:1–108, 1959.

Lin S-R, Crane MD, Lin ZS, et al: Characteristics of calcification in tumors of the pineal gland. *Radiology* 126:721–726, 1978.

Lingeman CH: Etiology of cancer of the human ovary: A review. *J Natl Cancer Inst* 53:1603–1618, 1974.

Lipton JS, Petterborg LJ, Steinlechner S, Reiter RJ: *In vivo* responses of the pineal gland of the Syrian hamster to isoproterenol or norepinephrine. In Reiter RJ (ed): *The Pineal and Its Hormones*. New York, Alan R. Liss, 1982, pp 107–115.

Lipton JS, Petterborg LJ, Reiter RJ: Influence of propranolol, phenoxybenzamine of phentolamine in the *in vivo* nocturnal rise of pineal melatonin levels in the Syrian hamster. *Life Sci* 28:2377–2382, 1981.

Logothetis CJ, Samuels ML, Trindade A: The management of brain metastases in germ cell tumors. *Cancer* 49:12–18, 1982.

Loken AC: On relation of atypical pinealomas to teratoid tumors. *Acta Pathol Microbiol Scand* 40:417–424, 1957.

London WT, Houff SA, Madden DL, Fuchillo DA, Gravell M, Wallen WC, Palmer AE, Sever JL: Brain tumors in owl monkeys inoculated with a human polyomavirus (JC virus). *Science* 201:1246–1249, 1978.

Lowenstein O: Alternating contraction anisocoria: Pupillary syndrome of anterior midbrain. *Arch Neurol* 72:742–757, 1954.

Lowenthal A, Flament-Durand J, Karcher D, Noppe M, Brion JP: Glial cells identified by anti-α-albumin (anti-GFA) in human pineal gland. *J Neurochem* 38:863–865, 1982.

Luccarelli G: Ectopic pinealomas of the optic nerve and chiasm. Report of two personal cases. *Acta Neurochir* (Wien) 27:205–221, 1972.

Lynch GR, Sullivan JK, Heath HW, Tamarkin L: Daily melatonin rhythms in photoperiod sensitive and insensitive white-footed mice (*Peromyscus leucopus*). In Reiter RJ (ed): *The Pineal and Its Hormones*. New York, Alan R. Liss, 1982, pp 67–73.

Lynch GR: Effect of simultaneous exposure to differences in photoperiod and temperature on the seasonal molt and reproductive system of the white-footed mouse, *Peromyscus leucopus*. *Comp Biochem Physiol* 53C:67–68, 1973.

Lynch H: Assay methodology. In Relkin R (ed): *The pineal gland*. New York, Elsevier, 1983, pp 129–150.

Lynch HJ: Diurnal oscillations in pineal melatonin content. *Life Sci* 10:791–795. 1971.

Lynch HJ, Wang P, Wurtman RJ: Increase in rat pineal melatonin content following L-DOPA administration. *Life Sci* 12:145–151, 1973.

Lynch HL, Rivest RW, Ronsheim PM, Wurtman RJ: Light intensity and the control of melatonin secretion in rats. *Neuroendocrinology* 33:181–186, 1981.

Lynch HJ, Wurtman RJ, Moskovitz MA, Archer MC, Ho MH: Daily rhythm in human urinary melatonin. *Science* 187:169–170, 1975.

Magee K, Basinska J, Quarrington B, Stancer HC: Blindness and menarche. *Life Sci* 9:7–12, 1970.

Mahour G, Wooley M, Trivedi S, et al: Sacrococcygeal teratoma: A 33 year experience. *J Pediatr Surg* 10:183–188, 1975.

Maier JG, Dejong D: Pineal body tumors. *Am J Roentgenol* 99:826–832, 1967.

Marburg O: Zur Kenntnis der normalen und pathologischen Histologie der Zirbeldruse. Die Adipositas cerebralis. *Arb Neurol Inst Wien Univ* 17:217–279, 1909.

Marburg O: Die adipositas cerebralis. Ein Beitrag zur pathologie der zirbeldrüse. *Wien Med Wochenschr* 28:2617–2622, 1908.

Markesbery WR, Brooks WH, Milsow L, Mortara RH: Ultrastructural study of the pineal germinoma *in vivo* and *in vitro*. *Cancer* 37:327–337, 1976.

Markesbery WR, Haugh RM, Young AB: Ultrastructure of pineal parenchymal neoplasms. *Acta Neuropathol* 55:143–149, 1981.

Markey SP, Buell PE: Pinealectomy abolishes 6-hydroxymelatonin excretion by male rats. *Endocrinol-*

ogy 111:425–426, 1982.

Marshall AHE, Dayan AD: An immune reaction in man against seminomas, dysgerminoas, pinealomas, and the mediastinal tumors of similar histological appearance? *Lancet* 2:1102–1104, 1964.

Marshall LF, Rorke LB, Schut L: Teratocarcinoma of the brain—A treatable disease? *Childs Brain* 5:96–102, 1979.

Martin GR: Teratocarcinomas as a model system for the study of embryogenesis and neoplasia: A review. *Cell* 5:229–243, 1975.

Martini N, Golbey RB, Hajdu SI, et al: Primary mediastinal germ cell tumors. *Cancer* 33:763–769, 1974.

Martins AN, Johnston JS, Henry JM, Stoffel TJ, Chiro GD: Delayed radiation necrosis of the brain. *J Neurosurg* 47:336–345, 1977.

Marx P, Kleihues P, Zülch KJ: Normale und pathologische Anatomie des Mittelhirns. *Radiologe* 8:335–347, 1968.

Mata MM, Schaier BK, Klein DC, Weller JL, Chiou CY: On GABA function and physiology in the pineal gland. *Brain Res* 118:383–397, 1976.

Matson DD: Neurosurgery of infancy and childhood. Springfield, IL, Charles C Thomas, 1969.

Matthews CD, Kenneway DJ, Fellenberg AJG, Phillipou G, Cox LW, Seamark, RF: Melatonin in man. In Birau N, Schloot W (eds): *Melatonin—Current Status and Perspectives.* New York, Pergamon, 1981, pp. 371–381.

Matthews SA, Evans KL, Morgan WW, Petterborg LJ, Rieter RJ: Pineal indoleamine metabolism in the cotton rat, *Sigmodon hispidus*: Studies on norepinephrine, serotonin, *N*-acetyltransferase and melatonin. In Reiter RJ (ed): *The Pineal and Its Hormones.* New York, Alan R. Liss, 1982, pp 35–44.

McCormack T, Plassche WM, Lin Shu-Ren: Ruptured teratoid tumor in the pineal region. *J Comput Assist Tomogr* 2:499–501, 1978.

McDonnell DE: Pineal epidermoid cyst: Its surgical therapy. *Surg Neurol* 7:387–391, 1977.

McGovern VJ: Tumors of the epiphysis cerebri. *J Pathol* 61:1–9, 1949.

McIsaac WM, Taborsky RG, Farrell G: 5-Methoxytryptophol: Effect on estrus and ovarian weight. *Science* 145:63–64, 1964.

McIsaac WM, Farrell G, Toborsky RG, Taylor AN: Indole compounds: Isolation from pineal tissue. *Science* 148:102–103, 1965.

McLean AJ: Pineal teratomas. With report of a case of operative removal. *Surg Gynecol Obstet* 61:523–533, 1935.

Megyeri L: Cystische Veränderungen des Corpus pineale. *Frankfurt Z Pathol* 70:699–704, 1960.

Messina AV, Potts DG, Sigel RM, Liebeskind AL: Computed tomography: Evaluation of the posterior third ventricle. *Radiology* 119:581–592, 1976.

Miller FP, Maickel RP: Fluorometric determination of indole derivatives. *Life Sci* 9:747–752, 1970.

Miller NR: *Walsh and Hoyt's Clinical Neuro-Ophthalmology*, ed 4. Baltimore, Williams & Wilkins, 1982, vol 1, pp 175–211.

Minger F, Meltzer J, Botstein C: Pinealoma. A report of twelve irradiated cases. *Cancer* 37:2713–2718, 1976.

Mintz B, Illmensee K: Normal genetically mosaic mice produced from malignant teratocarcinoma cells.

Proc Natl Acad Sci USA 72:3585–3589, 1975.

Misugi K, Liss L, Bradel EJ, et al: Electron microscopic study of an ectopic pinealoma. *Acta Neuropathol* 9:346–356, 1967.

Moller M, Gjerris F, Hansen HJ, Johnson E: Calcification in a pineal tumour studied by transmission electron microscopy, electron diffraction and X-ray microanalysis. *Acta Neurol Scand* 59:178–187, 1979.

Møller M: Presence of a pineal nerve (nervus pinealis) in the human fetus; a light and electron microscopical study of the innervation of the pineal gland. *Brain Res* 154:1–12, 1978.

Møller M: The ultrastructure of the human fetal pineal gland. I. Cell types and blood vessels. *Cell Tissue Res* 152:13–30, 1974.

Møller M: The ultrastructure of the human fetal pineal gland. II. Innervation and cell junctions. *Cell Tissue Res* 169:7–21, 1976.

Moore-Ede MC, Czeisler CA, Richardson GS: Circadian timekeeping in health and disease. Part I. Basic properties of circadian pacemakers. *N Engl J Med* 309:469–476, 1983; Part II. Clinical implications of circadian rhythmicity. *N Engl J Med* 309:530–536, 1983.

Moore RY: The retinohypothalamic tract, suprachiasmatic hypothalamic nucleus and central neural mechanisms of circadian rhythm regulation. In Suda M, Hayaishi O, Nakagawa H (eds): *Biological Rhythms and Their Central Mechanisms.* Amsterdam, Elsevier/North Holland, 1979, pp 343–354.

Moore RY: The innervation of the mammalian pineal gland. In Reiter RJ (ed): *The Pineal and Reproduction.* Basel, Karger, 1978, pp. 1–29.

Moser RP, Backlund EO: Stereotactic radiosurgery in the management of pineal region tumors. American Association of Neurological Surgeons Meeting, Hawaii, 1982.

Mostofi FK: Pathology of germ cell tumors of testis. *Cancer* 45:1735–1754, 1980.

Mostofi FK, Price Jr, EB: Tumors of the male genital system. Atlas of Tumor Pathology 2nd Series. *Washington DC Armed Forces Inst Pathol*, Fasc. 8, 1973.

Mullen PE, Linsell CR, Leone RM, Silman RE, Smith I, Hooper RJC, Finnie M, Parrot J: Melatonin and 5-methoxytryptophol, and 24 hour pattern of secretion in man. In Birau N, Schloot W (eds): *Melatonin—Current Status and Perspectives.* New York, Pergamon, 1981, pp 337–343.

Muller W, Schaefer HE, Kruger G: Beitrag zur kenntnis der intrakraniellen germinome. In Zellinger K, Gross H (eds): *Current Topics in Neuropathology.* Facultas, Vienna, 1978, vol 4.

Mundinger F: CT-Stereotactic biopsy of brain tumors. In Voth D, Gutjahr P, Langnaid C (eds): *Tumors of the Central Nervous System in Infancy and Childhood.* Berlin, Springer-Verlag, 1981, pp 334–346.

Murovic J, Ongley JP, Parker JC, Page LK: Manifestations and therapeutic considerations in pineal yolk-sac tumors. Case report. *J Neurosurg* 55:303–307, 1981.

Naffziger HC: Brain surgery with special reference to exposure of the brain stem and posterior fossa, the principle of intracranial decompression, and the relief of impactions in the posterior fossa. *Surg Gynecol Obstet* 46:240–248, 1928.

Nakano T: Studies on influence of synthetic LH-RH and dbcAMP on normal chorionic villi and BeWo cells. *Nippon Sanka Fujinka-Gakkai Zasshi* 33:2105–2114, 1981.

Nakazato Y, Ishida Y, Kawabuchi J: Ganglioneuroblastic differentiation in a pineocytoma. 8th International Congress Neuropathology, Abstract #255.

Nashold BS, Gills JP: Ocular signs from brain stimulation and lesions. *Arch Ophthalmol* 77:609–618, 1967.

Nassetti F: Dell' operabilita delle vie di accesso ai tumori della ghiandola pineale. *Il Policlinico Sez Chir* 20:497–501, 1913.

Negrin Jr, J: A new approach in the surgical treatment of tumors of the pineal region. The posterior coroneal flap. *Am J Surg* 80:581–583, 1950.

Neuwelt EA, Frenkel E: Is there a therapeutic role for blood brain barrier disruption? *Ann Intern Med* 93:135–137, 1980.

Neuwelt EA, Smith RG: Presence of lymphocyte membrane surface markers on "small cells" in a pineal germinoma. *Ann Neurol* 6:133–136, 1979.

Neuwelt EA, Batjer H: Surgical management of pineal region tumors. *Contemp Neurosurg* 4:1–5, 1982.

Neuwelt E, Glasberg M, Frenkel E, et al: Malignant pineal region tumors: A clinicopathologic study. *J Neurosurg* 6:133–136, 1979.

Neuwelt EA, Lewy A: Disappearance of plasma melatonin after removal of a neoplastic pineal gland. *N Engl J Med* 308:1132–1135, 1983.

Neuwelt EA, Clark WK: Unique aspects of central nervous system immunology. *Neurosurgery* 3:419–430, 1978.

Neuwelt EA, Maravilla KR, Frenkel EP, Barnett P, Hill S, Morse RJ: Use of enhanced computerized tomography to evaluate osmotic blood-brain barrier disruption. *Neurosurgery* 6:49–56, 1980.

Neuwelt EA, Frenkel EP, Smith RG: Suprasellar germinoma (ectopic pinealoma): Aspects of immunologic characterization and successful chemotherapeutic responses in recurrent disease. *Neurosurgery* 7:352–358, 1980.

Neuwelt EA: Treatment of central nervous system neoplasms. In Rosenberg RN (ed): *The Treatment of Neurological Diseases.* New York, Spectrum Publications, 1979, pp 205–229.

Neuwelt EA, Clark K: *Clinical Aspects of Neuroimmunology.* Baltimore, Williams & Wilkins, 1978, pp 93–94.

Neuwelt EA, Clark WK: Clinical Aspects of Neuroimmunology. Baltimore, Williams & Wilkins, 1978, pp 277.

Newton THH, Potts DG: Radiology of the skull and brain. St. Louis, Mosby, 1974, vol 2/3.

Nielsen SL, Wilson CB: Ultrastructure of a "pineocytoma." *J Neuropathol Exp Neurol* 34:148–158, 1975.

Nishiyama RH, Batsakis JG, Weaver DK, Simrall JH: Germinal neoplasms of the central nervous system. *Arch Surg* 93:342–347, 1966.

Nisonoff A, Wissler FC, Lipman LN, Woernley DL: Separation of univalent fragments from bivalent rabbit antibody molecule by reduction of disulfide bonds. *Arch Biochem Biophys* 89:230–244, 1960.

Norbut AM, Mendelow H: Primary glioblastoma multiforme of the pineal region with leptomeningeal metastases: A case report. *Cancer* 47:592–596, 1981.

Norgaard-Pedersen B, Landholm J, Albrechtsen R, et al: Alpha-fetoprotein and human chorionic gonadotropin in a patient with a primary intracranial germ cell tumor. *Cancer* 41:2315–2320, 1978.

Norlund JJ, Lerner AB: Melatonin: Its effects on skin color, pituitary trophic hormones and its toxicity in human subjects. *J Clin Endocrinol Metab* 45:152–158, 1977.

Norris DG, Bruce DA, Byrd RL, Schut L, Littman P, Bilaniuk LT, Zimmerman RA, Capp R: Improved relapse-free survival in medulloblastoma utilizing modern technique. *Neurosurgery* 9:661–662, 1981.

Nothnagel H: The diagnosis of diseases of the corpora quadrigemina. *Brain* 1889;12:21–35.

Nugent JL, Bunn Jr, PA, Matthews MJ, Ihde DC, Cohen MH, Gazdar A, Minna JD: CNS metastases in small cell bronchogenic carcinoma: Increasing frequency and changing pattern with lengthening survival. *Cancer* 44:1885–1893, 1979.

Oberman HA, Libcke JH: Malignant germinal neoplasms of the mediastinum. *Cancer* 17:498–507, 1964.

Obrador S, Soto M, Gutierrez-Diaz JA: Surgical management of tumours of the pineal region. *Acta Neurochir* 34:159–171, 1976.

Ochs AL, Stark L, Hoyt WF, D'Amico D: Opposed adducting saccades in convergence-retraction nystagmus—A patient with sylvian aqueduct syndrome. *Brain* 102:497–508, 1979.

Ojikuta NA: The pathology and clinical history of pineal teratoma. *West Afr Med J* 17:130–135, 1968.

Oksche A: Sensory and glandular elements of the pineal organ. In Wolstenholme GEW, Knight J (eds): *The Pineal Gland.* Edinburgh-London, Churchill Livingstone, 1971, pp 127–146.

Olivecrona H: Acoustic tumors. *J Neurosurg* 26:6–13, 1967.

Olivecrona H: The surgical treatment of intracranial tumors. In *Handbuch der Neurochirurgie, Vol IV/4.* Berlin, Springer-Verlag, 1967, pp 48–68.

Onoyama Y, Abe M, Takahashi M, Yabumoto E, Sakamoto T: Radiation therapy of brain tumors in children. *Radiology* 115:687–693, 1975.

Onoyama Y, Ono K, Nakajima T, Hiraoka M, Abe M: Radiation therapy of pineal tumors. *Radiology* 130:757–760, 1979.

Oppenheim H, Krause F: Operative Erfolg bei Seschwülsten der Sehhügel-und Vierhügelgegend. *Berl Klin Wochenschr* 50:2316–2322, 1913.

Ortega P, Malamud N, Shimkin MB: Metastasis to the pineal body. *Arch Pathol* 52:518–528, 1951.

Orton ST: A pathological study of a case of hydrocephalus. *Am J Insan* 65:229–278, 1908.

Ostrand-Rosenberg S, Cohan VL: H-2 negative teratocarcinoma cells become H-2 positive when passaged in genetically resistant host mice. *J Immunol* 126:2190–2193, 1981.

Ostrand-Rosenberg S, Cohn A: H-2 antigen expression on teratocarcinoma cells passaged in genetically resistant mice is regulated by lymphoid cells. *Proc Natl Acad Sci USA* 78:7106–7110, 1981.

Ozaki Y, Lynch HJ: Presence of melatonin in plasma and urine of pinealectomized rats. *Endocrinology* 99:641–644, 1976.

Pachtman H, Hilal SK, Wood EH: The posterior choroidal arteries. *Radiology* 112:343–352, 1974.

Page LK: The infratentorial-supracerebellar exposure of tumors in the pineal area. *Neurosurgery* 1:36–40, 1977.

Palma L, DiLorenzo N, Guidetti B: Lymphocytic infiltrates in primary glioblastomas and recidivous gliomas: Incidence, fate, and relevance to prognosis in 228 operated cases. *J Neurosurg* 49:854–861, 1978.

Palumbo LT, Cross KR, Smith AN, et al: Primary teratomas of the lateral retroperitoneal spaces. *Surgery* 26:149–159, 1949.

Pang SF, Brown GM, Grota LJ, Chambers JW, Rodman RL: Determinations of N-acetylserotonin and melatonin activities in the pineal gland, retina, Harderian gland, brain and serum of rats and chickens. *Neuroendocrinology* 23:1–13, 1977.

Panke ES, Reiter RJ, Rollag MD, Panke TW: Pineal serotonin N-acetyltransferase activity and melatonin concentrations in prepubertal and adult Syrian hamsters exposed to short daily photoperiods. *Endocrinol Res Commun* 5:311–324, 1978.

Panke ES, Rollag MD, Reiter RJ: Pineal melatonin concentrations in the Syrian hamster. *Endocrinology* 104:194–197, 1979.

Papaioannou VE, McBurney MW, Gardner RL, et al: Fate of teratocarcinoma cells injected into early mouse embryos. *Nature* 258:70–73, 1975.

Papasozomenos S, Shapiro S: Pineal astrocytoma: Report of a case, confined to the epiphysis, with immunocytochemical and electron microscopic studies. *Cancer* 47:99–103, 1981.

Pappenheim AM: Uber Seschwülste der Corpora pineale. *Virchows Arch [Pathol Anat]* 200:122–141, 1910.

Parfitt A, Weller JL, Klein DC: β-adrenergic-blockers decrease adrenergically stimulated N-acetyltransferase activity in pineal glands in organ culture. *Neuropharmacology* 15:353–358, 1976.

Parinaud H: De la neurite optique dans les affections cérébrales. *Ann d'Ocul* 82:5–47, 1879.

Parinaud H: Paralysie des mouvements associes der yeux. *Arch Neurol* 5:149–172, 1883.

Parinaud H; Paralysis of the movement of convergence of the eyes. *Brain* 9:330–341, 1886.

Partlow WR, Taybi T: Teratomas in infants and children. *Am J Roentogen* 112:155–166, 1971.

Pasik P, Pasik T, Bender MB: The pretectal syndrome in monkeys. I. Disturbances of gaze and body posture. *Brain* 92:521–534, 1969.

Pastori G: Ein bis jetzt hoch nicht beschriebenes sympathetisches Ganglion zum nervus conari sowie zur Vena magna Galeni. *Z Gesamte Neurol Psychiat* 123:81–90, 1930.

Pavel S: Arginine vasotocin as a pineal hormone. *J Neural Transm [Suppl]* 13:135–156, 1978.

Pearson JC, Spaulding JT, Friedman MA: Testicular cancer: Role of biological tumor markers. *Cancer Treat Rev* 6:217–221, 1979.

Pecker J, Scarabin JM, Vallee B, Brucher JM: Treatment of tumours of the pineal region: Value of stereotaxic biopsy. *Surg Neurol* 12:341–348, 1979.

Peeters FLM: The vertebral angiogram in patients with tumors in or near the midline. *Neuroradiology* 5:53–58, 1973.

Pelham RW, Ralph CL, Campbell IM: Mass spectral identification of melatonin in blood. *Biochem Biophys Res Commun* 46:1236–1241, 1972.

Pelham RW, Vaughan GM, Sandock KL, Vaughan MK: Twenty-four-hour cycle of melatonin-like substance in the plasma of human males. *J Clin Endocrinol Metab* 37:341–346, 1973.

Pellizzi GB: La syndrome epifisaria "macrogenitosomia precoce." *Riv Ital Neuropat* 3:193–250, 1910.

Pendl G: Mikrotopographische Untersuchunger über die operativen Zugänge zur Mittelhirn-Pinealis-Region. Thesis, University of Vienna Medical Faculty, 1981.

Pendl G: Infratentoria approach to mesencephalic tumors. In Koos WTh, Böck F, Spetzler RF (eds): *Clinical Microneurosurgery.* Stuttgart, Thieme Verlag, 1976, pp 143–150.

Pendl G, Koos W, Witzmann A: Surgical approach to pineal tumours in childhood. *Z Kinderchir* 34:203–204, 1981.

Perlow MJ, Reppert SM, Tamarkin L, Wyatt RJ, Klein DC: Photic regulation of the melatonin rhythm: Monkey and man are not the same. *Brain Res* 182:211–216, 1980.

Pernkopf E: Topographische Anatomie des Menschen. Urban and Schwarzenberg, München, 1960.

Perry JH, Rosenbaum AE, Lundsford LD, Swink CA, Zosul DS: Computed tomography-guided stereotactic surgery: Conception and development of a new stereotactic methodology. *Neurosurgery* 7:376–381, 1980.

Pertuiset B, Visot A, Metzger J: Diagnosis of pinealoblastomas by positive response to cobalt-therapy. *Acta Neurochir* (Wien) 34:151–152, 1976.

Peters A, Palay SL, Webster HDF: The Fine Structure of the Nervous System. *The Neurons and Supporting Cells.* Philadelphia, WB Saunders, 1976.

Petterborg LJ, Philo RC, Reiter RJ: The pineal body and pinealectomy in the cotton rat, *Sigmodon hispidus. Acta Anat* 107:108–113, 1980.

Petterborg LJ, Reiter RJ: Effect of photoperiod and pineal indoles on the reproductive system of young female white-footed mice. *J Neural Transm* 55:149–155, 1982.

Petterborg LJ, Richardson BA, Reiter RJ: Effect of long or short photoperiod on pineal melatonin content in the white-footed mouse, *Peromyscus leucopus. Life Sci* 29:1623–1627, 1981.

Pevet P, Haldar-Misra C: Morning injections of large doses of melatonin, but not 5-methoxytryptamine, prevent in the hamster the antigonadotrophic effect of 5-methoxytryptamine administered late in the afternoon. *J Neural Transm* 55:85–94, 1982.

Pia HW: Klinik, Differenzialdiagnose und Behandlung der Vierhügelgeschwülste. *Dtsch Z Nervenh* 172:12–32, 1954.

Piatt Jr, JH, Campbell GA: Pineal region meningioma: Report of two cases and literature review. *Neurosurgery* 12:369–376, 1983.

Pierce GB: Ultrastructure of human testicular tumors. *Cancer* 19:1963–1983, 1966.

Pierce GB, Abell MR: Embryonal carcinoma of the testis. *Pathol Ann* 5:27–60, 1970.

Pierrot-Deseilligny C, Chain F, Gray F, Serdaru M, Escourolle R, Lhermitte F: Parinaud's syndrome-electro-oculographic and anatomical analysis of six vascular cases with deductions about vertical gaze organization in the premotor structures. *Brain* 105:667–697, 1982.

Plaut HF: Size of the tentorial incisura related to

cerebral herniation. *Acta Radiol* 1:916–998, 1963.

Plotka ED, Seal US, Verme LJ: Morphologic and metabolic consequences of pinealectomy in deer. In Reiter RJ (ed): *The Pineal Gland Vol 3 Extra-Reproductive Effects.* Boca Raton, CRC Press, 1982, pp 153–170.

Poppen JL: The right occipital approach to a pinealoma. *J Neurosurg* 25:706–710, 1966.

Poppen JL, Marino Jr, R: Pinealomas and tumors of the posterior portion of the third ventricle. *J Neurosurg* 28:357–364, 1968.

Poppen JL: An atlas of neurosurgical techniques. WB Saunders, Philadelphia, 1960.

Posner M, Horrax G: Eye signs in pineal tumors. *J Neurosurg* 3:15–24, 1946.

Poth M, Tetsuo M, Markey S: Excretion patterns of 6-hydroxymelatonin in pubertal and pre-pubertal children. *Pediatr Res* 15:513–517, 1981.

Pratt DW, Brooks EF: Successful excision of a tumor of the pineal gland. *Can Med Assoc J* 39:240–243, 1938.

Preissig SH, Smith MT, Huntington HW: Rhabdomyosarcoma arising in a pineal teratoma. *Cancer* 44:281–284, 1979.

Preud'homme JL, Seligman M: Surface bound immunoglobulins as a cell marker in human lymphoproliferative diseases. *Blood* 40:777–794, 1972.

Prioleau G, Wilson CB: Endodermal sinus tumor of the pineal region. A case report. *Cancer* 38:2489–2493, 1976.

Prozialeck WC, Boehme DH, Vogel WH: The fluorometric determination of 5-methoxytryptamine in mammalian tissues and fluid. *J Neurochem* 30:1471–1477, 1978.

Prus J: Untersuchungen über elektrische Reizung der Vierhügel. *Wien Klin Wochenschr* 12:1124–1130, 1899.

Puschett JB, Goldberg M: Endocrinopathy associated with pineal tumor. *Ann Intern Med* 69:203–219, 1968.

Pussep L: Die operative entfernung einer zyste der glandula pinealis. *Neurol Centralbl* 33:560–563, 1914.

Quast P: Beiträge zue Histologie und Cytologie der normalen Zirbeldrüse des Menschen. II. Zellen und Pigment des interstitiellen Gewebes der Zirbeldrüse. *Z Mikrosk Anat Forsch* 24:38–100, 1931.

Quay WB: Circadian rhythm in rat pineal serotonin and its modulation by estrous cycle and photoperiod. *Gen Comp Endocrinol* 3:473–479, 1963.

Quay WB, Ma Y-H, Varakis Jn, ZuRhein GM, Padgett BL, Walker DL: Modification of hydroxyindole-o-methyltransferase activity in experimental pineocytomas induced in hamsters by a human papovavirus (JC). *J Natl Cancer Inst* 58:123–126, 1977.

Quest DO, Kleriga E: Microsurgical anatomy of the pineal region. *Neurosurgery* 6:385–390, 1980.

Raff MC, Steinberg M, Taylor RB: Immunoglobulin determinants on the surface of mouse lymphoid cells. *Nature* 225:553–554, 1970.

Raghavan D, Jelikovsky T, Fox RM: Father-son testicular malignancy. Does anticipation occur? *Cancer* 45:1005–1009, 1980.

Raimondi AJ, Tomita T: Pineal tumors in childhood. *Childs Brain* 9:239–266, 1982.

Ralph CL, Firth BT, Gern WA, Owens DW: The pineal complex and thermoregulation. *Biol Rev* 54:41–72, 1979.

Ramsey HJ: Ultrastructure of a pineal tumor. *Cancer* 18:1014–1025, 1965.

Rand RW, Lemmen LJ: Tumors of the posterior portion of the third ventricle. *J Neurosurg* 10:1–18, 1953.

Rao YTR, Medini E, Haselow RE, Jones TK, Levitt SH: Pineal and ectopic pineal tumors: The role of radiation therapy. *Cancer* 48:708–713, 1981.

Rapaport E, Schroeder EW, Black PH: Retinoic acid-promoted expansion of total cellular ATP pools in 3T3 cells can mediate its stimulatory and growth inhibitory effects. *J Cell Physiol* 110:318–322, 1982.

Rapoport SI: Blood-Brain barrier in physiology and medicine. New York, Raven Press, 1976, pp 77–78.

Rappaport R, Brauner R, Czernichow P, Thibaud E, Renier D, Zucker JM, Lemerle J: Effect of hypothalamic and pituitary irradiation on pubertal development in children with cranial tumors. *J Clin Endocrinol Metab* 54:1164–1168, 1982.

Ray P, Olson MH, Sarivar M, Wright AE, Wu J, Allam AA: Pinealoma: Analysis of treatment and failure. Proceedings of the American Society of Therapeutic Radiologists. *Int J Radiat Oncol Biol Phys* (Suppl) 1:144, 1976.

Reid WS, Clark WK: Comparison of the infratentorial and transtentorial approaches to the pineal region. *Neurosurgery* 3:1–8, 1978.

Reigel DH, Scarff TB, Woodford JE: Biopsy of pediatric brainstem tumors. *Child's Brain* 5:329–340, 1979.

Reiter RJ: Chronobiological aspects of the pineal gland. In Mayersback HV, Scheving LE, Pauly JE (eds): *Biological Rhythms in Structure and Function.* New York, Alan R. Liss, 1981, pp 223–333.

Reiter RJ: The mammalian pineal gland: Structure and function. *Am J Anat* 162:287–313, 1981.

Reiter RJ: Morphological studies on the reproductive organs of blinded male hamsters and the effects of pinealectomy or superior cervical ganglionectomy. *Anat Rec* 160:13–24, 1968.

Reiter RJ: Evidence for refractoriness of the pituitary-gonadal axis to the pineal gland in golden hamsters and its possible implications in annual reproductive rhythms. *Anat Rec* 173:365–372, 1975.

Reiter RJ: Comparative physiology: Pineal gland. *Ann Rev Physiol* 35:305–328, 1973.

Reiter RJ, Golovko V: Failure of duration of inbreeding to influence the rate of pineal-induced gonadal regression in short day exposed Syrian hamsters. *Arch Androl* 10:39–44, 1982.

Reiter RJ: Circannual reproductive rhythms in mammals related to photoperiod and pineal function: A review. *Chronobiologia* 1:365–395, 1974.

Reiter RJ: The pinal and its hormones in the control of reproduction in mammals. *Endocr Rev* 1:109–131, 1980.

Reiter RJ, Rudeen PK, Sackman JW, Vaughan MK, Johnson LY, Little JC: Subcutaneous melatonin implants inhibit reproductive atrophy in male hamsters induced by daily melatonin injections. *Endocr Res Commun* 4:35–44, 1977.

Reiter RJ, Hester RJ: Interrelationships of the pineal gland, the superior cervical ganglia and the photoperiod in regulation of the endocrine systems of hamsters. *Endocrinol* 79:1168–1170, 1966.

Reiter RJ, Craft CM, Johnson Jr, JE, King TS, Richardson BA, Vaughan GM, Vaughan MK: Age-asso-ciated reduction in nocturnal pineal melatonin levels in female rats. *Endocrinology* 109:1295–1297, 1981.

Reiter RJ, Vriend J, Brainard GC, Matthews SA, Craft CM: Reduced pineal and plasma melatonin levels and gonadal atrophy in old hamsters kept under winter photoperiods. *Exp Aging Res* 8:27–30, 1982.

Reiter RJ, Johnson LY: Pineal regulation of immu-noreactive luteinizing hormone and prolactin in light-deprived female hamsters. *Fertil Steril* 25:958–964, 1974.

Reiter RJ: Pineal function in long term blinded male and female golden hamsters. *Gen Comp Endocrinol* 12:460–468, 1969.

Reiter RJ, Johnson LY: Depressant action of the pineal gland, the superior cervical ganglia and the photoperiod on pituitary luteinizing hormone and prolactin in male hamsters. *Horm Res* 5:311–320, 1974.

Reiter RJ, Rollag MD, Panke ES, Banks AF: Mela-tonin: Reproductive effects. *J Neural Transm* [Suppl] 13:209–224, 1978.

Reiter RJ, King TS, Richardson BA, Hurlbut EC: Studies on pineal melatonin levels in a diurnal species, the eastern chipmunk (*Tamias striatus*): Effects of light at night, propranolol administration of superior cervical ganglionectomy. *J Neural Transm* 54:275–284, 1982a.

Reiter RJ: Changes in the reproductive organs of cold-exposed and light-deprived female hamsters. *J Re-prod Fertil* 16:217–222, 1968.

Reiter RJ: Interactions of the photoperiod, pineal and seasonal reproduction as exemplified by findings in the hamster. In Reiter RJ (ed): *The Pineal and Reproduction*. Basel, Karger, 1978, pp 169–190.

Reiter RJ, Richardson BA, Matthews SA, Lane SJ, Ferguson BN: Rhythms in immunoreactive mela-tonin in the retina and Harderian gland of rats: Persistence after pinealectomy. *Life Sci* 32:1229–1236, 1983.

Reiter RJ, Steinlechner S, Richardson BA, King TS: Differential response of pineal melatonin levels to light at night in laboratory-raised and wild-captured 13-lined ground squirrels (*Spermophilus tridecem-lineatus*). *Life Sci*, in press.

Reiter RJ, King TS, Richardson BA, Hurlbut EC, Karasek MA, Hansen JT: Failure of room light to inhibit pineal *N*-acetyltransferase activity and me-latonin content in a diurnal species, the Eastern chipmunk (*Tamias striatus*). *Neuroendocrinol Lett* 4:1–6, 1982b.

Reiter RJ: The effect of pinealectomy, pineal grafts and denervation of the pineal gland on the repro-ductive organs of male hamsters. *Neuroendocrinol-ogy* 2:138–146, 1967.

Reiter RJ: Influence of pinealectomy on the breeding capability of hamsters maintained under natural photoperiod and temperature conditions. *Neuroen-docrinology* 13:366–370, 1973/74.

Reiter RJ, Blask DE, Johnson LY, Rudeen PK, Vaughan MK, Waring PJ: Melatonin inhibition of reproduction in the male hamster: Its dependency on time of day of administration and on an intact and sympathetically innervated pineal gland. *Neu-roendocrinology* 22:107–116, 1976.

Reiter RJ, Richardson BA, Hurlbut EC: Pineal, retinal and Harderian gland melatonin in a diurnal species, the Richardson's ground squirrel (*Spermophilus ri-chardsonii*). *Neurosci Lett* 22:285–288, 1981.

Reiter RJ, Johnson LY, Steger RW, Richardson BA, Petterborg LJ: Pinal biosynthetic activity and neu-roendocrine physiology in the aging hamster and gerbil. *Peptides* 1:69–77, 1980.

Reiter RJ: Reproductive effects of the pineal gland and pineal indoles in the Syrian hamster and the albino rat. In Reiter RJ (ed): *The Pineal Gland, Vol 2, Reproductive Effects*. Boca Raton, CRC Press, 1982, pp 45–82.

Reiter RJ: Reproductive involution in male hamsters exposed to naturally increasing daylengths after the winter solstice. *Proc Soc Exp Biol Med* 163:264–266, 1980.

Reiter RJ: The pineal gland: A regulator of regulators. *Prog Psychobiol Physiol Psychol* 9:323–356, 1980.

Reiter RJ: Neuroendocrine effects of the pineal gland and of melatonin. In Ganong WR, Martini L (eds): *Frontiers in Neuroendocrinology, Vol 7*. New York, Raven Press, 1982, pp 278–316.

Reiter RJ, Vaughan MK, Blask DE, Johnson LY: Melatonin: Its inhibition of pineal antigonado-trophic activity in male hamsters. *Science* 185:1169–1171, 1974.

Reiter RJ, Richardson BA, Johnson LY, Ferguson BN, Dinh DT: Pineal melatonin rhythm: Reduction in aging Syrian hamsters. *Science* 210:1372–1373, 1980.

Reiter RJ, Hurlbut EC, Richardson BA, King TS, Wang LCH: Studies on the regulation of pineal melatonin production in the Richardson's ground squirrel (*Spermophilus richardsonii*). In Reiter RJ (ed): *The Pineal and Its Hormones*. New York, Alan R Liss, 1982, pp 57–65.

Reiter RJ: Pineal interaction with the central nervous system. *Waking Sleeping* 1:253–258, 1977.

Relkin R: Pineal-hormonal interactions. In Relkin R (ed): *The Pineal Gland*. New York, Elsevier, 1983, pp 225–246.

Rhines R, Windle WR: Early development of fascic-ulus longitudinalis medialis and associated second-ary neurons in the rat, cat, and man. *J Comp Neurol* 75:165–189, 1941.

Rhoton AL, Yamamoto I, Peace DA: Microsurgery of the third ventricle: Part 2. Operative approaches. *Neurosurgery* 8:357–373, 1981.

Ringertz N, Nordenstam H, Flyger G: Tumors of the pineal region. *J Neuropathol Exp Neurol* 13:540–561, 1954.

Rivest RW, Lynch HJ, Ronsheim PM, Wurtman RJ: Effect of light intensity on regulation of melatonin secretion and drinking behavior in the albino rat. In Birau N, Schloot W (eds): *Melatonin—Current Status and Perspectives*. New York, Pergamon, 1981, pp 119–121.

Robinson RG: A second brain tumour and irradiation. *J Neurol Neurosurg Psychiatry* 41:1005–1012, 1978.

Roda JM, Perez-Higueras A, Oliver B, Alvarez MP, Blazquez MG: Pineal region meningiomas without dural attachment. *Surg Neurol* 17:147–151, 1982.

Roessmann U, Velasco ME, Gambetti P, Autilio-Gam-betti L: Neuronal and astrocytic differentiation in human neuroepithelial neoplasms. An immunohistochemical study. *J Neuropathol Exp Neurol* 42:113–121, 1983.

Rollag MD, Stetson MH: Ontogeny of the pineal melatonin rhythm in golden hamsters. *Biol Reprod* 24:311–314, 1981.

Rollag MD: Methods for measuring pineal hormones. In Reiter R (ed): *The Pineal Gland: Anatomy and Biochemistry.* Boca Raton, CRC Press, 1981, Vol 1, pp 273–302.

Rollag MD, Chen JH, Ferguson BN, Reiter RJ: Pineal melatonin content throughout the hamster estrous cycle. *Proc Soc Exp Biol Med* 160:211–213, 1979.

Rollag MD, Panke ES, Reiter RJ: Pineal melatonin content in male hamsters throughout the seasonal reproductive cycle. *Proc Soc Exp Biol Med* 165:330–334, 1980.

Rollag MD, Stetson MH: Melatonin injection into Syrian hamsters. In Reiter RJ (ed): *The Pineal and Its Hormones.* New York, Alan R Liss, 1982, pp 143–151.

Roman B: Zur Kenntnis des Neuroepithelioma gliomatosum. *Virchows Arch Pathol Anat* 211:126–140, 1913.

Romero JA, Axelrod J: Regulation of sensitivity to β-adrenergic stimulation in induction of pineal *N*-acetyltransferase. *Proc Natl Acad Sci USA* 72:1661–1665, 1975.

Romshe CA, Sotos JF: Intracranial human chorionic gonadotropin-secreting tumor with precocious puberty. *J Pediatr* 86:250–252, 1975.

Rorschach H: Zur Pathologie und Operabilität der Tumoren der Zirbeldrüse. *Bruns Beitr* 83:451–474, 1913.

Rosenberg R, Neuwelt EA, Kirkpatrick J, Kohler P: Encephalopathy associated with cryoprecipitable australia antigen. *Ann Neurol* 1:298–300, 1977.

Rougier A, DaSilva NN, Cohadon F: Tumoral volume assessment: Contributions of SEEG. In Szikla G (ed): *Stereotactic Cerebral Irradiation. Inserm Symposium No. 12,* 1979, pp 63–68.

Roussas GG: *A First Course in Mathematical Statistics.* Addison-Wesley, 1973, pp 306–308.

Roussy G, Mosinger M: L'hypothalamus chez l'homme et chez le chien. *Revue Neurol* (Paris) 63:1–35, 1935.

Rozario R, Adelman L, Prager RJ, Stein BM: Meningiomas of the pineal region and third ventricle. *Neurosurgery* 5:489–495, 1979.

Rozencweig M, von Hoff DD, Slavik M, Muggia FM: *Cis*-diamminedichloro-platinum (II): A new anticancer drug. *Ann Intern Med* 86:803–812, 1977.

Rubery ED, Wheeler TK: Metastases outside the central nervous system from a presumed pineal germinoma. *J Neurosurg* 53:562–565, 1980.

Rubin P, Kramer S: Ectopic pinealoma: A radiocurable neuroendocrinologic entity. *Radiology* 85:512–523, 1965.

Rubinstein LJ: Tumors of the Central Nervous System. Atlas of Tumor Pathology, 2nd series, Fascicle 6. Washington, DC, Armed Forces Institute of Pathology, 1972.

Rubinstein LJ: Tumors of the Central Nervous System. Atlas of Tumor Pathology, 2nd series, Fascicle 6, Supplement. Washington, DC, Armed Forces Institute of Pathology, 1982.

Rubinstein LJ: Cytogenesis and differentiation of pineal neoplasms. *Hum Pathol* 12:441–448, 1981.

Rubinstein LJ: Cytogenesis and differentiation of primitive central neuroepithelial tumors. *J Neuropathol Exp Neurol* 31:7–26, 1972.

Rubinstein LJ, Okazaki H: Gangliogliomatous differentiation in a pineocytoma. *J Pathol* 102:27–32, 1970.

Rudeen PK, Reiter RJ, Vaughan MK: Pineal serotonin-*N*-acetyltransferase in four mammalian species. *Neurosci Lett* 1:225–229, 1975.

Rusak B: Circadian organization in mammals and birds: Role of the pineal gland. In Reiter RJ (ed): *The Pineal Gland, Vol 3 Extra-Reproductive Effects.* Boca Raton, CRC Press, 1982, pp 27–52.

Russel DS, Sachs E: Pinealoma. A clinicopathologic study of 7 cases with a review of literature. *Arch Pathol* 35:869–888, 1943.

Russell DS: The pinealoma: Its relationship to teratoma. *J Pathol* 56:145–150, 1944.

Russell DS: "Ectopic pinealoma": Its kinship to atypical teratomas of the pineal gland. *J Pathol* 68:125–129, 1954.

Russell DS, Rubinstein LJ: *Pathology of Tumors of the Nervous System,* ed 4. Baltimore, Williams & Wilkins, 1977, pp 287–290.

Rydygier RV: Erfahrungen über die Dekompressiv-Trepanation und der Balkenstich nach Anton v. Bramann beim Gehirndruck. *Dtsch Z Chir* 117:344–474, 1912.

Sakashita S, Loyanagi T, Tsuji I, et al: Congenital anomalies in children with testicular germ cell tumors. *J Urol* 124:889–891, 1980.

Sakata K, Yamada H, Sakai N, Hosono Y, Kawasako T, Sasaoka I: Extraneural metastasis of pineal tumor. *Surg Neurol* 3:49–54, 1975.

Salazar OM, Castro-Vita H, Bakos RS, Feldstein ML, Keller B, Rubin P: Radiation therapy for tumors of the pineal region. *Int J Radiat Oncol Biol Phys* 5:491–499, 1979.

Salus R: Über erworbenc retraktionsbervegungen der augen. *Arch Kinderkeilk* 47:61–76, 1910.

Sambasivan M, Nayar A: Epidermoid cyst of the pineal region. *J Neurol Neurosurg Psychiatry* 37:1333–1335, 1974.

Sanders MD, Bird AC: Supranuclear abnormalities of the vertical ocular motor system. *Trans Ophthalmol Soc UK* 90:433–450, 1970.

Sano K: Diagnosis and treatment of tumors in the pineal region. *Acta Neurochir* 34:153–157, 1976.

Sano K: Pinealomas in children. *Childs Brain* 2:67–72, 1976.

Sano K, Matsutani M: Pinealoma (germinoma) treated by direct surgery and postoperative irradiation: A long-term follow-up. *Childs Brain* 8:81–97, 1981.

Sano K, Matsutani M: Pinealoma (germinoma) treated by direct surgery and postoperative irradiation. *Childs Brain* 8:81–97, 1981.

Sano K, Nagai M, Mayanagi Y, Basugi N: Ectopic pinealoma in the chiasmal region in childhood. *Dev Med Child Neurol* 10:258–259, 1968.

Sano K, Hoshino T, Nagai M: Radiosensitization of brain tumor cells with a thymidine analogue (Bromouridine). *J Neurosurg* 28:530–538, 1968.

Saper CB, Loewy AB, Swanson LW, et al: Direct hypothalamic-autonomic connections. *Brain Res* 117:305–312, 1976.

Saxena RC, Beg MAQ, Das AC: The straight sinus. *J Neurosurg* 41:724–727, 1974.

Schaefer M, Lapras C, Thomalske G, Grau H, Schober R: Sarcoidosis of the pineal gland. *J Neurosurg* 47:630–632, 1977.

Schaltenbrand G, Bailey P: Introduction to stereotaxis with an atlas of the human brain. Thieme Verlag, Stuttgart, 1959.

Schindler E: Enzephalographische Befunde bei Tumoren der Pinealisregion. *Radiologe* 16:405–411, 1976.

Schmidek HH, Sweet WH: *Current Techniques in Operative Neurosurgery.* New York, Grune & Stratton, 1977.

Schmidek HH: Suprasellar germinomas (ectopic pinealomas). In Schmidek H (ed): *Pineal Tumors.* New York, Masson Publishing (USA), 1977, pp 115–126.

Schmidek HH (ed): *Pineal Tumors.* New York, Masson Publishing USA, 1977, pp 1–138.

Schold SC, Vurgrin D, Golbey RB, Posner JB: Central nervous system metastases from germ cell carcinoma of testis. *Semin Oncol* 6:102–108, 1979.

Schottenfeld D, Warshauer ME, Sherlock S, et al: The epidemiology of testicular cancer in young adults. *Am J Epidemiol* 112:232–246, 1980.

Schürmann K: Die Neurochirurgie der intrakraniellen Tumoren der Mittellinie. *Radiologe* 5:459–473, 1965.

Scully RE, Galdabini JJ, McNeely BU: Case records of the Massachusetts General Hospital (Case 38-1975). *N Engl J Med* 293:653–660, 1975.

Scully RE: Tumors of ovary and maldeveloped gonads. *Atlas of Tumor Pathology.* Washington DC, Armed Forces Institute of Pathol, Fasc 16, 1979.

Seaber JH, Nashold BS: Comparison of ocular motor effect of unilateral stereotaxtic midbrain lesions in man. *Neuro Ophthalmol* 1:95–99, 1980.

Seegal RF, Goldman BD: Effects of photoperiod on cyclicity and serum gonadotrophins in the Syrian hamster. *Biol Reprod* 12:223–231, 1975.

Seeger W: *Atlas of Topographical Anatomy of the Brain and Surrounding Structures.* Wien, Springer Verlag, 1978.

Selhorst JB, Hoyt WF, Feinsod M, Hosobuchi Y: Midbrain coectopia. *Arch Neurol* 33:193–195, 1976.

Sevitt S, Schorstein J: A case of pineal cyst. *Br Med J* 11:490–492, 1947.

Seybold ME, Yoss RE, Hollenhorst RW, Moyer NJ: Pupillary abnormalities associated with tumors of the pineal region. *Neurology* 21:232–237, 1971.

Shalet SM, Beardwell CG, Aarons BM, Pearson D, Jones PHM: Growth impairment in children treated for brain tumors. *Arch Dis Childhood* 53:491–494, 1978.

Sharan VM: Management of pineal tumors by radiation therapy and CT scanning. (Meeting Abstract) *Int J Radiat Oncol Biol Phys* 2(2):154, 1978.

Sheline GE: Radiation therapy of tumors of the central nervous system in childhood. *Cancer* 35:957–964, 1975.

Shih CJ: Intracranial tumors in Taiwan. A cooperative study of 1,200 cases with special reference to the intracranial tumors of childhood. *J Formosan Med Assoc* 76:515–528, 1977.

Shinomiya T, Toya S, Iwata T, Hosoda Y: Radioimmunoassay of alpha-fetoprotein in children with primary intracranial tumors. *Child's Brain* 5:450–458, 1979.

Sidell N: Retinoic acid-induced growth inhibition and morphologic differentiation of human neuroblastoma cells in vitro. *J Natl Cancer Inst* 68:589–596, 1981.

Siiteri PK, Febres F, Clemens LE, et al: Progesterone and the maintenance of pregnancy. Is progesterone nature's immunosuppressant? *Ann NY Acad Sci* 286:384–387, 1977.

Silman RE, Leone RM, Hooper RJL, Preece MA: Melatonin, the pineal gland and human puberty. *Nature* 282:301–303, 1979.

Simson LR, Lampe I, Abell MR: Suprasellar germinomas. *Cancer* 22:533–544, 1968.

Sizonenko PC, Moore DC, Pauneir L, Beaumanoir A, Nahory A: Melatonin secretion in relation to sleep in epileptics. *Prog Brain Res* 52:549–551, 1979.

Sklar CA, Grumback M, Kaplan SL, et al: Hormonal and metabolic abnormalities associated with central nervous system germinoma in children and adolescents and the effect of therapy: Report of 10 patients. *J Clin Endocrinol Metab* 52:9–16, 1981.

Skrzypczak J: Zur Symptomatologie, Diagnostik und Therapie der Vierhügeltumoren. *Neurochirurgia* 10:128–142, 1967.

Slawson RG: Radiation therapy for germinal tumors of the testes. *Cancer* 42:2216–2223, 1978.

Smith JA, Mee TJ, Padwick DP, Spokes EG: Human postmortem pineal enzyme activity. *Clin Endocrinol* 14:75–81, 1981.

Smith JA: The biochemistry and pharmacology of melatonin. In Birau N, Schloot W (eds): *Melatonin—Current Status and Perspectives.* New York, Pergamon, 1981, pp 135–147.

Smith JL, Zieper I, Gay AJ, Cogan DG: Nystagmus retractorius. *Arch Ophthalmol* 62:864–867, 1959.

Smith JL, David NJ, Ktintworth G: Skew deviation. *Neurology* 14:96–105, 1964.

Smith MS, Laguna JF: Upward gaze paralysis following unilateral pretectal infarction. *Arch Neurol* 38:127–129, 1981.

Smith NJ, El-Mahdi AM, Constable WC: Results of irradiation of tumors in the region of the pineal body. *Acta Radiol Oncol Radiat Phys Biol* 15:17–22, 1976.

Smith WT, Hughes B, Ermocilla R: Chemodectoma of the pineal region, with observations on the pineal body and chemoreceptor tissue. *J Pathol* 92:69–76, 1966.

So SC: Pineal tumours: A clinical study of 23 cases. *Aust NZ J Surg* 46:75–79, 1976.

Sobel RA, Trice JE, Neilsen SL, Ellis WG: Pineoblastoma with ganglionic and glial differentiation. *Acta Neuropathol* 55:243–246, 1981.

Sohn AP, Pittman JG: Multiple hypothalamic disorders produced by a suprasellar germinoma. *Rocky Mtn Med J* 68:23–27, 1971.

Solarski A, Panke ES, Panke TW: Craniopharyngioma in the pineal gland. *Arch Pathol Lab Med* 102:490–491, 1978.

Sones Jr, PJ, Hoffman Jr, JC: Angiography of tumors involving the posterior third ventricle. *Am J Roentgenol* 124:241–249, 1975.

Sonntag VKH, Waggener JO, Kaplan AM: Surgical removal of a hemangioma of the pineal region in a

4-week-old infant. *Neurosurgery* 8:586–588, 1981.

Spatz H: Anatomie des Mittelhirns. In Bumke O, Foerster O (eds): *Handbuch der Neurologie.* Berlin, Springer Verlag, 1935, vol I/1, pp 474–540.

Spiegel AM, Di Chiro G, Gorden P, Ommaya AK, Kolins J, Pomeroy TC: Diagnosis of radiosensitive hypothalamic tumors without craniotomy. *Ann Int Med* 85:290–293, 1976.

Stachura I, Mendelow H: Endodermal sinus tumor originating in the region of the pineal gland. *Cancer* 45:2131–2137, 1980.

Stavrou D, Anzil AP, Wiedenback W, et al: Immunofluorescence study of lymphocytic infiltration in gliomas. Identification of T-lymphocytes. *J Neurol Sci* 33:275–282, 1977.

Stefanko SZ, Manschot WA: Pinealoblastoma with retinoblastomatous differentiation. *Brain* 102:321–332, 1979.

Stefanko SZ, Manschot WA: Pinealoblastoma with photoreceptor differentiation. 8th International Congress Neuropathology, Abstract #341.

Stein B, Post KO: Current management of pituitary and pineal tumor. *Curr Concepts Oncol.* Winter 1982, pp 3–17.

Stein B: Personal communication, 1979.

Stein BM: Surgical treatment of pineal tumors. *Clin Neurosurg* 26:490–510, 1979.

Stein BM: Pineal region tumors. In *Pediatric Neurosurgery,* Surgery of the Developing Nervous System, ed. Section of Pediatric Neurosurgery, AANS. New York, Grune & Stratton, 1982, pp 469–485.

Stein BM: Supracerebellar approach for pineal region neoplasms. In Schmidek HH, Sweet WH (eds): *Operative Neurosurgical Techniques.* New York, Grune & Stratton, 1982, Vol 1.

Stein BM, Fraser RAR, Tenner MS: Tumours of the third ventricle in children. *J Neurol Neurosurg Psychiatry* 35:776–778, 1972.

Stein BM: The infratentorial supracerebellar approach to pineal lesions. *J Neurosurg* 35:197–202, 1971.

Stein BM: Supracerebellar-infratentorial approach to pineal tumors. *Surg Neurol* 11:331–337, 1979.

Steinbok P, Dolman C, Kaan K: Pineocytomas presenting as subarachnoid hemorrhage. Report of two cases. *J Neurosurg* 47:776–780, 1977.

Stevens LC: Origin of testicular teratomas from primordial germ cells in mice. *J Natl Cancer Inst* 38:549–552, 1967.

Stevenson GC, Hoyt WF: Metastasis to the midbrain from mammary carcinoma. *JAMA* 186:160–162, 1963.

Stolinsky DC: Prolonged survival after cerebral metastasis of testicular carcinoma. *Cancer* 47:978–981, 1981.

Stowell RE, Sachs E, Russell Wo: Primary intracranial chorionepithelioma with metastases to the lung. *Am J Pathol* 21:787–801, 1945.

Strang RR, Tovi D, Schiano G: Teratomas of the posterior cranial fossa. *Zentralbl Neurochir* 20:359–372, 1960.

Strauss JF: Testicular germ cell tumors. *Med Grand Rounds* Oct:1–30, 1980.

Strickland S, Mahdavi V: Induction of differentiation in teratocarcinoma stem cells by retinoic acid. *Cell* 15:393–403, 1978.

Strickland S: Mouse teratocarcinoma cells: prospects for study of embryogenesis and neoplasia. *Cell* 24:277–278, 1981.

Strickland S, Sawey MJ: Studies on the effect of retinoids on the differentiation of teratocarcinoma stem cells *in vitro* and *in vivo. Dev Biol* 78:76–85, 1980.

Sung D, Harisiadis L, Chang CH: Midline pineal tumors and suprasellar germinomas: Highly curable by radiation. *Radiology* 128:745–751, 1978.

Sung DI: Suprasellar tumors in children. A review of the clinical manifestations and managements. *Cancer* 50:1420–1425, 1982.

Suzuki J, Iwabuchi T: Surgical removal of pineal tumors (pinealomas and teratomas). *J Neurosurg* 23:565–571, 1965.

Suzuki J, Hori S: Evaluation of radiotherapy of tumors in the pineal region by ventriculographic studies with iodized oil. *J Neurosurg* 30:595–603, 1969.

Sweet WH: A review of dermoid, teratoid, and teratomatous intracranial tumors. *Dis Nerv Syst* 1:228–238, 1940.

Swischuk LE, Byan RN: Double midline intracranial atypical teratomas. *Am J Roentgenol* 122:517–524, 1974.

Snyder SH, Axelrod J: A sensitive assay for 5-hydroxytryptophan decarboxylase. *Biochem Pharmacol* 13:805–806, 1964.

Szymendera JJ, Zborzic J, Sikorowa L, et al: Evaluation of five tumor markers (AFP, CEA, hCG, hPL, and SPl) in monitoring therapy and follow-up of patients with testicular germ cell tumors. *Oncology* 40:1–10, 1983.

Tabuchi K, Tanigawa M, Baba Y, et al: Primary intracranial choriocarcinoma in the pineal region, a case report and review of the literature. *Acta Mee Okayama* 27:125–132, 1973.

Tabuchi K, Yamada O, Nishimoto A: The ultrastructure of pinealomas. *Acta Neuropathol* 24:117–127, 1973.

Takahashi M: *Atlas of Vertebral Angiography.* München, Urban and Schwarzenberg, 1974.

Takaku A, Mita R, Suzuki J: Intracranial teratomas in early infancy. *J Neurosurg* 38:265–268, 1973.

Takakura K, Matsutani M, Koyama K, Sing OK: Intrathecal BAR therapy for malignant brain tumors. *Brain Nerve* (Tokyo) 24:585–593, 1972.

Takei Y, Pearl GS: Ultrastructural study of intracranial yolk sac tumor: With special reference to the oncologic phylogeny of germ cell tumors. *Cancer* 48:2038–2046, 1981.

Takei Y, Mirra SS, Miles ML: Primary intracranial yolk sac tumor: Report of three cases and an ultrastructural study. *J Neuropathol Exp Neurol* (Abstract) 36:633, 1977.

Takeuchi J, Handa H, Nagata I: Suprasellar germinoma. *J Neurosurg* 49:41–48, 1978.

Takeuchi J, Handa H, Otsuka S, et al: Neuroradiological aspects of suprasellar germinoma. *Neurology* 17:153–159, 1979.

Takeuchi J, Mori K, Moritake K, et al: Teratomas in the suprasellar region, report of 5 cases. *Surg Neurol* 3:247–255, 1975.

Takeuchi J, Handa H, Oda Y, Uchida Y: Alphafetoprotein in intracranial malignant teratoma. *Surg Neurol* 12:400–404, 1979.

Tamaki N, Fujiwara K, Matsumoto S, Takeda H: Veins draining the pineal body. An anatomical and neuroradiological study of "pineal veins." *J Neurosurg* 39:448–454, 1973.

Tamarkin L, Cohen M, Roselle D, Reichert C, Lippman M, Chabner B: Melatonin inhibition and pinealectomy enhancement of 7,12-dimethylbenz (a)anthracene-induced mammary tumors in the rat. *Cancer Res* 41:4432–4436, 1981.

Tamarkin L, Hutchinson JS, Goldman BD: Regulation of serum gonadotropins by photoperiod and testicular hormone in the Syrian hamster. *Endocrinology* 99:1528–1533, 1976.

Tamarkin L, Westrom WK, Hamill AI, Goldman BD: Effect of melatonin on the reproductive system of male and female Syrian hamsters: A diurnal rhythm in sensitivity to melatonin. *Endocrinology* 99:1534–1541, 1976.

Tamarkin L, Reppert SM, Klein DC: Regulation of pineal melatonin in the Syrian hamster. *Endocrinology* 104:385–389, 1979.

Tamarkin L, Danforth D, Lichter A, DeMoss E, Cohen M, Chabner B, Lippman M: Decreased nocturnal plasma melatonin peak in patients with estrogen receptor positive breast cancer. *Science* 216:1003–1005, 1982.

Tamura H, Kury G, Suzuki K: Intracranial teratomas in fetal life and infancy. *Obstet Gynecol* 27:134–141, 1966.

Tanaka R, Ueki K: Germinomas in the cerebral hemisphere. *Surg Neurol* 12:239–241, 1979.

Tandler J, Ranzi E: Chirurgische Anatomie und Operationstechnik des Zentralnervensystems. In Kirschner M, Normann O (eds): *Die Chirurgie.* Berlin, Springer Verlag, 1920.

Tani E, Ikeda K, Kudo S, Yamagata S, Nishiura M, Higashi N: Specialized intercellular junctions in human intracranial germinomas. *Acta Neuropathol* 27:139–151, 1974.

Tapp E, Skinner RG, Phillips V: Radioimmunoassay for melatonin. *J Neural Transm* 48:137–141, 1980.

Tapp E: The pineal gland in malignancy. In Reiter RJ (ed): *The Pineal Gland, Vol 3 Extra-Reproductive Effects.* Boca Raton, CRC Press, 1982, pp 171–188.

Tavcar D, Robboy SJ, Chapman P: Endodermal sinus tumor of the pineal region. *Cancer* 45:2646–2651, 1980.

Teilum G: Classification of endodermal sinus tumor (mesoblastoma vitellinum) and so-called "embryonal carcinoma" of the ovary. *Acta Pathol Microbiol Scand* 64:407–429, 1965.

Tetsuo M, Perlow MJ, Mishkin N, Markey SP: Light exposure reduces and pinealectomy virtually stops urinary excretion of 6-hydroxymelatonin by rhesus monkeys. *Endocrinology* 110:997–1003, 1982.

Tetsuo M, Polinsky RJ, Markey SP, Kopin IJ: Urinary 6-hydroxymelatonin excretion in patients with orthostatic hypotension. *J Clin Endocrinol Metab* 53:607–610, 1981.

Thomas JB, Pizzarello PJ: Blindness, biologic rhythms, and menarche. *Obstet Gynecol* 30:507–509, 1967.

Thomson AF: Surgery of the third ventricle. In Walker AE (ed): *A History of Neurological Surgery.* New York, Hafner Publishing Co, 1967, pp 136–141.

Timonen S, Franzas B, Wichman K: Photosensibility of the human pituitary. *Ann Chir Gynaecol* 53:165–172, 1964.

Timonen S, Carpen E: Multiple pregnancies and photoperiodicity. *Ann Chir Gynaecol* 57:135–138, 1968.

Tompkins VN, Haymaker W, Campbell EH: Metastatic pineal tumors. A clinico-pathologic report of two cases. *J Neurosurg* 7:159–169, 1950.

Tonnies W: Behandlung der geschülste im hinteren teil des 3.ventrikels. Langenbecks. *Arch Klin Chir* 183:426–429, 1935.

Torkildsen A: A new palliative operation in cases of inoperable occlusion of the Sylvian aqueduct. *Acta Chir Scand* 82:117–124, 1939.

Torkildsen A: Should extirpation be attempted in cases of neoplasm in or near the third ventricle of the brain. Experiences with a palliative method. *J Neurosurg* 5:249–275, 1948.

Tottori K, Takahasi T, Hanaoka J, Sato Y, Takeuchi S: Approach to the early diagnosis of brain metastasis by the serum/CSF HCG and β-HCG ratio in patients with choriocarcinoma. In *Proceedings of the 38th Annual Meeting of the Japanese Cancer Association,* Tokyo, Japan, Sept. 1979, p 321, Tokyo, Japanese Cancer Association, 1979 (Abstr).

Travers PJ, Arklie JL, Trowsdale J, et al: Lack of expression of HLA-ABC antigens in choriocarcinoma and other human tumor cell lines. *Natl Cancer Inst Monogr* 60:175–180, 1982.

Trojanowski JQ, Tascos NA, Rorke LB: Malignant pineocytoma with prominent papillary features. *Cancer* 50:1789–1793, 1982.

Trojanowski JQ, Wray SH: Vertical gaze ophthalmoplegia: Selective paralysis of downgaze. *Neurology* 30:605–610, 1971.

Tschabitscher M: Die Venen des menschlichen Kleinhirns. *Acta Anat* 105:344–366, 1979.

Tso MOM, Fine BS, Zimmerman LE: The nature of retinoblastoma. I. Photoreceptor differentiation: A clinical and histopathologic study. *Am J Ophthalmol* 69:339–349, 1970.

Tso MOM, Fine BS, Zimmerman LE: The nature of retinoblastoma. II. Photoreceptor differentiation: An electron microscopic study. *Am J Ophthalmol* 69:350–359, 1970.

Tso MOM, Fine BS, Zimmerman LE, Vogel MH: Photoreceptor elements in retinoblastoma. *Arch Ophthalmol* 82:57–59, 1969.

Tsuchida T, Tanaka R, Kobayashi K, et al: A case of two cell pattern pinealoma developed 15 years after removal of pineal teratoma. *Brain Nerve* 28:893–899, 1976.

Tucker WG, Leong ASY, McCulloch GAJ: Tumours of the pineal region—neuroradiological aspects. *Aust Radiol* 21:313–324, 1977.

Turek FW, Alvis JD, Elliott JA, Menaker M: Temporal distribution of serum levels of LH and FSH in adult male golden hamsters exposed to long or short days. *Biol Reprod* 14:630–637, 1976.

Ueki K, Tanaka R: Treatments and prognoses of pineal tumors—experience of 110 cases. *Neurol Med Chir* 20:1–26, 1980.

Ueki K, Tanaka K: Study on treatment and prognosis of pineal neoplasms. *Seara Med Neurochir* 7:279–315, 1978.

Utz DC, Baucemi MF: Extragonadal testicular tumors. *J Urol* 105:271–274, 1971.

Valdiserri RO, Yunis EJ: Sacrococcygeal teratoma. A review of 68 cases. *Cancer* 48:217–221, 1981.

Van Wagenen WP: A surgical approach for the removal of certain pineal tumors. *Surg Gynecol Obstet*

53:216–220, 1931.

VanHaelen CPV, Fisher RI, Appello E, et al: Lack of histocompatibility antigens on a murine ovarian teratocarcinoma. *Cancer Res* 41:3186–3191, 1981.

Vaquero J, Carrillo R, Casezudo J, Leunda G, Villoria F, Bravo G: Cavernous angiomas of the pineal region. Report of two cases. *J Neurosurg* 53:833–835, 1980.

Varakis JN, ZuRhein GM: Experimental pineocytoma of the Syrian hamster induced by a human papovavirus (JC). A light and electron microscopic study. *Acta Neuropathol* 35:243–264, 1976.

Vaughan GM, Pelham RW, Pang SF, Laughlin LL, Wilson KM, Sandock KL, Vaughan MK, Koslow SH, Reiter RJ: Nocturnal elevation of plasma melatonin and urinary 5-hydroxyindole acetic acid: Attempts at modification by brief changes in environmental lighting and sleep and by autonomic drugs. *J Clin Endocrinol Metab* 42:752–754, 1976.

Vaughan GM, Allen JP, Tullis W, Siler-Khodr TM, de la Pena A, Sackman JW: Overnight plasma profiles of melatonin and certain adenohypophyseal hormones in man. *J Clin Endocrinol Metab* 47:566–572, 1978.

Vaughan GM, McDonald SA, Bell R, Stevens EA: Melatonin, pituitary function and stress in humans. *Psychoneuroendocrinol* 4:351–362, 1979.

Vaughan GM, Meyer GG, Reiter RJ: Evidence for a pineal-induced relationship in the human. In Reiter RJ (ed): *The Pineal and Reproduction*. Basel, Karger, 1978, pp 191–223.

Vaughan GM, Allen J, de la Pena A: Rapid melatonin transients. *Waking Sleeping* 3:169–179, 1979.

Vaughan MK, Reiter RJ, Vaughan GM, Bigelow L, Altschule MD: Inhibition of compensatory ovarian hypertrophy in the mouse and vole: A comparison of Altschule's pineal extract, pineal indoles, vasopressin, and oxytocin. *Gen Comp Endocrinol* 18:372–377, 1972.

Vaughan MK: The pineal gland—A survey of its antigonadotrophic substances and their actions. In McCann SM (ed): *International Review of Physiology, Vol 24 Endocrine Physiology III*. Baltimore, University Park Press, 1981, pp 41–95.

Vaughan MK, Vaughan GM, Klein DC: Arginine vasotocin: Effect on development of reproductive organs. *Science* 186:938–939, 1974.

Vejjajiva A, Sitprija V, Shuangshoti S: Chronic sustained hypernatremia and hypovolemia in hypothalamic tumor: A physiologic study. *Neurology* 19:161–166, 1969.

Ventureyra ECG: Pineal region: Surgical management of tumours and vascular malformations. *Surg Neurol* 16:77–84, 1980.

Volpe R, Knowlton T, Foster AD, et al: Testicular feminization: A study of two cases, one with a seminoma. *Can Med Assoc J* 98:438–445, 1968.

Vriend J: Evidence for pineal gland modulation of the neuroendocrine-thyroid axis. *Neuroendocrinology* 36:67–78, 1983.

Vugrin D, Cvitkovic E, Posner J, Hajdu S, Golbey RB: Neurological complications of malignant germ cell tumors of testis. *Cancer* 44:2349–2353, 1979.

Vuia O: Embryonic carcinosarcoma (mixed tumour) of the pineal gland. *Neurochirurgia* 23:47–54, 1980.

Wackenheim A, Braun JP: *Angiography of the Mesencephalon*. Berlin, Springer Verlag, 1970.

Waddington MM: *Atlas of Cerebral Angiography with Anatomic Correlation*. Boston, Little, Brown & Co, 1974.

Waga S, Handa H, Yamashita J: Intracranial germinomas: Treatment and results. *Surg Neurol* 11:167–172, 1979.

Wainwright SD: Role of the pineal gland in the vertebrate master biological clock. In Reiter RJ (ed): *The Pineal Gland, Vol 3 Extra-Reproductive Effects*. Boca Raton, CRC Press, 1982, pp 53–80.

Wakai S, Segawa H, Kitahara S, Asano T, Sano K, Ogihara R, Tomita S: Teratoma in the pineal region in two brothers. Case reports. *J Neurosurg* 53:239–243, 1980.

Wald SL, Fogelson H, McLaurin RL: Cystic thalamic gliomas. *Child's Brain* 9:381–393, 1982.

Waldbaur H, Gottschaldt M, Schmidt H, Neuhäuser G: Medulloblastom des Kleinhirns und Pineoblastom bei eineiigen Zwillingen. *Klin Padiatr* 188:366–371, 1976.

Wallen EP, Jachim JM: Rhythm function of pineal hydroxyindole-*O*-methyltransferase during the estrous cycle: An analysis. *Biol Reprod* 10:461–466, 1974.

Walsh FB, Hoyt WF: *Clinical Neuro-Ophthalmology*. Baltimore, Williams & Wilkins, 1969, pp 2240–2246.

Walsh FB, Hoyt WF: *Clinical Neuro-Ophthalmology*. Baltimore, Williams & Wilkins, 1969, pp 228–232.

Wara WM, Jenkin RDT, Evans A, Ertel I, Hittle R, Ortega J, Wilson CB, Hammond D: Tumors of the pineal and suprasellar region: Childrens cancer study group treatment results 1960–1975. *Cancer* 43:698–701, 1979.

Wara WM, Sheline GE: Radiation therapy of malignant brain tumors. *Clin Neurosurg* 25:397–402, 1978.

Wara WM, Fellows CF, Sheline GE, Wilson CB, Townsend JJ: Radiation therapy for pineal tumors and suprasellar germinomas. *Radiology* 124:221–223, 1977.

Weaver EN, Coulon RA: Excision of a brainstem epidermoid cyst. Case report. *J Neurosurg* 51:254–257, 1979.

Weber G: Tumoren der Glandula pinealis und ektopische Pinealocytome. *Schweiz Arch Neurol Neurochir Psychiatr* 91:473–509, 1963.

Weber G: Midbrain Tumours. In Vinken PJ, Bruyn GW (eds): *Handbook of Clinical Neurology*. Amsterdam, North Holland Publ Co, 1974, vol 17/II, pp 620–647.

Weigel K, Ostertag CB, Mundinger F: Interstitial long-term irradiation of tumors in the pineal region. Stereotactic cerebral irradiation. *Inserm Symp No. 12*, pp 283–292, 1979.

Weigert C: Zur lehre von den tumoren der hirnanhänge. *Virchows Arch [Pathol Anat]* 65:212–219, 1875.

Weinberg U, D'Eletto RD, Weitzman ED, Erlich S, Hollander CS: Circulating melatonin in man: Episodic secretion throughout the light-dark cycle. *J Clin Endocrinol Metab* 48:114–118, 1979.

Weinberg U, Weitzman ED, Fukushima DK, Cancel GF, Rosenfeld RS: Melatonin does not suppress the pituitary luteinizing hormone response to luteinizing hormone-releasing hormone in men. *J Clin Endocrinol Metab* 51:161–162, 1980.

Weissbach H, Redfield BG, Axelrod J: Biosynthesis

of melatonin: Enzymic conversion of serotonin to N-acetylserotonin. *Biochim Biophys Acta* 43:352–353.

Wende S, Ciba K: Die pneumographische Darstellung des Mittelhirns und seiner Nachbarschaft. *Radiologe* 8:347–354, 1968.

Wetterberg L, Arendt J, Paunier L, Sizonenko PC, van Donselaar W, Heyden T: Human serum melatonin changes during the menstrual cycle. *J Clin Endocrinol Metab* 42:185–188, 1976.

Wetterberg L: Melatonin in humans. Physiological and clinical studies. *J Neural Transm [Suppl] 13* pp 289–310, 1978.

Wheler GHT, Weller JL, Klein DC: Taurine: Stimulation of pineal N-acetyltransferase activity and melatonin production via a β-adrenergic mechanism. *Brain Res* 166:65–74, 1979.

Wilkinson M, Ardendt J, Bradtke J, de Ziegler D: Determination of a dark-induced increase in pineal N-acetyltransferase activity and simultaneous radioimmunoassay of melatonin in pineal, serum and pituitary tissue of the male rat. *J Endocrinol* 72:243–244, 1977.

Williams SD, Einhorn LH: Brain metastases in disseminated germinal neoplasms. *Cancer* 44:1514–1516, 1979.

Williams SD, Einhorn LH, Greco A, Oldham R, Fletcher R: VP-16-213 salvage therapy for refractory germinal neoplasms. *Cancer* 46:2154–2158, 1980.

Willis RA: Nervous tissue in teratomas. In Minckler J (ed): *Pathology of the Nervous System.* New York, McGraw-Hill, 1971, Vol 2, pp 1937–1943.

Wilner HI, Crockett J, Gilroy J: The Galenic venous system: A selective radiographic study. *Am J Roentgenol* 115:1–13, 1972.

Wilson BW, Lynch JH, Ozaki Y: 5-methoxytryptophol in rat serum and pineal: Detection, quantitation, and evidence for daily rhythmicity. *Life Sci* 23:1019–1024, 1978.

Wilson CB: Diagnosis and surgical treatment of childhood brain tumors. *Cancer* 35:950–956, 1975.

Wilson ER, Takei Y, Bikoff WT, O'Brien M, Tindall GT: Abdominal metastases of primary intracranial yolk sac tumors through ventriculoperitoneal shunts: Report of three cases. *Neurosurgery* 5:356–364, 1979.

Wilson SAK: Ectopia pupillae in certain mesencephalic lesions. *Brain* 29:524–536, 1906.

Winfree AT: Human body clocks and the timing of sleep. *Nature* 297:23–27, 1982.

Witschi E: Migration of germ cells of human embryos from the yolk sac to the primitive gonadal folds. *Contrib Embryol Carnegie Inst* 209:67–80, 1948.

Wollner N, Exelby PR, Woodruff JM, et al: Malignant ovarian tumors in childhood: Prognosis in relation to initial therapy. *Cancer* 37:1953–1964, 1976.

Wollschlager PB, Wollschlager G, Meyer PG: Die postmortale Angiographie des Mesencephalon und seiner direkten Umgebung. *Radiologe* 8:377–381, 1968.

Wood BP, Haller JO, Berdon WE, Lin SR: Shunt metastases of pineal tumors presenting as pelvic mass. *Pediatr Radiol* 8:108–109, 1979.

Wood JH, Zimmerman RA, Bruce DA, Bilaniuk LT, Norris DG, Schut L: Assessment and management

of pineal-region and related tumors. *Surg Neurol* 16:192–210, 1981.

Wray S: The neuro-ophthalmic and neurologic manifestations of pinealomas. In Schmidek HH, Brady LW and DeVita VT (eds): *Pineal Tumors.* New York, Masson Publishing USA, 1977, pp 21–59.

Wurtman RJ, Axelrod J, Kelly DE: *The Pineal.* New York, Academic Press, 1968, p 31.

Wurtman RJ: The pineal as a neuroendocrine transducer. *Hosp Pract* Jan:82–92, 1980.

Wurtman RJ, Ozaki Y: Physiological control of melatonin synthesis and secretion: Mechanisms generating rhythms in melatonin, methoxytryptophol, and arginine vasotocin levels and effects of the pineal of endogenous catecholamines, the estrous cycle, and environmental lighting. *J Neural Transm* [Suppl 13]:59–70, 1978.

Wurtman RJ, Shein HM, Larin F: Mediation by beta-adrenergic receptors of effect of norepinephrine on pineal synthesis of ^{14}C-serotonin and ^{14}C-melatonin. *J Neurochem* 18:1683–1687, 1971.

Wurtman RJ, Moskowitz MA: The pineal organ (Part I). *N Engl J Med* 296:1329–1333, 1977.

Wurtman RJ, Kammer H: Melatonin synthesis by an ectopic pinealoma. *N Engl J Med* 274:1233–1237, 1966.

Wurtman RJ, Moskowitz MA: The pineal organ (Part II). *N Engl J Med* 296:1383–1386, 1977.

Wurtman RJ, Axelrod J: Demonstration of hydroxyindole-O-methyltransferase, melatonin, and serotonin in a metastatic parenchymatous pinealoma. *Nature* 204:1323–1324, 1964.

Yamamoto I, Kageyama N: Microsurgical anatomy of the pineal region. *J Neurosurg* 53:205–221, 1980.

Yamamoto I, Rhoton AL, Peace DA: Microsurgery of the third ventricle: Part 1. Microsurgical anatomy. *Neurosurgery* 8:334–356, 1981.

Yasargil MG, Kasdaglis K, Jain KK, Weber HP: Anatomical observation of the subarachnoid cisterns of the brain during surgery. *J Neurosurg* 44:298–302, 1976.

Yoshiki T, Itoh T, Shirai T, Noro T, Tomino Y, Hamajima I, Takeda T: Primary intracranial yolk sac tumor. Immunofluorescent demonstration of alpha-fetoprotein synthesis. *Cancer* 37:2343–2348, 1976.

Young IM, Silman RE: Pineal methoxyindoles in the human. In Reiter RJ (ed): *The Pineal Gland, Vol 3 Extra-Reproductive Effects.* 1982, pp 189–218.

Yu HS, Pang SF, Tang PL, Brown GM: Persistence of circadian rhythms of melatonin and N-acetylserotonin in the serum of rats after pinealectomy. *Neuroendocrinology* 32:262–265, 1981.

Yuwiler A, Klein DC, Buda M, Weller JL: Adrenergic control of pineal N-acetyltransferase activity: Developmental aspects. *Am J Physiol* 233:E141–E146, 1977.

Zacharias L, Wurtman RJ: Blindness and menarche. *Obstet Gynecol* 33:603–608, 1969.

Zapletal B: Ein neuer operativer Zugang zum Gebiet der Incisura tentorii. *Zentralbl Neurochir* 16:64–69, 1956.

Zatz M: The role of cyclic nucleotides in the pineal gland. *Handbook Exp Pharmacol* 58:691–710, 1982.

Zatz M, Kebabian JW, Romero JA, Lefkowitz RJ, Axelrod J: Pineal adrenergic receptor: Correlation of binding of ^{3}H-alprenolol with stimulation of adenylate cyclase. *J Pharmacol Exp Ther* 196:714–722, 1976.

Zatz M: Pharmacology of the rat pineal gland. In Reiter RJ (ed): *The Pineal Gland, Vol 1 Anatomy and Biochemistry.* Boca Raton, CRC Press, 1981, pp 229–242.

Zeal AA, Rhoton AL: Microsurgical anatomy of the posterior cerebral artery. *J Neurosurg* 4:534–559, 1978.

Zimmerman BL, Tso MOM: Morphologic evidence of photoreceptor differentiation of pinealocytes in the neonatal rat. *J Cell Biol* 66:60–75, 1975.

Zimmerman RA, Bilaniuk LT, Wood JH, Bruce DA, Schut L: Computed tomography of pineal, parapineal, and histologically related tumors. *Radiology* 137:669–677, 1980.

Zimmerman RA, Bilaniuk LT: Age-related incidence of pineal calcification detected by computed tomography. *Radiology* 142:659–662, 1982.

Zondek H, Kaatz A, Unger H: Precocious puberty and chorionepithelioma of the pineal gland with report of a case. *J Endocrinol* 10:12–16, 1953b.

Zucker I, Johnston PG, Frost D: Comparative, physiological and biochronometric analyses of rodent seasonal reproductive cycles. In Reiter RJ, Follett BK (eds): *Seasonal Reproduction in Higher Vertebrates.* Basel, Karger, 1980, pp 102–133.

Zülch KJ: Die Pathologie und Biologie der Tumoren des dritten Ventrikels. *Acta Neurochir* 9:277–296, 1961.

Zülch KJ: Reflections on the surgery of the pineal gland (A glimpse into the past). *Neurosurg Rev* 4:152–162, 1981.

Zülch KJ: *Brain Tumors: Their Biology and Pathology,* New York, Springer Publishing Co, 1965, p 326.

Zülch KJ: Biologie und Pathologie der Hirngeschwülste. In Oliverona H, Tönnis J (eds): *Handbuch der Neurochirurgie.* Berlin, Springer Verlag, 1965, p 348.

Index

Page numbers in *italics* denote figures; those followed by "t" or "f" denote tables or footnotes, respectively.